Contemporary Topics in Immunobiology

VOLUME 14

Regulation of Leukocyte Function

Contemporary Topics in Immunobiology

General Editor:
M. G. Hanna, Jr.
Litton Institute of Applied Biotechnology
Rockville, Maryland

Editorial Board:
Max D. Cooper
University of Alabama
Birmingham, Alabama

John J. Marchalonis
Medical University of South Carolina
Charleston, South Carolina

G. J. V. Nossal
The Walter & Eliza Hall Insitute of Medical Research
Victoria, Australia

Victor Nussenzweig
New York University School of Medicine
New York, New York

George W. Santos
Johns Hopkins University
Baltimore, Maryland

Ralph Snyderman
Duke University Medical Center
Durham, North Carolina

Osias Stutman
Sloan-Kettering Institute for Cancer Research
New York, New York

Noel L. Warner
Becton Dickinson & Co.
Mountain View, California

William O. Weigle
Scripps Clinic and Research Foundation
La Jolla, California

A Continuation Order Plan is available for this series. A continuation order will bring delivery of each new volume immediately upon publication. Volumes are billed only upon actual shipment. For further information please contact the publisher.

Contemporary Topics in Immunobiology

VOLUME 14

Regulation of Leukocyte Function

Edited by
Ralph Snyderman
Howard Hughes Medical Institute and
Duke University Medical Center
Durham, North Carolina

Springer Science+Business Media, LLC

Library of Congress Cataloging in Publication Data

Main entry under title:

Regulation of leukocyte function.

(Contemporary topics in immunobiology; v. 14)
Includes bibliographical references and index.
1. Leukocytes. 2. Immune response — Regulation. 3. Cellular control mechanisms. I.
Snyderman, Ralph. II. Series. [DNLM: 1. Leukocytes — drug effects. 2. Leukocytes —
physiology. W1 CO77 v.14/WH 200 R344]
QR180.C632 vol. 14   574.2′9 s [616.07′9]   84-9889
[QP95]

Library of Congress Card Catalog Number 79-179761
ISBN 978-1-4757-4864-2   ISBN 978-1-4757-4862-8 (eBook)
DOI 10.1007/978-1-4757-4862-8
© 1984 Springer Science+Business Media New York
Originally published by Plenum Press, New York in 1984.
Softcover reprint of the hardcover 1st edition 1984

Contributors

Marco Baggiolini
Research Institute Wander
A Sandoz Research Unit
Wander Ltd.
CH-3001 Berne, Switzerland
Present address:
Theodor Kocher Institute
University of Berne
CH-3000 Berne 9, Switzerland

Beatrice Dewald
Research Institute Wander
A Sandoz Research Unit
Wander Ltd.
CH-3001 Berne, Switzerland
Present address:
Theodor Kocher Institute
University of Berne
CH-3000 Berne 9, Switzerland

John I. Gallin
Bacterial Diseases Section
Laboratory of Clinical Investigation
National Institute of Allergy and Infectious Diseases
National Institutes of Health
Bethesda, Maryland 20205

Ira M. Goldstein
Rosalind Russell Arthritis Research Laboratory
Medical Service
San Francisco General Hospital
Department of Medicine
University of California
San Francisco, California 94110

Harry R. Hill
Departments of Pathology and Pediatrics
University of Utah School of Medicine
Salt Lake City, Utah 84132

Tony E. Hugli
Department of Immunology
Scripps Clinic and Research Foundation
La Jolla, California 92037

Algirdas J. Jesaitis
Department of Immunology
Scripps Clinic and Research Foundation
La Jolla, California 92037

Linda C. McPhail   *Laboratory of Immune Effector Function*
                       Howard Hughes Medical Institute and
                       Division of Rheumatic and Genetic Diseases
                       Department of Medicine
                       Duke University Medical Center
                       Durham, North Carolina 27710

Edward L. Morgan   *Department of Immunology*
                       Scripps Clinic and Research Foundation
                       La Jolla, California 92037

Richard G. Painter   *Department of Immunology*
                       Scripps Clinic and Research Foundation
                       La Jolla, California 92037

Marilyn C. Pike   *Laboratory of Immune Effector Function*
                       Howard Hughes Medical Institute and
                       Division of Rheumatic and Genetic Diseases
                       Departments of Medicine and Microbiology and Immunology
                       Duke University Medical Center
                       Durham, North Carolina 27710

Bruce E. Seligmann   *Bacterial Diseases Section*
                       Laboratory of Clinical Investigation
                       National Institutes of Allergy and Infectious Diseases
                       National Institutes of Health
                       Bethesda, Maryland 20205

Larry A. Sklar   *Department of Immunology*
                       Scripps Clinic and Research Foundation
                       La Jolla, California 92037

Ralph Snyderman   *Laboratory of Immune Effector Function*
                       Howard Hughes Medical Institute and
                       Division of Rheumatic and Genetic Diseases
                       Departments of Medicine and Microbiology and Immunology
                       Duke University Medical Center
                       Durham, North Carolina 27710

John K. Spitznagel   *Department of Microbiology and Immunology*
                       School of Medicine
                       Emory University
                       Atlanta, Georgia 30322

Jay C. Unkeless   *Department of Cellular Physiology and Immunology*
                       Rockefeller University
                       New York, New York 10021

Frank H. Valone   *Cancer Research Institute*
                       University of California School of Medicine
                       San Francisco, California 94143

Samuel D. Wright   *Department of Cellular Physiology and Immunology*
                       Rockefeller University
                       New York, New York, 10021

Foreword

There was a time, not all that long ago, when scientific study of the cell was called cytology, and the workers in the field named themselves cytologists. When I was a medical student, lectures in cytology were a special, segregated part of the curriculum in the histology course, given along with general anatomy, and they were, as I recall, the surest of cures for insomnia. I still possess Cowdry's three-volume set entitled *Special Cytology*, published in 1934, and leafing through these books today is rather like examining a medieval manuscript. You could never have guessed what was going to happen to the field. At that time it was all structure, and all guesswork about the structure. When cells were packed together in various tissues, how did the geometry of packing work? How many sides did a liver cell have, in real life? What on earth were all those granules inside, and what were the best stains for looking at them? One thing about those granules, they never moved. Indeed, nothing moved.

Cytology turned into cell biology much later on, and suddenly came alive. As has been the case in so many disciplines in biology, it was brought to life by *techniques*. New instruments and cytochemical methods were devised for looking at cells, manipulating cells, more or less *in vivo*. It had been recognized since Metchnikoff's early studies, around the turn of the century, that leukocytes were wonderful creatures in their own right, undoubtedly important for the defense of their parent organism, capable of moving from place to place in response to various stimuli and capacitated for engulfing anything in their path, but for decades nobody could think of anything to do with them beyond observing their behavior in wonder. The time for asking direct, penetrating, reductionist questions about the cells did not arrive until other questions about immune responses, complement, lysosomes, free radicals, cell surface markers, microbial antigens, and the like had been raised and, provisionally, answered. Now, just in the past several years, the leukocyte has become the best of all models—working models at that—for cells in general.

The chapters in this volume are of the most practical, down-to-earth usefulness, for they bring us up to date on everything that is now known about the role of leukocytes in defense against tumors and microbial invaders. But the information in these chapters carries us farther along, into the profoundest depths of general cell biology. If you are interested in the everyday problem of keeping invaders out, the new facts are here at hand with lots more still to come. But if you are also interested in how cells work *qua* cells, in how extraordinarily intelligent a single cell can be, and in how marvelous, nothing in the world is as engrossing as a leukocyte.

Lewis Thomas

Chancellor
Memorial Sloan-Kettering Cancer Center
New York, New York

Preface

> The broad fact that the invasion of the organism by microbes most often induces, on the one hand, an inflammatory reaction with its associated immigration of leukocytes, and that, on the other hand, the phagocytes are capable of including and destroying the invaders, leads us to admit that the afflux of phagocytes to the invaded region, and their bactericidal properties, are mechanisms which serve to ward off bacterial attack and maintain the integrity of the organism.
>
> Elias Metchnikoff, Lecture on Phagocytosis and Immunity
> delivered at the Institute Pasteur, December 29, 1890

Approximately one hundred years ago, Metchnikoff outlined his phagocytic theory of host defense and focused attention on the importance of leukocytes in immunological reactions. It is appropriate that at the centennial of Metchnikoff's most important observations, a volume be dedicated to detailing the current concepts concerning the regulation of leukocyte function. This particular volume of the *Contemporary Topics in Immunobiology* series represents such an attempt and is dedicated to our many colleagues whose contributions have brought the field to the point where the study of leukocyte function is a major focus of biomedical research. This volume attempts to summarize our understanding of leukocyte chemotaxis, lysosomal secretion, and microbicidal activity, as well as clinical disorders of leukocyte function. It is hoped that the contributions in this volume will convey to the reader the excitement of research dealing with leukocyte activation, as well as the rapid advances that have been made during the past five years.

Ralph Snyderman

ix

Contents

Chapter 3

**Neutrophil Chemoattractant fMet-Leu-Phe Receptor Expression and
Ionic Events Following Activation**

John I. Gallin and Bruce E. Seligmann

Chapter 4

Mechanisms of Leukocyte Regulation by Complement-Derived Factors

  Tony E. Hugli and Edward L. Morgan

Chapter 5

Regulation of Human Leukocyte Function by Lipoxygenase Products of Arachidonic Acid

  Frank H. Valone

Chapter 6

Structure and Modulation of Fc and Complement Receptors

Jay C. Unkeless and Samuel D. Wright

Chapter 7

Neutrophil Degranulation

Ira M. Goldstein

Chapter 8

Exocytosis by Neutrophils

   Marco Baggiolini and Beatrice Dewald

Chapter 9

Mechanisms of Regulating the Respiratory Burst in Leukocytes

   Linda C. McPhail and Ralph Snyderman

Chapter 10

Nonoxidative Antimicrobial Reactions of Leukocytes

John K. Spitznagel

Chapter 11

Clinical Disorders of Leukocyte Function

    Harry R. Hill

Chapter 1

Transductional Mechanisms of Chemoattractant Receptors on Leukocytes

Ralph Snyderman and Marilyn C. Pike

Laboratory of Immune Effector Function
Howard Hughes Medical Institute and
Division of Rheumatic and Genetic Diseases
Departments of Medicine, and Microbiology and Immunology
Duke University Medical Center
Durham, North Carolina 27710

I. INTRODUCTION

The ability of phagocytic cells to migrate to chemical signals emanating from sites of intrusion of foreign substances was recognized more than a century ago and formed the basis of Metchnikoff's phagocytic theory of host defense (Metchnikoff, 1968). While the chemotactic migration of leukocytes was noted during the nineteenth century, it was not until 1962 that quantification of leukocyte chemotaxis *in vitro* became possible. The modern era of chemotaxis was spurred by the development of a method (Boyden, 1962) to quantify the migration of leukocytes across microporous filters. In his initial studies, Boyden demonstrated that the incubation of serum with immune complexes led to the formation of chemotactic activity. The production of this activity was blocked by preheating the serum at 56°C for 30 minutes before the addition of the immune complexes. These observations not only provided the groundwork for future quantitative studies of humoral and cellular mechanisms of leukocyte chemotaxis, but also suggested that serum complement might be a source of chemoattractants after activation by immune complexes.

Initial studies of leukocyte chemotaxis were largely performed by immunologists interested in the nature of substances generated by immunological reactions, which led to the accumulation of inflammatory cells. The first chemoattractant to be identified was C5a, a cleavage product derived from the fifth component of complement (Shin et al., 1968; Snyderman et al., 1968, 1969; Ward and Neuman, 1969). This peptide was shown to have both chemotactic and anaphylatoxic activities (Shin et al., 1968; Jensen et al., 1969) and to be the major source of chemotactic activity derived from complement activation (Snyderman et al., 1969, 1970). Subsequently, this molecule has been purified to homogeneity, and sequenced, and important structure-function relationships have been determined (Fernandez et al., 1978; Hugli and Müller-Eberhard, 1978). These are reviewed in Chapter 4. Other biologically relevant chemoattractants include chemotactic lymphokines (Ward et al., 1969; Snyderman et al., 1972; Cohen et al., 1979) a cell-derived chemotactic factor produced by polymorphonuclear leukocytes (PMNs) (Spillberg et al., 1976), eosinophilotactic tetrapeptides contained in mast cells (Goetzl and Austen, 1975), and neutrophil chemotactic factors contained in mast cells (Wasserman et al., 1977). More recently, products of arachidonic acid metabolism have been shown to be chemoattractants, the most potent of which appears to be leukotriene B4 (LTB4) (Ford-Hutchinson et al., 1980; Goetzl and Pickett, 1980; Palmer et al., 1980; reviewed Chapter 5).

What has become apparent over the past decade is that chemoattractants initiate a series of coordinated biochemical and cellular events in leukocytes including alterations in ion fluxes (Gallin and Rosenthal, 1974; Boucek and Snyderman, 1976; Naccache et al., 1977; Weissmann et al., 1982), morphological polarization (Smith et al., 1979; Cianciolo and Snyderman, 1981), locomotion, secretion of lysozomal contents (Goldstein et al., 1973), and production of superoxide anions (Klebanoff and Clark, 1978); see also Chapter 9. Chemoattractants are therefore not only responsible for the accumulation of leukocytes, but also can stimulate the cells to degranulate and to produce toxic oxygen radicals. The biological responses of leukocytes to chemoattractants can be divided into two groups: (1) those responses related to cellular motility, and (2) those responses related to the toxic or microbiocidal potential of leukocytes, i.e., lysozomal enzyme secretion and superoxide anion production. Interestingly, the two groups of responses initiated by chemoattractants appear to be regulated differently and can be divergently modified by pharmacological agents. Chemotaxis-related functions occur at low doses of chemoattractants, whereas the toxic responses of leukocytes generally require 10-fold higher concentrations of chemoattractants (Table I).

This chapter reviews work from the authors' laboratory characterizing a chemotactic factor receptor on leukocytes. This work has demonstrated that the affinity of the receptor is heterogeneous and is modified by guanine nucleotides and by prior agonist exposure. Transmethylation reactions mediated by S-adenosyl-methionine are important for the transduction of chemoattractant-related signals; pharmacological agents can be used to clearly dissect the transduction signals from the chemoattractant receptor into two groups.

Table I. Chemotactic and Secretory Functions of the
Oligopeptide Receptor

Effects	Chemotactic functions	Secretory functions
EC_{50} for fMet-Leu-Phe	~ 1 nM	~ 10 nM
Cytochalasin B	Inhibits	Enhances
Aliphatic alcohols	Enhances	Inhibits
Polyene antibiotics	Inhibits	Enhances

II. THE LEUKOCYTE OLIGOPEPTIDE CHEMOATTRACTANT RECEPTOR

A. N-Formylated Peptide Receptor Binding in Intact Leukocytes

The contention that leukocytes recognized chemoattractants via receptors was suggested by the strict structure–function relationships of synthetic N-formylated oligopeptides for initiating chemotactic and secretory activities by polymorphonuclear leukocytes (PMNs) (Showell et al., 1976). These observations as well as the availability of well-defined potent chemoattractants spurred us to develop fMet-Leu-[^{3}H]-Phe as a radioligand (Williams et al., 1977).

Initial studies defining the presence of specific N-formylated peptide receptors were done by measuring the direct binding of this radiolabeled peptide to human PMNs. The fMet-Leu-[^{3}H]-Phe used had a high specific activity (~ 46 Ci/mmol) as well as biological activity that exactly paralleled that of the unlabeled peptide (Williams et al., 1977). The binding of fMet-Leu-[^{3}H]-Phe to PMNs was saturable, and the number of binding sites per cell determined subsequently ranged from 40,000 to 60,000. The average equilibrium disassociation constant (K_D) for the interaction of the labeled peptide with human PMNs was 10–14 nmol. The binding was rapid with a half-time of 2.5–3.0 min at 37°C and was rapidly dissociable in the presence of a 1000-fold excess of unlabeled fMet-Leu-Phe, indicating that a portion of the peptide was bound to the exterior portion of the cell surface. The specificity of the N-formylated peptide receptor on human PMNs was demonstrated by showing that the relative potencies of a series of N-formylated peptides for producing a chemotactic response were reflected in the specificity of their binding to the fMet-Leu-[^{3}H]-Phe receptor. The order of potencies of the peptides for producing inhibition of fMet-Leu-[^{3}H]-Phe binding and for producing a chemotactic response was fMet-Leu-Phe > fMet-Met-Met > fMet-Phe > fMet-Leu > fMet. Linear regression analysis of a plot of the effective concentrations of peptides that produced a half-maximal (EC_{50}) chemotactic response vs. the EC_{50} for inhibition of fMet-Leu-[^{3}H]-Phe binding showed excellent correlation ($r = 0.999$) between these two activities. Direct binding techniques using radiolabeled N-formylated peptides have also demonstrated the presence of receptors for these substances on intact rabbit PMNs (Aswanikumar *et al.*, 1977), horse PMNs (Snyderman and Pike, 1980), rat PMNs (Marasco *et al.*, 1983), guinea pig peritoneal macrophages (Snyderman and Fudman, 1980), and human monocytes (Weinberg *et al.*, 1981; Benyunes and Snyderman, 1984). Development of direct binding of radiolabeled chemo-attractants to intact cells has also permitted the demonstration of distinct, specific receptors for C5a (Chenoweth and Hugli, 1978), a biologically active cleavage product derived from the fifth component of complement (C). The receptor for C5a is a separate entity from the *N*-formylated peptide receptor, since it has been shown that C5a does not compete for fMet-Leu-[^{3}H]-Phe binding on human PMNs (Williams *et al.*, 1977; Chenoweth and Hugli, 1978). Specific receptors have also been described for a crystal-induced chemotactic factor (CCF) released by PMNs upon phagocytosis of monosodium urate or calcium pyrophosphate dehydrate crystals (Spilberg and Mehta, 1979). For these studies, [^{125}I]-CCF binding to human PMNs was not displaced by the *N*-formylated peptides, or by activated plasma whose chemotactic activity is largely attributable to C5a (Snyderman *et al.*, 1970). Specific receptors for LTB4 have also been demonstrated on the surface of human PMNs (Goldman and Goetzl, 1982; Kreisle and Parker, 1983).

B. Cellular Models for the Study of Chemoattractant Receptor Transduction Mechanisms

Quantification of *N*-formylated peptide receptors using the direct binding techniques led to the finding that equine PMNs, despite containing on their surface specific high-affinity receptors for the *N*-formylated peptides, lacked chemotactic responses to these substances (Snyderman and Pike, 1980). The equine cells, however, responded to other chemotactic agents such as C5a and zymosan-activated horse serum. Interestingly, the *N*-formylated peptides did induce the release of lysosomal enzymes and stimulated the production of superoxide anion by equine PMNs. These data pointed out an important phenomenon concerning chemotactic factor receptor-mediated functions in mammalian cells. The transductional signals that transmit information from occupied receptors are different for various biological functions. This contention is further supported by the ability to dissect pharmacologically the chemotactic versus secretory responses in leukocytes (see Section III). It is nonetheless clear from the study of equine PMNs that transduction of secretory signals from the oligopeptide receptor does not require an intact chemotactic response pathway. It should now be possible, by comparing human and equine PMNs, to dissect the biochemical events following *N*-formylated peptide receptor binding that result in the various biological activities mediated by this receptor.

Several studies have shown that myeloid precursor cell lines lack specific receptors for fMet-Leu-[^{3}H]-Phe in the undifferentiated state but develop them when treated with agents which induce differentiation into PMNs and mononuclear phagocytes. The human monocytelike cell line, U937, can be stimulated to differentiate into macrophages *in vitro* in the presence of culture supernatants from lectin-stimulated lymphocytes (lymphokines) (Fischer *et al.*, 1980). Experiments using direct binding of fMet-Leu-[^{3}H]-Phe to U937 cells showed that undifferentiated cells possessed undetectable numbers of N-formylated chemoattractant receptors on their surface, as reflected by their inability to exhibit functional responses to these agents, including chemotaxis and lysosomal enzyme release. When the cells were incubated for 24–72 hr with lymphokine, however, the U937 cells developed increasing numbers of N-formylated peptide receptors, the appearance of which paralleled the acquisition of both chemotactic and secretory responses (Pike *et al.*, 1980).

Considering the heterogeneous nature of stimulated lymphocyte supernatants, attempts were made to identify well-defined agents that could reproducibly induce U937 cells to differentiate (Kay *et al.*, 1983). Both DMSO and dibutyryl cyclic adenosine monophosphate (cAMP) for the N-formylated oligopeptide chemoattractants in U937 cells. After exposure to 1 mM dibutyryl cAMP, 1.3% dimethyl sulfoxide, or 5% conditioned medium for 72 hr, the average number of oligopeptide chemoattractant receptors per cell was 33,000, 4000, and 3400, respectively. An average of 790 receptors per cell were detected on cells cultured in medium alone. Covalent affinity labeling methods were used to identify the N-formylated oligopeptide binding proteins on U937 cells treated with dibutyryl cAMP, conditioned medium, or DMSO, respectively. Normal human monocytes contained an oligopeptide binding protein of ~66,000 M_r. No specifically labeled proteins were detected on U937 cells grown in medium alone. Chemoattractant binding proteins with molecular weights similar to that of the monocyte receptor were expressed within 24 hr after exposure of U937 cells to 1 mM dibutryryl cAMP. Longer times were needed with DMSO treatment.

The receptors on dibutyryl cAMP-treated cells effectively initiated chemotaxis and lysosomal enzyme secretion in response to chemoattractants but not the formation of superoxide anion. Cells treated with DMSO responded chemotactically to fMet-Leu-Phe and did secrete lysosmal enzymes but also did not produce superoxide anion. Cells exposed to conditioned medium responded chemotactically, secreted lysosomal enzymes, and formed superoxide anion when incubated with fMet-Leu-Phe. These investigations demonstrated the usefulness of the U937 cell line as a source of reproducibly available cells with distinct responses to chemoattractants.

Studies by Niedel *et al.* (1980) have shown that another human myeloid precursor cell line, HL-60, can be induced to express increased numbers of N-formylated peptide receptors. This cell line develops into a neutrophil-like cell upon treatment with DMSO. Concomitant with this development is an increase in the percentage of cells expressing chemoattractant receptors from 2–3% to

30% in DMSO-treated HL-60 cells. Cyclic nucleotides also induce maturation of the HL-60 cells (Chaplinski and Niedel, 1982). Thus direct binding techniques employing high specific radioactivity chemotactic peptides has permitted the definition of continuous cell lines that can be induced to differentiate and to express receptors for N-formylated peptides. These cell lines are proving a useful tool not only for the characterization of such receptors, but also for the delineation of regulatory mechanisms involved in cellular differentiation and the chemotactic response.

C. N-Formylated Peptide Receptors in Leukocyte Membranes

Major advances have been made in the characterization of various cellular receptors, such as the adrenergic (Williams and Lefkowitz, 1978) and acetylcholine (Burgisser *et al.*, 1982) receptors primarily because of the availability of techniques to study these molecules in isolated membrane systems. Since ongoing cellular metabolic events interfere with accurate quantitative and qualitative measurement of receptor function in intact cells, we developed methods to measure receptors in isolated cellular membranes. For more precise quantification of binding parameters, the experimental data were subjected to a computer modeling techinque based on the law of mass action which allows analysis of the binding of multiple ligands to multiple classes of receptors. The computer pro-

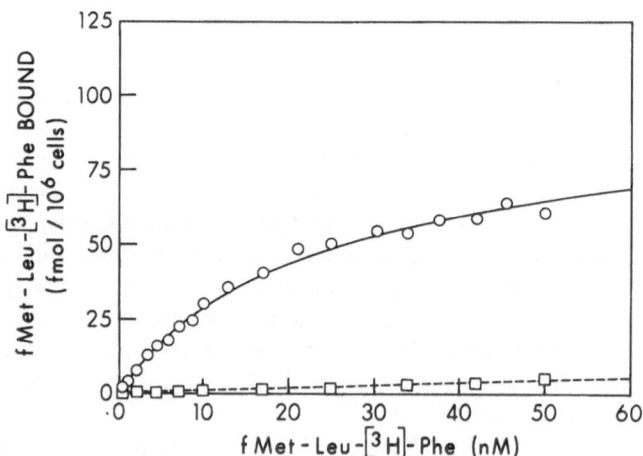

Figure 1. FML-[^{3}H]-P binding isotherms of intact polymorphonuclear leukocytes (PMNs). (○) Total ligand bound; (□) nonspecific binding (defined as the amount of radioligand bound in the presence of 1000-fold excess of unlabeled ligand). (——) Computer-fitted line for the total binding. (- - -) Nonspecific component. (From Koo *et al.*, 1982.)

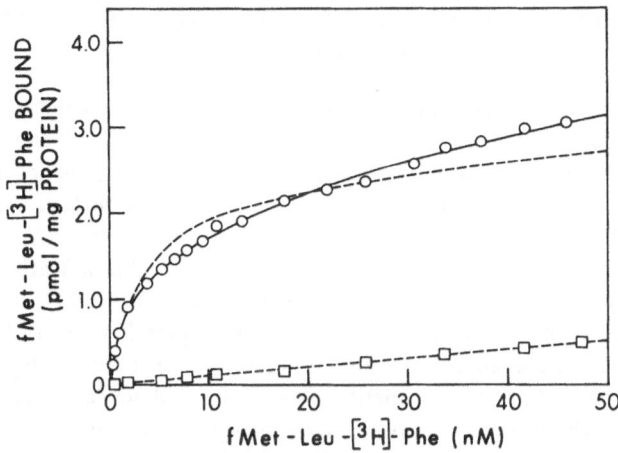

Figure 2. FML-[³H]-P binding isotherms of polymorphonuclear leukocyte membrane preparations. (——) Two-site fit to the data. (- - -, upper) One-site fit to the same data. The two-site fit was the significantly better treatment of the data with $P < 0.001$. (- - -, lower) Nonspecific binding. (o) Total binding; (□) nonspecific binding. (From Koo *et al.*, 1982.)

gram termed SCFIT permits determination of the affinity constants and concentration of each class of receptors (Hancock *et al.*, 1979; DeLean *et al.*, 1982*a*). A binding isotherm of the radiolabeled chemotactic peptide, fMet-Leu-[³H]-Phe to intact human PMNs is shown in Figure 1 (Koo *et al.*, 1982). Computer analysis showed a single class of receptor sites; no statistical improvement was found for a two-site fit. The average K_D and number of sites per PMN obtained from 25 experiments were 22.3 ± 2.4 nM and 55,700 ± 4800, respectively. In contrast, data derived from the binding of fMet-Leu-[³H]-Phe to PMN membranes fit significantly ($P < 0.001$) better to a model employing two classes of receptor sites (Fig. 2). The K_D values of these sites derived from the average of 20 experiments were 0.53 ± 0.01 n*M* and 24.4 ± 1.2 n*M*, respectively. The concentration of high-affinity receptors in different membrane preparations varied from 10% to 30% and the K_D of the low-affinity site did not differ significantly from the K_D of the receptors identified on intact PMNs. Dissociation kinetics of the receptor in membrane preparations in the presence and absence of excess cold ligand were identical, favoring an interpretation of heterogeneity of sites rather than negative cooperativity of one class of receptors. In contrast to intact viable PMNs, Formalin-fixed PMNs also demonstrated heterogeneity of binding sites with K_D of $K_H = 0.55 ± 0.3$ n*M* and $K_L = 18.6 ± 3.1$ n*M*, results in good agreement with those found in isolated membranes. These findings suggested that some ongoing metabolic process(es) in intact viable PMNs allow(s) receptor interconversion and thus permits detection of only a single affinity state of the chemoattractant receptor.

D. Guanine Nucleotides as Regulators of Binding Affinity of the Oligopeptide Receptor

In certain receptor systems, including the α- and β-adrenergic (Stadel *et al.*, 1982), glucagon (Lad *et al.*, 1977), muscarinic cholinergic (Burgisser *et al.*, 1982) and dopaminergic (DeLean *et al.*, 1982*b*) receptors, gaunine nucleotides play an important role in regulating the hormone–receptor interaction. In some instances, such as the β-adrenergic receptor, guanine nucleotides are required for transduction of the hormonal signal, which leads to the activation of adenyl cyclase (Stadel *et al.*, 1982; Verghese and Snyderman, 1983). Regulation of receptor-ligand interactions by guanine nucleotides has been shown to be associated with their ability to cause interconversion between high- and low-affinity receptor states. Experiments were performed to determine the effects of guanine nucleotides on the *N*-formylated peptide chemoattractant receptor. The nonhydrolysable analogue of GTP, p-[NH]-ppG, was incubated with PMN membranes and the binding of fMet-Leu-[³H]-Phe determined. Figure 3 illustrates that p-[NH]-ppG reduced the binding of the ligand when compared with membranes incubated with buffer alone. Analysis of the data indicated that the decreased binding was explained by a reduction in the number of high-affinity receptors. In seven experiments, it was found that membranes incubated in buffer alone expressed an average of $21.3 \pm 0.13\%$ high-affinity receptors, but when 10^{-4} *M* p-[NH]-ppG was included in the incubation mixture, only $11.8 \pm 0.05\%$

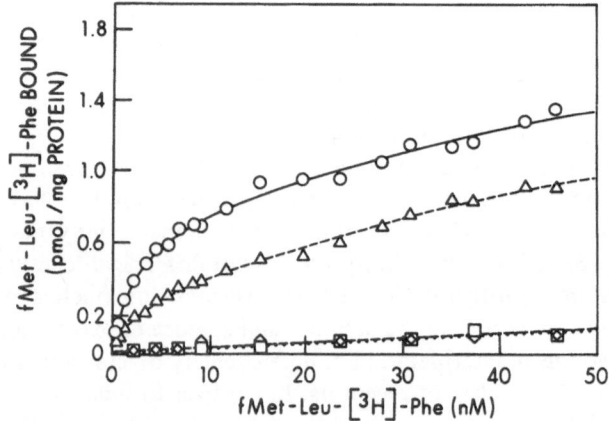

Figure 3. (A) FML-[³H]-P binding isotherms to human polymorphonuclear leukocyte (PMN) membrane preparations. PMN membranes, treated with buffer (o) or 10^{-4} *M* p-[NH]-ppG(Δ) were incubated with varying concentrations of FML[³H]-P at 25°C for 30 min. Both isotherms represent two-site fits to the data, which were significantly better than one-site fits ($P < 0.01$). The symbols □ and ◊ represent nonspecific binding in the presence of buffer or 10^{-4} *M* p-[NH]-ppG, respectively. (From Koo *et al.*, 1983.)

of the receptors were in the high-affinity state. The total number of receptors present under both incubation conditions was identical (0.435 ± 0.07 nM for buffer, 0.425 ± 0.06 nM for p-[NH]-ppG treated membranes). Since under both conditions, data modeled significantly better to a two-site fit, and since K_H and K_L were the same regardless of whether membranes were incubated with buffer or p-[NH]-ppG, the effect of the guanine nucleotide is thus to convert receptors originally present in the high-affinity state to a low-affinity state.

The effects of guanine nucleotide were dose dependent, in that a half-maximal effect of p-[NH]-ppG was observed at a concentration of 10^{-6} M, while that of GTP was 5×10^{-6} M and that of GDP was 5×10^{-5} M. The specificity of the guanine nucleotide effect on the fMet-Leu-[^{3}H]-Phe receptor was such that only GDP, GTP, and the nonhydrolysable analogues of GTP such as p-[NH]-ppG and GTP$_\gamma$S decreased the percentage of high-affinity receptors. ATP, ADP, AMP, cAMP, p-[NH]-ppA, GMP, and cGMP produced no effect on binding (Koo et al., 1983a).

The effects of guanine nucleotides on the fMet-Leu-[^{3}H]-Phe receptor are not limited to human PMN membranes, since similar results were noted in guinea pig macrophages membranes (Snyderman et al., 1984). Binding data from guinea pig macrophage membrane preparations indicated the presence of two classes of binding sites with K_D values 0f 1.5 ± 0.4 nM and 25.5 ± 11.0 nM. In the presence of p-[NH]-ppG, the number of high-affinity receptors was reduced from 29.4 to 8.7%, with a concomitant increase in low-affinity receptor sites and no significant change in the total number of binding sites.

The aforementioned findings share some similarities to the effects of guanine nucleotides on the binding of β-adrenergic agonists to their β-receptors on frog and turkey erythrocyte membranes (Stadel et al., 1982). Biochemical transduction of the β-adrenergic receptor signal has been shown to be mediated by a nucleotide regulatory protein (N protein), which activates adenylate cyclase. A model involving a guanine nucleotide regulatory unit can be applied to the fMet-Leu-[^{3}H]-Phe binding data presented herein. Figure 4 presents a ternary

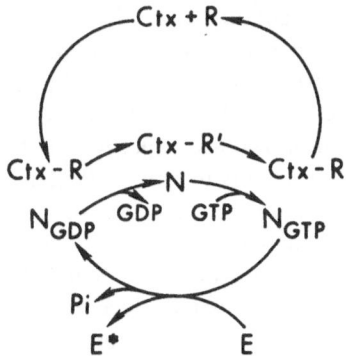

Figure 4. Postulated model for the interaction of guanine nucleotides with a nucleotide regulatory protein and the chemoattractant (Ctx)–receptor complex. It is proposed that the affinity of the receptor is affected by its coupling to a regulatory unit N, which binds guanine nucleotides. The transient high-affinity state R' may occur when the receptor is bound to free N. (From Snyderman et al., 1984.)

complex model in which receptor occupancy by fMet-Leu-[^{3}H]-Phe facilitates the substitution of GDP by GTP on a nucleotide regulatory subunit, thereby providing a N-GTP to activate an effector molecule(s) or reaction(s). When coupled to the N-unit carrying GDP or GTP, the receptor expresses a low-affinity state. We postulate that the high-affinity state of the receptor is manifest when the receptor is bound to N in the absence of any guanine nucleotide.

The effector(s) for the chemoattractant receptor is as yet unknown, but likely candidates would include a phospholipase, protein kinase, methyltransferase, or perhaps adenylate cyclase. Recent studies have shown that adenylate cyclase activation or inhibition by certain hormones in guinea pig macrophage membranes require the presence of guanine nucleotides (Verghese and Snyderman, 1983). Activation of adenylate cyclase by β-adrenergic agonists and prostaglandins as well as inhibition of cyclase activation by a-adrenergic agonists has an absolute requirement for guanine nucleotide triphosphates. The chemoattractants fMet-Leu-Phe and C5a, however, neither activated nor inhibited the stimulation of adenylate cyclase in these membranes. Therefore, although guanine nucleotide regulation of the N-protein is involved in activation of adenylate cyclase in many receptor systems, the chemoattractant receptor–guanine nucleotide-N-protein model may be independent of adenylate cyclase regulation. Indeed, it has been shown that light activation of a photoreceptor 3',5'-c GMP phosphodiesterase in retinal rods requires the binding of GTP to a specific protein (Wheeler and Bitensky, 1977). This phenomenon suggests that GTP-activated protein–receptor complexes may be generally important for biochemical activation of several transduction systems independent of adenylate cyclase.

E. Agonist Preincubation Enhances the Fraction of High-Affinity Binding Sites That Are Not Regulated by Guanine Nucleotides

Only a portion of the high-affinity receptors in PMN membranes were interconvertible to the low-affinity state by guanine nucleotides. It was therefore important to better characterize the nonconvertible high-affinity receptors, since high-affinity states have been associated with both activation as well as desensitization processes in nonchemotactic factor receptors. Preexposure of PMNs with agonists alters their biological responsiveness, so we investigated the effect of prior agonist exposure on the equilibrium binding characteristics of chemoattractants to human PMN membranes (Koo *et al.*, 1983). Preincubation of PMN membranes with fMet-Leu-Phe followed by extensive washing to remove the ligand-enhanced subsequent fMet-Leu-[^{3}H]-Phe binding. Computer analysis of such data indicated that PMN membranes incubated in buffer alone contained 16% high-affinity receptors. This fraction was increased to 35% ($P < 0.01\%$) and 45% when the membranes were preincubated with 10^{-7} and 10^{-6} *M* fMet-Leu-

Phe for 30 min at 25°C, respectively. The dose of fMet-Leu-Phe used in the preincubation with the membranes was critical in regard to the enhancement of subsequent binding. Preincubation with 10^{-9} M fMet-Leu-Phe had no observable effect on subsequent binding while 10^{-8} M fMet-Leu-Phe increased binding to 180% of control values, 10^{-7} M fMet-Leu-Phe to 230% of control values and 10^{-6} M fMet-Leu-Phe to 280% of control values. Agonist-induced enhancement of binding was also time and temperature dependent. At 0°C no enhancement by agonist preincubation could be seen. At 25°C, with 10^{-8} M fMet-Leu-Phe, the maximum of approximately 200% of controlled binding was seen after 30 min. At 37°C, however, the same dose of fMet-Leu-Phe enhanced binding to 300% of control by 5 min, the earliest time tested.

The specificity of agonist-induced receptor conversion to the high-affinity state is seen in Table II. C5a did non enhance subsequent binding of fMet-Leu-Phe and fMet-Leu-Phe-induced conversion was blocked by 10^{-5} M of the pentapeptide t boc-Phe-Leu-Phe-Leu-Phe (boc PLPLP). While guanine nucleotides interconvert receptors from the high to low-affinity state in untreated membranes, guanine nucleotides had no effect on the high-affinity receptors induced by fMet-Leu-Phe preincubation. Experiments were also performed to determine whether the high-affinity state induced by agonist exposure could be reverted to the low-affinity state after guanine nucleotide incubation. This was found not to be the case. Once high-affinity receptors induced by agonists were formed, they were no longer susceptible to guanine nucleotide regulation.

Thus, the high-affinity state of the chemoattractant receptor on PMN membranes exists in two forms: a guanine nucleotide-sensitive form convertible to the low-affinity state and a guanine nucleotide-insensitive form induced by prior receptor occupancy. The high-affinity state induced by agonist exposure follows a dose–response curve similar to that required for secretion or superoxide anion

Table II. Agonist Preincubation Enhances Guanine Nucleotide Independent High-Affinity Binding

Preincubation Condition[a]	Percent high affinity fMet-Leu-Phe receptors
Buffer alone	17
10^{-8} M C5a	19
10^{-8} M fMet-Leu-Phe	38
10^{-7} M fMet-Peu-Phe	48
10^{-7} M fMet-Leu-Phe + 10^{-5} M bocPLPLP	16
10^{-7} M fMet-Leu-Phe + 10^{-4} M p-[NH]-ppG	43

[a]PMN membranes were preincubated with the indicated attractants at 25°C for 30 min, washed extensively, and assayed for radioligand binding under equilibrium conditions. Binding data were subjected to computer analysis; percentages of high-affinity receptors are shown. (From Koo and Snyderman, 1983.)

production (Yuli *et al.*, 1982). The high-affinity non-guanine nucleotide-sensitive form of the receptor could represent an intermediate form associated with the rapid receptor internalization, since it is not expressed on cells preincubated with agonist at 37°C, but is expressed on cells incubated with agonist at 15°C. The latter condition prevents internalization. It can be hypothesized that when formation of this receptor state exceeds internalization rates, this form of the receptor transmits signals for O_2^- production and secretion. Jerisaitis *et al.* (1983) recently described an apparent high-affinity form of the oligopeptide chemo-attractant receptor that appears to mediate its internalization after interaction with cytoskeletal elements (see Chapter 2). The high-affinity binding site in-duced by agonist preexposure and not regulated by guanine nucleotides could represent the high-affinity receptor described by Jerisaitis *et al.* (1983).

III. INDEPENDENT REGULATION OF CHEMOTACTIC AND SECRETORY FUNCTIONS OF THE OLIGOPEPTIDE RECEPTOR

A. Effects of Pharmacologically Induced Alterations in Membrane Fluidity on Functions Mediated by the *N*-Formylated Chemoattractant Receptor

In several cellular systems, changes in membrane fluidity have been shown to alter receptor–hormone interactions and resultant metabolic processes (Heron *et al.*, 1980). Alterations in membrane microviscosity and/or lipid composition in leukocyte membranes can be achieved with aliphatic alcohols (Yuli *et al.*, 1982) and polyene antibiotics such as amphotericin B or nystatin (Lampen, 1969; Andreoli, 1973). Studies were therefore performed to evaluate the effects of these agents on *N*-formylated chemoattractant receptor function. Aliphatic alcohols, such as *n*-pentanol and *n*-butanol, which increase membrane fluidity nonspecifically, were tested for their effects on fMet-Leu-[^{3}H]-Phe binding to intact human PMNs (Yuli *et al.*, 1982). Cells were incubated with concentrations of *n*-pentanol (0.1%) and *n*-butanol (0.25%), which maintained cellular viability and produced equivalent decreases in the membrane microviscosity parameter measured using diphenylhexatriene fluorescence polarization. Figure 5 shows isotherms of fMet-Leu-[^{3}H]-Phe binding to cells treated with the alcohols, which produced a shift in the receptor affinities ($K_D \pm$ SEM) from 25.7 ± 7.6 nM for the untreated cells to 5.2 ± 0.9 and 6.0 ± 0.9 nM for the *n*-butanol and *n*-pen-tanol-treated cells, respectively. No significant changes in the total number of receptors per cell was produced by incubation with alcohols. Thus, under con-ditions in which membrane fluidity was increased, *N*-formylated chemoattractant receptor affinity was augmented. To determine whether the change in affinity of the receptor was reflected in its biological activity, the effects of *n*-butanol and *n*-pentanol on PMN chemotaxis were studied. When chemotaxis was assessed by

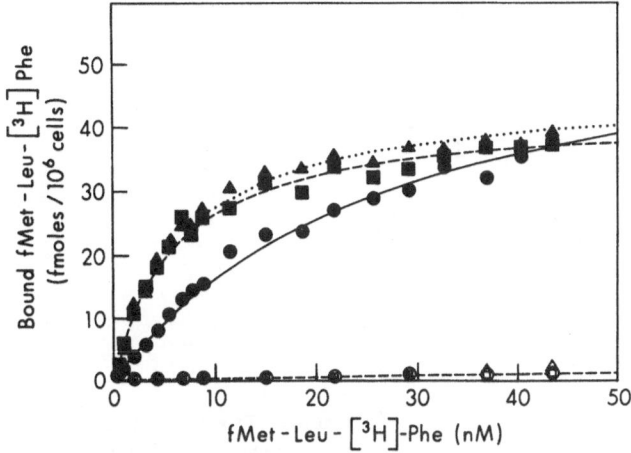

Figure 5. Total and nonspecific binding of fMet-Leu-[³H]-Phe ([³H]-FMLP) to PMNs in the absence (○) and the presence of either 0.25% *n*-butanol (□) or 0.1% *n*-pentanol (△). Binding was performed in the absence (filled symbols) and in the presence (open symbols) of 10 μ*M* FMLP at 25°C for 60 min. The curves were produced by computerized fitting of the data to a monoaffinity receptor model. Paired Student's *t* test of the data obtained from three duplicated experiments revealed no significant difference between the *n*-butanol- and *n*-pentanol-treated systems ($P \gg 0.5$), both of which are significantly different from the control system ($P < 0.01$ up to 20 n*M* [³H]-FMLP). (From Yuli *et al.*, 1982.)

the leading front-migration method (Zigmond and Hirsch, 1973), it was found that PMNs treated with *n*-butanol and *n*-pentanol increased the sensitivity of the cells to submaximal stimulating doses of fMet-Leu-Phe.

The effects of the alcohols on chemoattractant-stimulated superoxide anion production and lysosomal enzyme secretion were also determined (Yuli *et al.*, 1982). In contrast to their effects on migration, these two functions mediated by the chemoattractant receptor were greatly decreased in the presence of the alcohols. Figure 6A demonstrates that *n*-butanol concentration of 0.1% and 0.25% inhibited stimulated O_2^- production by 50% and 85%, respectively. *n*-Pentanol produced similar effects. Phorbol myristate acetate (PMA)-stimulated O_2^- production was however not altered by *n*-butanol (Fig. 6B), indicating that the enzymes necessary for the respiratory burst were not affected; rather, the effect was due to a change in the chemoattractant receptor's transduction mechanism for O_2^- production. Lysosomal enzyme secretion was also markedly depressed by treatment of the cells with *n*-butanol. Lysozyme secretion was inhibited by 0.25% *n*-butanol with a pronounced EC_{50} shift of more than an order of magnitude to higher fMet-Leu-Phe concentrations (data not shown).

These data demonstrate that a decrease in PMN membrane microviscosity produced by aliphatic alcohols is accompanied by an increase in the affinity of

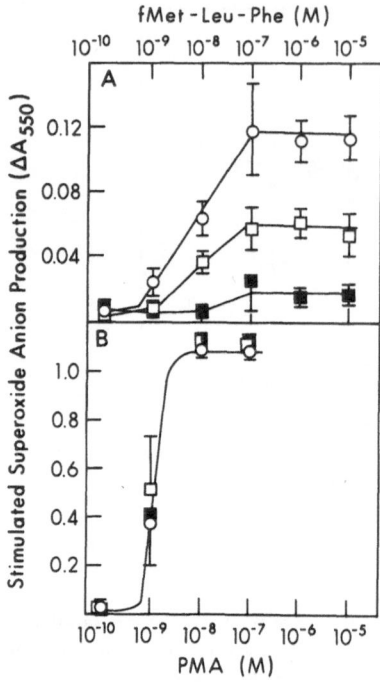

Figure 6. Effect of *n*-butanol on superoxide anion production. Polymorphonuclear leukocytes (PMNs) preincubated with either buffer (o), 0.1% (□), or 0.25% (■) *n*-butanol were stimulated by either fMet-Leu-Phe (FMLP) (A) or phorbol myristate acetate (PMA) (B). The stimulated O_2^- production is expressed by the increased 550 nm absorbance of experimental minus control, and presented as the mean and SD of four experiments performed in duplicates. (From Yuli *et al.*, 1982.)

the *N*-formylated peptide receptor. These changes are accompanied by altered biological responses of the cells to the chemoattractants, including increased sensitivity of the chemotactic response to lower concentrations of fMet-Leu-Phe, but depressed superoxide generation and lysosomal enzyme secretion. Thus, it appears that the transduction mechanisms of the chemoattractant receptor can be divided into at least two categories: (1) those such as chemotaxis, which require low doses of chemoattractants and are augmented by conditions that increase the affinity of the receptor and (2) those such as lysosomal enzyme secretion and superoxide production that are depressed when the higher average affinity of the receptor predominates.

B. Differential Effects of Polyene Antibiotics on Chemoattractant-Receptor-Mediated Functions

Studies performed with the polyene antibiotics, amphotericin B and nystatin, support the contention that various chemoattractant-mediated functions are regulated differently and that transduction mechanisms are affected by the affinity state of the receptor (Lohr and Snyderman, 1982). Amphotericin B, which is known to inhibit chemotaxis (Bjorksten *et al.*, 1976), binds to sterols in membranes and thus disrupts normal phospholipid–cholesterol interactions (Andreoli, 1973; Lampen, 1969). Since cholesterol synthesis is required for chemotaxis (Pike and Snyderman, 1980) and chemoattractants alter phospholipid metabolism in leukocytes (Pike et al., 1979); Ishizaka et al., 1980), it was hypothesized that amphotericin B produces its effects in leukocytes by altering the lipid environment surrounding the chemotactic factor receptor (Lohr and Snyderman, 1982). Incubation of human PMNs with 2 or 4 μM amphotericin B inhibited chemotaxis in a dose-dependent fashion without affecting cell viability. The less potent polyene antibiotic, nystatin, also inhibited the chemotactic response at concentrations ranging from 10 to 40 μM. The nonpolyene antifungal agent, griseofulvin, had no effect on chemotaxis even at concentrations 25-fold higher than those of amphotericin B, which inhibited chemotaxis.

To determine whether the decreases in the chemotactic response in the presence of amphotericin B could be explained by altered receptor function, intact PMNs and isolated membranes were incubated with concentrations of the drug ranging from 1 to 10 μM. Amphotericin B caused a dose-dependent decrease in fMet-Leu-[^{3}H]-Phe binding in both cell and membrane preparations. Nystatin in concentrations of 5 and 10 μM also inhibited fMet-Leu-[^{3}H]-Phe binding to intact cells, but griseofulvin was without effect. Amphotericin B did not affect the specificity of the N-formylated peptide receptor because it did not alter the order to potency of the various N-formylated peptides for inhibition of fMet-Leu-[^{3}H]-Phe binding. The effects of 2 μM amphotericin B on fMet-Leu-[^{3}H]-Phe binding to PMNs were analyzed using the computer modeling method and were shown to lower the K_D value from 13 to 44 nM. There was a slight but statistically insignificant increase in total receptor number in the presence of the drug.

In contrast to the effects on chemotaxis, amphotericin B increased lysozyme secretion initiated by the oligopeptide chemoattractant. It was found that the drug accelerated stimulated lysozyme release at 5 min at both 2 and 4 μM concentrations, whereas at 15 min only the 4-μM dose produced a small increase. Both doses had no significant effect on the release of β-glucuronidase, an azurophilic granule enzyme. The cytoplasmic enzyme marker, lactic dehydrogenase, was not released by amphotericin B treatment, and there was no release of lysosomal contents in the presence of drug alone without fMet-Leu-Phe. Amphotericin B produced no effect on fMet-Leu-Phe-induced superoxide radical production at concentrations of 2 μM and 4 μM. These data show that a decrease in the affinity of the chemoattractant receptor is accompanied by depressed chemotaxis, an increase in specific granule enzyme secretion, and no inhibition of superoxide anion production. Take together with the effects of the alcohols on chemoattractant oligopeptide receptor affinity and function, the data obtained with amphotericin B and nystatin provide further support for the contention that the affinity state of the receptor reflects transduction of different signals.

The oligopeptide chemotactic factor receptor in human PMNs and guinea pig macrophage membranes thus exists in two affinity states that are interconvertible and regulated in part by guanine nucleotides and in part by agonist exposure. The high-affinity state of the receptor is not detected in untreated intact cells presumably because of the high intracellular concentration of guanine nucleotides as well as rapid internalization of the agonist-induced high-affinity state. The average affinity of the receptor in intact cells can, however, be modified by agents that alter the physical state of the PMN membrane. Decreased membrane microviscosity produced by aliphatic alcohols increases the average affinity of the receptor and favors transduction of chemotactic signal but suppresses lysosomal enzyme release and superoxide production. These latter functions are favored when the average affinity state of the receptor is lowered by polyene antibiotic treatment. The implication from these studies is that one can differentially modify the biological functions of human PMNs by exposing them to agents that affect physical parameters of membranes, and thus receptor function. Differential pharmacological manipulation of the various functional responses of leukocytes will have important therapeutic implications for inflammatory, neoplastic, and immunodeficiency diseases.

IV. ROLE OF TRANSMETHYLATION REACTIONS AND MEMBRANE PHOSPHOLIPID METABOLISM IN CHEMOATTRACTANT RECEPTOR-LIGAND INTERACTIONS

The foregoing studies underscore the importance of the oligopeptide chemoattractant receptor's affinity in reflecting its ability to initiate various functional activities of leukocytes. In addition, studies with amphotericin B and the alcohols suggest that membrane fluidity and/or lipid composition are instrumental in regulating receptor affinity and activity. The precise endogenous biochemical reactions that control chemoattractant receptor affinity and subsequent transduction of functional signals through the membrane are unknown at this time. Transmethylation reactions using S-adenosyl-L-methionine (AdoMet) as the methyl donor are required for many functions of eukaryotic cells initiated by plasma membrane receptors. Included in these are the release of histamine by mast cells and basophils in response to (Ishizaka et al., 1980), the blastogenesis of lymphocytes in response to mitogens (Hirata et al., 1980), the capping of IgG in lymphocytes (Braun et al., 1980), and phagocytosis by macrophages (Leonard et al., 1978; Snyderman et al., 1980). Work from this laboratory as well as others have implicated a role for methylation reactions in the chemotaxis of leukocytes (O'Dea et al., 1978; Pike et al., 1978; Snyderman et al., 1980).

The treatment of intact cells with EHNA (erythro-9,2(hydroxy-3-nonyl-adenine), an inhibitor of adenosine deaminase, plus adenosine and L-homocysteine thiolactone produces an increase in intracellular S-adenosyl-L-homosteine (AdoHcy), a competitive inhibitor of AdoMet-mediated methylation reactions (Kredich and Martin, 1977). Other agents such as 3′-deaza-adenosine with or without L-homocysteine derivatives also inhibit transmethylation reactions (Chiang et al., 1977). Chemotaxis of leukocytes as measured in modified Boyden chambers is inhibited when the cells are incubated with these compounds (Pike et al., 1978). The level of chemotaxis inhibition correlated well with the degree to which methylation reactions were depressed. In addition, it appears that some methylation reaction is required for the early cytoskeletal alterations that permit the cell shape changes manifested during the chemotactic response. This was suggested by experiments showing that the morphological polarization of monocytes by chemoattractants is inhibited by conditions that inhibit methylation reactions (Pike and Snyderman, 1981a).

The effects of methylation inhibition on superoxide anion production by chemoattractants were also investigated since this reaction occurs within seconds of receptor occupancy. Guinea pig macrophages were preincubated with buffer or with EHNA and various concentrations of adenosine in the presence or absence of L-homocysteine thiolactone (Pike and Snyderman, 1982). Superoxide production was monitored by measuring the reduction of ferricytochrome C spectrophotometrically. Increasing concentrations of adenosine in the presence of EHNA inhibited fMet-Leu-Phe-stimulated superoxide production by a maximum of 59%. The further addition of 0.1 mM L-homocysteine thiolactone to the cells increased the inhibition of methylation and depressed superoxide release by 95%. The depression of superoxide production by methylation inhibitors was not due to increased superoxide dismutase activity in cells treated with methylation inhibitors.

The foregoing studies suggested that transmethylation reactions are required for early transductional events after chemoattractant receptor occupancy. Studies were performed to clarify further the role of transmethylation reactions in the regulation of the chemoattractant receptor (Pike and Snyderman, 1982). Intact guinea pig macrophages were incubated with EHNA, adenosine, and L-homocysteine thiolactone and the binding of fMet-Leu-[^{3}H]-Phe was quantified. These conditions, which inhibited cellular AdoMet-mediated methylation reactions by 90%, caused the affinity of the receptor to be reduced by a factor of 2.6. Figure 7 shows that the K_D for the interaction of fMet-Leu-[^{3}H]-Phe with cellular receptors was 2.9 ± 0.2 nM and the number of receptor sites per cell was 11,082 ± 533 in the absence of methylation inhibitors. In the presence of EHNA, adenosine, and L-homocysteine, however, the K_D value was increased to 7.5 ± 0.6 nM and there was a slight but significant increase in the receptor number (12,709 ± 431 sites per cell). The specificity of methylation inhibition for producing a reduction in the affinity of the fMet-Leu-[^{3}H]-Phe receptor was investigated. Incubation of cells with EHNA and adenosine in the absence of L-homocysteine, conditions that favor suboptimal inhibition of methylation reactions, had no effect on the affinity of the fMet-Leu-[^{3}H]-Phe receptor.

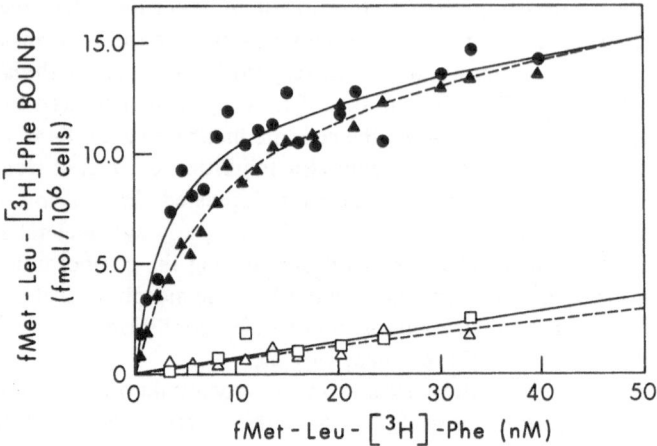

Figure 7. Effects of erythro-9,2(hydroxy-3-nonyl-adenine (EHNA), adenosine, and L-homocysteine thiolactone on the binding of fMet-Leu-[³H]-Phe to intact guinea pig macrophages.
Guinea pig macrophages were preincubated in the presence or absence of 10 μM EHNA, 0.5
mM adenosine, and 0.1 mM L-homocysteine thiolactone and then added to tubes containing various concentrations of fMet-Leu-[³H]-Phe in the presence or absence of 10 μM unlabeled fMet-Leu-Phe. Total and nonspecific binding after 60 min at 25°C was then measured by vacuum filtration, and the results were subjected to computer analysis. Closed
symbols represent total binding and open symbols represent nonspecific binding. Circles are
results obtained from cells incubated in buffer alone, and triangles are results obtained from
cells incubated with EHNA, adenosine, and L-homocysteine thiolactone. (From Pike and
Snyderman, 1982.)

Another agent known to inhibit methylation reactions in intact cells, 3'-deaza-
adenosine, was also tested for its effects on fMet-Leu-[³H]-Phe binding to guinea
pig macrophages. This agent is both a substrate and inhibitor of S-adenosyl-
L-homocysteine hydrolase in intact cells (Chiang et al., 1977). Treatment of
cells with this compound leads to an accumulation of both AdoHcy and S-3'-
deaza-adenosyl homocysteine, both of which can inhibit AdoMet-mediated
methylation reactions. The formation of these inhibitors within cells in the presence of 3' deaza-adenosine is augmented by L-homocysteine thiolactone. Incubation of macrophages with this adenosine analogue and L-homocysteine
thiolactone produced a dose-dependent decrease in the affinity of the fMet-Leu-
[³H]-Phe receptor (Pike and Snyderman, 1982). A concentration of 1.0 mM
3'-deaza-adenosine in the presence of 0.1 mM L-homocysteine thiolactone increased the K_D value of the fMet-Leu-[³H]-Phe receptor from 3.1 ± 5 nM to
5.4 ± 0.8 nM and 0.5 mM 3'-deaza-adenosine increased it to 4.9 ± 0.9 nM without significantly altering the receptor number.
    It has been reported that the combination of EHNA, adenosine, and L-
homocysteine thiolactone increases concentrations of cAMP in murine lympho-

cytes by enhancing adenylate cyclase activity and decreasing cAMP phospho-diesterase activity (Zimmermann *et al.*, 1980). This mechanism of action cannot explain the effects of EHNA, adenosine and L-homocysteine thiolactone on the macrophage fMet-Leu-[^{3}H]-Phe receptor because agents known to increase cAMP in these cells, i.e., isoproterenol (0.1 mM) and theophylline (0.1 mM), produced no effect whatsoever on the binding of the chemoattractant. Other studies have suggested that the pharmacological agents used to inhibit methyl-tion in these studies decrease protein synthesis (Backlund and Cantoni, 1983). It has therefore been postulated that inhibition of protein synthesis is the mech-anism for inhibition of chemotaxis by EHNA, adenosine, and L-homocysteine. We have shown, however, that conditions that inhibit up to 90% of protein syn-thesis in human leukocytes have no effect on the directed migration of these cells (Pike *et al.*, 1978). These results further support the interpretation that EHNA, adenosine, and L-homocysteine thiolactone inhibit chemoattractant-mediated functions by curtailing methylation reactions.

It appears from the above studies that some ongoing methylation reaction is required to maintain the oligopeptide chemoattractant receptor in a func-tionally active state and that inhibition of methylation lowers receptor affinity. We hypothesize that the lower average receptor affinity caused by inhibition of methylation reflects an alteration in the receptor and is associated with its being uncoupled from its transduction apparatus. The nature of the transduction unit is unknown, but a nucleotide regulatory unit is an obvious possibility. Inhibition of methylation results in decreased mononuclear cell morphological polarization, chemotaxis, secretion, O_2^- production, and arachidonate release from phospho-lipids in response to chemoattractants. It is unknown at this time which specific methylation reaction(s) is involved in the stimulus–response coupling of the chemoattractant receptor.

Interestingly, chemotactic factors themselves, when incubated with macro-phages, depress one type of transmethylation reaction, the formation of methyl-ated derivatives of phosphatidyl ethanolamine (PE) (Pike *et al.*, 1979). This inhibition cannot be explained by an increased destruction of methylated phos-pholipids, and chemotactic factors do not alter total phospholipid synthesis in these cells. Because of this, one would expect to increase the ratio of PE to methylated phospholipids in the newly synthesized membrane lipids of such cells. Changes in the ratio of PE to methylated lipids could alter the biophysical characteristics in focal areas of the membrances of chemotactically responsive cells, particularly at the leading front membrane, where the greatest degree of chemotactic factor receptor occupancy would be expected to occur. These changes in phospholipid ratios may serve to regulate the affinity of the chemo-attractant receptor and thus facilitate transduction of the chemotactic signal. We tested this hypothesis directly by measuring PE to total methylated phospholipid (PL) ratios in plasma membranes from guinea pig macrophages treated with chemotactic factors (Pike and Snyderman, 1981*b*). Cells were incubated with [methyl-^{3}H] methionine and [^{14}C] ethanolamine in buffer alone or containing the chemotactic factors fMet-Leu-Phe, fNle-Leu-Phe, or C5a. The plasma membranes were then isolated and the amount of newly synthesized methylated PL (labeled with tritium) and PE (labeled with carbon-14) were determined. The three chemotactic agents increased the ratio of newly synthesized PE : total methylated PL in the plasma membrane by 53 to 111% (Fig. 8). The PE : phos-

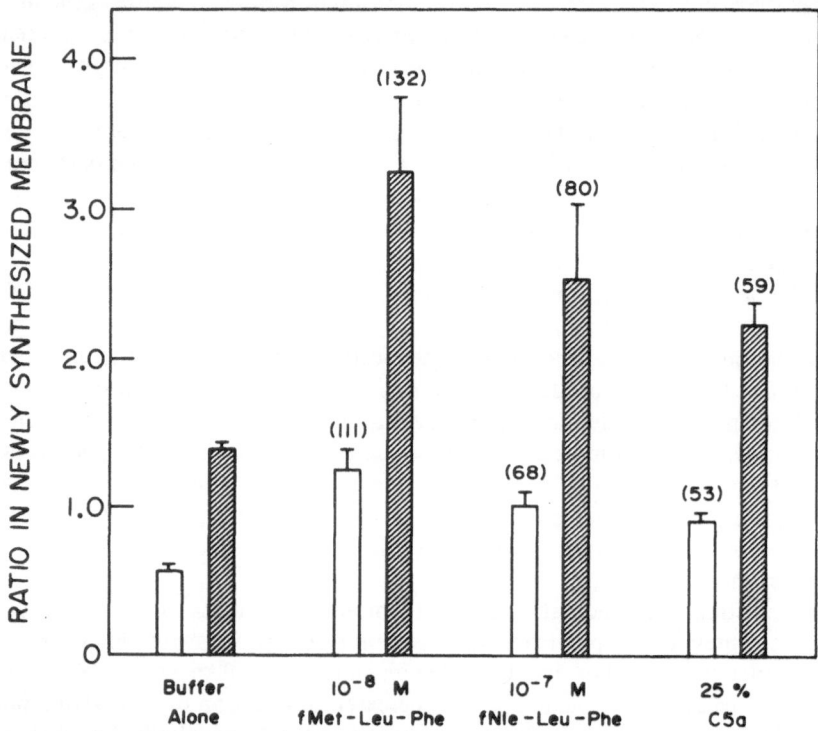

Figure 8. Effects of chemotactic factors on newly synthesized phosphatidyl ethanolamine : methylated phospholipid ratios in macrophage plasma membranes. Duplicate samples of intact macrophages were incubated for 1 hr at 37°C in the presence or absence of chemotactic factors in medium containing [^{3}H-methyl]methionine and [^{14}C]ethanolamine. The plasma membranes were then isolated and extracted with chloroform : methanol, and the labeled phospholipids were analyzed by thin-layer chromatography. Ratios (±SD) were calculated by dividing the number of [^{14}C]-cpm incorporated into phosphatidyl ethanolamine (PE) by the number of [^{3}H]-cpm incorporated into the total methylated phospholipids (□) or into phosphatidyl choline (PC) alone (▨). Percentage increase (represented by the numbers in parentheses) in the PE : total methylated phospholipid ratio = $(E_C - 1) \times 100$, where E is the ratio obtained in the presence of fMet-Leu-Phe and C is the ratio obtained when cells were incubated with buffer alone. (From Pike and Snyderman, 1981*b*.)

phatidyl choline (PC) ratio was similarly increased in the plasma membranes by 59 to 132%. This increase was due to decreased synthesis of methylated PL and not to altered formation of PE or activation of phospholipases that degrade PE.

Methylated PL ratios were also studied in the leading front lamellipodia isolated from macrophages migrating under chemotactic and nonchemotactic conditions. The ratios of PE : total methylated PL and PE : PC were increased 2- to 4-fold in lamellipodia derived from macrophages that had responded to zymosan activated serum, C5a or fMet-Met-Met when compared with those from cells responding to buffer alone (Pike and Snyderman, 1981b). It has recently been shown by Wright (1983) that secondary granules contain a greater PE : PC ratio as compared to primary granules and plasma membranes of leukocytes. In addition, low concentrations of chemoattractants cause fusing of lysosomal granules to the plasma membrane, which results in increased chemoattractant binding (Fletcher and Gallin, 1980). The integration of secretory granule membrane into leading front lamellipodia in cells responding to chemoattractant substances with a subsequent increase in PE : PC ratios may be required for sustained directed migration and subsequent alterations in chemoattractant receptor function.

Another mechanism by which methylation reactions could control membrane phospholipid composition, and thus receptor function, is through regulation of leukocyte phospholipases. Many hormone–receptor interactions in different cell types have been shown to release free arachidonic acid from membrane phospholipids through the activation of phospholipase C and phospholipase A (Maino et al., 1975; Rittenhouse-Simmons, 1979; Kennerly et al., 1979). Indeed, we and others have found this to occur in both PMNs and mononuclear leukocytes (Hirata et al., 1979; Pike and Snyderman, 1981a). We have also found, that inhibition of methylation reactions in mononuclear cells effectively inhibits chemoattractant-mediated activation of phospholipases (Pike and Snyderman, 1981a). When human monocytes are incubated with chemoattractants, arachidonate is released, and it can be shown from phospholipid analyses that the source of this free fatty acid is phosphatidyl inositol (PI). Levels of this phospholipid are decreased by 35% in monocytes treated with 10^{-7} M fMet-Leu-Phe, while there are no significant changes detected in PE and PC (Table III). Methylation inhibitors reduced the chemoattractant-mediated degradation of PI to only 14%. Interestingly, in the absence of chemottractant, methylation inhibition selectively increased the total amount of PI in monocytes, suggesting that the activity of the phospholipase that normally metabolizes this phospholipid requires an ongoing methylation reactions. The enhanced turnover of PI induced by chemoattractants in monocytes suggests that phospholipase C activation may be involved in this process. Diacylglycerol produced as a result of PI breakdown as well as the release of membrane Ca^{2+} by chemoattractants could lead to the activation of protein kinase C (Castagna et al., 1982). Protein kinase C has recently been shown to be directly activated by PMA (Castagna et al., 1982;

Table III. Effects of fMet-Leu-Phe and Methylation Inhibition on
^{3}H-Arachidonic Acid-Labeled Cellular Lipids

Cellular incubation medium[a]	Residual cpm ($\times$ 10^{-3})[b]			
	PC	PI	PE	AA
Buffer	26.7 ± 1.4[c]	31.6 ± 0.8	12.2 ± 1.0	30.6 ± 2.1
100 nM fMet-Leu-Phe	23.1 ± 1.9 (–13)[d]	20.6 ± 0.3 (–35)	13.5 ± 2.9 (+11)	29.7 ± 4.9 (–3)
EHNA + Ado + homocysteine	28.7 ± 2.0	39.5 ± 0.1	11.2 ± 0.4	28.4 ± 1.3
EHNA + Ado + homocysteine + 100 nM fMet-Leu-Phe	27.1 ± 0 (–6)	34.1 ± 0.1 (–14)	12.4 ± 1.1 (+11)	28.2 ± 0.6 (–1)

Source: Pike and Snyderman (1981*a*).
Abbreviations: AA, arachidonic acid; cpm, counts per minute; EHNA, erythro-9, 2 (hydroxy-3-nonyl-adenine; PC, phosphatidyl choline; PE, phosphatidyl ethanolamine; PI, phosphatidyl inasitol.
[a] Monocyte-enriched cells (65% peroxidase positive) were labeled with 0.5 μCi/ml [^{3}H] arachidonic acid for 30 min at 37°C, washed three times, and resuspended in buffer alone or containing 10 μM EHNA, 0.5 mM adenosine, and 0.1 mM homocysteine thiolactone. After an incubation for 15 min at 37°C, buffer or 100 nM fMet-Leu-Phe was added for an additional 15 min at 37°C.
[b] Cellular lipids were extracted with chloroform : methanol and applied to a silica gel plate, which was developed in chloroform : methanol : acetic acid : water(65 : 25 : 4 : 2). Spots of reference lipids were visualized with iodine, and 0.5-cm fractions were counted for radioactivity. The numbers represent the sum of counts per minute in each individual peak of radioactivity that migrated with the indicated reference lipid.
[c] ± SD of duplicate samples. The experiment was performed three times with similar results.
[d] Numbers in parentheses indicate the percentage change in residual counts per minute due to incubation with fMet-Leu-Phe.

Niedel *et al.*, 1983), a substance that is a potent secretogogue and inducer of O$_2^-$ production by leukocytes. Taken as a whole, these findings suggest that binding of chemoattractants to their receptors in leukocytes activate phospholipase C, thereby providing free Ca^{2+}, diacyglycerol, and presumably phosphatidylserine for the activation of protein kinase C, which in turn is involved in activating the secretory and respiratory burst mechanisms of the cell. An ongoing methylation reaction appears to be required for the activation of phospholipase C, an early step in this process (Fig. 9).

V. SUMMARY

Phagocytic leukocytes contain receptors for chemoattractants on their cell surface. Binding of chemotactic factors to these receptors initiates a number of coordinated cellular responses in a strict dose-dependent manner. Motility-

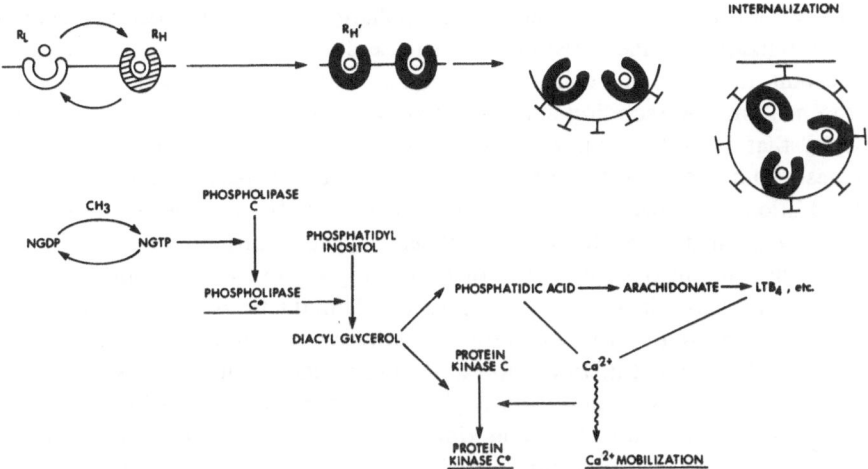

Figure 9. Model for the activation of transduction mechanisms of a chemoattractant receptor on leukocytes. Binding of the chemoattractant to its receptor leads to the formation of
a reversible high-affinity state regulated by guanine nucleotides. At high concentrations of
the chemoattractant, a non-guanine nucleotide-sensitive high-affinity receptor is formed. This
receptor is rapidly internalized. Associated with receptor occupancy is activation of phospholipases and increase of intracellular cyclic adenosine monophosphate (cAMP). Portrayed
is one of the pathways that appears to be activated by chemoattractants in leukocytes. A
role for methylation (CH_3) and a nucleotide regulatory protein in activation of phospholipase C are suggested by data presented in this review.

related functions such as shape change, cytoskeletal rearrangement, and chemotaxis are stimulated by relatively low doses of chemoattractants, while microbiocidal or cytotoxic functions (i.e., secretion of lysosomal enzymes or stimulation of the respiratory burst), require ~10- to 50-fold higher concentrations of
these agents. The receptor for oligopeptide chemotactic factors on leukocytes
has provided an important model for the study of stimulus-response coupling in
phagocytic cells. This receptor on human polymorphonuclear leukocytes exists
in two affinity states that are partially interconvertible. Guanine nucleotides
regulate the convertibility between a portion of the high- and low-affinity states,
thereby suggesting that a nucleotide regulatory protein allosterically modifies
receptor affinity and participates in its transduction mechanisms. A fraction of
the high-affinity receptors in PMN membranes is not subject to guanine nucleotide regulation and appears to be formed by prior exposure of the receptors to
specific agonists. This high-affinity form of the oligopeptide chemoattractant
receptor is rapidly internalized at 37°C, and its formation may be dependent on
aggregation or covalent modification of the receptor. The chemotaxis and
microbiocidal functions of PMNs can be divergently manipulated by pharmacological agents indicating that the transduction mechanisms for these two types of

processes are independently regulated. Aliphatic alcohols at doses that induce mild fluidization of PMN membranes increase the average affinity of the chemo-attractant receptor and enhance chemotactic functions but markedly depress lysosomal enzyme secretion and the respiratory burst. In contrast, polyene anti-biotics that bind to membrane cholesterol lower the receptor's affinity and depress chemotactic functions but enhance secretion of specific granule enzymes. In addition, transmethylation reactions mediated by S-adenosyl-methionine appear to regulate receptor affinity. When such reactions are blocked pharma-cologically, the oligopeptide receptor on macrophages reverts to a lower average affinity form and is ineffective in transducing chemotactic as well as microbicidal functions. Among the stimulus–response pathways that appear to be involved in regulating leukocyte function is the activation of phospholipase C, as well as the production of products such as diacylglycerol and arachidonate, which are likely to stimulate the activity of protein kinase C. Activation of the protein kinase C and the cAMP-dependent protein kinase pathways by the chemoattractant re-ceptor may provide both positive and negative stimuli for the numerous func-tions of phagocytic cells.

VI. REFERENCES

Andreoli, T. E., 1973, On the anatomy of amphotericin β-cholesterol pores in lipid bilayer membranes, *Kidney Int.* 4:337.

Aswanikumar, S., Corcoran, B., Schiffman, E., Day, A. R., Freer, R. J., Showell, H. J., and Pert, C. B., 1977, Demonstration of a receptor on rabbit neutrophils for chemotactic peptides, *Biochem. Biophys. Res. Commun.* 74:810.

Backlund, P., and Cantoni, G. L., 1983, Chemotaxis and methylation reactions in a mouse macrophage cell line, *Proceedings of the Fifth Phagocyte Workshop, Washington, D.C.*

Benyunes, M. C., and Snyderman, R., 1984, Characterization of an oligopeptide chemo-attractant receptor on human blood monocytes using a new radioligand, *Blood* in press.

Bjorksten, B., Ray, C., and Quie, P. G., 1976, Inhibition of human neutrophil chemotaxis and chemiluminescence by amphotericin β, *Infect. Immun.* 14:315.

Boucek, M. M., and Snyderman, R., 1976, Calcium influx requirement for human neutrophil chemotaxis:Inhibition by lanthanum chloride, *Science* 193:905.

Boyden, S., 1962, The chemotactic effect of mixtures of antibody and antigen on poly-morphonuclear leukocytes, *J. Exp. Med.* 115:453.

Braun, J., Rosen, F. S., and Unanue, E. R., 1980, Capping and adenosine metabolism, *J. Exp. Med.* 151:174.

Burgisser, G., DeLean, A., and Lefkowitz, R. J., 1982, Reciprocal modulation of agonist and antagonist binding to muscarinic cholinergic receptor by guanine nucleotides, *Proc. Natl. Acad. Sci. (USA)* 79:1732.

Castagna, M., Yoshima, T., Kaibachi, S., Kikkawa, U., and Nishizuka, Y., 1982, Direct acti-vation of calcium activated phospholipid dependent protein kinase by tumor-promoting phorbol esters, *J. Biol. Chem.* 257:7847.

Chaplinski, T. J., and Niedel, J. E., 1982, Cyclic nucleotide induced maturation of human promyelocytic leukemia cells, *J. Clin. Invest.* 70:953.

Chenoweth, D. E., and Hugli, T. E., 1978, Demonstration of a specific C5a receptor on in-tact polymorphonuclear leukocytes, *Proc. Natl. Acad. Sci. (USA)* 75:3943.

Chiang, P. K., Richards, H. H., and Cantoni, G. L., 1977, S-adenosyl-L-homocysteine hydrolase: Analogues of S-adenosyl-L-homocysteine as potential inhibitors, *Mol. Pharmacol.* **13**:939.

Cianciolo, G. J., and Snyderman, R., 1981, Monocyte responsiveness to chemotactic stimuli is a property of a subpopulation of cells which can respond to multiple chemoattractants, *J. Clin. Invest.* **67**:60.

Cohen, S., Pick, E., and Oppenheim, J. J., 1979, *The Biology of the Lymphokines*, Academic Press, New York.

DeLean, A., Hancock, A. A., and Lefkowitz, R. J., 1982*a*, Validation and statistical analysis of computer modeling method for quantitative analysis of radioligand binding data for mixtures of pharmacological receptor subtypes, *Mol. Pharm.* **21**:5.

DeLean, A., Kilpatrick, B. F., and Caron, M. G., 1982*b*, Dopamine receptor of the porcine anterior pituitary gland, *Mol. Pharm.* **22**:290.

Fernandez, H. N., Henson, P. M., Otani, A., and Hugli, T. E., 1978, Chemotactic response to human C3a and C5a anaphylatoxins: I. Evaluation of C3a and C5a leukotaxis in vitro and under simulated in vivo conditions, *J. Immunol.* **120**:109.

Fischer, D. G., Pike, M. C., Koren, H. S., and Snyderman, R., 1980, Chemotactically responsive and non-responsive forms of a continuous human monocyte cell line, *J. Immunol.* **125**:463.

Fletcher, M. P., and Gallin, J. I., 1980, Degranulating stimuli increase the availability of receptors on human neutrophils for the chemoattractant fMet-Leu-Phe, *J. Immunol.* **124**:1585.

Ford-Hutchinson, A. W., Bray, M. A., Doig, M. V., Shipley, M. E., and Smith, M. J. H., 1980, Leukotriene B, a potent chemokinetic and aggregating substance released from polymorphonuclear leukocytes, *Nature* **286**:264.

Gallin, J. I., and Rosenthal, A. S., 1974, The regulatory role of divalent cations in human granulocyte chemotaxis: Evidence for an association between calcium exchanges and microtubule assembly, *J. Cell. Biol.* **62**:594.

Goetzl, E. J., and Austen, K. F., 1975, Purification and synthesis of eosinophilic tetrapeptides of human lung tissue: Identification as eosinophil chemotactic factor of anaphylaxis, *Proc. Natl. Acad. Sci. (USA)* **72**:4123.

Goetzl, E. J., and Pickett, W. C., 1980, The human PMN leukocyte chemotactic activity of complex hydroxy-eicosatetraenoic acids (HETES), *J. Immunol.* **125**:1789.

Goldman, D. W., and Goetzl, E. J., 1982, Specific binding of leukotriene B4 to receptors on human polymorphonuclear leukocyes, *J. Immunol.* **129**:1600.

Goldstein, I., Hoffstein, S., Gallin, J., and Weissmann, G., 1973, Mechanisms of lysosomal enzyme release from human leukocytes: Microtubule assembly and membrane fusion induced by a component of complement, *Proc. Natl. Acad. Sci. (USA)* **70**:2916.

Hancock, A. A., DeLean, A., and Lefkowitz, R. J., 1979, Quantitative resolution of beta-adrenergic receptor subtypes by selective ligand binding. Application of a computerized model fitting technique, *Mol. Pharm.* **16**:1.

Heron, D. S., Shinitzky, M., Hershkowitz, M., and Samuel, D., 1980, Lipid fluidity markedly modulates the binding of serotonin to mouse brain membranes, *Proc. Natl. Acad. Sci. (USA)* **77**:7463.

Hirata, F., Corcoran, B. A., Venkatasubramanian, K., Schiffmann, E., and Axelrod, J., 1979, Chemoattractants stimulate degradation of methylated phospholipids and release of arachidonic acid in rabbit leukocytes, *Proc. Natl. Acad. Sci. (USA)* **76**:2640.

Hirata, F., Togoshima, S., Axelrod, J., and Waxdal, M. J., 1980, Phospholipid methylation: A biochemical signal modulating lymphocyte mitogenesis, *Proc. Natl. Acad. Sci. (USA)* **77**:862.

Hugli, T. E., and Müller-Eberhard, H. J., 1978, Anaphylatoxins, *Adv. Immunol.* **26**:1.

Ishizaka, T., Hirata, F., Ishizaka, K., and Axelrod, J., 1980, Stimulation of phospholipid methylation, Ca^{2+} influx, and histamine release by bridging of IgE receptors on rat mast

mast cells, *Proc. Natl. Acad. Sci. (USA)* 77:1903.

Jensen, J. A., Snyderman, R., and Mergenhagen, S. E., 1969, Chemotactic activity, a property of guinea pig C′5-anaphylatoxin, *Proceedings of the Third International Symposium on Cellular and Humoral Mechanisms in Anaphylaxis and Allergy*, p. 265, Karger, Basel.

Jerisaitis, A. J., Naemura, J. R., Sklar, L. A., Cochrane, C. G., and Painter, R. G., 1983, *N*-formyl-met-leu-phe is found in transient association with detergent-insoluble, cytoskeleton-rich structure of stimulated granulocytes, *Fed. Proc.* (in press).

Kay, G. E., Lane, B. C., and Snyderman, R., 1984, Induction of selective biological responses to chemoattractants in a human monocyte like cell line, *Infect. Immun.* 41:1166–1147.

Kennerly, D. A., Sullivan, T. J., Sylvester, P., and Parker, C. W., 1979, Diacylglycerol metabolism in mast cells: A potential role in membrane fusion and arachidonic acid release, *J. Exp. Med.* 150:1039.

Klebanoff, S. J., and Clark, R. A., 1978, *The Neutrophil: Function and Clinical Disorders*, North-Holland, New York.

Koo, C., and Snyderman, R., 1983, The oligopeptide chemoattractant receptor on human neutorphils converts to an irreversible high affinity state subsequent to agonist exposure, *Clin. Res.* 31(2):491A.

Koo, C., Lefkowitz, R. J., and Snyderman, R., 1982, The oligopeptide chemotactic factor receptor on human polymorphonuclear leukocyte membranes exists in two affinity states, *Biochem. Biophys. Res. Commun.* 106:442.

Koo, C., Lefkowitz, R. J., and Snyderman, R., 1984, Guanine nucleotides modulate the binding affinity of the oligopeptide chemoattractant receptor on human polymorphonuclear leukocytes, *J. Clin. Invest.* 72:748–753.

Kredich, N. M., and Martin, D. W., Jr., 1977, Role of *S*-adenosyl-homocysteine in adenosine mediated toxicity in cultured mouse T lymphoma cells, *Cell* 12:931.

Kreisle, R. A., and Parker, C. W., 1983, Specific binding of leukotriene B4 to a receptor on human polymorphonuclear leukocytes, *J. Exp. Med.* 157:628.

Lad, P. M., Welton, A. F., and Rodbell, M., 1977, Evidence for distinct guanine nucleotide sites in the regulation of the glucagon receptor and of adenylate cyclase activity, *J. Biol. Chem.* 252:5942.

Lampen, J. O., 1969, Amphotericin B and other polyenic antifungal antibiotics, *Am. J. Clin. Pathol.* 52:138.

Leonard, E. J., Skeel, A., Chiang, P. K., and Cantoni, G. L., 1978, The action of the adenosylhomocysteine hydrolase inhibitor, 3-deazaadenosine on phagocytic function of mouse macrophages and human monocytes, *Biochem. Biophys. Res. Commun.* 84:102.

Lohr, K. M., and Snyderman, R., 1982, Amphotericin B alters the affinity and functional activity of the oligopeptide chemotactic factor receptor on human polymorphonuclear leukocytes, *J. Immunol.* 129:1594.

Maino, V. C., Hayman, M. J., and Crumpton, M. J., 1975, Relationship between enhanced turnover of phosphatidylinositol and lymphocyte activation by mitogens, *Biochem. J.* 146:247.

Marasco, W.A., Fantone, J. C., Freer, R. J., and Ward, P. A., 1983, Characterization of the rat neutrophil formyl peptide chemotaxis receptor, *Am. J. Pathol.* 111:373.

Metchnikoff, E., 1968, *Lectures on the Comparative Pathology of Inflammation*, Dover, New York.

Naccache, P. H., Showell, H. J., Becker, E. L., and Shaa′fi, R. I., 1977, Transport of sodium, potassium, and calcium across rabbit polymorphonuclear leukocyte membranes: Effect of chemotactic factor, *J. Cell. Biol.* 73:428.

Niedel, J., Kahane, I., Lachman, L., and Cuatrecasas, P., 1980, A subpopulation of cultured human promyelocytic leukemia cells (HL-60) displays the formyl peptide chemotactic receptor, *Proc. Natl. Acad. Sci. (USA)* 77:1000.

Niedel, J. E., Kuhn, L. J., and Vandenbark, G. R., 1983, Phorbol diester receptor copurifies with protein kinase C, *Proc. Natl. Acad. Sci. (USA)* 80:36.

O'Dea, R. F., Viveros, O. H., Aswanikumar, S., Schiffmann, E., Chiang, P. K., Cantoni, G. L., and Axelrod, J., 1978, A protein carboxymethylation stimulated by chemotactic peptides in leukocytes, *Fed. Proc.* 37:1656.

Palmer, R. M. J., Steprey, R. J., Higgs, G. A., and Eakins, K. E., 1980, Chemotactic activity of arachidonic acid lipoxygenase products in leukocytes from different species, *Prostaglandins* 20:411.

Pike, M. C., and Snyderman, R., 1980, Lipid requirements for leukocyte chemotaxis and phagocytosis: Effects of inhibitors of phospholipid and cholesterol synthesis, *J. Immunol.* 124:1963.

Pike, M. C., and Snyderman, R., 1981a, Transmethylation reactions are required for initial morphologic and biochemical responses of human monocytes to chemoattractants, *J. Immunol.* 127:1444.

Pike, M. C., and Snyderman, R., 1981b, Alterations of new methylated phospholipid synthesis in the plasma membranes of macrophages exposed to chemoattractants, *J. Cell. Biol.* 91:221.

Pike, M. C., and Snyderman, R., 1982, Transmethylation reactions regulate affinity and functional activity of chemotactic factor receptors on macrophages, *Cell* 28:107.

Pike, M. C., Kredich, N. M., and Snyderman, R., 1978, Requirement of S-adenosyl-L-methionine-mediated methylation for human monocyte chemotaxis, *Proc. Natl. Acad. Sci. (USA)* 75:3928.

Pike, M. C., Kredich, N. M., and Snyderman, R., 1979, Phospholipid methylation in macrophages is inhibited by chemotactic factors, *Proc. Natl. Acad. Sci. (USA)* 76:2922.

Pike, M. C., Fischer, D. G., Koren, H. S., and Snyderman, R., 1980, Development of specific receptors for N-formylated chemotactic peptides in a human monocyte cell line stimulated with lymphokines, *J. Exp. Med.* 152:31.

Rittenhouse-Simmons, S., 1979, Production of diglyceride from phosphatidylinositol in activated human platelets, *J. Clin. Invest.* 63:580.

Shin, H. S., Snyderman, R., Friedman, E., Mellors, A., and Mayer, M. D., 1968, Chemotactic and anaphylatoxic fragment, cleaved from the fifth component of guinea pig complement, *Science* 162:361.

Showell, H. J., Freer, R. J., Zigmond, S. H., Schiffmann, E., Aswanikumar, S., Corcoran, B. A., and Becker, E. L., 1976, The structure–activity relations of synthetic peptides as chemotactic factors and inducers of lysosomal enzyme secretion for neutrophils, *J. Exp. Med.* 143:1154.

Smith, C. W., Hollers, J. C., Patrick, R. A., and Hassett, 1979, Motility and adhesiveness in human neutrophils. Effects of chemotactic factors, *J. Clin. Invest.* 63:221.

Snyderman, R., and Fudman, E. J., 1980, Demonstration of a chemotactic factor receptor on macrophages, *J. Immunol.* 124:2754.

Snyderman, R., and Pike, M. C., 1980, N-formylmethionyl peptide receptors on equine leukocytes initiate secretion but not chemotaxis, *Science* 209:493.

Snyderman, R., Gewurz, H., and Mergenhagen, S. E., 1968a, Interactions of the complement system with endotoxic lipopolysaccharide. Generation of a factor chemotactic for polymorphonuclear leukocytes, *J. Exp. Med.* 128:259.

Snyderman, R., Shin, H. S., Phillips, J. K., Gewurz, H., and Mergenhagen, S. E., 1969, A neutrophil chemotactic factor derived from C5 upon interaction of guinea pig serum with endotoxin, *J. Immunol.* 103:413.

Snyderman, R., Phillips, J. K., and Mergenhagen, S. E., 1970, Polymorphonuclear leukocyte chemotactic activity in rabbit and guinea pig serum treated with immune complexes: Evidence for C5a as the major chemotactic factor, *Infect. Immun.* 1:521.

Snyderman, R., Altman, L. C., Hausman, M. S., and Mergenhagen, S. E., 1972, Human mononuclear leukocyte chemotaxis: A quantitative assay for mediators of humoral and cellular chemotactic factors, *J. Immunol.* 108:857.

Snyderman, R., Pike, M. C., and Kredich, N. M., 1980, Role of transmethylation reactions in cellular motility and phagocytosis, *Mol. Immunol.* 17:209.

Snyderman, R., Pike, M. C., Edge, S., and Lane, B. C., 1984, A chemoattractant receptor on macrophages exists in two affinity states regulated by guanine nucleotides, *J. Cell. Biol.* 98:(in press).

Spilberg, I., and Mehta, J., 1979, Demonstration of a specific neutrophil receptor for a cell derived chemotactic factor, *J. Clin. Invest.* 59:582.

Spilberg, I., Gallacher, A., Mehta, J., and Mandell, B., 1976, Urate crystal induced chemotactic factor, isolation and partial characterization, *J. Clin. Invest.* 58:815.

Stadel, J. M., DeLean, A., and Lefkowitz, R. J., 1982, Molecular mechanisms of coupling in hormone receptor-adenylate cyclase systems, *Adv. Enzymol.* 53:1.

Verghese, M. W., and Snyderman, R., 1983, Hormonal regulation of adenylate cyclase in macrophage membranes is regulated by guanine nucleotides, *J. Immunol.* 180:869.

Ward, P. A., and Newman, L. J., 1969, A neutrophil chemotactic factor from human C5, *J. Immunol.* 102:93.

Ward, P. A., Reinold, H. G., and David, J. R., 1969, Leukotactic factor produced by sensitized lymphocytes, *Science* 163:1079.

Wasserman, S. I., Sater, N. A., Center, D. M., and Austen, K. F., 1977, Cold urticaria: Recognition and characterization of a neutrophil chemotactic factor which appears in serum during experimental cold challenge, *J. Clin. Invest.* 60:189.

Weinberg, J. B., Muscato, J. J., and Niedel, J., 1981, Monocyte chemotactic peptide receptor, *J. Clin. Invest.* 68:621.

Weissmann, G., Serhan, C., Smolen, J. E., Korchak, H. M., Friedman, R., and Kaplan, H. B., 1982, Stimulus–secretion coupling in the human neutrophil: The role of phosphatidic acid and oxidized fatty acids in the translocation of calcium, *Adv. Prostaglandin Thromboxane Leukotriene Res.* 9:259.

Wheeler, G. L., and Bitensky, M. W., 1977, A light-activated GTPase in vertebrate photoreceptors: Regulation of light-activated cyclic GMP phosphodiesterase, *Proc. Natl. Acad. Sci. (USA)* 74:4238.

Williams, L. T., and Lefkowitz, R. J., 1978, *Receptor Binding Studies in Adrenergic Pharmacology*, Raven Press, New York.

Williams, L. T., Snyderman, R., Pike, M. C., and Lefkowitz, R. J., 1977, Specific receptor sites for chemotactic peptides on human polymorphonuclear leukocytes, *Proc. Natl. Acad. Sci. (USA)* 74:1204.

Wright, D., 1983, Cytoplasmic granules of human neutrophils: Differences in the membrane lipids of primary and secondary granules, *Proceedings of the Fifth Phagocyte Workshop, Washington, D.C.*

Yuli, I., Tomonaga, A., and Snyderman, R., 1982, Chemoattractant receptor functions in human polymorphonuclear leukocytes are divergently altered by membrane fluidizers, *Proc. Natl. Acad. Sci. (USA)* 79:5906.

Zigmond, S. H., and Hirsch, J. G., 1973, Leukocyte locomotion and chemotaxis: New methods for evaluation and demonstration of a cell-derived chemotactic factor, *J. Exp. Med.* 137:387.

Zimmerman, T. P., Schmitges, C. J., Walberg, G., Deeprose, R. D., Duncan, G. S., Cuatrecasas, P., and Elion, G. B., 1980, Modulation of cyclic AMP metabolism by S-adenosyl-homocysteine and S-3-deazaadenosyl-homocysteine in mouse lymphocytes, *Proc. Natl. Acad. Sci. (USA)* 77:5639.

Chapter 2

The Neutrophil N-Formyl Peptide Receptor: Dynamics of Ligand–Receptor Interactions and Their Relationship to Cellular Responses

Larry A. Sklar, Algirdas J. Jesaitis, and Richard G. Painter

Department of Immunology
Scripps Clinic and Research Foundation
La Jolla, California 92037

I. INTRODUCTION

A. Overview

The *N*-formyl peptides, as a class, evoke in neutrophils *in vitro* an array of responses that mimic the biological functions of these cells in the inflammatory process. Because these peptides can be prepared synthetically, it has been possible to correlate extensively the structure–function relationships of a variety of amino acid sequences in both stimulatory and inhibitory peptides. Moreover, this diversity in available sequences has permitted the development not only of numerous radiolabeled ligands, but of photoaffinity and fluorescent molecules as well. During the short period since *N*-formyl-methionyl peptides were first identified as chemoattractants derived from bacteria, the *N*-formyl peptides receptor has been catapulted into a position of prominence as a model, not only for studies of neutrophil stimulation but for receptor-mediated cell stimulation in general.

A number of features of neutrophil activation and formyl peptide–formyl peptide receptor interaction have combined to make this an attractive model system in which to elucidate the entire sequence of biochemical events initiated at the receptor and responsible for several cellular responses:

An addendum to this chapter begins on page 395.

1. The neutrophil responses are diverse (including protease secretion, generation of free radicals of oxygen, production of bioactive metabolites of arachidonate, phagocytosis and killing of bacteria and other particles, and chemotaxis).
2. The responses of the cells are relatively rapid and are tightly connected, both temporally and physically, to the occupancy of cell-surface receptors.
3. The development of new methods (in conjunction with the array of available ligands) that permit the real-time analysis of ligand–receptor interactions and their quantitative relationships to cellular responses will promote rapid progress in this system.

We will emphasize in this review those aspects of ligand–receptor interaction and cellular response pathways in which quantitative analysis hold special promise. We have also made an effort to draw upon examples from other receptor systems in which parallel analyses have already been developed.

B. The Ligand

During the past decade, it has been recognized that a variety of presumably monovalent ligands were not only chemoattractants for neutrophils, but that they also stimulated a battery of associated cellular responses. The ligands include activated complement (C5a), arachidonate metabolites (the leukotrienes), and additional factors derived from host cells and tissues (platelet activating factor, N-formylated mitochondrial proteins) as well as bacterial cells. Schiffmann *et al.* (1975) set into motion the present interest in formyl peptides by demonstrating that the chemoattractants of bacterial cultures were N-formyl-methionyl oligopeptides. Shortly thereafter, a specific receptor for these peptides in human neutrophils was identified (Aswanikumar *et al.*, 1977; Williams *et al.*, 1977).

During the ensuing years, remarkable progress in elucidating the structural requirements for ligand binding and cellular stimulation has been accomplished, largely through the efforts of Becker and Freer, their colleagues, and other investigators (Showell *et al.*, 1976; Niedel *et al.*, 1979a; Freer *et al.*, 1980, 1982). The salient features of this work have been recently reviewed by Becker (1979).

By way of summary, we note that the most active tripeptide, N-fMet-Leu-Phe, is the "parent" of these ligands in widest use. A systematic study of different amino acid sequences has demonstrated a requirement for hydrophobic residues adjacent to the formyl group. Studies of peptides of different lengths, i.e., N-fMet-Leu-Phe, N-fMet-Leu-Phe-Met, and N-fMet-Leu-Phe-Met-Tyr, suggest that at least five residues can contribute to the binding and imply that the size of the binding site is sufficient to accommodate a peptide of this size (Niedel *et al.*, 1979a). Freer *et al.* (1982) summarize these observations in a model of the binding pocket (Fig. 1). The model specifies several points:

1. The requirement for the formyl group and its irreplaceability by an acetyl group are consistent with a prerequisite for H-bonding to the receptor.
2. The requirement for methionine in position 1 and its replaceability by norleucine (but not residues with longer side chains) is consistent with a hydrophobic pocket of defined size and with a positively charged region in the binding site.
3. The efficacy of leucine in position 2, and its replaceability by valine, suggests that the hydrophobic interactions are less restricted than in position 1.
4. The requirement for the phenylalanine side chain precludes charged residues at position 3.
5. A variety of nonpolar substituents at position 4 (and potentially at position 5) enhance the binding of the peptide and are consistent with additional hydrophobic interactions in or near the binding pocket.

The structure and activity of inhibitors are in contrast with the peptides themselves. Replacing the formyl group by t-butyloxy often gives rise to inhibitory ligands, but there is as yet no simple correlation of the amino acid sequence with inhibitory action. Thus the tripeptides $t$boc-Met-Leu-Phe and $t$boc-Phe-Leu-Phe are comparable ($ID_{50} \sim 6 \times 10^{-7}$ M) while the tetrapeptide $t$boc-Leu-Phe-Leu-Phe and the pentapeptide $t$boc-Phe-Leu-Phe-Leu-Phe are also comparable ($ID_{50} \sim 3 \times 10^{-7}$ M). In Sections III.C, D we consider some characteristics of

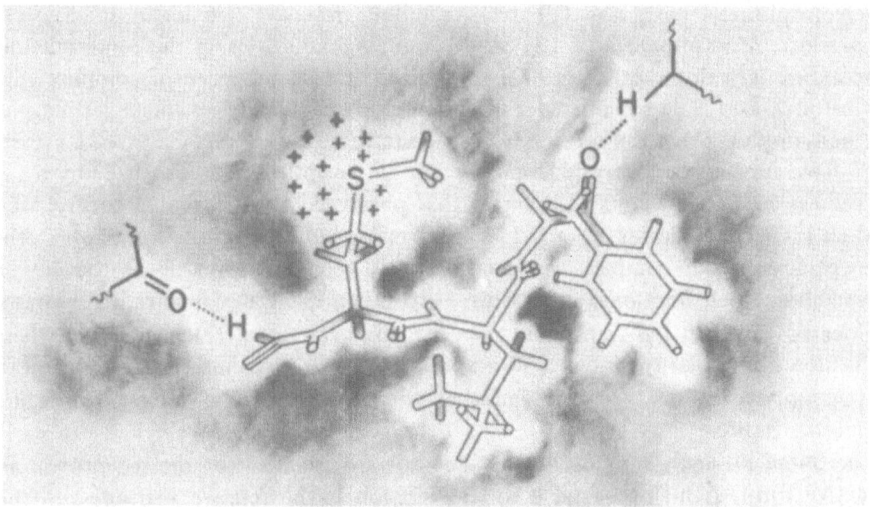

Figure 1. Model of N-fMet-Leu-Phe in the binding pocket of the N-formyl peptide receptor on rabbit neutrophils. (Reprinted with permission from Freer $et\ al.$, 1982, $Biochemistry$ 21:257–263, Fig. 4. (The print was kindly supplied by Dr. R. J. Freer, Virginia College of Medicine.)

the ligand–receptor interaction that may give rise to inhibitory or stimulatory capabilities of different peptides.

C. Molecular Characterization of the *N*-Formyl Peptide Receptor

The neutrophil receptor for *N*-formyl peptides was first characterized by Niedel and co-workers, who showed that the hexapeptide *N*-fNle-Leu-Phe-Nle [^{125}I]-Tyr-Lys, when bound to membrane fractions isolated from neutrophils, could be crosslinked to the receptor with any of several bifunctional reagents. While the crosslinking was specific and saturable, less than 1% of the receptor were labeled (Niedel *et al.*, 1980). SDS-PAGE analysis revealed a specifically labeled species of ~55–70 kd. Since the apparent molecular weight was not affected by disulfide reducing agents, the absence of intermolecular disulfide bonds was inferred.

These workers also reported the synthesis of a photoactivatable derivative of the hexapeptide that crosslinked with a low efficiency ($<$0.1%), but which was not suitable for labeling the receptor in intact neutrophils. More recently, Schmitt *et al.* (1983) described crosslinking studies with the hexapeptide derivatized with a longer "spacer" arm, nitroazidohexanoate. We were able to crosslink the ligand to up to 40% of the available receptors in intact neutrophils under conditions in which cell viability was maintained. Two-dimensional gel electrophoresis using the O'Farrell technique revealed two major species: (1) pI = 6.5, M_r = 60,000, and (2) pI = 6.0, M_r = 50,000. Using the same labeling conditions, Painter *et al.* (1982) solubilized the ligand–receptor complex with Triton X-100. The solubilized complex bound specifically to wheat germ agglutinin, implying that the receptor is a glycoprotein.

We further demonstrated that the labeled receptor was internalized by living cells at 37°C in a manner similar to that observed for the ligand *N*-formyl-Met-Leu-[^{3}H]-Phe (Jesaitis *et al.*, 1983). In subcellular fractionation studies, the peptide–receptor complex was quantitatively recovered, initially in the plasma membrane-rich fractions, and within 5–10 min at 37°C was quantitatively translocated to galactosyl transferase-rich, Golgilike fractions. Taken together, these studies imply that the labeled 50- to 60-kd species represents, at least, the binding moiety of the receptor, and that the receptor is the vehicle for ligand internalization.

Some progress has now been made toward isolation of the receptor in an active form. A major obstacle to its isolation is the relative sparseness of the receptor. Starting with 10^9 cells containing 10^5 univalent receptors per cell, one could obtain at most 0.17 nmole receptor (i.e., ~ 10 µg). Goetzl *et al.* (1981) described a partial purification using the nonionic detergent NP-40 to solubilize the receptors from the plasma membrane followed by two purification steps. The first was affinity chromatography on *N*-fMet-Leu-Phe–Sepharose and the second was gel filtration. SDS-PAGE analysis revealed three polypeptides of 94, 68, and 40 kd. The 68-kd species accounted for 74-93% of the total protein and represented about 30% of the theoretical yield. It appeared that a fraction of the isolated receptor remained active in that 0.2–0.3 moles of N-fMet-Leu-Phe bound per mole of receptor with an affinity of $K_d = 10^{-9}$ M.

Niedel (1981) has also reported a solubilization of the receptor binding activity after digitonin treatment of the membrane fractions of human neutrophils. In this procedure 60-70% of the membrane-binding sites were recovered. Using a rapid gel filtration binding assay, Niedel found saturable, high-affinity binding of the hexapeptide to the solubilized receptor. Moreover, the ligand binding showed comparable pH and sulfhydryl reagent sensitivity in both the soluble and membrane-bound cases. When the ligand was crosslinked to the solubilized receptor, the same 55- to 70-kd species was identified by SDS-PAGE. This disparity between the characterization of the receptor based on crosslinking studies compared to the purification procedures has yet to be resolved.

Only preliminary information is available concerning the interaction of the receptor or the ligand–receptor complex with membrane components that could play a role in the generation of the signal for cellular response. While these issues are considered in more detail in Section II, it is worth noting that the receptor appears to be able to interact directly with the guanosine-5'-triphosphate (GTP) binding protein/adenylate cyclase system in a manner parallel to the β-adrenergic receptor. This conclusion is based on ligand binding studies in membrane preparations of neutrophils and macrophages in which the presence of the nonhydrolysable GTP analogue (GPPNHP) reduces the affinity of the N-formyl peptide receptor for its ligand (Koo et al., 1982; Snyderman et al., 1982).

Of considerable importance is the recent observation by Jesaitis et al. (1982b) that the activated ligand–receptor complex interacts with the neutrophil cytoskeleton in a transient fashion. Whether this linkage is a prerequisite for chemotaxis by the neutrophil or merely part of the mechanism by which the receptors are internalized or downregulated is not yet clear.

D. Physiological Roles of the N-Formyl Peptide Receptor

The N-formyl peptide receptor is presumed to be capable of initiating neutrophil responses to bacterial invasion of the host. While the synthetic N-formyl peptides are analogues of natural chemoattractants derived from bacteria, the in vivo function of this system awaits verification. On the basis of the observation that neutrophils respond chemotactically to N-formylated proteins derived from bovine mitochondria, Carp (1982) postulated that mitochondria liberated at sites of tissue damage or necrosis in infection or inflammatory disease could signal the accumulation of inflammatory cells at these sites. Potentially, the receptors could also play a role in phagocytosis of the degenerating mitochondria.

The physiological significance of the interaction of neutrophils with chemo-attractants dwarfs these putative roles however if the interaction is viewed as a model for the study of the role of neutrophils in host defense and inflammation. The physiological role of neutrophils can be grouped into events proximal and distal to the site of injury or infection. Functions involved in the distal events mediate migration of leukocytes toward the sites and involve the entry of the cells into the bloodstream, transport to vessels near the sites, margination or adherence to vessel walls, and migration through the tissues. These events may involve the complement component C3b, which has a neutrophil receptor and induces leukocytosis (Ghebrehiwet and Müller-Eberhard, 1979), prostaglandins that stimulate vascular permeability (Vane, 1976), C5a, leukotrienes, and the *N*-formyl peptides, which mediate margination (O'Flaherty and Ward, 1978; Craddock *et al.*, 1979) and chemotaxis (Chenoweth and Hugli, 1978; Petrone *et al.*, 1980; Niedel and Cuatrecasas, 1980).

Migration through the tissues and endothelium may involve a physical movement accompanied by secretion of granule contents that contain proteases such as elastase and collagenase (Olsson and Venge, 1980) and a basic metal chelating protein, lactoferrin (Ainscough *et al.*, 1980). These granule components could therefore facilitate migration from the bloodstream to the tissues by first mediating adherence to the vascular endothelium (Oseas *et al.*, 1981). After attachment, noninjurious movement through the endothelial tight junctions and extracellular matrix (Cramer and Milks, 1982) might be accomplished by the controlled release of specific granules containing specific collagen and lactoferrin but no non-specific proteases. Release of the contents of both granules to the neutrophil-tissue interface, however, could produce a more severe proteolysis, perhaps leading to tissue and basement membrane damage (Cochrane, 1977).

As the cells approach the origin of chemoattractants, they are probably bombarded by a multiplicity of stimuli in addition to the elevated levels of chemoattractant. These include immune complexes (Cochrane, 1977; Johnson and Ward, 1982) products of complement activation (Müller-Eberhard, 1981), anaphylatoxins such as arachidonate metabolites (Robinson *et al.*, 1982), antibody and complement-coated particles, as well as the invading organisms and damaged tissue. These agents mediate inflammatory activation of neutrophils variously causing them to produce active oxygen species, to secrete contents of granules adhered to, and to phagocytose, digest, and oxidize opsonized particles (Olsson and Venge, 1980). Thus the neutrophil executes a microbicidal role, enhances complement action, and produces toxic oxygen species, and probably participates in a clearing function, removing foreign matter, toxins, and endogenous agents that would tend to amplify the inflammatory response (Jesaitis and Cochrane, 1983). Consequently, not only does the neutrophil serve as a front-line defense against invasion of foreign organisms and tissues, but is poised in a balance between processes both beneficial and injurious to the host.

II. KINETICS OF CELLULAR RESPONSE

A. Temporal Framework

Before embarking on our description of the quantitative relationship between ligand–receptor interaction and the stimulation of cellular response, we will describe the time frame of cellular responses and the likely biochemical mechanisms that contribute to transduce the occupancy of the formyl peptide receptor into signals for cellular response. We shall emphasize the idea that since many of the transducing events and cellular responses overlap in a temporal sense, even a very detailed analysis of the relative timing of all these events may ultimately yield an incomplete scheme for the sequence of steps in cell triggering. We direct the reader to the review by Weissmann *et al.* (1981), in which the events leading to neutrophil secretion stimulated by various secretagogues are discussed, and to the review by Becker *et al.* (1981), in which additional mechanistic details particularly relating to ionic events and arachidonate metabolism are considered. The involvement of methylation reactions among the early events of neutrophil activation by formyl peptides is dealt with in detail in the recent review by Pike and Snyderman (1982*a*).

1. General Notions Concerning Ligand–Receptor Interaction and Cell Activation

There are several known mechanisms by which receptors initiate cellular responses. For example, the acetylcholine receptor is a stimulus-activated ion channel. Both the β-adrenergic receptor and rhodopsin (the visual photoreceptor) activate a diffusible GTP-binding protein that in the former case activates an adenylate cyclase (Limbird, 1981) and in the latter a phosphodiesterase (Stryer *et al.*, 1981). A third general mechanism, exemplified by the mast cell immunoglobulin E (IgE) receptor, requires antigen-mediated receptor crossbridging (Delisi and Siraganian, 1979*a,b*), which appears to lead to a Ca^{2+} influx required in stimulation of the cell (Ishizaka, 1982). While a dimerization event may participate in the activation of cells sensitive to insulin, epidermal growth factor, and nerve growth factor (Schreiber *et al.*, 1983), the subsequent transduction events are not unequivocally identified. It has been suggested, however, that clustered receptors may serve as ion channels (Young *et al.*, 1982) or may, in addition, become crosslinked to cytoskeletal elements (Nicolson and Painter, 1973; Bourguignon and Singer, 1977; Flanagan and Koch, 1978).

In many instances, the occupied receptors appear to undergo an alteration of affinity for the ligand generally taken to reflect a conformational change in the receptor (Corin and Donner, 1982). Such a structural change may permit interaction of the receptor with particular membrane components such as activatable enzymatic species. Alternatively, a conformational change could permit expression of a latent enzymatic activity in the receptor. For example, the EGF receptor appears to be a protein kinase that is autophosphorylated upon activation (Cohen *et al.*, 1980). Unfortunately, changes in affinity of the receptor for ligand do not provide unambiguous evidence of a conformational change. Generally the change in affinity must be distinguished both from internalization and clustering events which may give rise to an altered dissociation rate for the ligand.

Whatever the mechanism of receptor activation, it is presumed that a transducing species and/or second messenger is generated. On the basis of evidence derived from a wide variety of cell types, Ca^{2+} and cyclic adenosine monophosphate (cAMP) have been suggested to act as interacting or "synarchic" messengers (Rasmussen, 1981). However, signals could in principle also involve fluxes of monovalent cations, activation of protein kinases by mechanisms independent of the control of Ca^{2+} or cAMP, and some aspects of lipid metabolism such as arachidonate metabolism, phospholipid methylation, or turnover of phosphatidyl inositol. The identification of these second messengers is the essence of the biochemistry of cell activation; several criteria for their identification have been accepted (Rasmussen, 1981):

1. The intracellular level of a second messenger changes when the cell is stimulated.
2. The cellular responses are inhibited when the signal is blocked.
3. The application of the signaling species from an exogenous source (e.g., dibutyryl cAMP for cAMP) mimics the ligand in inducing the response.
4. A biochemical pathway connecting receptor occupancy to the generation of the signal and ultimately to the generation of the response can be described.

It will become clear in Section II.B that no single species fits all these criteria in the neutrophil, nor is there as yet a thorough scheme that meets the fourth criterion for any of the cellular responses. Nonetheless, it is worthwhile to set forth the most attractive candidates and to place these events within an overall temporal framework for cellular response.

B. Kinetics of Intracellular Biochemical Events

1. Cyclic Nucleotides

In the following discussion we have elected to place particular emphasis on the potential roles of cyclic nucleotides in neutrophil stimulation. The reason for this decision is that the biochemistry controlling the levels of cyclic nucleotides is among the best understood. cAMP bears at least some of the characteristics of a second messenger in the stimulation of neutrophils via the formyl peptide receptor. There is a transient elevation (a doubling or tripling of the basel level), which is half-maximal within 5 sec and which reaches a maximal level 10–20 sec after the cells are exposed to formyl peptides (Simchowitz *et al.*, 1980*a,b*; Smolen and Weissmann, 1981) (Fig. 2). Recovery of the basal cAMP levels requires ~3 min). The kinetics of the responses are only slightly dependent on the stimulus concentration.

In the neutrophil, the cAMP system is likely to be coupled to the formyl peptide receptor in a manner parallel to the coupling of the cAMP system in the β-adrenergic receptor of the turkey hen erythrocyte, i.e., a catalytic unit that is a GTP binding protein appears to be present. When this G protein is

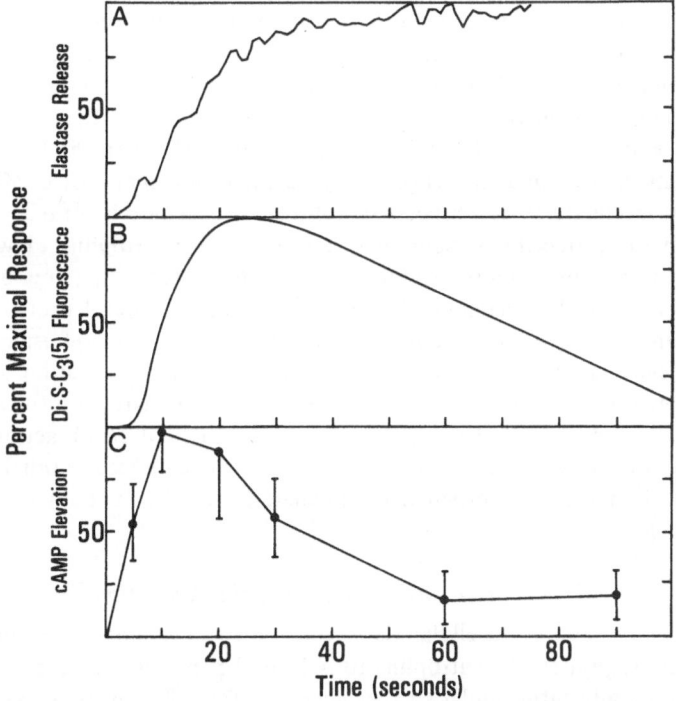

Figure 2. Several early responses of neutrophils to *N*-formyl peptides. The data are plotted as the percentage maximal response *vs.* time (in seconds). The responses are (A) elastase release; (B) the fluorescence response of the membrane potential-sensitive dye Di-S-C$_3$-(5); (C) the transient elevation of intracellular cyclic adenosine monophosphate (cAMP). The responses were to 10 n*M* *N*-formyl-Nle-Leu-Phe-Nle-Tyr-Lys-FL at 37°C. Details for (A) are given in Sklar *et al.* (1982*a*); details for (B) are given in Sklar *et al.* (1981*a*). cAMP levels were measured essentially as described in Smolen and Weissmann (1981) and Simchowitz *et al.* (1980*a*).

occupied by the nonhydrolyzable GTP analogue (GPPNHP) and is bound to the receptor, the affinity of the receptor for the ligand is reduced. Koo *et al.* (1982) reported that GPPNHP reduced the affinity of the formyl peptide receptor for formyl peptides in a neutrophil membrane preparation by increasing the dissociation rate. Furthermore, their results are consistent with the notion that the interaction of a G protein with the formyl peptide receptor is responsible for the apparent heterogeneity of ligand–receptor binding in some neutrophil plasma membrane preparations.

The picture of cAMP as a second messenger is complicated by the fact that dibutyryl cAMP, an exogenous precursor for cAMP, does not mimic the action of the ligand. Furthermore, phosphodiesterase inhibitors, which elevate intracellular cAMP, alter the kinetics of cellular response to ligand (Simchowitz *et al.*, 1980*a*). While the overall responses are amplified in the presence of elevated cAMP levels, the latency periods for the initiation of the responses are elongated. In contrast, while cGMP levels are apparently unaffected by ligand, the elevation of intracellular cGMP (derived from dibutyryl cGMP) modulates the orientational response of neutrophils (Stephens and Snyderman, 1982).

These studies suggest that neither cAMP nor cGMP alone fully meets the requirement as a second messenger. However, it is apparent that cAMP in particular can modulate several aspects of cell response. There is little direct information on the intracellular locus of cAMP action in neutrophils. However, on the basis of the precedents established in other systems, it is reasonable to postulate the cAMP-dependent phosphorylation of neutrophil proteins whose activities are related to their extent of phosphorylation. If these phosphorylation reactions cause activation in some enzyme systems and inactivation of others, one can envision that intracellular cAMP levels can modulate both the initiation and the sensitivity of cellular responses. Since the sites of cAMP action and its mechanism of production and catabolism are well characterized in other systems, we believe that dramatic progress in elucidating its roles in the neutrophil are forthcoming.

2. The Role of Ca^{2+} in Neutrophil Activation

Intracellular and extracellular Ca^{2+} contribute to the time course and magnitude of the responses of neutrophils to *N*-formyl peptides. However, it appears that whereas only intracellular Ca^{2+} is necessary for cell activation, extracellular Ca^{2+} modulates the level of the responses (Smolen *et al.*, 1981; see also reviews by Becker *et al.*, 1981; Weissmann *et al.*, 1981). A stimulated transmembrane influx of ^{45}Ca appears to be largely complete within 30–60 sec following exposure of the cells to peptide (Naccache *et al.*, 1977*a*). An intracellular dislocation, detected by the Ca^{2+}-sensitive chelator chlortetracycline (CTC), is initiated within 5 sec and also appears to be maximal within 30–60 sec (Naccache *et al.*, 1979). Since CTC is membrane permeable and only weakly discriminates between Ca^{2+} or Mg^{2+}, a detailed analysis of intracellular Ca^{2+} concentration or the kinetics of its elevation and depletion is not yet complete. A more detailed analysis, using the new Ca^{2+}-sensitive probes Quin 2AM described by Tsien *et al.* (1982) should be forthcoming.

The mechanism by which receptor occupancy leads to Ca^{2+} fluxes and dislocation has not been defined. In fact, general mechanisms based on precedents derived from other receptor systems have not yet been established. The Ca^{2+} influx has been speculatively related to specific ion channels, the turnover of phosphatidyl inositol, and arachidonic acid metabolism. Moreover, intracellular regulation could depend on calmodulin, as suggested by the fact that inhibitors of calmodulin inhibit neutrophil responses, or on the release of compartmentalized Ca^{2+}, which would require yet a different signal connecting the receptor to that compartment.

Even in the face of these uncertainties about mechanism, Ca^{2+} remains a viable candidate as a second messenger because intracellular Ca^{2+} chelators block cellular responses (criterion 2) (Smolen *et al.*, 1981) and Ca^{2+} ionophore mimics the ligand (criterion 3) (see Becker *et al.*, 1981).

3. Other Candidates as Transducing Events

A number of other events, which appear to contribute to signal transduction in other receptor systems, occur on a time scale consistent with their participation in neutrophil triggering. As is the case with Ca^{2+}, mechanisms by which the binding of the *N*-formyl peptide to its receptor lead to these events are not yet understood, so that a detailed discussion of their importance is not in order. For details concerning the roles of monovalent cations, anions, the arachidonic acid cascade, and transmethylation, consult the reviews of Weissmann *et al.* (1981), Becker *et al.* (1981), and Pike and Snyderman (1982*a,b*).

It is worthwhile to note that the fluxes of monovalent ions, as measured directly (Naccache *et al.*, 1977*a,b*), with the lipophilic cation TPMP$^+$ (Korchak and Weissmann, 1980; Seligmann and Gallin, 1980) or by fluorescent membrane-potential sensitive dyes, are very rapid. For example, the fluorescent responses of the dye di-S-C$_3$-(5) is initiated within 5 sec of exposure to the peptides (Fig. 2). The maximal response occurs after $\sim$30 sec, and the kinetics of the dye responses are weakly dependent on the stimulus concentration (Sklar *et al.*, 1981*a*). However, it seems apparent that these monovalent cations are not second messengers, since ion fluxes initiated with the ionophores monensin and valinomycin do not lead to cell activation.

C. Kinetics of Cell Response

1. Generation of Free Radicals of Oxygen

In response to *N*-formyl peptides, neutrophils in suspension generate free radicals of oxygen, predominantly superoxide anion, O_2^-. O_2^- is detected within $\sim$10 sec after the cells are exposed to *N*-formyl peptides and the generation continues for 2-3 min at 37°C. In cytochalasin B-treated cells, the onset may be delayed 5-10 sec. The latency period is only weakly dependent on the concentration of the ligand (Smolen *et al.*, 1980; Sklar *et al.*, 1981a).

The biochemistry of the system has been investigated (Badwey and Karnovsky, 1979). The system is sensitive to calmodulin and to drugs that inhibit calmodulin (Jones *et al.*, 1982). Moreover, the activity of the system is modulated in whole cells when the cAMP levels are altered (Simchowitz *et al.*, 1980a). A sequence relating occupancy of the *N*-formyl peptide receptors to the subsequent activation of the NADPH oxidase has not been formulated. The stimulation appears to be a localized phenomenon in that superoxide is generated at sites proximal to the binding of particulate stimuli (Ohno *et al.*, 1982a). Considerable effort has gone into the analysis of the production and significance of several oxygen radicals, reviewed elsewhere (De Chatelet, 1978).

2. Secretion of Proteases

Neutrophils can secrete a significant fraction (>10%-20%) of their granule contents in response to *N*-formyl peptides or other monovalent ligands only after the cells have been treated with cytochalasin B (1-5 μg/ml). While cytochalasin B is known to inhibit the elongation of actin filaments (Brenner and Korn, 1979; Lin *et al.*, 1980; Brown and Spudich, 1981), neither the mechanism of its action nor its relationship to physiological degranulation is clear.

In order to define the kinetics of secretion in neutrophils stimulated by *N*-formyl peptides or other secretagogues, four general protocols are now available. A centrifugation assay involves stimulating a cell suspension, separating cells and supernatant by a rapid centrifugation step, and assaying the supernatant for activity. In such a system, β-glucuronidase, lysozyme, and lactoferrin are all detected in the supernatants of cells stimulated by formyl peptides with a latency of ~5 sec (Smolen *et al.*, 1980; Brentwood and Henson, 1980). Secretion was complete within 30-60 sec at 37°C. Similar results have been observed with C5a and platelet activating factor (Smolen *et al.*, 1980; Shaw *et al.*, 1981).

Two spectroscopic procedures have recently been described. We have used a fluorogenic substrate that is specific for elastase, MeO-Succ-Ala-Ala-Pro-Val-MCA, to examine elastase release (Sklar *et al.*, 1982a). Elastase, a component of azurophilic granules, is released with kinetics similar to those above: after a latency period of ~5 sec or less, elastase secretion is essentially complete within 30 sec. The kinetics of release were found to be nearly independent of the concentration of *N*-formyl peptide. Smolen *et al.* (1982) have also examined the fluorescence intensity neutrophils labeled with acridine orange, a histochemical marker for granules. They detected fluorescence increases in stimulated cell suspensions over a similar time frame consistent with and attributed to the release of the granules and the subsequent relief of the fluorophore self-quenching.

In contrast, these latter workers reported latencies of ~30 sec for the release of lysozyme and lactoferrin from neutrophils stimulated by *N*-formyl peptides using a flow dialysis assay system (Smolen *et al.*, 1980). In this assay, the latency period was described as the lag time between the detection of inulin in the effluent (added to the cell suspension at the time of stimulation) compared with the detection of the secreted component of interest.

3. Rapid Cytoskeletal and Morphological Responses

Rapid changes in the organization of the neutrophil cytoskeleton occur after stimulation by formyl peptides. White *et al.* (1982) have shown an increase in actin recovered in a Triton-insoluble cytoskeletal pellet that appears to represent a *de novo* polymerization of G-actin monomers to F-actin filaments (Rao and Varani, 1982). A kinetic analysis showed that the decrease in G actin from 60% to 30% was completed within 10–15 sec—the earliest time tested. The polymerization was blocked by cytochalasin D, which acts *in vitro* by binding to the barbed end of the growing filament (Brenner and Korn, 1979; Lin *et al.*, 1980; Brown and Spudich, 1981). The peptides also induce an increase in microtubule numbers (Goldstein *et al.*, 1973; Hoffstein *et al.*, 1977) and average length (Anderson *et al.*, 1982). These reactions appear to correlate with the tyrosinylation of tubulin (Nath *et al.*, 1982).

N-formyl peptide also induces interactions between its receptor and the cell cytoskeleton. By 5 sec at 37°C, ligand becomes associated with the Triton cytoskeleton (Jesaitis *et al.*, 1984). Incorporation of radioactive ligand into the actin-rich pellet increases with time reaching a maximum, steady-state level of ~7500 molecules per cell equivalent by 5–6 min and was inhibited by dehydrocytochalasin B. Pulse-chase studies suggested that the observed association with the cytoskeleton was transient, decaying with a half-life of 50 sec. The association was absent at 4°C. Interestingly, at 15°C, where internalization of peptide is essentially blocked (see Section III.C), the association of the ligand with the cytoskeleton exactly paralleled in a quantitative way, the amount bound to the cell surface before Triton lysis. This result implies that cytoskeleton–receptor interactions occur at the surface membrane before internalization and dissociate shortly after endocytosis.

Such interactions can be demonstrated in plasma membrane fractions isolated from peptide-treated neutrophils (Jesaitis *et al.*, 1983). We have shown that when membranes were isolated from cells stimulated at 37°C with ligand, the ligand was resistant to solubilization with Triton X100. When a Triton lysate of such membranes was chromatographed on Sepharose 4B column, the tightly bound ligand eluted in the void volume. Free peptide was found in the salt volume as expected. In view of recent reports showing the presence of a submembranous cytoskeleton in isolated plasma membranes (Mescher *et al.*, 1981; Luna *et al.*, 1981) this result suggests that the receptor–ligand complex may be associated with the underlying membrane cytoskeleton. This putative interaction appears to be induced by formyl peptide binding at 37°C, since the complex of the receptor at 4°C with a photoaffinity peptide is a relatively low-molecular-weight species (Stokes radius <50 Å) (Painter *et al.*, 1982).

In a manner that is not yet clear, these cytoskeletal events may be connected to morphological changes in the cell. For example, pseudopods and blebs are extended within 5-10 sec after the stimulus is presented, either in the form of a gradient (Zigmond and Sullivan, 1979), in the bulk phase solution, or from a micropipette positioned near the cell (Gerish and Keller, 1981). If the stimulus is retained for more than 60 sec, the cells adopt a polarized or oriented morphology that is relatively refractory to stimulation from a new direction (Section IV.D).

D. Summary of Kinetics

Within 5 sec, cells exposed to formyl peptides begin to respond in a variety of ways. Intracellular levels of cAMP, Ca^{2+}, and Na^+ are all elevated. Reorganization occurs in the cytoskeleton, and degranulation begins in cytochalasin B-treated cells. O_2^- is detected within 10 sec. By 20 sec, cAMP has achieved its maximal levels. Within 1 min, Ca^{2+} and Na^+ are approaching or have attained their maximal levels and degranulation is nearly complete. While O_2^- generation will continue for several minutes, its rate of production at this time is optimal. Beyond 30-60 sec, the cAMP level begins to fall back to its basal level and the intracellular Ca^{2+} concentration and the permeability of the plasma membrane to Ca^{2+} and Na^+ fall to their basal level.

The kinetics of most of these responses (except O_2^-) are weakly dependent of the concentration of the ligand to which the cells had been initially exposed. All these observations suggest that the binding of the *N*-formyl peptide, which contribute to the initiation of the responses (<5 sec) and the maximal responses (<30 sec) of everything but O_2^- production, must be rather rapid and must occur before binding equilibrium is established. In Section III we consider the data available concerning ligand–receptor interactions, as well as new techniques that make possible the analysis of ligand–receptor interaction on a time scale consistent with the initiation of the cell responses.

III. LIGAND–RECEPTOR INTERACTIONS AND CELLULAR RESPONSE

A. Which Parameters of Ligand–Receptor Interaction Are Relevant to Cellular Response?

It is a common notion that in the activation of cells by specific ligands—be they *N*-formyl peptides, hormones, or drugs—there is a correlation between ED_{50}, K_d, and the equilibrium occupancy of the receptors by the ligand. In the neutrophil, it is now clearly documented that the activity of a series of peptides in evoking cellular responses (e.g., chemotaxis, secretion) is strongly correlated with the affinity of the ligand for the receptor (as measured in competitive binding assays with either N-formyl-Nle-Leu-[^{3}H]-Phe-OH or N-formyl-Nle-Leu-Phe-Nle-[^{125}I]-Tyr-Lys) (Showell et $al.$, 1976; Freer et $al.$, 1980, 1982). Freer et $al.$ (1982) noticed, however, that the peptides of highest activity ($ED_{50} < 10^{-10}$ M) that were modified in the Phe-OH group bind less avidly than predicted by their biological activity. These observations suggest the involvement of additional, perhaps structural, factors that contribute to the efficacy of the various ligands.

We suggested above that many cellular responses were maximally elicited within 30–60 sec after exposure of cells to a dose of stimulatory peptide. While there is only sketchy published information concerning ligand-binding kinetics under stimulatory conditions, these short periods required for evoking cellular responses would seem to preclude, a $priori$, the possibility that cell responses were governed entirely by receptor occupancy, hence the K_d of the ligand alone. In the following discussion, we show that the cell responses depend on the dynamics of ligand–receptor interaction, particularly the on and off rate constants for binding, and the number of receptors occupied as a function of time.

In order to understand the quantitative relationship between the time course of receptor occupancy and the time course of cellular response we described a format of pulse stimulation (Sklar et $al.$, 1981b). Cell suspensions were placed in a sample chamber (in our case, a stirred cuvette) in which responses to a stimulatory ligand could be monitored. The stimulation process could be interrupted at any time after the initial exposure of cells to ligand by the addition of an agent that blocked the binding of the ligand to the receptor.

We found particularly useful in this regard a pulse protocol in which the stimulus was the fluoresceinated (FL) hexapeptide N-fNle-Leu-Phe-Nle-Tyr-Lys-FL and the blocker was a high-affinity antibody to fluorescein. Under optimal conditions, the antibody binds the haptenated ligand in solution with a half-time of <1 sec ($k_{on} \sim 10^{10}$ M^{-1} min^{-1}), but does not bind receptor-associated ligand. Since the complex of the peptide and the antibody is itself nonstimulatory to the cell, the antibody addition has the effect of limiting receptor occupancy to that which occurred only during the period before its addition. The extent of receptor occupancy in such a pulse is a function of the concentration of the ligand and the period of uninterrupted binding (Fig. 3).

We have now measured four cellular responses under such pulse conditions: elastase release (Fig. 4), cAMP elevation, carbocyanine dye response ("membrane depolarization"), and O_2^- production (Sklar et $al.$, 1983c). For near-optimal concealtrations of stimulus, the three former responses all required binding that occurred within a few seconds of exposure of the cells to ligand. Shorter periods of binding were needed for higher (saturating) stimulus doses. In contract, the O_2^- production generally required periods of binding >1 min.

A comparable procedure using N-formyl peptide and competitive antagonists

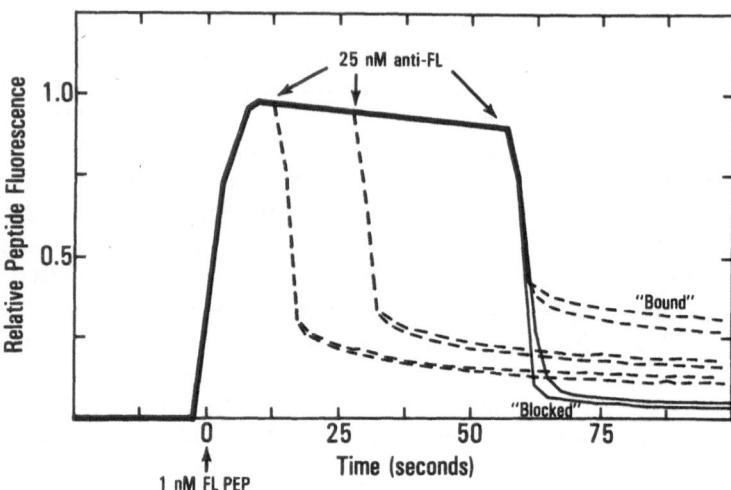

Figure 3. Pulse stimulation of neutrophils and spectrofluorimetric assay of ligand binding. The data are plotted as the fluorescence intensity of the peptide, N-formyl-Nle-Leu-Phe-Nle-Tyr-Lys-FL (FLPEP) versus time. The cell suspensions contained 10^7 neutrophils/ml and were thermostatted to $37°C$ in a stirred cuvette. Fluorescence conditions are provided in Sklar *et al.* (1983*b*). However, in these experiments, the fluorescence signal was averaged for 2.5 sec giving rise to the boxey appearance of the curves (see Fig. 7). The pulse consists of the administration of 1 nM FLPEP at time 0, followed at the times indicated by the arrows by 25 nM anti-FL IgG. In the blocked curves (solid lines throughout), the binding of the FLPEP to the cell receptor was blocked by 1 μM nonfluorescent hexapeptide. The number of receptors occupied in a pulse is related to the level of residual fluorescence at the times of antibody addition. The decay of the residual fluorescence after antibody addition reflects, in part, dissociation of FLPEP from the cells (see Fig. 5).

rather than the antibody is also possible. The inhibitors work by blocking the binding of the ligand to the receptor rather than by complexing the ligand in solution as does the antibody. In order to be effective, inhibitor concentrations (10^{-5} M cbz-Phe-Met and 10^{-6} M *t*boc-Phe-Leu-Phe-Leu-Phe) were based on their ability to stop cell responses as *rapidly and effectively* as the antibody (Sklar *et al.*, 1981*b*). (For reasons discussed in Section III.D, we presume that the concentration of antagonist and its on rate constant, were such that the available receptors were equilibrated with inhibitor in about a second or so, a time comparable to the action of antibody in solution.)

Using this inhibitor pulse procedure, Radin *et al.* (1982) verified the conclusion that secretion was an early response, while O_2^- generation was a late response. In addition, they suggested further that Ca^{2+} influx depended on early ligand binding, while cell aggregation depended on the entire time course of ligand binding. A complete understanding of these pulse experiments hinges on both an analysis of the number or receptors occupied in such a pulse, and moreover, the time frame of ligand dissociation from the receptor that occurs

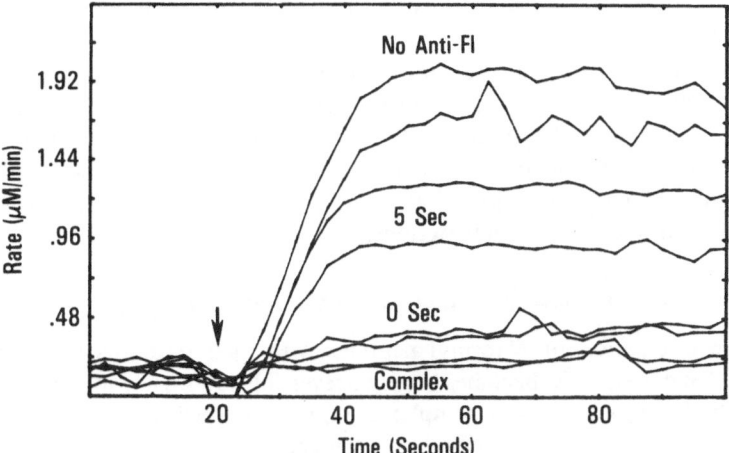

Figure 4. Release of elastase at 37°C from neutrophils after pulse stimulation. The data are plotted as the rate of cleavage of the substrate MeO-Succ-Ala-Ala-Pro-Val-MCA versus time. The cells were stimulated with 1.25 nM N-formyl-Nle-Leu-Phe-Nle-Tyr-Lys-FL at the time indicated by the arrow (20 sec). Duplicate curves are shown. The antibody (25 nM anti-FL) was either preadded to the stimulus (complex), present at the time of stimulation (0 sec), was added 5 sec after stimulation, or was not added at all. Since the rate of substrate cleavage is proportional to the amount of elastase present, the time courses indicate that secretion is completed within 30 sec after stimulation, and that 5 sec of binding for a near-optimal stimulus concentration leads to ≃50% release. Experiments were performed in its presence of 1 μg/ml cytochalasin B. (Reprinted with permission from Sklar *et al.*, 1982a, *J. Biol. Chem.* **257**:5471–5475, Fig. 3a.)

after by the administration of the blocking agent. It is instructive to consider that the half-time for ligand dissociation (before internalization) in cells at 37°C ($t_{1/2\,off} > 1$ min) is long compared with the half-time for the shut off of the O_2^--generating system ($t_{1/2} \sim 12$ sec) once the blocker has been added. Moreover, parallel studies of binding and O_2^- production under pulse conditions (Section III.C) suggest that it is the *de novo* occupancy of additional receptors rather than the continuous occupancy of individual receptors that contributes to the time course of response.

Not only is the time frame of occupancy important, but when the stimulus is infused slowly into cell suspensions, the rate of receptor occupancy also plays a deciding role in cellular response (Sklar *et al.*, 1981a). An additional factor that may distinguish the stimulatory and inhibitory ligands is their residence time at the receptor. Taken together, all these observations point to our need to consider not only the equilibrium parameters of ligand–receptor interaction (K_d and the number of sites), but also to analyze and distinguish the kinetic parameters relating to the on and off rate constants for the ligands and the rate of down regulation of the receptors.

B. Dynamics of Ligand–Receptor Interaction

The dynamics of the interactions formyl peptides with their receptors on neutrophils have been considered in the reviews of Becker (1979), Becker *et al.* (1981), and Pike and Snyderman (1982*a*). In the following discussion, we briefly review the conclusions of those earlier studies, placing particular emphasis on the results of new techniques that permit a detailed and highly time-resolved analysis of ligand–receptor interactions.

1. Overview Based on Studies with Radioligands

The association of *N*-formyl peptides with their receptors on neutrophils at 37°C and even 24°C becomes largely irreversible after a few minutes primarily because the ligand–receptor complex is rapidly internalized and potentially because changes in receptor affinity may occur even while the ligand–receptor complex is present on the cell surface (Zigmond and Sullivan, 1979; Zigmond, 1981; Zigmond *et al.*, 1982; Niedel *et al.*, 1979*a,b*; Vitkauskas *et al.*, 1980; Jesaitis *et al.*, 1984; Sklar *et al.*, 1983*b*). Becker *et al.* (1981) have differentiated these processes as receptor modulation and downregulation, respectively. The interaction of the peptides with viable cells is further complicated because the receptor number varies due to the expression of cryptic receptors, the clearance of occupied receptors, the apparent recycling of internalized receptors, and because of the alterations in the topography of distribution of receptors on the membrane surface (see Section IV). Finally, the quantitation of free and bound radiolabel and its relationship to occupied receptors is confounded by the intracellular processing and degradation of the ligand leading to the release of peptide fragments as well as intact peptide (Niedel *et al.*, 1979*a*).

For these and other reasons, the most extensive characterization of the interaction of *N*-formyl peptides and their receptors has been performed at 4°C in cells or on membrane preparations. In detailed kinetic studies, Sullivan and Zigmond (1980) have defined the rate constants for association ($2 \times 10^7 \, M^{-1}$ min^{-1}) and dissociation ($0.4 \, min^{-1}$) of the ligand *N*-f Nle-Leu-[^{3}H]-Phe-OH. From a practical point of view, these rates mean that the half-time for binding for a ligand concentration near K_d ($2 \times 10^{-8} \, M$) is ~1 min. They observed that the ratio of the rate constants k_{off}/k_{on} is consistent with the value of the dissociation constant obtained directly from equilibrium binding studies. While different rate constants have been obtained by Dougherty *et al.* (1983) in human peripheral neutrophils compared with DMSO-differentiated HL-60 cells, the ratio of the rate constants is the same in both cases. Whereas both Zigmond and Freer (1983) fit their kinetic data as single exponential functions, Koo *et al.* (1982) and Mackin *et al.* (1982) suggested that in isolated membranes (from human neutrophils) and cells (rabbit peritoneal neutrophils), respectively, the steady-state binding data are more adequately fit by a heterogeneous population of receptors. The membrane binding data are consistent with the idea that the heterogeneity arises from the interaction of the receptor with a GTP-binding protein. Although it has been noted that formyl-peptide binding to membranes is reversible, with $t_{1/2 \; off}$ ~15 sec at either 4°C or 37°C (Vitkauskas et al., 1980), in cells the dissociation appears to be either nonexponential, i.e., not characterized by a single-rate constant, or not completely reversible, or both, even at 4°C.

At elevated temperatures (25°C and 37°C), internalization of the ligand and receptor plays a rapid and major role in the alteration of the receptor number and the dissociability and uptake of the ligand (Zigmond et al., 1982). Niedel et al. (1979b) demonstrated, by video intensification fluorescence microscopy, the onset of internalization of the rhodaminated hexapeptide within 2 min of the exposure of the cells to the ligand at 37°C. Using spectroscopic methods, we have identified a latency period of 30–45 sec for ligand internalization at 37°C (Sklar et al., 1982b; Finney and Sklar, 1983). The quantitative details of both long-term and short-term aspects of the internalization process are discussed in Section IV.C.

From these studies, one central notion emerges. Ligand binding, ligand dissociation, ligand–receptor processing, and cellular response occur in overlapping time domains. Clearly, in order to understand the contribution of the dynamics of ligand–receptor interaction to cellular responses over a time period of a few seconds to a few minutes, it is necessary to resolve and distinguish the impact of the various processes. In order to resolve these overlapping processes, the assays of ligand–receptor interaction must possess an adequate time resolution. We note that the time resolution of any radiolabel binding method is dependent on the time required for the step in which free ligand and receptor-bound ligand are separated. Any binding process occurring on a time scale similar to the separation step is likely to be obscured. Clearly, a homogeneous assay system requiring no separation step or a very rapid separation step would be advantageous. Second, in order to correlate binding and response, it would be preferable to have experimental conditions in which the desired cell response and the binding parameters could be examined at least in parallel, if not simultaneously. We describe in Section III.B.2 the development of two independent techniques that permit real-time, and in some cases, continuous analyses of ligand–receptor association, dissociation, and internalization. The methods permit parallel analyses of cell function under essentially identical experimental conditions.

2. Fluorimetric Assays of Ligand–Receptor Dynamics

We described the basis of a spectrofluorometric assay of ligand binding, which exactly parallels the protocol for the pulse stimulation of neutrophils (Sklar et al., 1981b, 1982b). A high-affinity antibody to fluorescein is used to discriminate between free ligand and receptor-bound ligand in a homogeneous assay system (Fig. 3). The antibody specifically, efficiently (>96%), and rapidly

($t_{1/2} < 1$ sec) quenches the fluorescence of the free fluoresceinated hexapeptide in solution, while the receptor–bound ligand is inaccessible to quenching by the antibody (Sklar and Finney, 1982). Temporal resolution is built into the binding assay because the interaction between the hapten (the fluoresceinated hexapeptide) and the antibody (to fluorescein) is rapid and because the fluorescence signals can be examined continuously and in real time. The temporal resolution of this system when applied to ligand dissociation is illustrated in Figure 5.

A separate fluorescence flow cytometry assay that we have described (Sklar and Finney, 1982) has been used independently by others (J. Niedel, personal communication; Seligmann *et al.*, 1982*a*) as well. The discrimination between free and receptor–bound ligand arises because the free ligand (<10 nM) is relatively dilute in the medium surrounding cells, while the concentration of the receptor (and thus the receptor–bound ligand) can be >100 nM in the volume containing the cell being analyzed. The application of this technique to an analysis of steady-state ligand binding and the number of sites are illustrated in Figure 6. Since the discrimination between free and bound ligand is built into the instrumental sampling procedure (i.e., analyses are triggered by the presence of a cell in the flow stream) this assay is intrinsically homogeneous and requires no separation step. Good temporal resolution is also intrinsic to the system be-

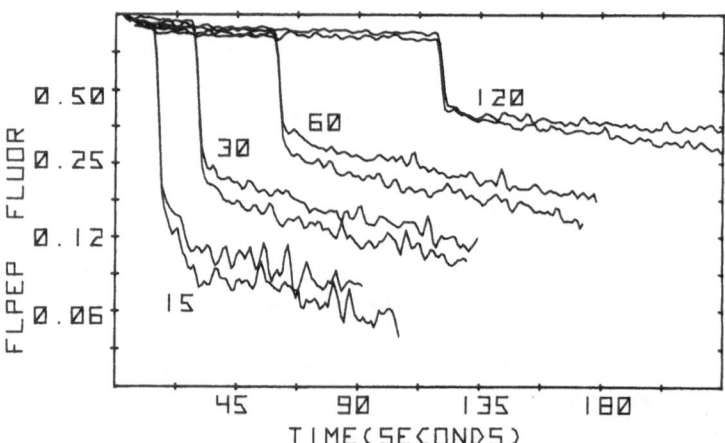

Figure 5. The dissociation of FLPEP *vs.* time after addition of antibody. The data are plotted as the fluorescence of FLPEP on a logarithmic scale versus time (in seconds). In these experiments cells (10^7/ml, 37°C) were exposed to 1 nM FLPEP at time 0. Antibody to fluorescein was added after 15, 30, 60, or 120 sec. The fluorescence data were acquired at 1-sec intervals. Duplicate determinations are shown. The decreasing fluorescence after antibody addition reflects the time dependence of dissocation. Two features are prominent. At early times (15 sec), there appears to be a fast and a slower component ($k_{off} \simeq 0.4$/min) of dissocation. The proportion of the slower component appears to increase in the 30- and 60-sec curves. In the 120-sec curves, the k_{off}^{app} is ~0.2/min because a substantial fraction of the ligand is already internalized (see Figs. 8, 9, and 10).

cause the analysis can be either continuous or periodic (with analyses at the desired time intervals), depending on the particular cytometric instrument and its computer system. A single sample can be repetitively analyzed over the entire course of ligand association and dissociation. The temporal resolution of the binding analysis is illustrated in Figure 7.

Methods for examining ligand internalization in conjunction with these fluorimetric methods, and with comparable temporal resolution, have also been described (Sklar *et al.*, 1982*b*; Finney and Sklar, 1983). The method is based on the well-known sensitivity of the fluorescence intensity of fluorescein (when excited at ~490 nm) to the pH of the environment. Lowering the pH to 4.0 has the effect of reducing the fluorescence intensity of fluorescein to less than 1% of its value at pH 7.4. A rapid alteration in the pH of a cell suspension and the observation of fluorescence intensity after that event permit a discrimination between intracellular and extracellular fluorescent ligand. In this case, the discrimination is based on differential rates of fluorescence quenching. While the extracellular ligand is quenched instantaneously, intracellular ligand protected from the medium is quenched much more slowly. The application of cytometric and fluorimetric techniques to the kinetics of ligand internalization are shown in Figures 8 and 9, respectively. A comparison of the features of the radioligand, fluorometric, and cytometric assays is provided in Table I.

3. Results of Spectroscopic Analyses of Ligand–Receptor Interaction

The number of binding sites available at 4° or 15°C, at equilibrium, as determined by the fluorimetric or cytometric procedures, is typically ~50,000 for neutrophils from normal human donors (Sklar and Finney, 1982; Sklar *et al.*, 1983*b* (Fig. 6). The binding kinetics at 4°C are characterized by an association rate constant ~4 × 10^8 M^{-1} min^{-1} for the fluoresceinated hexapeptide (Sklar and Finney, 1982; Sklar *et al.*, 1983*c*). While the number of immediately available receptors is somewhat larger at 37°C, the initial binding kinetics do not permit an unambiguous resolution of whether receptors are rapidly incorporated into the plasma membrane from a cryptic pool. For saturating concentrations of fluoresceinated ligand (>3 nM), an apparent binding plateau is obtained within 3 min (Fig. 7). If only the data of the earliest times are analyzed, k_{on} at 37°C is ~10^9 M^{-1} min^{-1}. For a ligand concentration (0.3 nM) that gives rise to approximately half-maximal cell responses, ~20% of the receptors are occupied in the first minute of binding.

The average off rate constant is ~0.5/min at 4°, 15°, or 25°C. At 37°C an apparent constant of similar magnitude is obtained (Fig. 5), but the dissociation at 37°C is obscured by the fact that internalization begins within the first minute and by 3 min ~60% of the receptor-bound ligand is internalized (Sklar *et al.*, 1983*b*; Finney and Sklar, 1983 (Fig. 10). Ligand dissociation is further complicated by the fact that the extent of dissociability appears to be both time and

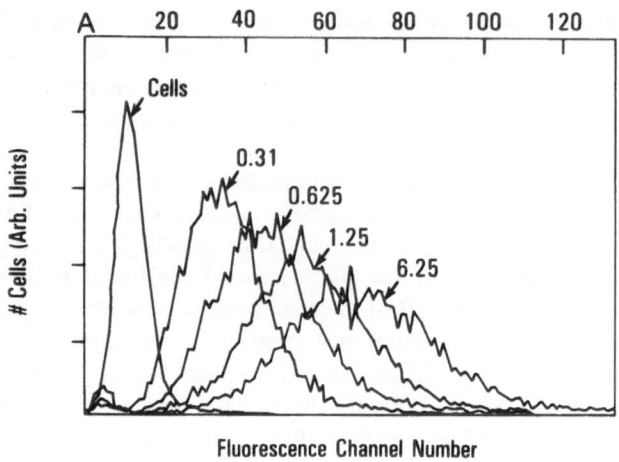

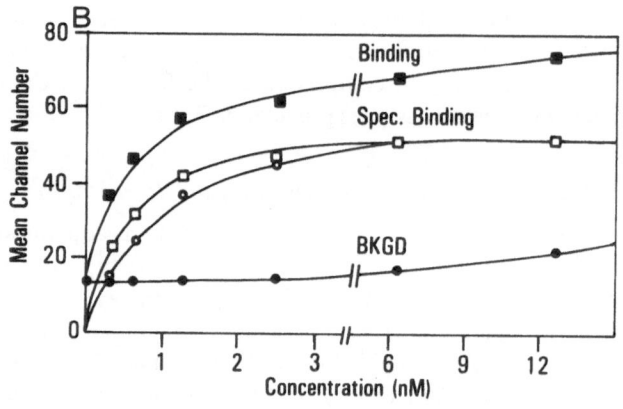

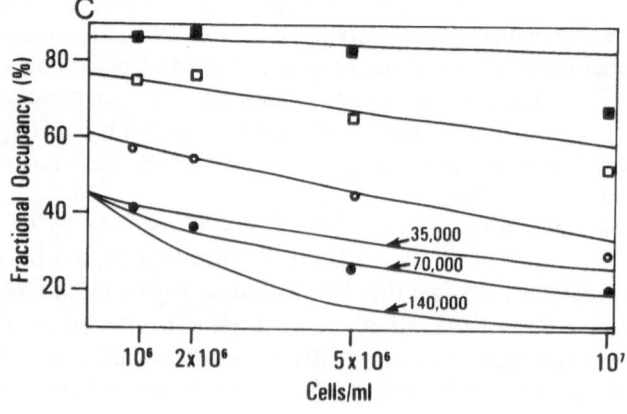

temperature dependent and because the resolution between intracellular *vs.* extracellular but irreversibly bound ligand has been difficult until now. For example, we have observed that ligand equilibrated with cells for more than 1 hr at 15°C is largely nondissociable or very slowly dissociable, but at the same time, this ligand appears to be extracellular, based on the criterion of its accessibility to quenching by a rapid alteration in pH (Sklar *et al.*, 1983*c*). Under similar conditions, but at 4°C, ligand is largely dissociable and extracellular (Sklar and Finney, 1982; Finney and Sklar, 1983). Since the dissociation process appears to be heterogeneous and time dependent, detailed analyses have not yet been completed. However, there is a possibility that there is a conversion of ligand affinity that occurs within seconds at 37°C, which is prior to ligand internalization, and which may reflect the linkage of the occupied receptor either with effector elements in the pathway of cell stimulation (Koo *et al.*, 1982) or with the cytoskeleton (Jesaitis *et al.*, 1984).

We have also obtained information concerning the temperature dependence of the kinetics of ligand internalization. Receptor-mediated ligand internalization appears to be considerably more temperature dependent than binding (Sklar *et al.*, 1983*c*). The rate at 25°C is one-half or one-third as fast at 37°C and is perhaps one-tenth as fast at 15°C. The latency period is at least several minutes at 25°C.

C. Quantitative Relationship Between Receptor Occupancy and Cellular Response

1. Pulse Stimulation

Several alternative approaches have been used to estimate the number of receptors that contribute to cellular response. If responses were governed by equilibrium receptor occupancy it would be reasonable to correlate dose–response curves with the equilibrium values of receptor occupancy. Given the fact that

←——

Figure 6. Equilibrium association of the FLPEP with neutrophils at 15°C as monitored in the fluorescence activated cell sorter. (A) Profiles of cellular fluorescence (number of cells/ channel) are shown for cells (10^6/ml) equilibrated with the indicated concentration (nM) of FLPEP. (B) Binding curves have been generated from plots of the mean fluorescence channel number (obtained as in A) versus the concentration of N-formyl-Nle-Leu-Phe-Nle-Tyr-Lys-FL (FLPEP). The specific binding (□, 10^6/ml; 5.0 × 10^6/ml) is obtained by subtracting the background (●) from the total cellular fluorescence (■, from A). The values of the background are obtained in the presence of 1 μM nonfluorescent peptide. (C) Fractional receptor occupancy as a function of the cell density and the ligand concentration. The symbols represent different concentrations of fluorescent peptide (■, 2.5 nM; □, 1.25 nM; ○, 0.625 nM; ●, 0.31 nM). The solid lines, except where noted, are the calculated values for 70,000 receptors/cell. (Additional details are provided in Sklar and Finney, 1982, *Cytometry* 3: 161–165, Fig. 1. Reprinted with permission.)

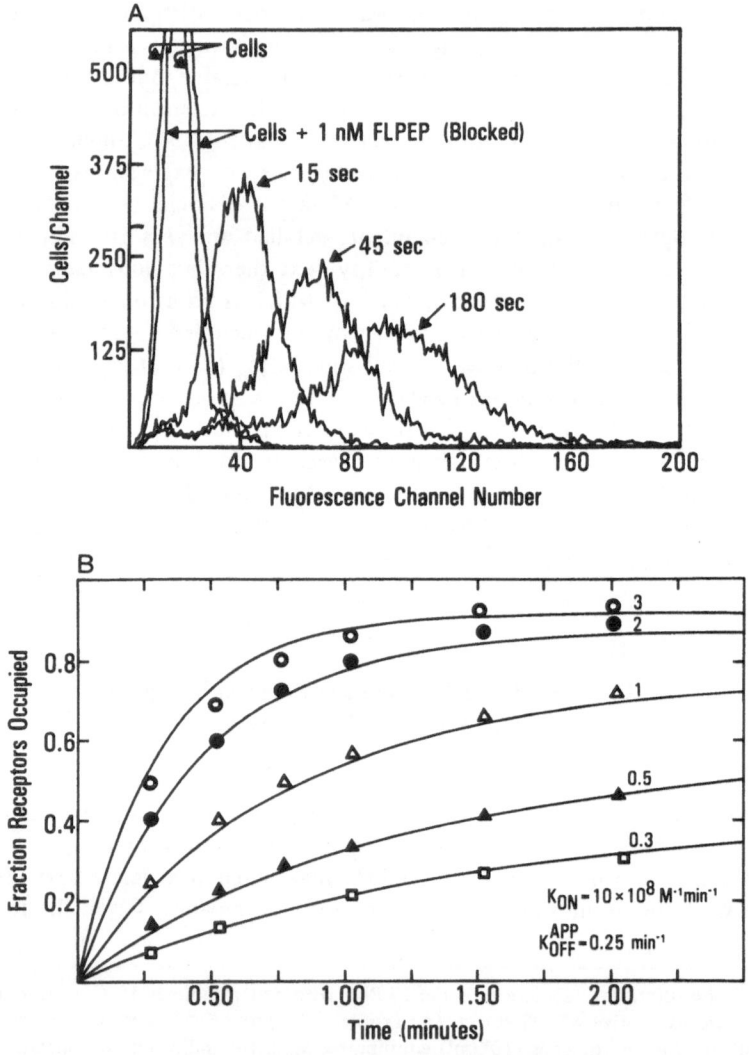

Figure 7. Kinetics of binding of *N*-formyl-Nle-Leu-Phe-Nle-Tyr-Lys-FL (FLPEP) to neutrophils at 37°C determined with the fluorescence cell sorter. (A) Profiles of cellular fluorescence of cells exposed to 1 n*M* FLPEP after 15, 45, or 180 sec and cells exposed to 1 n*M*
FLPEP in the presence of 1 μ*M* nonfluorescent peptide (blocked). (B) Fractional receptor
occupancy versus time for cells exposed to FLPEP at 37°C. The numbers above the curves
refer to the concentration (n*M*). The solid lines are calculated using the rate constants shown
(Sklar *et al.*, 1983c). The off-rate constant, k_{off}^{app}, is an apparent constant that reflects a
combination of the changing dissociability with time and the internalization (see Fig. 5).
(Data replotted with permission from Vitkauskas *et al.*, 1980.)

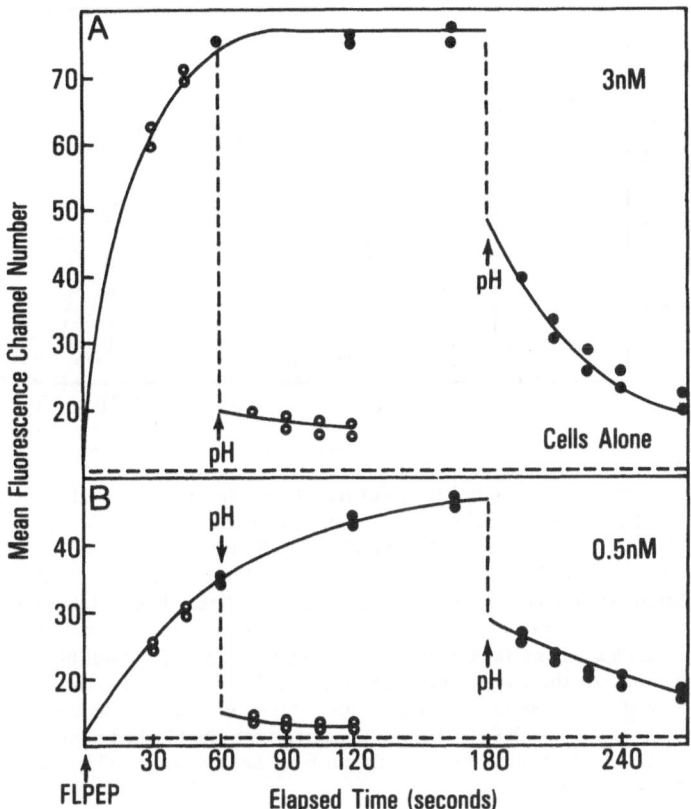

Figure 8. Binding and internalization of *N*-formyl-Nle-Leu-Phe-Nle-Tyr-Lys-FL (FLPEP) by neutrophils at 37°C. (A), (B) Neutrophils were exposed to 3 or 0.5 n*M* FLPEP at time 0, and fluorescence profiles were obtained during the course of binding (1 min, o; 3 min, ●). The pH of the suspension was lowered at the time indicated by the arrow. The data (duplicate determinations) are plotted as the mean fluorescence channel number *vs.* the elapsed time after the addition of FLPEP. (Reprinted with permission from Finney and Sklar, 1983, *Cytometry* 4:54–60, Fig. 4.)

cellular responses actually appear to be determined by pre-equilibrium binding and that the number of receptors is modulated by exposure to ligand, this approach becomes questionable, at best. A reasonable alternative would seem to be to correlate the comparative kinetics of cell responses with the kinetics of ligand binding. The basic problem with such an approach is that ligand binding and cell response occur simultaneously, and the simple comparison of the relative occupancy and the relative response at a particular time does not guarantee any correspondence between these parameters. This is best demonstrated by the results obtained in stimulus pulse experiments (Figs. 4 and 11). In cytochalasin

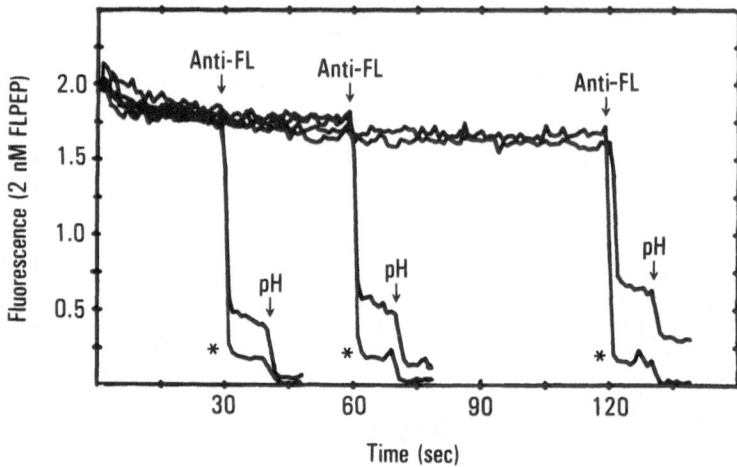

Time (sec)

Figure 9. Fluorimetric assay of the kinetics of receptor-mediated internalization of *N*-formyl-Nle-Leu-Phe-Nle-Tyr-Lys-FL (FLPEP) by human neutrophils at 37°C. The data are plotted as the fluorescence intensity of 2 n*M* FLPEP in the cell suspension (1.5 ml, 10^7 cells/ml) as a function of time. At 0 time, the cells were exposed to 2 n*M* FLPEP. At 30, 60, or 120 sec, 20 n*M* anti-fluorescein IgG was added; 10 sec following the antibody addition, i.e., 40, 70, or 120 sec elapsed, 15 µl of 0.33 *M* HCl was added to the suspensions (final pH 4.0). In the traces indicated by asterisks, the binding and internalization of FLPEP was blocked by 1 µ*M* unlabeled peptide. In these experiments the residual fluorescence after antibody addition, compared with the blocked controls, represents binding of the FLPEP to the receptors; the residual fluorescence after the pH change, compared with the blocked controls, represents internalized FLPEP. (Reprinted with permission from Sklar *et al.*, 1982*b*, *J. Cell Biochem.* **20**:193, Fig. 4.)

B-treated cells, elastase release is completed in ~30–40 sec after the addition of stimulus, and the time course is only slightly dependent on the stimulus concentration. If a near-optimal dose (~1 n*M* fluoresceinated hexapeptide) is administered, an optimal response is obtained even if the stimulus binding to the receptor is inhibited after 5 sec by administration of a high-affinity antibody to fluorescein or 10^{-6} *M* *t*boc-Phe-Leu-Phe-Leu-Phe (Fig. 11A). In other words, the response is determined by levels of receptor occupied before the measured optimal response. Thus, merely measuring ligand binding and cell response at times during the stimulation process can provide no direct information about their relationship.

Fortunately, the pulse format of stimulation provides a direct method for identifying those receptors that contribute to cellular response. As indicated in Section III.B.2, it has been possible to analyze the number of receptors occupied in a pulse (which depends on the ligand concentration, its on rate constant, and the period of uninterrupted binding to the receptor) as well as the magnitude of cellular response that results from that occupancy. Results from a series of pulse-

Table I.
Comparison of Methods of Analysis of Ligand–Receptor Interactions[a]

Parameter	Radioligand	Spectrofluorometry (using αFL-IgG)	Fluorescence flow cytometry
K_d	Yes	Yes	Yes
No. of sites	Yes	Yes	Yes
k_{on}	Individual points may require separate samples	Real time; individual samples required	Real time; same sample analyzed repetitively
k_{off}	Individual points may require separate samples	Real time: continuous analysis following antibody addition	Real time; same sample analyzed repetitively
Internalization	Requires subcellular fractionation	Real time using pH shift; individual samples required	Real time using pH shift; individual samples required
Competition with unlabeled ligand	Steady state	Steady state	Real-time kinetics can provide k_{on} and k_{off} of unlabeled ligand
Time resolution	Depends on separation step (5–10 sec or more)	Depends on times of mixing and binding of ligand by antibody (~1 sec)	Depends on rate of analysis and number of cells analyzed; can be 3 sec or less
Limitations	Accuracy depends on the magnitude of k_{off} and the time of the separation step	1. A significant fraction of ligand must bind to the receptor. 2. The antibody to fluorescein must discriminate between free and receptor-bound ligand.	If $K_d > 10^{-8}\ M$, then the number of receptors/cell must exceed ~100,000

[a]Data used with permission from Simchowitz et al. (1980b).
Abbreviations: K_d, dissociation constant; k_{on}, association-rate constant; k_{off}, dissociation-rate constant; αFL-IgG, high affinity polyclonal antibody against fluorescein.

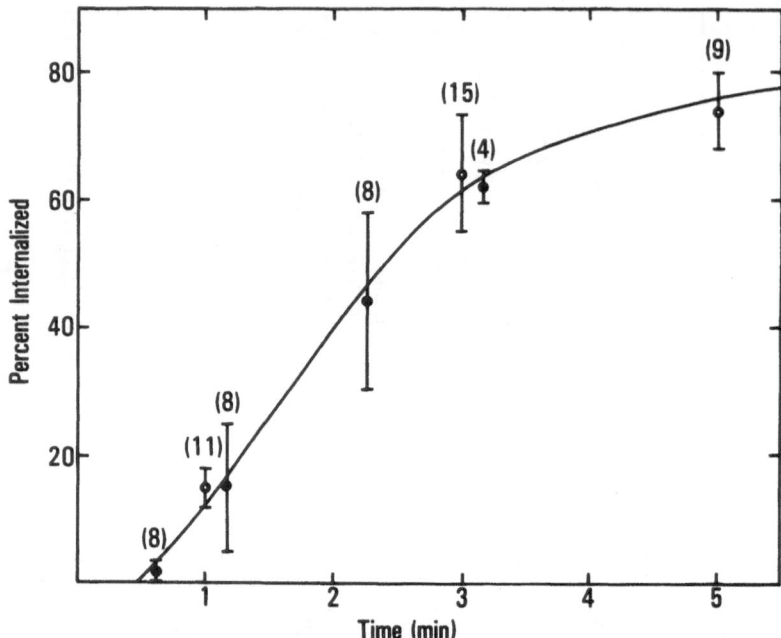

Figure. 10. Comparison of internalization at 37°C as measured by the flow cytometric and fluorimetric procedures. The data are plotted as the percent of occupied receptors internalized versus time. The cytometric data (o) are obtained from a compilation of data (FLPEP = 0.5, 1, 3, and 10 nM). The spectrofluorimetric data (•) using the SLM 4800 are obtained as in Figure 8. The numbers in parentheses represent the total number of determinations. (Reprinted with permission from Finney and Sklar, 1983, *Cytometry* 4:54–60, Fig. 6.)

degranulation experiments are shown in Figure 11. The time course of the degranulation response was shown in Figure 4 as a function of the time of the pulse width, i.e., the length of time between the addition of the fluoresceinated hexapeptide stimulus and the antibody to fluorescein. Figure 11A plots data from several experiments in terms of the percentage maximal response elicited for a given ligand concentration as a function of the period in which the ligand has been allowed to interact with the receptors, i.e., before the addition of the blocking agent. Using such response data and the binding data of Figure 7 or Figure 3 we then calculate the number of receptors occupied in such a pulse (Fig. 11B). We find that three early responses (cAMP elevation, the response of the carbocyanine dye di-S-C$_3$-5, and the release of elastase in cytochalasin B-treated cells) are elicited largely in response to the occupancy of about 10 percent of the receptors (Sklar *et al.*, 1981*b*, 1983*a*). In contrast, we find that the sustained generation of superoxide anion to its maximal level depends upon the occupancy of more than 50% of the receptors (Sklar *et al.*, 1981*b*, 1983*a*). More-

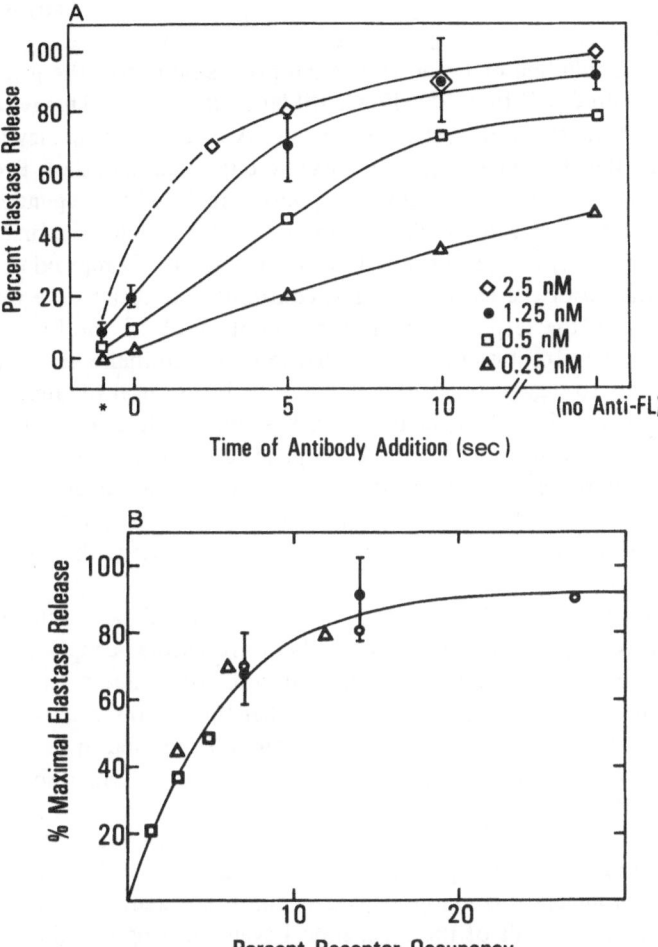

Figure 11. The dependence of elastase release on receptor occupancy. (A) Release of elastase under pulse stimulation (Figs. 3 and 4) as a function of the concentration of FLPEP
and the period of the pulse (in seconds). The data for 1.25 nM stimulus are averaged from
four experiments. The data for the other doses represent compilations from two experiments. Data are presented as the percentage of elastase released versus the time of antibody
addition. Asterisk represents addition of the antibody–peptide complex; the addition of
complex is displayed as −1 sec. The rationale for this is that when antibody is present at
time 0, the interaction of the peptide with the cells occurs during the 1–2 sec required for
the antibody to complex the peptide and interfere with its stimulation of the cells. (Reprinted with permission from Sklar *et al.*, 1982*a*, *J. Biol. Chem.* **257**:5471–5475, Fig. 3B.)
(B) The occupancy–response relationship for elastase release. The fractional receptor occupancy for the pulses (A) is calculated using the kinetics of binding in Figure 7B. While cytochalasin B affects FLPEP binding at occupancy greater than ≃70% or times longer than
1 min, the initial 30 sec of binding obtained under conditions in Figure 7B (but with 1 μg/ml
cytochalasin B) are similar to within about 25%. (◇) 2.5 n*M*; (●) 1.25 n*M*; (□) 0.5 n*M*; (△)
0.25 n*M*.

over, when the binding of ligand to the receptor is inhibited, the generation of O_2^- decays with a half-time of ~12 sec (Sklar *et al.*, 1981*b*). This result implies that both the transduction system that connects receptor occupancy to the O_2^- response and the O_2^- generating system itself are transient and short lived.

The kinetics of the other three responses are largely independent of the extent of receptor occupancy. Such a result suggests that for the first challenge of stimulus at least, that occupancy beyond that required (approximately 10%) for the initiation of the early responses, contributes neither to the time course or magnitude of the response nor, in the case of cAMP on the fluorescent dye response, to the restoration of these cellular responses to their basal levels.

If one were to suggest that cAMP was a second messenger required in the O_2^- generation, it would be difficult to rationalize that its elevation and restoration depend on 10% occupancy, while O_2^- depends on nearly complete occupancy unless a compartment of the cAMP response had an occupancy requirement parallel to O_2^-. Indeed, we believe that there must be an as yet undetermined species contributing to the signaling for the O_2^- response with a parallel occupancy requirement.

The magnitude of each of the responses in the initial part of the occupancy response curve, is proportional to the number of receptors occupied. While there is still theoretical debate about the implication of the shape of an occupancy-response relationship, it has been suggested that this relationship is sigmoidal at the outset if the clustering of occupied receptors is required in the initiation of cell activation (DeLisi and Siraganian, 1979*a*,*b*). Moreover, the response may be biphasic at extreme levels of receptor crosslinkage.

While this quantitative approach is rather recent with respect to *N*-formyl peptides and neutrophil receptors, it actually parallels precedents established in the visual photoreceptor (rhodopsin) system. In that system, remarkable progress in elucidating the details of the biochemical events linking the photoexcitation of rhodopsin to the response of the rod outer segment cell has been possible in part because of the ability to stimulate defined numbers of photoreceptors and to examine, in real time, the ensuing responses. We believe that similar progress in the neutrophil will be possible and that the linkage of biochemical events and their functional correlates in a quantitative and mechanistic manner can be accomplished in the near future.

2. Potential Relationship of Stimulus Infusion to Chemotaxis

Cellular responses (except chemotaxis) are generally measured after bolus addition of the ligand to the cells. It is clear that under these conditions the binding rate is maximal at the outset (Fig. 7B) and would be expected to approach equilibrium in a more or less exponential fashion, complicated, of course, by any receptor modulation. In a chemotactic gradient, however, cells may be exposed to an ever-increasing stimulus concentration.

Depending on the precise conditions, the rate of binding may be nearly constant or even increasing over long periods of time (Lauffenberger and Zigmond, 1981). While it has been proposed that the chemotactic gradient is detected spatially by the cell (Zigmond, 1977), we expect nonetheless that over the period of time during which cells move up a spatial gradient they are exposed to ever-increasing stimulus concentrations, i.e., a temporal gradient. Thus, it is relevant to differentiate the dependence of cellular responses on the rate of ligand binding as compared with the total number of receptors occupied. This question actually serves as the basis of a fundamental issue in receptor theory (Ariens, 1979; Birnbaumer et al., 1974). To wit: Do occupied receptor remain active (in which case the absolute number occupied is important), or do occupied receptors have a transient active lifetime (in which case the response can depend quite substantially on the rate of occupancy)?

For these reasons, we have examined cellular responses to a ramp or temporal gradient (Sklar et al., 1981a). The ramp was administered by infusing the ligand into the cell suspension over a period of minutes. We have observed that the magnitude of several cellular responses–O_2^- (Sklar et al., 1981b), carbocyanine dye, and elastase release (L. A. Sklar et al., unpublished observations)–were reduced when ligand concentrations that were less than optimal were infused over periods of several minutes. This adaptation of the cells during the course of the infusion seemed not to reflect desensitization because the cells could respond in an apparently normal fashion to a bolus injection of the ligand. The ligand itself so infused also had not lost activity because it was capable of stimulating previously unchallenged cells. On the basis of such experiments, we hypothesize distinct temporal regimes of cellular response. When binding is rapid, such as when the stimulus is added as a bolus, and the occupancy rate is greater than roughly 1%/minute, the relationship between occupancy and response is as described above. In contrast, when the binding is slow (<1%/min) the responses adapt in the sense that there is a reduced efficiency in the connection between occupancy and response.

Under conditions appropriate to chemotaxis, one might expect low rates of ligand binding over prolonged periods of time. For instance, in a Zigmond chamber, a cell chemotaxing at 5 μm/min into a gradient near the ligand K_d, (~0.5 nM for the fluoresceinated hexapeptide) can be calculated to experience an increase in ligand concentration with time of ~10^{-11} M^{-1} min[1], according to Lauffenberger and Zigmond (1981). In an infusion, in order to occupy receptors at about 1%/minute, the concentration of the ligand in the suspension needs to be increased at a roughly comparable rate. It is therefore remarkable that it is possible that the inflammatory components of the neutrophil function are diminished under conditions that promote optimal chemotaxis. While the physiological relevance of responses under infusion conditions is still uncertain, we believe that biochemical events that occur by sequential or parallel pathways may adapt in parallel, whereas events along independent pathways will adapt independently. Together, the pulse-response and infusion-response approaches may provide new insight into the biochemical mechanisms regulating neutrophil function. A more detailed consideration of adaptation and its relationship to receptor occupancy is provided in Section IV.

D. Inhibitors

Competitive inhibitors alter the rate and/or magnitude of receptor occupancy by ligand molecules. The classical view of their action is that a competitive inhibitor alters the equilibrium concentration of stimulatory ligand bound to the receptor. If cellular responses actually depended on equilibrium receptor occupancy by the stimulus, then it is reasonable to predict that the efficiency with which competitive inhibitors block cell response (ID_{50}) would exactly parallel their efficiency in blocking stimulus binding (K_d). Indeed, it has been pointed out that the K_d and ID_{50} of the inhibitor cbz-Phe-Met are identical ($\sim 10^{-5}$ M), but the inhibitor $t$boc-Phe-Leu-Phe has an apparent K_d 6.2×10^{-6} M and an ID_{50} for granule enzyme release of 6.1×10^{-7} M (Becker, 1979). We are confronted with something of a paradox. If the kinetic features of ligand binding control at least in some aspects of cell function, then the kinetic components of inhibitor–receptor interaction can play a role in the rate at which the stimulatory ligand gains access to "blocked" receptors. Little information about the kinetic parameters of inhibitor–receptor interaction is now available.

Another closely related question concerns the difference between the interaction of inhibitors and stimuli at the N-formyl peptide receptor. The available studies suggest that the residence time ($t_{1/2 \, off}$) of stimulatory ligands at the receptor in cells (~ 1 min) is long compared with the time required for the initiation of the cellular responses (at most a few seconds). The residence time may be required for an induced conformational change in the receptor or some diffusion-limited interaction of the occupied receptor with other membrane components. That inhibitors do not permit the required stimulatory events could depend in part on their residence time at the receptor. We have conducted preliminary competitive binding experiments with fluorescence flow cytometry based on a kinetic model of stimulus–receptor–inhibitor interactions (Sklar *et al.*, 1983c). Results from these studies suggest that the available inhibitors may have a short residence period (<1 sec) at the receptor.

Drugs that affect the cell membrane alter the binding of formyl peptides to their receptors (Lohr and Snyderman, 1982; Yuli *et al.*, 1982). Amphotericin B, a polyene antibiotic that complexes membrane cholesterol appears to decrease receptor affinity for the ligand and at the same time depresses chemotaxis without altering the generation of O_2^- or the release of proteases (Lohr and Snyderman, 1982). In contrast, aliphatic alcohols (such as butanol and pentanol, which are local anaesthetics) increase receptor affinity and enhance chemotaxis while inhibiting secretion and O_2^- generation (Yuli *et al.*, 1982). These experiments were taken to imply that there is a relationship between receptor affinity and transduction or cell function. The results could be consistent with the proposition that the high-affinity state of the receptor is associated with chemotaxis while the low-affinity receptor is associated with the secretory response and free radical generation. Alternatively, the conversion from low to high affinity could be associated with regulating the generation of free radicals and the release of proteases. The possible relationship of these results with the GTP- and methylation-dependent control of receptor affinity or heterogeneity is not yet known (Koo *et al.*, 1982; Mackin *et al.*, 1982; Pike and Snyderman, 1982*b*).

IV. LIGAND–RECEPTOR DYNAMICS AND LONG-TERM RESPONSIVENESS

A. Neutrophil Adaptation and Sensory Physiology

The host-defense function of the neutrophil rests on its ability to locate a site of injury and infection and unleash its oxidative, hydrolytic, and phagocytic arsenal at that site. Clearly, premature or spontaneous release would be detrimental to its host and thereby negate its function. Yet its chemotactic migration uses the same stimuli that can trigger activation of the cell. Thus during migration, the activation must be held in check without diminishing its potential to respond to other stimuli or to higher levels of the same stimulus. A biological mechanism that fulfills such a requirement is found in the well-studied sensory adaptation of photo- chemo-, or thigmo-responsive organisms and cells (Lowenstein, 1971; Hazelbauer, 1978). These systems have the ability to desensitize to a particular level of stimulation while retaining sensitivity to changes in that level. Examples of the most studied systems are animal vision (Autrum, 1981), bacterial chemotaxis (Koshland, 1981), and plant phototropism (Bergman *et al.*, 1969). The responses in these systems to their respective stimuli characteristically involve short latencies, transient responses, some relatively short refractory periods, and restoration (within minutes) of sensitivity to changes in stimulus level. Such a sensory adaptation mechanism endows vertebrates with discriminatory visual capacity operative over seven orders of magnitude of light intensity. It would also preclude response if the rate of change in stimulus level were sufficiently slow (Bergman *et al.*, 1969).

Neutrophils have the ability to "adapt" to stimuli such as N-formyl peptides and C5a in the sense that they exhibit graded, transient responses to changes in concentration of these chemoattractants within the dynamic response range of the cell, i.e., between $\sim 0.01 \ K_d$ and $100 \ K_d$, depending on the particular response. Within this range, the transient nature of the response is neither due to destruction of the stimulant (Zigmond and Sullivan, 1979) nor due to temporary impairment of the responsive system owing to the depletion of some biochemical intermediate or self-destructive process, since it can be stimulated equally well by other chemoattractants (Simchowitz *et al.*, 1980*b*), except perhaps at very high ligand concentrations (Henson *et al.*, 1981).

Thus the cells are capable of responding either morphologically or biochemically (Zigmond and Sullivan, 1979; Becker, 1979) to successive steps up or down in concentration, to pulsed exposure, or to continuous exposure in a gradient (Zigmond, 1978). In addition, many of the responses are diminished if the cells are exposed to an increase in concentration administered over a prolonged period of time (Sklar *et al.*, 1981*a*).

In order to begin an analysis of the mechanism of adaptation a systematic characterization of the response must be undertaken. This can begin with (1) the measurement of the refractory period; (2) the adaptation level, i.e., the concentration of stimulus to which the cell has become adapted (Bergmann *et al.*, 1969; Delbrück and Reichardt, 1956); or (3) the dynamic range of the response. Three types of stimulation regimes may be imposed: multiple step up, step down, and pulsed exposures. Of particular importance is the systematic investigation of the effect of duration and frequency of stimulation. Ultimately, it should be possible, using the antibody to fluorescein (Sklar *et al.*, 1981*b*) to quantitatively remove the free fluoresceinated ligand from the cell suspension and to mathematically describe the complete response capability of the neutrophil using a white noise analysis, as has been successfully done both in plant and animal visual systems (Lipson, 1975; Marmerelius and Naka, 1973).

At our current level of understanding, it appears that neutrophils "preexposed" to different levels of stimulus will respond to a subsequent saturating dose of N-formyl peptides only under certain conditions. It is instructive to replot the results obtained from several investigators using a format accepted for the analysis of adaptive responses. In Figure 12 the data of Simchowitz *et al.* (1980*b*) and Vitkauskas *et al.* (1980) are replotted. From Table I (Simchowitz *et al.*, 1980), the O_2^- response of human neutrophils to a 100-nM step up in fMet-Leu-Phe after a previous 5-min preincubation to different levels of the same chemoattractant are expressed, as a function of the proportion of surface receptors left after the preincubation period. The number of surface receptors was estimated from the calculations of Zigmond *et al.* (1982) from rabbit neutrophils assuming that receptor modulation in human and rabbit cells are comparable (see Section IV.C). Similarly, the fractional response, recalculated from Figure 7 (Vitkauskas *et al.*, 1980) for fMet-Leu-Phe-induced lysozyme release from rabbit neutrophils, is plotted as a function of the receptor availability after a 5-min preexposure to various levels of fMet-Leu-Phe. Since both plots are roughly linear as the logarithm of the surface receptor number, it would appear that receptor availability is the primary determinant of responsiveness and that there is minimal adaptation. However, it could be concluded from

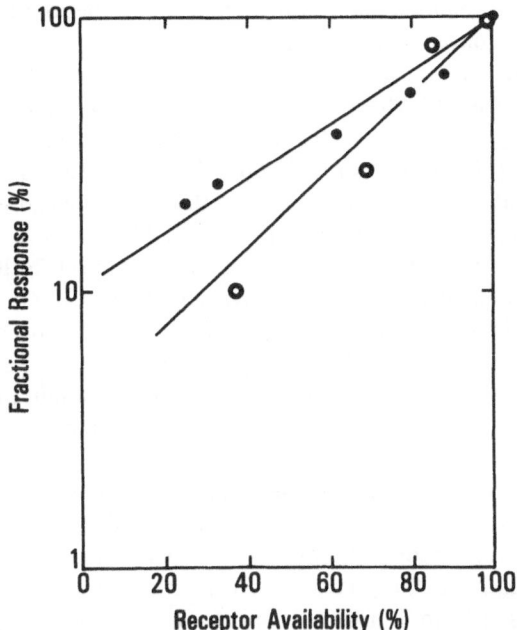

Figure 12. Dependence of response on receptor availability. The percentage of the maximum response of rabbit neutrophils (●—●) or human neutrophils (○—○) is plotted as a function of the measured or calculated receptor availability. Receptor levels were modulated by pre-exposure of neutrophils to differing concentrations of N-formyl-Met-Leu-Phe for 5 min at 37°C. Calculation of receptor levels in humans were based on the steady-state level of receptors postulated for rabbit cells from the calculations of Zigmond et al. (1982). Results were recalculated from Table I in Simchowitz et al. (1980); for O_2 response in human neutrophils, and from Figure 7 (Vitkauskas et al., 1980); for lysozyme release in rabbit neutrophils. (Data are replotted with permission from Simchowitz et al., 1980b, and from Vitkauskas et al., 1980.)

Figure 5A Sklar et al. (1981b) that the cells have not had sufficient time to become adapted to the first stimulus, since a full depolarization response is recovered only after ~10 min of preincubation with a concentration of chemoattractant that should reduce the receptor number approximately 50% ([stimulus] = $\sim K_d$) at steady state.

The analysis of adaptation of neutrophils to two sequential steps up in concentration of chemoattractant, (i.e., fMet-Leu-Phe, $K_d \sim 10^{-8}$ M, has been extended by Seligmann et al. (1982b). These investigators have measured the change in fluorescence of a membrane potential sensitive dye to monitor the response to a second step up in chemoattractant concentration as a function of the intervening time between the first step up or adapting concentration. Their results suggest a time dependent decrease in sensitivity to concentration changes at low levels of stimulus without impairment of the response capability of the cell to changes in concentration to higher levels.

We can define the dynamic response range of the cell as those concentration steps that produce a 10%–90% maximal response. From Figure 2 in Seligmann *et al.*, 1982*b*, the dynamic range of the unadapted cell is a step up in concentration spanning ~5 nM (10% response) to 1 μM (90%). The cell adapted for 12 min to a chemoattractant concentration of 25 nM shows an analogous range from 140 nM to 50 μM. The 50% response is shifted from 25 nM to 700 nM or a factor of ~30. This clearly shifts the response capability of the cell to higher concentration, as would be expected for an adaptive system. If we define the adaptation level of the unstimulated cell C_a as the highest concentration of stimulant that causes no response, in this case 1 nM, then again from Figure 2 and from Figure 4 (Seligmann *et al.*, 1982*b*) we can calculate a stimulus parameter S based on the Weber–Fechner law and on analysis of adaptation by Delbrück and Reichhardt (1956).

In Figure 13 the percentage of the maximum response is plotted as a function of the log of the stimulus parameter S defined as C_s/C_a, where C_s is the concentration of the second stimulus step. It is apparent that for responses of 50%–75% of maximum, the curves are linear with very similar slopes for adaptation levels, ranging from 1 nM (unstimulated) to 50 nM. At greater response levels, the curves flatten out, as might be expected as the cells approach the limit of their response capability and dynamic range. For higher adaptation levels (Fig. 3; Seligmann *et al.*, 1982*b*) the results are analogous, except that linearity is lost at lower response levels. Such behavior was also observed by Keller *et al.* (1977, 1978) and analyzed according to the Weber–Fechner Law or the more generalized Stevens' double-logarithmic power function (Stevens, 1971) with similar results. Thus, it appears that the neutrophil behaves as a classical sensory adaptive system able to discriminate logarithmic differences in concentration over a range spanning 1 nM to 50 μM or a dynamic range of 5×10^4.

Is it reasonable to explain this adaptive response by a change in affinity of the available receptors as proposed by Seligmann *et al.* (1982*b*)? For example, adaptive methylation has been shown to occur at the receptor level in bacterial chemotaxis. While methylation appears to regulate the affinity of the macrophage N-formyl peptide receptor (Pike and Snyderman, 1982*b*), the link between adaptation and receptor occupancy or receptor affinity remains obscure. Seligmann *et al.* (1982*b*) suggest that the receptors available (newly inserted) after a stimulus challenge have a reduced affinity. Zigmond *et al.* (1982), however, suggest that the affinity of the surface receptors after downregulation remains constant.

Another contributing factor in adaptation could involve receptor modulation (internalization of occupied receptors and expression of cryptic receptors). Zigmond *et al.* (1982) have shown that within 15 min after the administration of a ligand concentration at K_D, a steady-state level of receptors equal to 50% of the

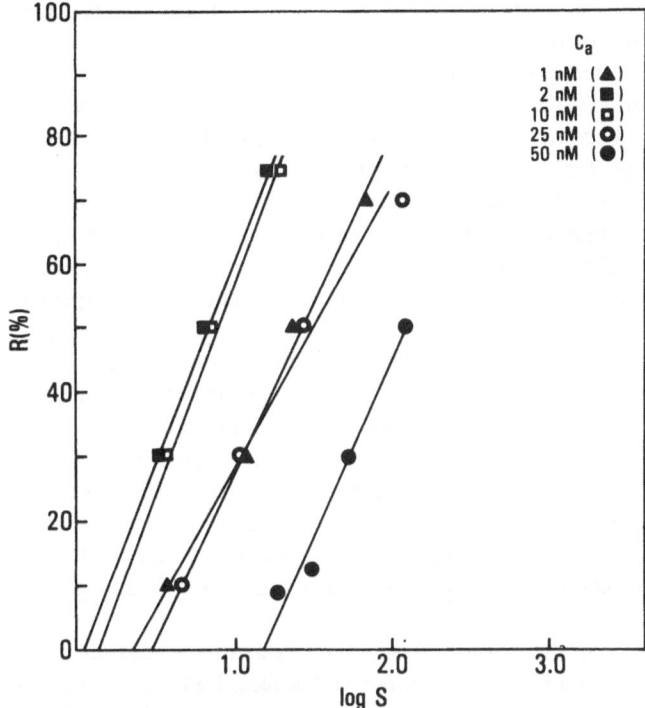

Figure 13. The fraction of the maximum response (percentage R) of human neutrophils preexposed to differing concentrations of N-fMet-Leu-Phe for 12–14 min at 37°C (from Figs. 2 and 3 of Seligmann et al., 1982) is plotted as a function of the log of the stimulus parameter S. $S = C_s/C_a$, where C_a is the adaptation level or concentration to which the cells had been adapted, i.e., S_1, and C_s is the concentration of the second stimulus dose S_2. C_a: (▲) 1 nM; (■) 2 nM; (□) 10 nM; (○) 25 nM; (●) 50 nM. (Replotted with permission from Seligmann et al., 1982b.)

initial level is achieved in rabbit neutrophils. It is as yet unknown whether these newly inserted receptors have the same intrinsic ability to trigger the cell, be it due to altered affinity or to the availability of the catalytic coupling factors, for instance, the GTP-binding protein in the adenylate cyclase activation system. We suggest that while it seems clear that the locus of the adaptation of the cell responsiveness is probably not at the "effector" or response level, it is not clear whether it is due to the number of receptors, their affinity, or their ability to trigger responses, or some combination of these factors.

B. Deactivation

More information is available about the stimulation of neutrophils outside of the putative "adaptive" dynamic range. At concentrations ranging about 5 to

10 times the ligand–receptor dissociation constant, the steady-state level of surface receptors is minimal, i.e., it is reduced to approximately $<20\%$ of its initial level. Thus, preexposure of cells at these chemoattractant levels results in a phenomenon variously called deactivation or desensitization. After deactivation, a neutrophil becomes unresponsive to the same or different stimuli.

Two important aspects of this phenomenon must be understood. The first is that deactivation usually refers to doses that saturate surface receptor rapidly and that are therefore outside the dynamic range of the neutrophil adaptation. In addition, the deactivation is not transient and cannot be explained by the temporary refractory period of the response. The second aspect is that these high doses of chemoattractants are capable of inactivating the response by destruction of the stimulus, by self-inflicted damage to the cell, or by immobilization of the cell (in the case of migratory responses) to the experimental substrate.

Ligand inactivation by the neutrophil response may be either hydrolytic or oxidative. The former involves the secretion of proteases by the neutrophil, which can degrade the formyl peptides (Gallin *et al.*, 1978). Oxidative inactivation of the ligand can proceed via direct oxidation of the thioester group of the methionyl residues of N-formyl-methionyl peptides (Tsan and Chen, 1980; Clark and Szot, 1982) involving the myeloperoxidase H_2O_2-halide system secreted by the activated cell.

Evidence for the "nonspecific" desensitization or deactivation of the neutrophil itself comes from a number of sources. Lane and Lamkin (1982) have measured the auto-oxidation of the receptors on the cells by the production of active O_2^- species, most likely H_2O_2, by the cells. H_2O_2 is derived from stimulation of the cells' hexose monophosphate shunt activity (Nelson *et al.*, 1980) or by dismutation of O_2^- produced at the surface (Ohno *et al.*, 1982b). Support for the involvement of nonspecific activation was provided by the observation that phagocytosis and chemotaxis were potentiated by H_2O_2 scavengers such as catalase (Baehner *et al.*, 1977) and inhibition of cellular H_2O_2 production (Nelson *et al.*, 1980, 1981). Further support for this hypothesis has come from studies of cells from patients who have chronic granulomatous disease. These cells lack the ability to generate an oxidative burst and show no deactivation in their migratory responses (Nelson *et al.*, 1979).

Another source of desensitization that does not fit into the adaptation framework is the interference of one response with another. For example, the stimulation of adherence of neutrophils impedes their migration (Gallin *et al.*, 1978; Fehr and Dahinden, 1979). Consequently neutrophils in suspension pretreated in a manner that would effect a deactivation of motile responses to a second heterologous stimulus show no deactivation of the morphological polarization response (Smith *et al.*, 1979).

To date there is very little evidence for the irreversible saturation of response capabilities of cells protected from auto-oxidation that cannot be interpreted in terms of receptor availability. For example, the aggregation of neutrophils, their changes in membrane potential, and cAMP levels, were not irreversibly perturbed in experiments in which the crossdeactivation of fMet-Leu-Phe responses by C5a and vice versa was examined (Simchowitz *et al.*, 1980*b*; O'Flaherty *et al.*, 1977).

It appears, therefore, that a significant degree of specific deactivation is due to changes in the receptor number. Receptor availability at the cell surface in turn is a function of the stimulation of endocytosis of occupied receptors and reexpression of receptors from internal stores or by recycling mechanisms. The relative rates of these processes therefore play a major role in adaptation and deactivation.

C. Internalization and Processing of Receptor

The *N*-formyl peptide receptors of granulocytes are under considerable cellular control. A number of studies have demonstrated that at physiological temperatures peptide is accumulated by these cells via a receptor-mediated internalization process (Niedel *et al.*, 1979*a,b*; Sullivan and Zigmond, 1980; Jesaitis *et al.*, 1983*a*, Sklar *et al.*, 1982*c*; Finney and Sklar, 1983). Recently we showed this internalization to involve physical translocation of the receptor–peptide complex to an internal compartment that has sedimentation properties similar to low-density Golgi (Jesaitis *et al.*, 1982*b*) or pinocytotic vesicles variously called receptosomes, endosomes, and receptor-mediated pinocytotic vesicles (Willingham and Pastan, 1980; Geisow, 1982; Schneider *et al.*, 1979; Courtoy *et al.*, 1982). Autoradiography at the electron microscopic level has confirmed this passage demonstrating translocation of $[^{125}I]$-peptide from the plasma membrane to the perinuclear Golgi complex (Painter *et al.*, 1984*a*). This translocation therefore provides a mechanism for the downregulation of receptors at the surface (Zigmond *et al.*, 1982; Jesaitis *et al.*, 1983) by which the sensitivity of the cell may be controlled (Zigmond, 1981).

In rabbit cells the steady-state rate of peptide uptake is directly proportional to the occupancy of the receptors, and the uptake proceeds at a rate of 0.125 occupied receptors per minute or in a cell with 50,000 receptors at 6250 receptors per minute at saturation (Zigmond *et al.*, 1982). In human cells, we have calculated similar rates by two independent methods using different peptides (Jesaitis *et al.*, 1983; Sklar *et al.*, 1982*c*; Finney and Sklar, 1983). With fMet-Leu-Phe, the rate at saturation is ~8000–10,000 molecules/min-cell. With the hexapeptide the initial rate was measured to be 12,500/min. Since internalization begins only after a delay of ~0.5 min, it is probably too slow to be involved in the initiation of many of the rapid neutrophil responses.

Internalization rates are compatible with prolonged peptide uptake, extended chemotaxis, and continued sensitivity only if receptors are reexpressed at the plasma membrane. Indeed, if cells are given a saturating dose of peptide, then within 5–10 min the receptor-binding activity on cells (Zigmond *et al.*, 1982) and isolated membrane (Jesaitis *et al.*, 1983*a*) drops to 20%–30% of the original level in unstimulated cells. If these downregulated cells are observed at subsequent times after the excess peptide has been removed, the receptor binding activity reappears at the cell surface in a manner dependent on the original dose. Zigmond *et al.* (1982) reported that at concentrations of ligand at least 10 times the dissociation constant in the resulting system a recovery of receptor number of 100%–150% was observed. Therefore, the cell must have a source of receptor over and above the original fraction at the cell surface.

Gallin *et al.* (1978, 1979) and Fletcher *et al.* (1982) have postulated that the cryptic receptors are not necessarily synthesized, but are stored in an intracellular pool that is translocated to the surface after stimulation. We have demonstrated intracellular localization of receptor by analytical subcellular fractionation (Jesaitis *et al.*, 1982*a*). Approximately equivalent amounts of receptor were localized to fractions coenriched in specific granules and galactosyl transferase. Recently, Fletcher and Gallin (1982) confirmed the localization to subcellular fractions enriched in specific granules. However, they estimate a value for the receptor number (1.5×10^6) that differs significantly from our estimates. Functionally, secretory Golgi vesicles or specific granules are equivalent candidates for intracellular reserves of receptors. Therefore, assignment of receptor to either organelle must await resolution of the markers.

In a number of hormone receptor systems, including those for insulin, epidermal growth factor, asialoglycoprotein, and transferrin, receptors are reutilized or recycled after internalization (King and Quatrecasas, 1982). In a terminally differentiated cell such as the mature granulocyte, this process may be crucial for its long-term receptor-dependent processes. Zigmond *et al.* (1982) calculated the kinetics of receptor reexpression in rabbit polymorphonuclear leukocytes and have found that the rate of recovery after downregulation depends on the size of the internalized pool or the number of surface vacancies. This type of regulation is consistent with receptor recycling or with mobilization of an internal pool of spare receptors.

We have attempted to follow the internal fate of the *N*-formyl peptide receptor in stimulated human granulocytes in two ways. The first method measured the receptor binding activity in subcellular fractions obtained from pre- and post-peptide-stimulated cells. We have estimated that after cells are stimulated for 5 min with 500 n*M* fMet-Leu-Phe ($>10 K_d$) at 37°C, approximately 20% of the binding activity that has been lost from the surface is recovered in the subcellular fractions corresponding to the dense granule fractions. These fractions showed only trace amounts of internalized peptide. Complementary electron microscopic studies with the hexapeptide labeled with ^{125}I confirmed the observation that peptide and receptor are transferred from a fraction enriched in Golgi complex to a lysosomal fraction (resembling azurophil granules).

Internalized receptor that had been photoaffinity labeled at the cell surface with a radioactive and aryl azido derivative of a chemotactic hexapeptide was used as another tracer of the internal fate of the receptor (Jesaitis *et al.*, 1982*b*; Painter *et al.*, 1982; Schmitt *et al.*, 1983). Subcellular fractionation studies indicated that after it was internalized more than 95% of the tracer remained in the low-density (ρ = 1.10–1.11) subcellular fractions enriched in the Golgi marker galactosyl transferase. This result therefore suggests that when the peptide was covalently bound to the receptor (in a presumably irreversible manner), the receptor was apparently not efficiently transferred to another compartment.

Subsequent steps of recycling of granuloctye receptors remains to be analyzed. Our results, which suggest only a limited pool of reserve receptors in the specific granule/Golgi fractions, therefore favor recycling as a way of explaining long-term peptide processing. A much larger number as suggested by Fletcher and Gallin (1982) might suggest that receptor recycling plays a less significant role.

The consequences of the receptor processing in granulocytes are significant. Zigmond (1981) has analyzed the ability of rabbit polymorphonuclear leukocytes to orient in artificial gradients of chemotactic factors as a function of the availability and fractional occupancy of surface receptors. This calculation suggests that the effect of receptor downregulation is a loss of sensitivity at high concentrations of peptide. The implications, however, could be even more far reaching. Several rapid responses of neutrophils depends very much on the rate of occupancy of a small number of receptors (approximately 5%–10%). Consequently the steady-state modulation of receptor numbers at the surface becomes a very pertinent issue for subsequent challenges to the stimulus, especially in a neutrophil adapted to a level within its dynamic range. For chemotaxis, receptor modulation may be crucial (Jesaitis and Cochrane, 1983).

D. Chemotactic Responses

1. Cell Orientation

While leukocyte chemotaxis has been extensively reviewed, (Zigmond, 1978; Gallin *et al.*, 1979; Snyderman and Goetzl, 1981; Schiffmann, 1982; Painter *et al.*, 1984*b*), the precise mechanism by which receptor–ligand interactions are coupled to chemotactic behavior are currently obscure. Recent evidence indicates that the response of neutrophils to gradients of *N*-formyl peptides is at a minimum biphasic (Gerish and Keller, 1981; Zigmond, 1981). Using a chamber in which defined linear gradients can be generated, it has been shown that cells first elongate or polarize by extension of pseudopodia in the direction of the gradient with a remarkable degree of precision (90% of the population oriented within ±30° of the correct direction). This so-called orientation phase is followed by amoeboid-like motility in a relatively straight line up the concentration gradient (Ramsey, 1972; Allan and Wilkinson, 1978; Zigmond *et al.*, 1981). Furthermore, the absolute rate of motility is accelerated (2- to 4-fold) over that observed in cells migrating in the absence of a chemoattractant.

Like other responses of the cell, the orientation response detects changes in concentration of stimulus best in the range of the dissociation constant. The polarization phase occurs over a several-minute period and can be itself separated into two distinct sequential phases. When cells are placed near micropipettes containing N-formyl peptide, the first noticeable response is the extension of a pseudopod(s) at that portion of the cell nearest the pipette (Gerish and Keller, 1981). This response is initiated within 5–10 sec after positioning of the micropipette which places it in the category of the fast biological response of neutrophils observed in response to N-formyl peptides. This response was reversible for at least 5–6 min. Upon repositioning the micropipette tip, the previously formed pseudopods retracted and new ones formed near the micropipette tip. This occurred even when placed near the tail or urapod of the migrating cell (Gerish and Keller, 1981).

Zigmond *et al.* (1981), using a different approach, have reported results that at first appear to conflict with the above observations. These workers found that cells preoriented for 15–30 min in a gradient of peptide could indeed reverse their direction of movement if the gradient was reversed. However, in contrast to the results of Gerish and Keller (1981), it was found that the cell always did so by executing a U-turn maneuver rather than by extending pseudopodia from the uroped region. The reasons for these discrepancies with regard to reversibility are unclear but could reflect the different methodologies employed by the laboratories, or perhaps the precise timing of the first and second stimulus. In view of new evidence showing dramatic changes in surface receptor number, surface receptor topography and adaptive changes that occur during incubation with N-formyl peptide, the precise timing of the gradient reversal could influence the experimental outcome.

2. Role of Microtubules in Directed Motility

In *Dictyostelium discoideum* amoebas, Taylor *et al.* (1981) have found that orientation toward micropipettes loaded with the chemoattractant cAMP is reversible, although an extended refractory lag period is observed for the second response. These same workers also found that when amoebas were cut into enucleated and nucleated fragments both cell fragments responded to cAMP-loaded pipettes by extending pseudopodia. Only the nucleated fragment was capable of directed motility. These workers suggested the possibility that an oganelle associated with the nucleus such as the Golgi complex and/or the microtubule-organizing body might be required for sustained directional motility. However, several reports indicated that neutrophils enucleated by treatment at 42°C still retained full chemotactic activity (Keller and Bessis, 1975; Malawista and Chevance, 1982). Furthermore, electron microscopic analysis of the enucleated fragments suggested that few, if any, organelles, including granules, organized Golgi, microtubules, or centrioles were apparent (Malawista and Chevance,

1982). These enucleated cell fragments appeared to contain only microfilaments and associated contractile proteins and glycogen particles. These findings would suggest that in neutrophils, at least, organized Golgi, microtubules, and the microtubule organizing center may play no obligatory role in chemotactic responsivity. These findings are somewhat at odds with a considerable body of literature, showing that pharmacological agents that affect microtubule assembly interfere with directed motility (Caner, 1965; Bandmann *et al.*, 1974; Malech *et al.*, 1976; Oliver *et al.*, 1978). This effect is not an inhibitory effect per se, however. Several laboratories have shown that colchicine interferes with chemotaxis by reducing the precision of cell orientation and subsequent migration, not the ability to sense the direction of the gradient. This suggests that intact microtubules may allow the cell to make more precise turns by simply organizing cytosolic organelles more efficiently (Zigmond, 1977; Allan and Wilkinson, 1978; Malawista and Chevance, 1982).

3. Effect of Receptor Modulation on Chemotactic Responses

Once the cell has oriented and directed migration has commenced, the cell can migrate up a gradient of chemoattractant over a period of several hours both *in vitro* and *in vivo*. Over this time scale, several processes occur that could serve to alter the baseline sensitivity of the system to chemoattractant concentration. First, the downregulation of surface receptors occurs probably in concert with their recycling and expression of cryptic intracellular receptors (Niedel *et al.*, 1979a; Sullivan and Zigmond, 1980). Second, an adaptive response occurs (Seligmann *et al.*, 1982b; Zigmond and Sullivan, 1979). Thus, in effect, surface-receptor number and sensitivity to ligand probably decrease during chemotaxis. Third, there is some evidence indicating that the distribution of surface markers becomes polarized. For example, Fc receptors and concanavalin A (Con A) receptors reorient at the leading edge of polarized neutrophils (Wilkinson *et al.*, 1980). *N*-formyl peptide receptors also appear to become concentrated at the leading cell edge (Walter *et al.*, 1980; Sullivan and Zigmond, 1982).

These results can be explained in at least three ways: (1) *N*-formyl peptide receptors that are occupied could be selectively internalized at the cell tail; (2) the occupied surface receptors could redistribute on the surface ("capping"); and (3) the cryptic and/or newly recycled receptors could be selectively introduced at the cell's leading edge. This last possibility is supported by evidence indicating that secretory vesicles or granules (Wright and Gallin, 1979) and elements of the Golgi apparatus (Kupfer *et al.*, 1982; Bergmann *et al.*, 1983) through which the receptor may recycle are selectively intercalated into the leading front of motile cells.

How might these modulations in surface-receptor number, affinity, and surface distributions affect the way in which the cell senses the gradient? Adaptation would be expected to extend the dynamic concentration range of the cellular response. Thus, as a cell migrated into concentrations above the initial K_d of the receptor, migration would continue rather than be suppressed. If receptor occupancy is the parameter by which cells sense the gradient, however, then adaptation must somehow result from increasing the K_d of the receptor and/or resetting the detection level or response regulator (Koshland, 1981) of the transduction system so as to detect smaller differences in receptor occupancy.

Changes in the surface distribution of N-formyl peptide receptors could also modulate the way in which a cell senses a chemotactic gradient (Davis *et al.*, 1982). If newly expressed surface N-formyl peptide receptors are selectively expressed at the cell anterior membrane surface, then this could in effect amplify the absolute differences in global receptor occupancy at a given ligand concentration. This could propagate motility in the same direction as long as sufficient concentrations of chemoattractant were present. Biochemically this could be accomplished if, for example, the ligand–receptor complex were to result in local changes in the gel-sol state of the cytosol such that cytoplasmic flow in the forward direction was favored. Another possibility, based largely on proposals made by Abercrombie *et al.* (1970), is that the asymmetric intercalation of new surface membrane (from the Golgi apparatus?) into the cell anterior membrane would drive the motile process. This hypothesis could explain why so many different surface proteins are localized at the cell anterior after N-formyl peptide stimulation (Walter *et al.*, 1980; Wilkinson *et al.*, 1980; Davis *et al.*, 1982) and why particles attached to motile cells move backward toward the nucleus over the cell surface (Abercrombie *et al.*, 1970; Harris and Dunn, 1972).

4. Coupling of the Sensory Apparatus to the Motile Apparatus

Current research indicates that changes in the cytoskeletal organization and the resulting gel-sol state and contractile state of the cytoplasm are regulated by free Ca^{2+} ion. Such changes have been directly observed in motile eukaryotic cell types at several laboratories. Taylor *et al.* (1980*a*) have microinjected the Ca^{2+}-sensitive luminescent protein aequorin into living fibroblasts. Using quantitative fluorescent microscopic techniques, they have shown that free Ca^{2+} levels increase from $<10^{-7}$ M to 10^{-6}–10^{-5} M levels at the leading front or lamellipodial edges of locomoting cells. At this same laboratory, fluorescent actin has similarly been microinjected into fibroblast and actin has been shown to accumulate at such sites (Taylor *et al.*, 1980*b*). In chemotaxing neutrophils, Oliver *et al.* (1978) have shown with conventional immunofluorescent techniques that actin is concentrated at similar sites.

While microinjection has not yet been reported, several reports suggest that the local concentration of Ca^{2+} may change in response to chemotactic peptides. Naccache *et al.* (1979*a*) have shown that neutrophils labeled with the Ca^{2+}-sensitive fluorescent probe chlortetracycline show changes induced by N-formylated peptide probe fluorescence suggestive of alterations in membrane-bound

Ca^{2+}. More directly, Cramer and Gallin (1979) have histochemically localized plasma membrane bound Ca^{2+} using the pyroantimonate method and have demonstrated that Ca^{2+} staining is lost at the leading membrane regions of chemotaxing neutrophils. The lost Ca^{2+} is presumed to raise local concentrations of free Ca^{2+} transiently in the adjacent cytoplasm. While some doubt remains concerning the specificity and exact interpretation of such methods, the data do suggest the possibility that as in the fibroblast system, free Ca^{2+} ion may transiently increase at the leading edge of chemotaxing neutrophils.

Calcium ion in the micromolar range can affect the gel-sol properties of actin gels *in vitro* in at least two ways. First, increasing free Ca^{2+} can affect the interaction of actin binding and gelation proteins directly by regulating and then binding to F actin (Burridge and Feramisco, 1981; Rosenberg *et al.*, 1981) or by binding to proteins like gel-solin, thereby affecting the state of actin (Yin *et al.*, 1981; Stossel *et al.*, 1981). Second, Ca^{2+} can indirectly affect the function of cytoskeletal proteins by means of calmodulin-dependent protein kinases. For example, in nonskeletal muscle, the binding of actin to myosin and the myosin ATPase activities require obligatory phosphorylation of its light chain. These processes are regulated by a calmodulin-dependent protein kinase (Adelstein and Eisenberg, 1980). In addition, phosphorylation of several other cytoskeletal proteins, including vinculin (Sefton *et al.*, 1981) and actin-binding protein (filamin) (Wallach *et al.*, 1978; Carroll and Gerrard, 1982), have been documented, although the relationship between their actin-binding properties and their state of phosphorylation is unclear. If an asymmetric occupancy of receptor on the cell surface is required for generation of a chemotactic signal, then the directional motility could possibly be controlled by locally altering the gel-sol state of the cytosol in an asymmetric manner.

At least three distinct models have been proposed to explain motility in eukaryotic cells (Abercrombie *et al.*, 1970; Huxley, 1973; Stossel, 1978; Taylor *et al.*, 1979). A complete understanding of how a chemotactic signal might generate a directional response must await a more thorough understanding of the biochemistry and biomechanics of the motile process itself.

ACKNOWLEDGMENTS

This work was supported by grants AI-17354 and AI-19032 from the National Institutes of Health. L.A.S. is a recipient of an Established Investigator Award from the American Heart Association. R.G.P. is a recipeint of an NIH Research Career Development Award AM-00437. We would like to thank Mrs. Monica Bartlett for typing the manuscript. We would like to thank Dr. Paul Hyslop for helpful discussions concerning adaptation and desensitization and Charles G. Cochrane, M.D. for his support and encouragement. This work is publication #2976-IMM from the Research Institute of Scripps Clinic.

V. REFERENCES

Abercrombie, M., Heaysman, J. E. M., and Pegrum, S. M., 1970, The locomotion of fibroblasts in culture. III. Movements of particles on the dorsal surface of the leading lamella, *Exp. Cell Res.* 62:389.

Adelstein, R. S., and Eisenberg, E, 1980, Regulation and kinetics of the actin–myosin–ATP interaction, *Annu. Rev. Biochem.* 49:921.

Ainscough, E. W., Brodie, A. M., Plowman, J. E., Bloor, S. J., Loehr, J. S., and Loehr, T. M., 1980, Studies in human lactoferrin by electron paramagnetic resonance, fluorescence, and resonance raman spectroscopy, *Biochemistry* 19:4072.

Allan, R. B., and Wilkinson, P. C., 1978, A visual analysis of chemotactic and chemokinetic locomotion of human neutrophilic leucocytes. Use of a new chemotaxis assay with *Candida albicans* as a gradient source, *Exp. Cell Res.* 111:191.

Anderson, D. C., Wible, L. J., Hughes, B. J., Smith, C. W., and Brinkley, B. R., 1982, Cytoplasmic microtubles in polymorphonuclear leukocytes: Effect of chemotactic stimulation and colchicine, *Cell* 31:719.

Ariens, E. J., 1979, Receptors: From fiction to fact, *TIPS* 1:11.

Aswanikumar, S., Corcoran, B., Schiffmann, E., Day, A. R., Freer, R. J., Showell, H. J., Becker, E. L., and Pert, C. B., 1977, Demonstration of a receptor on rabbit neutrophils for chemotactic peptides, *Biochim. Biophys. Res. Commun.* 74:810.

Autrum, H., 1981, Light and dark adaptation in invertebrates, in: *Handbook of Sensory Physiology* (H. Autrum, ed.), Vol. VIIC, Springer-Verlag, Berlin.

Badwey, J. A., and Karnovsky, M. L., 1979, Production of superoxide and hydrogen peroxide by an NADH oxidase in guinea pig polymorphonuclear leukocytes, *Biochemistry* 254:11530.

Baehner, R. L., Boxer, L. A., Allen, J. M., and Davis, J., 1977, Autooxidation as a basis for altered function by polymorphonuclear leukocytes, *Blood* 50:327.

Bandmann, U., Rydgren, L., and Norberg, B., 1974, The difference between random movement and chemotaxis, *Exp. Cell Res.* 88:63.

Becker, E. L., 1979, A multifunctional receptor on the neutrophil for synthetic chemotactic oligopeptides, *J. Reticuloendothel. Soc.* 26:701.

Becker, E. L., Naccache, P. H. Showell, H. J., and Walenga, R. W., 1981, Early events in neutrophil activation: Receptor stimulation, ionic fluxes, and arachidonic acid metabolism, in: *Lymphokines*, Vol. 4, pp. 297–334, Academic Press, New York.

Bergman, K., Burke, P. V., Cerda-Olmedo, E., David, C. N., Delbrück, M., Foster, K. W., Goodell, E. W., Heisenberg, M., Meissner, G., Zalokar, M., Dennison, D. S., and Shropshire, V., Jr., 1969, Phycomyces, *Bacteriol. Rev.* 33:99.

Bergmann, J. E., Kupfer, A., and Singer, S. J., 1983, Membrane insertion at the leading edge of motile fibroblasts, *Proc. Natl. Acad. Sci. (USA)* 80:1367.

Birnbaumer, L., Pohl, S. L., and Kaumann, A. J., 1974, Receptors and acceptors: A necessary distinction in hormone binding studies, *Adv. Cyclic Nucleotide Res.* 4:239.

Bourguignon, L. Y. W., and Singer, S. J., 1977, Transmembrane interactions and mechanism of capping of surface receptors by their specific ligands, *Proc. Natl. Acad. Sci. (USA)* 74:5031.

Brenner, S. L., and Korn, E. D., 1979, Substoichiometric concentrations of cytochalasin D inhibit actin polymerization, *J. Biol. Chem.* 254:9982.

Brentwood, B. J., and Henson, P. M., 1980, The sequential release of granule constituents from human neutrophils, *J. Immunol.* 124:855.

Brown, S. S., and Spudich, J. A., 1981, Mechanism of action of cytochalasin: Evidence that it binds to actin filament ends, *J. Cell Biol.* 88:487.

Burridge, K., and Feramisco, J. R., 1981, α-Actinin and vinculin from non-muscle cells: Calcium sensitive interactions with actin, *Cold Spring Harb. Symp. Quant. Biol.* **46**:587.

Caner, J. E. Z., 1965, Colchicine inhibition of chemotaxis, *Arthritis Rheum.* **8**:757.

Carp, H., 1982, Mitochondrial N-formyl methionyl proteins as chemoattractants for neutrophils, *J. Exp. Med.* **155**:264.

Carroll, R. C., and Gerrard, J. M., 1982, Phosphorylation of platelet actin binding protein during platelet activation, *Blood* **59**:466.

Chenoweth, D. E., and Hugli, T. E., 1978, Demonstration of specific C5a receptor on intact human polymorphonuclear leukocytes, *Proc. Natl. Acad. Sci. (USA)* **75**:3943.

Clark, R. A., and Szot, S., 1982, Chemotactic factor inactivation by stimulated human neutrophils mediated by a myeloperoxidase-catalyzed methionine oxidation, *J. Immunol.* **128**:1507.

Cochrane, C. G., 1977, Role of granulocytes in immune complex-induced tissue injuries, *Inflammation* **2**:319.

Cohen, S., Carpenter, G., and King, L., 1980, Epidermal growth factor–receptor–protein kinase interactions. Co-purification of receptor and epidermal growth factor-enhanced phosphorylation activity, *J. Biol. Chem.* **255**:4834.

Corin, R. E., and Donner, D. B., 1982, Insulin receptors convert to a higher affinity state subsequent to hormone binding, *J. Biol. Chem.* **257**:104.

Courtoy, P. J., Quinart, J., and Baudhuin, P., 1982, Shift in the equilibrium density of subcellular organelles containing peroxidase using the diaminobenzidine procedure, *J. Cell. Biol.* **95**:423a.

Craddock, P. R., Hammerschmidt, D. E., Moldow, C. F., Yamada, O., and Jacob, H. S., 1979, Granulocyte aggregates as a manifestation of membrane interaction of complement: Possible roles in leukocyte margination, microvascular occlusion and endothelial damage, *Semin. Hematol.* **16**:140.

Cramer, E. B., and Gallin, J. I., 1979, Localization of submembraneous cations to the leading end of human neutrophils during chemotaxis, *J. Cell Biol.* **82**:369.

Cramer, E. B., and Milks, L. C., 1982, Transepithelial migration of human neutrophils. II. Permeability studies, *Fed. Proc.* **41**:372.

Davis, B. H., Walter, R. J., Pearson, C. B., Becker, E. L., and Oliver, J. M., 1982, Membrane activity and topography of F-Met-Leu-Phe-treated polymorphonuclear leukocytes, *Am. J. Pathol.* **108**:206.

De Chatelet, L. R., 1978, Initiation of the respiratory burst in human neutrophils. A critical review, *J. Reticuloendothel. Soc.* **24**:73.

Delbrück, M., and Reichardt, W., 1956, System analysis for the light growth reactions of phycomyces, *Cell. Mechanisms Differentiation Growth* **14**:3.

DeLisi, C., and Siraganian, R. P., 1979a, Receptor crosslinking and histamine release. I. The quantitative dependence of basophil degranulation on the number of receptor doublets, *J. Immunol.* **122**:2286.

DeLisi, C., and Siraganian, R. P., 1979b, Receptor crosslinking and histamine release. II. Interpretation and analysis of anomalous dose response patterns, *J. Immunol.* **122**:2293.

Dougherty, R. W., Carchman, R. A., and Freer, R. J., 1983, Comparison of formyl peptide receptors in human neutrophils and HL-60 cells. Binding and secretion, *Fed. Proc.* **42**:1357.

Fehr, J., and Dahinden, C., 1979, Modulating influence of chemotactic factor-induced cell adhesiveness on granulocyte function, *J. Clin. Invest.* **64**:8.

Finney, D. A., and Sklar, L. A., 1983, Ligand/receptor internalization: A kinetic, flow cytometric analysis of the internalization of N-formyl peptides by human neutrophils, *Cytometry* **4**:54.

Flanagan, J., and Koch, C. L. E., 1978, Cross-linked surface Ig attached to actin, *Nature* **273**:278.

Fletcher, M. P., and Gallin, J. I., 1982, Human neutrophils contain an intracellular pool of putative receptors for the chemoattractant *N*-formyl methionylleucylphenylaline with a density of specific granules, *J. Cell Biol.* **95**:444a.

Fletcher, M. P., Seligmann, B. E., and Gallin, J. I., 1982, Correlation of human neutrophil secretion, chemoattractant receptor mobilization and enhanced functional capacity, *J. Immunol.* **128**:941.

Freer, R. J., Day, A. R., Radding, J. A., Schiffman, E., Aswanikumar, S., Showell, H. J., and Becker, E. L., 1980, Further studies on the structural requirements for synthetic peptide chemoattractants, *Biochemistry* **19**:2404.

Freer, R. J., Day, A. R., Muthukumaraswamy, N., Pinon, D., Wu, A., Showell, H. J., and Becker, E. L., 1982, Formyl peptide chemoattractants: A model of the receptor on rabbit neutrophils, *Biochemistry* **21**:257.

Gallin, J. I., Wright, D. G., and Schiffmann, E., 1978, Role of secretory events in modulating human neutrophil chemotaxis, *J. Clin. Invest.* **62**:1364.

Gallin, J. I., Gallin, E. K., and Schiffmann, E., 1979, Mechanism of leukocyte chemotaxis, in: *Advances in Inflammation Research* (G. Weissman, ed.), pp. 123–138, Raven Press, New York.

Geisow, M. J., 1982, Intracellular membrane traffic, *Nature* **295**:649.

Gerish, G., and Keller, H. U., 1981, Chemotactic reorientation of granulocytes stimulated with micropipettes containing F-Met-Leu-Phe, *J. Cell Sci.* **52**:1.

Ghebrehiwet, B., and Müller-Eberhard, 1979, C3e: An acidic fragment of human C3 with leukocytosis inducing activity, *J. Immunol.* **123**:616.

Goetzl, E. J., Foster, D. W., and Goldman, D. W., 1981, Isolation and partial characterization of membrane protein constituents of human neutrophil receptors for chemotactic formyl methioyl peptides, *Biochemistry* **20**:5717.

Goldstein, I., Hoffstein, S., Gallin, J., and Weissmann, G., 1973, Mechanisms of lysosomal enzyme release from human leukocytes: Microtubule assembly and membrane fusion induced by a component of complement, *Proc. Natl. Acad. Sci. (USA)* **70**:2916.

Harris, A., and Dunn, G., 1972, Centripetal transport of attached particles on both surfaces of moving fibroblasts, *Exp. Cell. Res.* **73**:519.

Hazelbauer, G. L. (ed.), 1978, Taxis and behavior, in: *Receptors and Recognition*, Ser. B, Vol. 5, Chapman and Hall, London.

Henson, P. M., Schwartzmann, N. A., and Zanolari, B., 1981, Intracellular control of human neutrophil secretion. II. Stimulus specificity of desensitization induced by six different soluble and particulate stimuli, *J. Immunol.* **127**:754.

Hoffstein, S., Godstein, I. M., and Weissmann, G., 1977, Role of microtubule assembly in lysosomal enzyme secretion from human polymorphonuclear leukocytes. A reevaluation, *J. Cell Biol.* **73**:242.

Huxley, H. E., 1973, Muscular contraction and cell motility, *Nature* **243**:445.

Ishizaka, T., 1982, Biochemical analysis of triggering signals induced by bridging of IgE receptors, *Fed. Proc.* **41**:17.

Jesaitis, A. J., and Cochrane, C. G., 1983, Receptor mediated endocytosis, host defense and inflammation, *Lab Invest.* **48**:117.

Jesaitis, A. J., Naemura, J. R., Painter, R. G., Sklar, L. A., and Cochrane, C. G., 1982*a*, Intracellular localization of *N*-formyl chemotactic receptor and Mg^{+2} dependent ATPase in human granulocytes, *Biophys. Biochim. Acta* **719**:556.

Jesaitis, A. J., Naemura, J. R., Painter, R. G., Schmitt, M., Sklar, L. A., and Cochrane, C. G., 1982*b*, The fate of the *N*-formylated chemotactic peptide receptor in stimulated human granulocytes: Subcellular fractionation studies, *J. Cell. Biochem.* **20**:143.

Jesaitis, A. J., Naemura, J. R., Painter, R. G., Sklar, L. A., and Cochrane, C. G., 1983, The fate of the *N*-formylated chemotactic peptide in stimulated human granulocytes: Subcellular fractionation studies, *J. Biol. Chem.* **258**:1968.

Jesaitis, A. J., Naemura, J. R., Sklar, L. A., Cochrane, C. G., and Painter, R. G., 1984, Rapid modulation of *N*-formyl chemotactic peptide receptors on the surface of human granulocytes: Formation of high affinity ligand-receptor complexes in transient association with cell cytoskeleton, *J. Cell. Biol.* (in press).

Johnson, K. J., and Ward, P. A., 1982, Newer concepts in the pathogenesis of immune complex induced tissue injury, *Lab. Invest.* **47**:218.

Jones, H. P., Ghai, G., Petrone, W. F., and McCord, J. M. 1982, Calmodulin-dependent stimulation of the NADPH oxidase of human neutrophils, *Biochim. Biophys. Acta* **714**:152.

Keller, H. U., and Bessis, M., 1975, Migration and chemotaxis of anucleate cytoplasmic leukocyte fragments, *Nature* **258**:73.

Keller, H. U., Wissler, J. H., Hess, M. W., and Cottier, H., 1977, Relation between stimulus intensity and neutrophil chemotactic response, *Experientia* **33**:534.

Keller, H. U., Wissler, J. H., Hess, M. W., and Cottier, H., 1978, Distant chemokinetic and chemotactic responses in neutrophil granulocytes, *Experientia* **8**:1.

King. A. C., and Cuatrecasas, P., 1981, Peptide hormone induced receptor mobility, aggregation and internalization, *N. Engl. J. Med.* **305**:77.

Koo, C., Lefkowitz, R. J., and Snyderman, R., 1982, The oligopeptide chemotactic factors on human PMN membranes exists in two affinity states, *Fed. Proc.* **41**:272.

Korchak, H. M., and Weissmann, G., 1980, Stimulus response coupling in the human neutrophil: Transmembrane potential and the role of extracellular Na^+, *Biochim. Biophys. Acta* **601**:180.

Koshland, D. E., Jr., 1981, Biochemistry of sensing and adaptation in a simple bacterial system, *Annu. Rev. Biochem.* **50**:765.

Kupfer, A., Louvard, D., and Singer, S. J., 1982, Polarization of the Golgi apparatus and the micotubule-organizaing center in cultured fibroblasts at the edge of an experimental wound, *Proc. Natl. Acad. Sci. (USA)* **79**:2603.

Lane, T. A., and Lamkin, G. E., 1982, Phagocytosis induced chemotaxis receptor cycling in neutrophils as mediated by thiol oxidation, *Blood* **59**:1337.

Lauffenberger, D. A., and Zigmond, S. H., 1981, Chemotactic factor concentration gradients in chemotaxis assay systems, *J. Immunol. Methods* **40**:45.

Limbird, L. E., 1981, Activation and attenuation of adenylate cyclase, *Biochem. J.* **195**:1.

Lin, D. C., Tobin, K. D., Grumet, M., and Lin, S., 1980, Cytochalasins inhibit nuclei-induced actin polymerization by blocking filament elongation, *J. Cell Biol.* **84**:455.

Lipson, E. D., 1975, White noise analysis of *Phycomyces* light growth response system, *Biophys. J.* **15**:989.

Lohr, K. M., and Snyderman, R., 1982, Amphotericin B alters the affinity and functional activity of the oligopeptide chemotactic receptor on human polymorphonuclear leukocytes, *J. Immunol.* **129**:1594.

Lowenstein, W. R. 1971, Principles of receptor physiology, in: *Handbook of Sensory Physiology*, Vol. 1 (W. R. Lowenstein, ed.), Springer-Verlag, Berlin.

Luna, E. J., Fowler, V. M., Swanson, J., Branton, D., and Taylor, D. L., 1981, A membrane cytoskeleton from *Dictyostelium discoideum*. I. Identification and partial purification of an actin binding activity, *J. Cell Biol.* **88**:396.

Mackin, W. M., Huang, C-K., and Becker, E. L., 1982, The formylpeptide chemotactic receptor and rabbit peritoneal neutrophils. I. Evidence for two binding sites with different affinities, *J. Immunol.* **129**:1608.

Malawista, S. E., and Chevance, A. de B., 1982, The cytokineplast: Purified, stable and functional motile machinery from human blood polymorphonuclear leukocytes, *J. Cell. Biol.* **95**:960.

Malech, H. C., Root, R. K., and Gallin, J. I., 1976, Centriole, microtubule and microfilament orientation during human polymorphonuclear leukocyte chemotaxis, *Clin. Res.* 24:314A.

Marmerelius, P. Z., and Naka, K. I., 1973, Nonlinear analysis and synthesis of receptor field responses in the cat fish retina, *J. Neurophys.* 36:605.

Mescher, M. F., Jose, M. J. L., and Balk, S. P., 1981, Actin-containing matrix associated with the plasma membrane of murine tumor and lymphoid cells, *Nature* 289:139.

Müller-Eberhard, H. J., 1981, The human complement protein C3: Its unusual function and structural versatility in host defense and inflammation, in: *Advances in Immunopathology* (W. O. Weigle, ed.), pp. 141–160, Elsevier-North Holland, New York.

Naccache, P. H., Showell, H. J., Becker, E. L., and Sha'afi, R. I., 1977a, Changes in ionic movements across rabbit leukocyte membranes during lysosomal enzyme release, *J. Cell Biol.* 76:635.

Naccache, P. H., Showell, H. J., Becker, E. L., and Sha'afi, R. I., 1977b, Sodium, potassium, and calcium transport across rabbit polymorphonuclear leukocyte membranes. Effect of chemotactic factor, *J. Cell Biol.* 73:428.

Naccache, P. H., Volpi, M., Showell, H. J., Becker, E. L., and Sha'afi, R. I., 1979, Chemotactic factor-induced release of membrane calcium in rabbit neutrophils, *Science* 203:461.

Nelson, R. D., McCormack, R. T., Fiegel, V. D., Herron, M., Simmons, P. L., and Quie, P. G., 1979, Chemotactic deactivation of human neutrophils: Possible relationship to stimulation of oxidative metabolism, *Infect. Immun.* 23:282.

Nelson, R. D., Fiegel, V. D., Herron, M. J., Gracyk, J. M., Bauman, M. P., McCormack, R. T., and Simmons, R. L., 1980, Chemotactic deactivation of human neutrophils: Role of stimulation of hexose monophosphate shunt activity in nonspecific deactivation, *Acta Physiol. Scand. (Suppl.)* 492:31.

Nelson, R. D., Gracyk, J. M., Fiegel, V. D., Herron, M. J., and Chenoweth, D. E., 1981, Chemotactic deactivation of human neutrophils: Protective influence of phenylbutazone, *Blood* 58:752.

Nicolson, G. L., and Painter, R. G., 1973, Anionic sites of human erythrocyte membranes. II. Antispectrin-induced transmembrane aggregation of the binding sites for positively charged colloidal particles, *J. Cell. Biol.* 59:395.

Niedel, J. E., 1981, Detergent solubilization of the formyl peptide chemotactic receptor, *J. Biol. Chem.* 256:9295.

Niedel, J. E., and Cuatrecasas, P., 1980, Formyl peptide chemotactic reception of leukocytes and macrophages, *Curr. Top. Cell Res.* 17:137.

Niedel, J., Wilkinson, S., and Cuatrecasas, P., 1979a, Receptor-mediated uptake and degradation of ^{125}I-chemotactic peptide by human neutrophils, *J. Biol. Chem.* 254:10700.

Niedel, J. E., Kahane, I., and Cuatrecasas, P., 1979b, Receptor mediated internalization of fluorescent chemotactic peptide by human neutrophils, *Science* 205:1412.

Niedel, J. E., Davis, J., and Cuatrecasas, P., 1980, Covalent affinity labelling of the formyl peptide chemotactic receptor, *J. Biol. Chem.* 255:7063.

O'Flaherty, J. T., and Ward, P. A., 1978, Leukocyte aggregation induced by chemotactic factors. A review, *Inflammation* 3:177.

O'Flaherty, J. T., Showell, H. J., and Ward, P. A., 1977, Influence of extracellular Ca^{2+} and Mg^{2+} on chemotactic factor-induced neutrophil aggregation, *Inflammation* 2:265.

Ohno, Y-I, Hirai, K-I, Kanoh, T., Uchino, H., and Ogawa, K., 1982a, Subcellular localization of H_2O_2 production in human neutrophils stimulated with particles and an effect of cytochalasin B on the cells, *Blood* 60:253.

Ohno, Y-I, Hirai, K-I, Kanoh, T., Haruto, U., and Ogawa, K, 1982b, Subcellular localization of hydrogen peroxide production in human polymorphonuclear leukocytes stimulated with lectins, phorbol myristate acetate, and digitonin: An electron microscopic study using $CeCl_3$, *Blood* 60:1195.

Oliver, J. M., Krawiec, J. A., and Becker, E. L., 1978, The distribution of actin during chemotaxis in rabbit neutrophils, *J. Reticuloendothel. Soc.* **24**:697.

Olsson, I., and Venge, P., 1980, The role of the human neutrophil in the inflammatory reaction, *Allergy* **35**:1.

Oseas, R., Yang, H-H, Baehner, R. L., and Boxer, L. A., 1981, Lactoferrin: A promoter of polymorphonuclear leukocyte adhesiveness, *Blood* **57**:939.

Painter, R. G., Schmitt, M., Jesaitis, A. J., Sklar, L. A., Preissner, K., and Cochrane, C. G., 1982, Photoaffinity labeling of the *N*-formyl peptide receptor of human polymorphonuclear leukocytes, *J. Cell. Biochem.* **20**:193.

Painter, R. G., Allen, R. A., Sklar, L. A., Schmitt, M., Cochrane, C. G., and Jesaitis, A. J., 1984a, Intracellular processing of *N*-formulated chemotactic peptide receptors by human neutrophil (submitted).

Painter, R. G., Jesaitis, A. J., and Sklar, L. A., 1984b, Mobilization of the motile apparatus by *N*-formyl chemotactic peptides. Neutrophil chemotaxis: Mobilization of the motile apparatus by *N*-formyl chemotactic peptides, in: *Cell Membranes: Methods and Reviews*, Vol. 1 (E. L. Elson, W. A. Frazier, and L. Glaser, eds.), Plenum Press, New York (in press).

Painter, R. G., Jesaitis, A. J., and Sklar, L. A., 1983b, Mobilization of the motile apparatus by *N*-formyl chemotactic peptides (submitted).

Petrone, W. F., English, D. K., Wong, K., and McCord, J. M., 1980, Free radicals and inflammation: Superoxide dependent activation of neutrophil chemotactic factor in plasma, *Proc. Natl. Acad. Sci. (USA)* **77**:1159.

Pike, M. C., and Snyderman, R., 1982a, Chemoattractant–receptor interaction in leukocytes, in: *Advances in Inflammation Research* (M. Ziff, P. Giampaolo, and S. Gorini, eds.), pp. 109–130, Raven Press, New York.

Pike, M. C., and Snyderman, R., 1982b, Transmethylation reactions regulate affinity and functional activity of chemotactic factor receptors on macrophages, *Cell* **28**:107.

Radin, R. A., Korchak, H. M., Wilkenfeld, C., Rutherford, L. E., and Weissmann, G., 1982, Differential requirements for receptor occupancy in neutrophil responses to chemoattractant, *Clin. Res.* **30**:520A.

Ramsey, W. S., 1972, Analysis of individual leukocyte behavior during chemotaxis, *Exp. Cell. Res.* **70**:129.

Rao, K. M. K., and Varani, J., 1982, Actin polymerization induced by chemotactic peptide and concanavalin A in rat neutrophils, *J. Immunol.* **129**:1605.

Rasmussen, H., 1981, *Calcium and cAMP as Synarchic Messengers*, Wiley–Interscience, New York.

Robinson, D. R., Curran, D. P., and Hamer, P. J., 1982, Prostaglandins and related compounds in inflammatory rheumatic diseases, in: *Advances in Inflammation Research*, Vol. 3, (M. Ziff, P. Giampaolo, S. Gorini, eds.), pp. 17–27, Raven Press, New York.

Rosenberg, S., Stracher, A., and Burridge, K., 1981, Isolation and characterization of a calcium-sensitive α-actinin-like protein from human platelet cytoskeletons, *J. Biol. Chem.* **256**:12986.

Schiffmann, E., 1982, Leukocytes chemotaxis, *Annu. Rev. Physiol.* **44**:553.

Schiffmann, E., Corcoran, B. A., and Wahl, S. M., 1975, *N*-formyl methionyl peptides as chemoattractants for leukocytes, *Proc. Natl. Acad. Sci. (USA)* **72**:1059.

Schmitt, M., Painter, R. G., Jesaitis, A. J., Preissner, K., Sklar, L. A., and Cochrane, C. G., 1983, Photoaffinity labeling of the *N*-formyl peptide receptor binding site of intact human polymorphonuclear leukocytes. Evaluation of a label as suitable to follow the fate of the receptor–ligand complex, *J. Biol. Chem.* **258**:649.

Schneider, Y. J., Tulkens, P., de Duve, C., and Touet, A., 1979, Fate of plasma membrane during endocytosis, *J. Cell. Biol.* **82**:466.

Schreiber, A. B., Liberman, T. A., Lax, I., Yarden, Y., and Schlessinger, J., 1983, Biological role of experimental growth factor–receptor clustering, *J. Biol. Chem.* **258**:846.

Sefton, B. M., Hunter, T., Ball, E. H., and Singer, S. J., 1981, Vinculin: A cytoskeletal target of the transforming protein of Rous sarcoma virus, *Cell* **24**:165.

Seligmann, B. E., and Gallin, J. I., 1980, Use of lipophilic probes of membrane potential to assess human neutrophil activation. Abnormality in chronic granulomatous disease, *J. Clin. Invest.* **66**:493.

Seligmann, B., Chused, T., and Gallin, J. I., 1982a, Binding of fluoresceinated chemotactic peptide to human neutrophil is heterogeneous and correlates with the heterogeneous stimulation of membrane potential changes, *J. Cell. Biol.* **95**:444a.

Seligmann, B. E., Fletcher, M. P., and Gallin, J. I., 1982b, Adaptation of human neutrophil responsiveness to the chemoattractant *N*-formylmethionylleucylphenylalanine, *J. Biol. Chem.* **257**:6280.

Shaw, J. O., Pinckard, R. N., McManus, L. M., and Hanahan, D. J., 1981, Activation of human neutrophils with 1-*O*-hexadecyl/octadecyl-2-acetyl-*Sn*-glycerol-3-phosphate (platelet activating factor), *J. Immunol.* **127**:1250.

Showell, H. J., Freer, R. J., Zigmond, S. H., Schiffmann, E., Aswanikumar, S., Corcoran, B., and Becker, E. L., 1976, The structure–activity relations of synthetic peptides as chemotactic factors and inducers of lysozomal enzyme secretion for neutrophils, *J. Exp. Med.* **143**:1154.

Simchowitz, L., Fishbein, L. C., Spilberg, I., and Atkinson, J. P., 1980a, Induction of a transient elevation in intracellular levels of adenosine-3′,5′-cyclic monophosphate by chemotactic factors: An early event in human neutrophil activation, *J. Immunol.* **124**:1482.

Simchowitz, L., Atkinson, J. P., and Spilberg, I., 1980b, Stimulus-specific deactivation of chemotactic factor-induced cyclic AMP response and superoxide generation by human neutrophils, *J. Clin. Invest.* **66**:736.

Sklar, L. A., and Finney, D. A., 1982, Analysis of ligand–receptor interactions with the fluorescence activated cell sorter, *Cytometry* **3**:161.

Sklar, L. A., Jesaitis, A. J., Painter, R. G., and Cochrane, C. G., 1981a, The kinetics of neutrophil activation: The response to chemotactic peptides depends upon whether ligand–receptor interaction is rate-limiting, *J. Biol. Chem.* **256**:9909.

Sklar, L. A., Oades, Z. G., Jesaitis, A. J., Painter, R. G., and Cochrane, C. G., 1981b, Fluoresceinated chemotactic peptide and high affinity antibody to fluorescein as a probe of the temporal characteristics of neutrophil stimulation, *Proc. Natl. Acad. Sci. (USA)* **78**:7540.

Sklar, L. A., McNeil, V. M., Jesaitis, A. J., Painter, R. G., and Cochrane, C. G., 1982a, A continuous, spectroscopic analysis of the kinetics of elastase secretion by neutrophils. The dependence of secretion upon receptor occupancy, *J. Biol. Chem.* **257**:5471.

Sklar, L. A., Jesaitis, A. J., Painter, R. G., and Cochrane, C. G., 1982b, Ligand/receptor internalization: A spectroscopic analysis and a comparison of ligand binding, cellular response, and internalization by human neutrophils, *J. Cell. Biochem.* **20**:193.

Sklar, L. A., Jesaitis, A. J., Painter, R. G., and Cochrane, C. G., 1983a, Quantitative analysis of the relationship between receptor occupancy and cellular response in the human neutrophil, *Biophys. J.* **41**:132a.

Sklar, L. A., Jesaitis, A. J., Painter, R. G., and Cochrane, C. G., 1983b, The dynamics of ligand–receptor interactions. Real time fluorimetric analyses of association, dissociation, and internalization of an *N*-formyl peptide and its receptors on human neutrophils, *J. Biol. Chem.* (in press).

Sklar, L. A., McNeil, V. M., and Finney, D. A., 1983c, Competitive binding kinetics in ligand–receptor–inhibitor systems: Theoretical and experimental approaches, *Circulation* **66**, Supplement III, page F.

Smith, C. W., Hollers, J. C., Patrick, R. A., and Harrett, C., 1979, Motility and adhesiveness in human neutrophils, *J. Clin. Invest.* **63**:221.

Smolen, J. E., and Weissmann, G., 1981, Stimuli which provoke secretion of azurophil enzymes from human neutrophils induce increments in adenosine cyclic 3′-5′-monophosphate, *Biochim. Biophys. Acta* **672**:197.

Smolen, J. E., Korchak, H. M., and Weissmann, G., 1980, Initial kinetics of lysozomal enzyme secretion and superoxide anion generation by human polymorphonuclear leukocytes, *Inflammation* **4**:145.

Smolen, J. E., Korchak, H. M., and Weissmann, G., 1981, The roles of extracellular and intracellular calcium in lysozomal enzyme release and superoxide generation by human neutrophils, *Biochim. Biophys. Acta* **677**:512.

Smolen, J. E., Korchak, H. M., and Weissmann, G., 1982, The kinetics of lysosomal degranulation of human neutrophils as measured by 9-amino acridine self-quenching, *J. Cell. Biol.* **95**:397a.

Snyderman, R., and Goetzl, E. J., 1981, Molecular and cellular mechanisms of leukocyte chemotaxis, *Science* **213**:830.

Snyderman, R., Edge, S., and Pike, M. C., 1982, Macrophage chemotactic factor receptor exists in two interconvertible affinities modulated by guanine nucleotides, *Clin. Res.* **30**:521A.

Stephens, C. G., and Snyderman, R., 1982, Cyclic nucleotides regulate the morphologic alterations required for chemotaxis in monocytes, *J. Immunol.* **126**:1192.

Stevens, S. S., 1971, Sensory power functions and neutral events, in: *Handbook of Sensory Physiology*, Vol. 1 (W. E. Lowenstein, ed.), p. 226, Springer-Verlag, Berlin.

Stossel, T. P., 1978, The mechanism of leukocyte locomotion, in: *Leukocyte Chemotaxis: Methods, Physiology and Clinical Implications* (J. I. Gallin and P. G. Quie, eds.), p. 143, Raven Press, New York.

Stossel, T. P., Hartwig, J. H., Yin, H-L, and Zaner, K. S., 1981, Structure of the cortical cytoplasm, *Cold Spring Harb. Symp. Quant. Biol.* **46**:569.

Stryer, L., Hurley, J. B., and Fung, B. K-K., 1981, Transducin: An amplifier protein in vision, *Trends Biol. Sci.* **6**:245.

Sullivan, S. J., and Zigmond, S. H., 1980, Chemotactic peptide receptor modulation in polymorphonuclear leukocytes, *J. Cell. Biol.* **85**:703.

Sullivan, S. J., and Zigmond, S. H., 1982, Asymmetric receptor distribution on PMNs, *J. Cell. Biol.* **95**:418a.

Taylor, D. L., Hellewell, S. B., Virgin, H. W., and Heiple, J. M., 1979, The solation–contraction coupling hypothesis of cell movements, in: *Cell Motility: Molecules and Organization* (S. Hatano, H. Ishikawa, and H. Sato, eds.), p. 363, University of Tokyo Press, Tokyo.

Taylor, D. L., Wang, Y. L., and Heiple, J., 1980a, The contractile basis of ameboid movement. VII. The distribution of fluorescently labeled actin in living amoebas, *J. Cell. Biol.* **86**:590.

Taylor, D. L, Blinks, J. R., and Reynolds, G., 1980b, Contractile basis of ameboid movement. VIII. Aequorin luminescence during ameboid movement, endocytosis and capping, *J. Cell. Biol.* **86**:599.

Taylor, D. L, Heiple, J., Wang, Y-L, Luna, E. J., Tanasugarn, L., Brier, J., Swanson, J., Fecheimer, M., Amato, P., Rockwell, M., and Daley, G., 1981, Cellular and molecular aspects of amoeboid movement, *Cold Spring Harb. Symp. Quant. Biol.* **XLVI**:101.

Tsan, M-F, and Chen, J. W., 1980, Oxidation of methionine by human PMNs, *J. Clin. Invest.* **65**:1041.

Tsien, R. Y., Pozzan, T., and Rink, T. J., 1982, Calcium homeostasis in intact lymphocytes:

Cytoplasmic free calcium monitored with a new, intracellularly trapped fluorescent indicator, *J. Cell. Biol.* **94**:325.

Vane, J. R., 1976, Prostaglandins as mediators of inflammation, in: *Advances in Prostaglandin and Thromboxane Research* (B. Samuelsson and R. Paoletti, eds.), pp. 791–801, Raven Press, New York.

Vitkauskas, G., Showell, H. J., and Becker, E. L., 1980, Specific binding of synthetic chemotactic peptides to rabbit peritoneal neutrophils: Effects on dissociability of bound peptide, receptor activity and subsequent biologic responsiveness (deactivation), *Mol. Immunol.* **17**:171.

Wallach, D., Davies, P. J. A., and Pastan, I., 1978, Cyclic AMP dependent phosphorylation of filamin in smooth muscle, *J. Biol. Chem.* **253**:4739.

Walter, R. J., Berlin, R. D., and Oliver, J. M., 1980, Asymmetric Fc receptor distribution of human PMN oriented in a chemotactic gradient, *Nature* **286**:724.

Weissmann, G., Smolen, J., Korchak, H., and Hoffstein, S., 1981, The secretory code of the neutrophil in cellular interactions, in: *Research Monographs in Cell and Tissue Physiology* (J. T. Dingle and J. L. Gordon, eds.), pp. 15–31, Elsevier North-Holland Biomedical Press, New York.

White, J. R., Naccache, P. H., and Sha'afi, R. I., 1982, The synthetic chemotactic peptide formyl-methionyl-leucyl-phenylalanine causes an increase in actin associated with the cytoskeleton in rabbit neutrophils, *Biochem. Biophys. Res. Commun.* **108**:1144.

Wilkinson, P. C., Michl, J., and Silverstein, S. C., 1980, Receptor distribution in locomoting neutrophils, *Cell Biol. Int. Rep.* **4**:736.

Williams, L. T., Snyderman, R., Pike, M. C., and Lefkowitz, R. J., 1977, Specific receptor sites for chemotactic peptides on human polymorphonuclear leukocytes, *Proc. Natl. Acad. Sci. (USA)* **74**:1204.

Willingham, M. C., and Pastan, I., 1980, The receptosome: An intermediate organelle of receptor mediated endocytosis in cultured fibroblasts, *Cell* **21**:67.

Wright, D. G., and Gallin, J. I., 1979, Secretory responses of human neutrophils: Exocytosis of specific (secondary) granules by human neutrophils during adherence *in vitro* and during exudation *in vivo*, *J. Immunol.* **123**:285.

Yin, H. L, Albrecht, J. H., and Faltoum, A., 1981, Identification of gel-solin, a Ca^{2+} dependent regulatory protein of actin gel-sol transformation and its intracellular distribution in a variety of cells and tissues, *J. Cell. Biol.* **91**:901.

Young, J. D-E., Young, T. M., Kaback, H. R., Cohn, Z. A., and Unkeless, J. C., 1982, The IgG Fc receptor is a ligand activated ion channel, *J. Cell. Biol.* **95**:443a.

Yuli, I., Tomonago, A., and Snyderman, R., 1982, Chemoattractant receptor functions in human polymorphonuclear leukocytes are divergently altered by membrane fluidizers, *Proc. Natl. Acad. Sci. (USA)* **79**:5906.

Zigmond, S. H., 1977, Ability of polymorphonuclear leukocytes to orient in gradients of chemotactic factors, *J. Cell. Biol.* **75**:606.

Zigmond, S. H., 1978, Chemotaxis by polymorphonuclear leukocytes, *J. Cell. Biol.* **77**:269.

Zigmond, S. H., 1981, Consequences of chemotactic peptide receptor modulation for leukocyte orientation, *J. Cell. Biol.* **88**:644.

Zigmond, S. H., and Sullivan, S. J., 1979, Sensory adaptation of leukocytes to chemotactic peptides, *J. Cell. Biol.* **82**:517.

Zigmond, S. H., Levitsky, H. J., and Kreel, B. J., 1981, Cell polarity: An examination of its behavioral expression and its consequences for polymorphonuclear leukocyte chemotaxis, *J. Cell. Biol.* **89**:585.

Zigmond, S. H., Sullivan, S. J., and Lauffenburger, D. A., 1982, Kinetic analysis of chemotactic receptor modulation, *J. Cell. Biol.* **92**:34.

Chapter 3

Neutrophil Chemoattractant fMet-Leu-Phe Receptor Expression and Ionic Events Following Activation

John I. Gallin and Bruce E. Seligmann

Bacterial Diseases Section
Laboratory of Clinical Investigation
National Institute of Allergy and Infectious Diseases
National Institutes of Health
Bethesda, Maryland 20205

I. INTRODUCTION

The identification of receptors for chemotactic factors on neutrophils opened a new era in the investigation of these cells. The first chemoattractant receptor defined was for the synthetic peptide N-formyl-methionylleucyl-phenylalanine (fMet-Leu-Phe) (Aswanikumar *et al.*, 1977; Williams *et al.*, 1977), which had been discovered by Schiffmann *et al.* (1975). This receptor was linked to chemoattractant-elicited events of directed locomotion, activation of the respiratory burst, and degranulation of lysosomal enzymes (Becker, 1979). Subsequently receptors have been defined for numerous chemoattractants (Chenoweth and Hugli, 1978; Spilberg and Mehta, 1979; Wilkinson and Allan, 1978), although the best studied receptor is for fMet-Leu-Phe and closely related analogues.

The dynamics of the fMet-Leu-Phe receptor appear to have an important modulatory role in neutrophil responsiveness. A schematic diagram of the events currently thought to be important in fMet-Leu-Phe receptor modulation is shown in Figure 1. On the basis of studies using N-formyl-blocked oligopep-tide chemoattractants, modulation of neutrophils through receptor binding of chemoattractant is thought to involve differential occupancy of chemoattrac-tant receptors along the length of the cell, presumably to amplify the detection of low concentrations of chemoattractant. Such asymmetric receptor occupancy

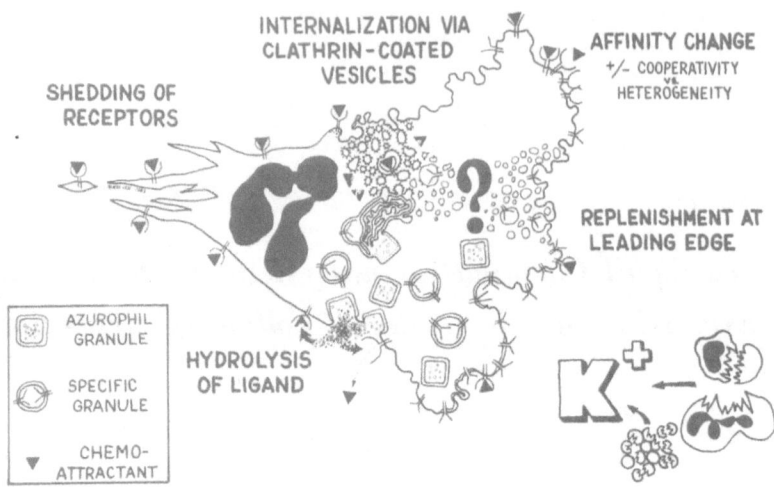

Figure 1. Hypothetical model of the dynamics of the fMet-Leu-Phe receptor on human neutrophils. (Adapted from Gallin *et al.*, 1983.)

has been shown to occur (Sullivan and Zigmond, 1982). It has been speculated to result from several processes, including capping of receptors to the front end of the cell and/or shedding, or internalization or downregulation of receptors probably via clathrin-coated vesicles, which have been shown to be in the rear of the cell (Davis *et al.*, 1982). Replenishment of receptors at the leading edge of the cell, possibly by recycling of used receptors (Zigmond *et al.*, 1982) and/ or by translocation of a pool of spare receptors (Fletcher *et al.*, 1982) is also thought to contribute to the mechanism for sensing a chemoattractant gradient (J. I. Gallin, 1982). Clearance of ligand from receptors may also occur by chemoattractant hydrolysis, since the potency of synthetic peptide chemoattractants is related to their ability to be hydrolyzed by the cell and agents that block peptide hydrolysis inhibit chemotaxis (Aswanikumar *et al.*, 1976).

Sensing a gradient of chemoattractant may involve changes in the affinity of the receptor for its ligand. Heterogeneity and/or negative cooperative interaction of the fMet-Leu-Phe receptor is thought to be the mechanism for the different affinity states of the receptor (Seligmann *et al.*, 1982a). Chemotaxis has been postulated to relate to a high-affinity state of the receptor, while degranulation and superoxide production relate to a low-affinity state (Koo *et al.*, 1982; Lohr and Snyderman, 1982). The complexity of the fMet-Leu-Phe receptor is complicated by the demonstration of heterogeneity among peripheral blood human neutrophils in their expression of, and responsiveness to the receptor (Seligmann *et al.*, 1981). The purpose of this chapter is to summarize the current status of the fMet-Leu-Phe receptor and to review the earliest events (elicited changes in membrane potential) that follow its occupation by ligand.

II. DYNAMICS OF THE fMET-LEU-PHE RECEPTOR

A. Receptor Turnover

Recycling of the N-formylated chemotactic peptide receptor in neutrophils has been suggested from data indicating receptor-modified time-dependent and temperature-dependent endocytosis of ligand within minutes of binding to its receptor (Niedel et al., 1979; Sullivan and Zigmond, 1980) as well as ligand appearance in the cytosol and Golgi-like structures (Jesaitis et al., 1983). With internalization of ligand there is a decrease in expressed receptors, a process called downregulation. Subsequently upregulation of receptor expression occurs and, with continuous exposure to ligand 4- to 5-fold more chemoattractant, is taken up by the cell, via specific receptors, compared with the amount originally bound. The evidence of Jesaitis et al. (1982) suggests that receptor internalization occurs along with internalization of ligand. The ligand is ultimately separated from the receptor upon entering an acidic intracellular compartment. Since surface binding is maintained at a steady state during this process, it appears that there is either a recycling of used receptors or a large reservoir or pool of cryptic receptors (Zigmond et al., 1982; Fletcher et al., 1982). The data for recycling are indirect as are the data for internalization of the receptor, which are based on studies in which ligand is crosslinked to the putative receptor and its fate followed. From the published data on ligand internalization (Niedel et al., 1979a,b), it is not clear whether the intact ligand or just a labeled piece of the parent peptide is internalized. Neutrophils continue to accumulate ligand into a nondisplaceable, i.e., internalized, pool even after the number of surface receptors has attained a steady state (Sullivan and Zigmond, 1980). By analysis of kinetic studies of down regulation, receptor-mediated peptide uptake, and receptor recovery, Zigmond et al. (1982) have suggested that the plateau of surface receptor number that is reached when cells are incubated with a formyl peptide chemoattractant represents a steady state in which receptor-mediated internalization of binding sites is approximately equal to the rate of receptor recovery, although no direct evidence was presented for formyl peptide receptor recycling. A recent study by Niedel indicated that after proteolytic marking of the surface fMet-Leu-Phe receptor, the proteolytically labeled receptor failed to reappear on the cell surface after internalization (Niedel and Dolmatch, 1983). This could be interpreted to indicate recycling of receptor does not occur. Thus the data strongly indicate that if recycling of the fMet-Leu-Phe receptor occurs a storage pool of receptors probably exists as well. The use of a number of agents listed in Table I that modulate receptor expression as well as the application of recently available techniques including detergent solubilization of the receptor (Niedel, 1981), antibodies against the receptor (Marasco et al., 1982; Marasco and Becker, 1982; Goetzl et al., 1982), or photoaffinity labeling of the receptor (Schmitt et al., 1983) should be particularly useful in future studies.

Table I. Known Modulators of Neutrophil Oligopeptide Receptor Function

Modifying agent(s)[a]	Effects on binding and/or receptor function[b]	Proposed mechanism	Reference
Secretagogues (e.g., PMA, A32187, Ca^{2+})			
Low dose	↑ Number, ↓ affinity	Translocation of organelle membrane to the cell surface	J. I. Gallin et al. (1978); Fletcher and Gallin (1980); Fletcher et al. (1982)
High dose	↓ Binding	Destruction of receptor	
Aliphatic alcohols (e.g., butanol)	↑ Binding	Solvent effect	Liao and Freer (1980); Fletcher et al. (1982)
	↑ Number, ↑ affinity; ↑ ctx; ↓ O_2^-; ↓ secretion	Affinity change	Yuli et al. (1982)
Phospholipases A_2, C	↑ Binding		Schiffmann et al. (1980)
Amphotericin B Nystatin	↑ Number, ↓ affinity; ↓ ctx; no effect O_2^- or secretion	Altered membrane fluidity or affinity change	Lohr and Snyderman (1982)
Dimethyl sulfoxide Dimethylformamide	↑ Number and function	Stimulates differentiation of HL-60 cell line	Niedel et al. (1980b) Fontana et al. (1980)

Agent	Effect	Mechanism	Reference
Peptide attractants (e.g., fMet-Leu-Phe)			
Low dose	Increases FMLP response Km; no change in maximum response.	Negative cooperativity or receptor heterogeneity	Seligmann et al. (1983)
High dose	↓ Number	Downregulation; then receptor recovery	Koo et al. (1982)
	↓ Number then ↑ number		Donabedian and Gallin (1981)
Protease inhibitors (e.g., TPCK, PBET, TBET)	↓ Ligand uptake at 37°C	Blocks receptor-mediated ligand internalization	Niedel et al. (1980b)
	↑ Binding at 0°C	Proteolysis of peptide	Fletcher and Gallin (1980)
Glucocorticoids	↓ Affinity	↓ K_a; no change K_d	Skubitz et al. (1981)
Cytochalasin B (microfilament disrupter)	↓ Binding	Blocks receptor-mediated ligand internalization	Koo et al. (1980)
ETYA (inhibitor of cyclooxygenase and lipooxygenase pathways)	↓ Binding	Unclear; nonspecific effect on membrane	Atkinson et al. (1982)

Source: Modified from Fletcher and Gallin (1983).

[a]*Abbreviations:* A23187: Calcium ionophore A23187; ctx, chemotaxis; ETYA, 5,8,11,14-eicosatetraynoic acid; FMLP, fMet-Leu-Phe; O_2^-, superoxide generation; PBET: L-phenylalaninebenzyl ester-p-tosylate; PMA, phorbol myristate acetate; TBET, L-tyrosine-benzyl ester-p-tosylate; TPCK, 1-tosylamido-2-phenylethylchloromethylketone.

[b]I = increased, 0 decreased.

The downregulation of receptors after ligand–receptor interaction is associated with a decrease in functional responsiveness (chemotaxis) to the same concentration of stimulus; this inhibition of chemotaxis is preferential for the chemoattractant used (Sullivan and Zigmond, 1979; Zigmond and Sullivan, 1979; Zigmond, 1981; Donabedian and Gallin, 1981). Whether the downregulation of the fMet-Leu-Phe receptor after incubation with fMet-Leu-Phe reflects receptor internalization, hydrolysis of the receptor by secreted products, or shedding into the extracellular environment is not known. When the cell recovers receptors and actually has increased expressed receptors, the chemotactic response of the cells remains impaired when cells are tested against the same concentration of the chemoattractant. Clearly, the presence of adequate numbers of receptors is insufficient for a sustained chemotactic response, a point addressed in Section II.B.

1. Evidence for a Reservoir of fMet-Leu-Phe Receptors

Neutrophil chemotaxis and fMet-Leu-Phe receptor mobilization after ligand interaction are not affected by protein synthesis inhibitors at concentrations that block $[^3H]$ leucine incorporation into trichloroacetic acid (TCA) precipitable material by more than 90% (J. I. Gallin et al., 1978; Fletcher et al., 1982). Thus, if plasma membrane turnover is important for receptor replenishment and cell function, as originally suggested by Stossel (1979), it is unlikely that synthesis of new protein is required.

Receptor replenishment or enhancement at the leading edge of a locomoting neutrophil by translocation of a spare receptor pool is believed by our laboratory to play an important role in maintaining neutrophil responsiveness. This spare receptor pool may come from specific granules or other organelles (Gallin et al., 1979). This hypothesis has grown out of (1) studies demonstrating increased binding of the chemoattractant fMet-Leu-Phe to human neutrophils previously stimulated to release their specific granules preferentially (Fig. 2) and (2) the finding that preferential degranulation of specific granules occurs during exudation of neutrophils into experimentally induced sterile skin blisters in vivo and during migration of isolated neutrophils through Micropore filters toward a chemoattractant stimulus in vitro (Wright and Gallin, 1979). The degranulation occurs at the leading edge of migrating cells (Cramer and Gallin, 1979) and is associated with the addition of new plasma membrane (Hoffstein et al., 1982).

The enhanced fMet-Leu-Phe binding that occurs after specific granule discharge was shown by Scatchard analysis to be compatible with increased numbers of fMet-Leu-Phe receptors (Fletcher and Gallin. 1980). The binding affinity K_a, calculated from the Scatchard analyses, indicated that there was a small but significant decrease in the affinity of the receptors after degranulation ($K_a = 0.15$ nM^{-1} for control versus $K_a = 0.123$ nM^{-1} or stimulated, $P < 0.05$). More recently, as shown in Figure 2, we have demonstrated that the apparent increase

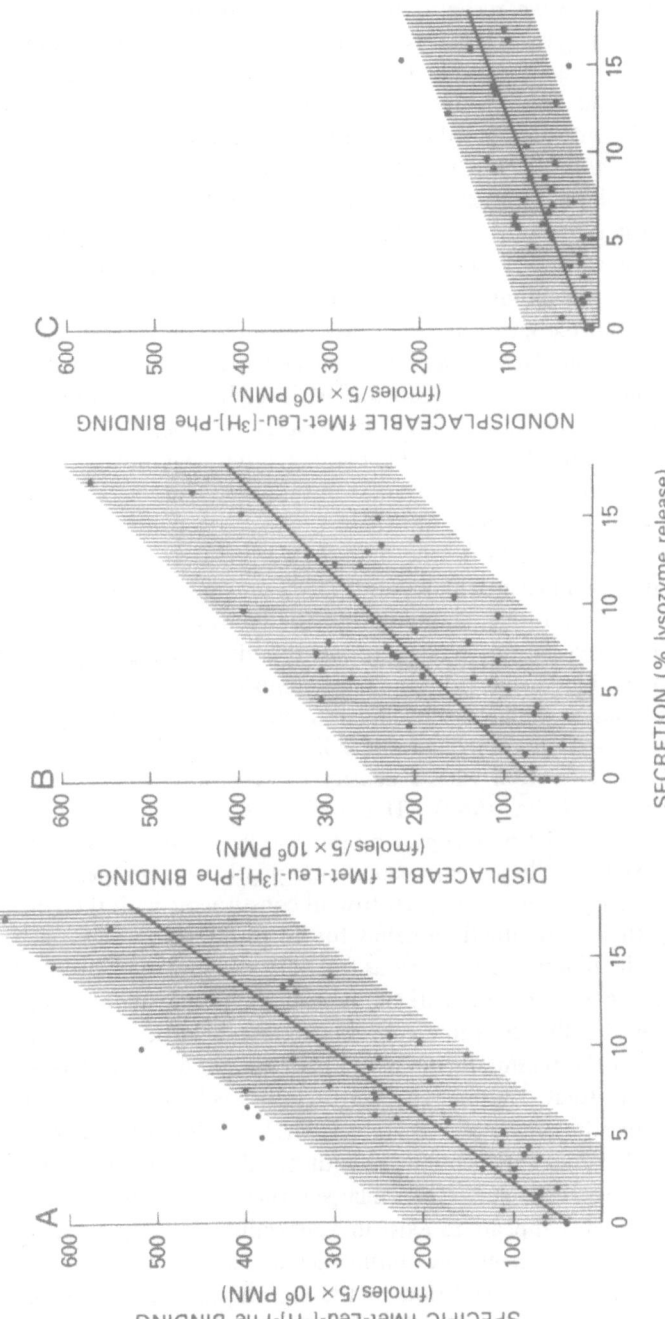

Figure 2. Relationship between secretion and subsequent specific fMet-Leu-[³H]-Phe binding. Pooled data from individual experiments in which polymorphonuclear leukocytes (PMNs) were exposed to varying conditions of stimulation (kept on ice, incubated at 37°C with or without A23187 or PMA) that resulted in a range of measured lysozyme release. The subsequent specific fMet-Leu-[³H]-Phe binding (30-min assay at 0°C) was plotted as a function of the degree of lysozyme release. (A) Plot of total specific binding versus secretion; (B) and (C) plot the displaceable and nondisplaceable components of that binding, respectively. In each case, the best fit line of the data by linear regression analysis demonstrates a significantly positive slope ($P < 0.001$ versus slope = 0, Student's t-test; null hypothesis: slope = 0). The hatched areas represent exact 95% confidence intervals around the regression lines. Each point represents the mean of triplicate and duplicate determinations of binding and lysozyme release, respectively. (From Fletcher et al., 1982, with permission.)

in the number of fMet-Leu-Phe receptors in neutrophils stimulated with low concentrations of secretagogues represents an increase in the number of binding sites from which fMet-Leu-Phe can be readily displaced as well as an increase in the nondisplaceable and presumably internalized pool of peptide. These increases cannot be explained solely on the basis of bulk pinocytosis of extracellular fluid (Fletcher *et al.*, 1982). The specificity of the receptor population made available by stimulation was similar to that of unstimulated neutrophils, as demonstrated by the same rank order of potency of a series of formyl peptide analogues in competing for fMet-Leu-$[^3H]$-Phe binding. The increased binding of fMet-Leu-Phe after limited degranulation was not dependent on protein synthesis, products of oxidative metabolism, or secreted lysozyme or lactoferrin acting on the cell. Similar increases in fMet-Leu-Phe binding have been demonstrated when neutrophils are incubated with high concentrations of chemoattractants (Donabedian and Gallin, 1981; Fletcher *et al.*, 1982). Cells demonstrating increased fMet-Leu-$[^3H]$-Phe binding after degranulation also demonstrate increased functional responsiveness in fMet-Leu-Phe-elicited superoxide and hydrogen peroxide production. These findings are compatible with those of Van Epps and Garcia (1980), who have shown increased metabolic responsiveness in polymorphonuclear leukocytes (PMNs) previously stimulated to chemotax through Micropore filters, and with those of Tsung *et al.* (1980), who have found increased formyl peptide binding to rabbit peritoneal exudate PMNs compared with peripheral blood cells from the same animal.

Direct binding studies to isolated subcellular fractions of disrupted PMNs indicate that human neutrophils contain an intracellular pool of additional fMet-Leu-Phe binding sites in a fraction with a density of specific granules (Gallin *et al.*, 1979; Fletcher and Gallin, 1983). This pool of receptors had the same specificity as the plasma membrane receptor on intact cells, as evidenced by the ability of a family of structurally similar chemotactic peptides to compete with fMet-Leu-$[^3H]$-Phe binding to the various neutrophil constituents with the same rank order shown by their chemotactic potency for intact cells. On the basis of Scatchard analyses of the binding to the various fractions and on the recovery of the neutrophil membrane and granule markers, it would appear that there may be up to 30 times more binding sites in a subcellular fraction with markers for specific granules than on the plasma membrane. Furthermore, when neutrophil plasma membranes were isolated after exposure of intact cells to the specific granule secretagogue phorbol myristate acetate (PMA), binding of fMet-Leu-$[^3H]$-Phe was increased significantly compared with membranes obtained from cells not exposed to the secretagogue. Thus, a large intracellular pool of reserve chemoattractant binding sites appears to exist in a subcellular fraction, which is incorporated into the plasma membrane during degranulation. Jesaitis *et al.* (1982) recently suggested that in addition to the specific granules the Golgi apparatus may also contain a spare pool of fMet-Leu-Phe receptors.

Other investigators have demonstrated that purification of cells from blood enhances formyl peptide binding (Fearon and Collins, 1983). In addition, prior exposure of neutrophils to short-chain aliphatic alcohols or phospholipases increases fMet-Leu-Phe binding (Liao and Freer, 1980; Schiffmann et al., 1980) (Table I). The mechanism(s) for enhancement of fMet-Leu-Phe receptor number by these agents is/are unknown and may vary for the different agents. Unmasking of cryptic receptors found in the membrane by changing membrane fluidity and mobilization of an intracellular receptor pool are possible sources of the receptor upregulation.

It is of interest that an intracellular pool of receptors for ligands other than fMet-Leu-Phe has also been described. Recently Fearon and Collins (1983) reported an intracellular pool of receptors for C3b that was mobilized during cell purification or exposure to chemotactic factors. Interestingly, although these investigators verified that the above procedures mobilized fMet-Leu-Phe receptors as well, they were unable to show enhancement of $C5a_{des\ Arg}$ receptor. Thus there may be fundamental differences between formyl peptide and complement-related chemoattractant receptor processing.

2. Studies in Cells Deficient in Specific Granules

One test of the validity of the hypothesis that neutrophil-specific granules are a source of new plasma membrane containing certain receptors would be to study neutrophils from patients with specific granule deficiency. Several such patients have been described each of whom has had recurrent pyrogenic infections. Recently we had the opportunity to study a patient with specific granule deficiency (Gallin et al., 1982). The patient had a severe deficiency of the specific granule markers lactoferrin and vitamin B_{12} binding proteins. Assessment of inflammation in vivo revealed an abnormal skin window response with diminished neutrophil accumulation into skin windows. Studies of neutrophil locomotion in vitro showed decreased neutrophil chemotaxis to a variety of stimuli relative to control cells, the difference becoming more pronounced with the length of assay. This was associated with significantly decreased fMet-Leu-[^{3}H]-Phe binding and failure to see appropriate increases in binding after exposure to the degranulating stimulus PMA. This evidence supported the concept that renewal of receptors from specific granules may be necessary for optimal sustained chemotaxis.

Preparations of normal neutrophils void of lysosomal granules and nuclei provide another useful model. We have recently used the method of Roos et al. (1983) to make such preparations, called neutrophil cytoplasts (Gallin et al., 1984). In our preparations more than 90% of specific and azurophil granule markers have been depleted. fMet-Leu-Phe binding to neutrophil cytoplasts is about one-half that of intact cells. After incubation with the specific granule secretagogue PMA, there was no increase in fMet-Leu-Phe binding in the cytoplasts. Scatchard analyses have also been performed, and the results indicate that cytoplasts have no change in number or affinity of fMet-Leu-Phe receptors after exposure to concentrations of PMA that will double the number of receptors in whole cells. Thus, the data with specific granule-deficient neutrophils and neutrophil cytoplasts support the concept that an intracellular pool of fMet-Leu-Phe receptors may exist on the specific granules or on a closely related organelle.

B. Adaptation to fMet-Leu-Phe

Although neutrophils can respond to as little as a 1% gradient of formyl peptide across their length (Zigmond, 1974), once they respond they adapt to the stimulus (Zigmond and Sullivan, 1979) with a decrease in the chemotactic responsiveness of the cell to the same concentration of stimulus. We recently suggested that a decrease in fMet-Leu-Phe receptor affinity, through either heterogeneity or negative cooperativity, is important in neutrophil adaptation to the chemoattractant (Seligmann *et al.,* 1982*b*). Such a mechanism for adaptation could permit the cell to sense very small changes in attractant concentration when the ambient peptide concentration was low (conditions required for sensing a gradient during directed locomotion) and still respond at high peptide concentrations with degranulation and respiratory burst activities—conditions expected when cells have arrived at an inflammatory focus. Such concepts are borne out by experimental data that demonstrate that the optimal chemotactic concentration of fMet-Leu-Phe is 1- to 2-fold lower than that for secretion or superoxide production. The data for our conclusions were based on dose-response studies of neutrophil responsiveness to fMet-Leu-Phe as monitored with the lipophilic cationic membrane potential sensitive fluorescent probe di-O-C$_5$(3) (Seligmann *et al.,* 1981). Addition of a nonsaturating initial S_1 stimulus of $2.5 \times 10^{-8} M$ fMet-Leu-Phe resulted in a characteristic loss of di-O-C$_5$(3) fluorescence (apparent depolarization), followed by a recovery of fluorescence (repolarization). The amount of fluorescence lost was the measurement of cell responsiveness used to assess the extent of adaptation. Exposure of cells to an initial S_1 stimulus of 2.5×10^{-8} M fMet-Leu-Phe resulted in a 75% maximal response; restimulation with 10^{-7} M fMet-Leu-Phe caused no additional depolarization, indicating that the cells had lost responsiveness. When, however, a higher S_2 concentration of 5×10^{-6} M was used, a response similar in magnitude to the maximum S_1 response was elicited, suggesting that the cells had undergone adaptation.

Through a series of dose–response experiments in which cells were exposed to varying S_1 concentrations of fMet-Leu-Phe and then the K_m determined for the S_2 or second response, the following conclusions regarding the adaptation of cells to fMet-Leu-Phe were reached:

1. Adaptation requires ~1.5-min exposure to fMet-Leu-Phe to reach a maximum.

2. Adaptation is completely reversible upon removal of fMet-Leu-Phe if 5×10^{-8} M fMet-Leu-Phe is used

3. Adaptation persists unaltered as long as fMet-Leu-Phe is present (up to 45 min).

4. It appears that adaptation represents a decrease in the affinity of the cell's responsiveness to fMet-Leu-Phe, with no effect on the maximal responsiveness of cells as long as the S_1 stimulus concentration is $<10^{-8}$ M. At concentrations $>10^{-8}$ M not only does the apparent affinity decrease, but the maximal responsiveness of the cells decreases as well.

Hill analysis of the adaptation data was performed to assist in assessing the nature of adaptation. The Hill coefficient for the functional response was found to be 0.68 ± 0.07, which was close to the Hill coefficients for binding to isolated plasma membranes (0.69 ± 0.07) or intact cells (0.64 ± 0.06) (Seligmann et al., 1982b). The Hill coefficient of <1 is compatible with heterogeneity or negative cooperative interaction of receptors as a basis for altered receptor affinity. Interestingly, Koo et al. (1982) and Mackin et al. (1982) have independently presented data indicating that the fMet-Leu-Phe receptor can exist in two affinity states. Goetzl et al. (1981) have also demonstrated heterogeneity to peptide binding proteins isolated from detergent-solubilized PMN membranes.

Further analysis of the data on adaptation of neutrophils to fMet-Leu-Phe as studied with di-O-C_5(3) provided insights into how cells adapt to a gradient of chemoattractant (Gallin et al., 1983). Studies of the dependence of the second (S_2) stimulus on the first (S_1) concentration indicated that with S_1 concentrations $<10^{-8}$ M small increases in S_2 were needed to elicit responses. However, with S_1 concentrations $>10^{-8}$ M, large increases in S_2 were required to give a subsequent response.

Allometric equations have been derived to describe the dependence of the concentrations of S_2 stimulus necessary to elicit an S_2 response (Seligmann et al., 1982) on the initial S_1 challenge stimulus (producing an S_1 response). If we assume that the cell response measured with di-O-C_5(3) relates to cell response in a chemotactic chamber we can use these equations, together with our knowledge that it takes $\sim$1.5 min to adapt to a chemoattractant stimulus, to predict the rate at which cells would have to move in a gradient of chemoattractant to keep up with, or just ahead of, the change in receptor affinity as they move up a gradient of stimulus (Fig. 3). By this analysis, when cells are exposed to low concentrations of chemoattractant they would have to move at rates of 3–10 μm/min, which are quite compatible with the actually measured rates of migration, and would provide a mechanism for cell sensing of a chemoattractant gradient. With higher concentrations of chemoattractant, encountered by cells as they enter depths of the filter closer to the chemoattractant source, the cells would have to move extremely fast in order to remain equivalently stimulated, rates they probably cannot achieve. Hence,

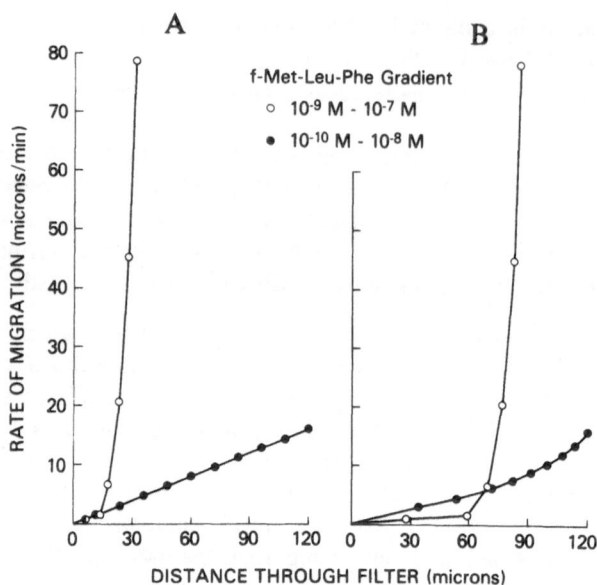

Figure 3. Calculated rates of neutrophil migration through a cellulose nitrate filter required for cells to respond continually to fMet-Leu-Phe using the di-0-C_5(3) adaptation model. (A) Linear decay; (B) exponential decay of chemoattractant gradient with the two gradients of chemoattractant indicated by (o) 10^{-7} M and (•) 10^{-8} M fMet-Leu-Phe below the chemoattractant filter. (From Gallin et al., 1983, with permission.)

the cells would stop moving at the higher concentrations of chemoattractant reached after migrating 30–40 μm into the filter (Gallin et al., 1983). This prediction fits closely with the well-demonstrated dose–response data for fMet-Leu-Phe-stimulated chemotaxis in which optimal chemotaxis is at 10^{-8} M fMet-Leu-Phe and inhibition occurs at higher concentrations. Thus, decreases in chemoattractant receptor affinity, by negative cooperative interaction and/or receptor heterogeneity, is a possible explanation for the characteristic rise and fall dose–response curves observed for neutrophil chemotaxis (Cramer and Gallin, 1979). It can account for such behavior independently or synergistically with other mechanisms, such as changes in cell adherence, degranulation, and depletion of an intracellular pool of receptors. This explanation also suggests that both adaptation and asymmetric distribution of receptors are important in neutrophil sensing of a chemoattractant gradient.

Two papers from Snyderman's laboratory have suggested that fMet-Leu-Phe receptor affinity regulates different neutrophil functions. Lohr and Snyderman (1982) showed that amphotericin B decreases the affinity of fMet-Leu-Phe binding up to 5-fold, inhibits chemotaxis responsiveness, but has no effect on lysosomal enzyme release or superoxide production. In contrast, Yuli et al. (1982)

showed that aliphatic alcohols increase fMet-Leu-Phe receptor affinity while increasing chemotaxis responsiveness and depressing fMet-Leu-Phe secretion and superoxide production (Table I). The possibility that pharmacological control of the neutrophil chemoattractant receptor can regulate neutrophil responsiveness has obvious implications with regard to treatment of certain inflammatory, immune, and neoplastic diseases.

The affinity of fMet-Leu-Phe for its receptor will influence the kinetics of fMet-Leu-Phe binding to the receptor and the duration of binding. Sklar, *et al.* (1981*a*,*b*) have shown that the functional responses to fMet-Leu-Phe binding depend in part on the duration of binding. For example, it is possible to elicit membrane potential changes by fMet-Leu-Phe (discussed in Section III.C) without initiating superoxide production by limiting the time neutrophils are exposed to fMet-Leu-Phe. If neutrophils are stimulated with chemoattractant for only 30 sec and the stimulus is then removed by addition of antibody or competitive antagonist, the membrane potential changes are stimulated normally, but superoxide production is severely reduced. Thus the temporal nature of the binding of fMet-Leu-Phe to its receptor is critical in determining the responses elicited.

C. Neutrophil Heterogeneity

Interpretation of the above binding studies assumes that neutrophils are homogeneous, but this is not correct (Gallin, 1984). Recent studies have indicated that mature neutrophils are not homogeneous with respect to expression of Fc receptors (Klempner and Gallin, 1978), alkaline phosphatase content (Fehr and Grossman, 1979) or responsiveness to fMet-Leu-Phe as monitored with the lipophilic cationic membrane potential-sensitive probe di-O-C_5(3) (Seligmann *et al.*, 1981). Studies of neutrophils using the fluorescence-activated cell sorter with di-O-C_5(3) indicate that whereas approximately 80 percent of neutrophils respond to fMet-Leu-Phe with a transient loss of fluorescence (an apparent membrane depolarization), 20 percent of the cells either do not respond or show an increase in dye fluorescence (apparent hyperpolarization).

We have recently studied the association of a formyl peptide chemoattractant with cells showing either a depolarization (80 percent of cells) or no change or having a small hyperpolarization of membrane potential (20 percent of cells). The studies were performed using fluorescein-labeled fMet-Leu-Phe-Lys with di-I-C_5(3), a recently described membrane potential-sensitive probe that fluoresces with a wavelength similar to that of rhodamine (Seligmann and Gallin, 1983*a*). Studies with di-I-C_5(3) and fMet-Leu-Phe-Lys-fluorescein permit double-label experiments in the cell sorter. The data indicate that cells responding with a loss of fluorescence (apparent depolarization) have more chemoattractant associated with them than cells showing no response (or apparent hyperpolarization). Addition of unfluoresceinated fMet-Leu-Phe to cells previously exposed to fluoresceinated peptide displaces a large portion of the fluoresceinated peptide from the cells that exhibited a depolarization of membrane potential, but does not displace peptide from neutrophils that showed either no change or a small hyperpolarization of membrane potential. This heterogeneity among cells may contribute to the apparent heterogeneity of binding of fMet-Leu-[^{3}H]-Phe seen by Scatchard analyses of studies using bulk cell populations. Thus, the data indicate that both structural and functional expression of formyl peptide receptors among cells is heterogeneous. It is noted, however, that the adaptation studies described in Section II.B. cannot be explained by delayed recruitment of a nonresponding cell population, since in studies using the cell sorter, repetitive stimulation did not result in recruitment of cells from the population of nonresponding cells. Instead, responding cells adapt and then reresponds to higher concentrations of stimulus.

III. INITIAL EVENTS FOLLOWING fMET-LEU-PHE BINDING

A. Ion Fluxes

From the above discussion of adaptation of the fMet-Leu-Phe receptor it should be apparent that interaction of fMet-Leu-Phe with receptors on neutrophils appears to alter the membrane potential. Since changes in membrane potential are rapid, occurring before alterations in cell shape, superoxide production, or degranulation, they may have a role in transduction of the signal for functional response and/or in modulating expression of the fMet-Leu-Phe receptor (Korchak and Weissmann, 1978). The membrane potential of cells is established by the distribution of ions across the membrane. Hence, this section reviews ionic changes seen in neutrophils after activation by chemoattractants.

Studies of ion composition and fluxes of resting and stimulated neutrophils, as well as functional requirements for specific ions, have produced an extensive body of literature that has already been well reviewed (Schiffmann and Gallin, 1979; Weissmann *et al.*, 1980; Becker *et al.*, 1981; Wilkinson, 1982). These findings will be summarized here.

Resting neutrophils have high permeability to potassium and sodium, as compared with either calcium or chloride. This is consistent with observations that the resting membrane potential of neutrophils is highly negative and potassium dependent, but less so than the potassium equilibrium potential (Cividalli and Nathan, 1974; Seligmann *et al.*, 1980; Simchowitz *et al.*, 1982). Stimulation of neutrophils with chemoattractants such as fMet-Leu-Phe leads to both influx and efflux of calcium, as well as to intracellular mobilization of calcium from previously bound pools (J. I. Gallin and Rosenthal, 1974; Boucek and Synderman, 1976; Naccache *et al.*, 1977). The net result is a rise in intracellular free calcium levels with an efflux of calcium. fMet-Leu-Phe also enhances the influx of sodium (reaching a maximum within 30 sec), followed by sodium efflux and potassium influx at 1 min (Naccache *et al.*, 1977; Simchowitz and Spilberg, 1979; Weissmann *et al.*, 1980; Becker *et al.*, 1981). These sodium and potassium flux changes are inhibited by ouabain and hence presumably result from the stimulation of Na–K-ATPase activity. Activation of the Na–K-ATPase may occur either as a result of stimulation by the raised intracellular sodium concentration or because of an actual activation of the Na–K-ATPase (Becker *et al.*, 1978). Cytochalasin B enhances the fMet-Leu-Phe-induced calcium and sodium fluxes.

Direct coupling between the sodium and calcium fluxes does not appear to occur, because inhibition of stimulated sodium influx does not inhibit either sodium efflux or calcium influx (Sha'afi *et al.*, 1981). However, the processes appear to be linked in some manner, because lowering the extracellular sodium concentration results in a lowered calcium influx (Simchowitz and Spilberg, 1979). The intracellular pH fluctuates (Levin *et al.*, 1976; Molski *et al.*, 1980; Becker *et al.*, 1981) and protons are released following stimulation, although it has been speculated that this process is not the result of actual proton transport across the plasma membrane (Van Zwieten *et al.*, 1981).

The calcium ionophore A23187 stimulates a large calcium influx and delayed potassium efflux (Becker *et al.*, 1981). This ionophore is referred to as a secretagogue because it stimulates secretion and oxidative metabolism, but not chemotaxis. Arachidonic acid and its metabolic cascade product leukotriene B_4 also stimulate the influx of calcium and sodium (Molski *et al.*, 1981). Leukotriene B_4 stimulates chemotaxis and the production of superoxide anion; recently it was reported to be a calcium ionophore (Weissmann *et al.*, 1982). The potassium ionophore valinomycin does not initiate any functions, but it may enhance chemotaxis, whereas the sodium ionophore monensin reportedly stimulates limited amounts of secretion and superoxide production (Becker *et al.*, 1981).

The dependence of particular functions on ions can also be demonstrated. Production of superoxide anion and stimulation of the respiratory burst, chemotaxis, aggregation, phagocytosis, and secretion are generally enhanced by external calcium. However, calcium does not enhance superoxide production stimulated by the secretagogue PMA (Lehmeyer *et al.*, 1979; Becker *et al.*, 1979). Lanthanum, which inhibits calcium influx, blocks chemotaxis (Boucek and Snyderman, 1976). Magnesium inhibits both superoxide production and chemotaxis in the presence of optimal amounts of calcium, whereas lowering the concentration of sodium inhibits secretion and superoxide production (Simchowitz and Spilberg, 1979) in response to fMet-Leu-Phe. Varying the potassium has no effect on stimulated superoxide production, but its removal results in some inhibition of chemotaxis and secretion of lysozyme (Weissman *et al.*, 1980; Becker *et al.*, 1981). Casein-induced guinea pig peritoneal exudate neutrophils spontaneously generate superoxide anion when suspended in high-potassium medium containing sodium, but not when suspended in high-sodium medium with no potassium or low potassium (Rossi *et al.*, 1981). These cells respond subsequently, regardless of suspension medium, to PMA. The requirement was shown to be a potassium effect, and in fact the amount of superoxide anion produced was directly proportional to potassium ion concentration.

Recently, Roberts and Gallin (1984) showed that high potassium (60 mM) will induce human neutrophil fMet-Leu-Phe shape changes and facilitates capping on concanavalin A receptors. The effects of high potassium were dependent on extracellular calcium and since high potassium depolarizes neutrophil membranes (Seligmann *et al.*, 1980) the data suggest that neutrophils may have a voltage-dependent calcium channel, which is important in signal transduction.

B. Chemoattractant Alteration of Surface Charge and Possible Relationship of Surface Charge and Ion Currents to Cell Adhesion and Membrane Changes

1. Surface Charge

The possible importance of surface charge and leukocyte chemotaxis was apparently first suggested by Dineur (1893; discussed in Abramson, 1927), who attempted to study the electrical charge of white blood cells. Dineur placed platinum wires into frog peritoneum and noted that leukocytes were attracted to the anodal capillary. Abramson (1927) thought that potential differences between inflammatory sites and blood vessels were important in leukocyte mobilization. However, the possibility that alterations of leukocyte surface charge are important in cell motility was not considered by these early investigators. More recent studies in the amoeba and fibroblasts showed that cell adhesiveness was dependent on surface charge (Jones, 1966; Ambrose and Forrester, 1968). Ambrose and Forrester (1968) related amoeba contraction and expansion with associated decreases or increases in negative surface charge, respectively. Lichtman and Weed (1972) reported a relationship between high negative surface charge, poor distensibility, low cell adhesiveness, and poor pseudopod formation in human bone marrow neutrophil precursor cells.

Gallin *et al.* (1975) reported that incubation of human peripheral blood neutrophils with three different chemotactic factors resulted in a small yet significant reduction in surface charge. These observations have been confirmed (Schaak *et al.*, 1980). More recently, it was shown that agents that cause release of intracellular granule contents potentiate the reduction in surface charge, and the reduction in surface charge has been temporally although not causally related to neutrophil aggregation and adhesiveness to other surfaces (Gallin *et al.*, 1980). Interestingly, concentrations of steroids that inhibited cell adhesiveness to nylon wool columns (MacGregor *et al.*, 1974; Clark *et al.*, 1979) and aggregation blocked chemotactic factor-induced reduction in surface charge (Gallin *et al.*, 1975), suggesting that steroid inhibition of neutrophil adhesiveness may involve this mechanism. Thus the data support the theory that modulation of cell-to-cell and cell-to-surface contact is under the influence of the net effect of attractive (primarily Van der Waal forces) and repulsive (primarily electrostatic) forces.

2. Ion Currents

In a recent review, Nuccitelli (1983) emphasized that transcellular ion currents are commonly found in cells and that the spatial pattern of these currents is intimately associated with the cell's polarity. It appears that most cells do not have a uniform distribution of plasma membrane ion channels and pumps, but instead separate these sites, generating transcellular currents. In some cases, these currents can play a causal role in determining cell polarity. There is no direct evidence for localized ion channels in phagocytic cells. However, Cramer and Gallin (1979) showed local accumulation of submembranous calcium at the leading edge of oriented human neutrophils, suggesting localized ion channels may be present. Orida and Feldman (1982) recently showed that extracellularly applied electric fields can cause murine macrophages to undergo directional protrusive pseudopodal activity toward the positive pole of the electric field, capping of concanavalin A receptors to the negative pole, and capping of PHA receptors to the positive pole. These data, together with the data summarized by Nuccitelli (1983), raise many interesting questions about the possible role of ion currents and surface charge in neutrophil orientation and in the expression and function of receptors in neutrophils and other phagocytic cells.

C. Membrane Potential and Neutrophil Function

The membrane potential of cells can be measured using three general methods: (1) directly, by the use of intracellular recording through microelectrodes penetrating into the intracellular spaces of the cell; (2) indirectly, using extracellular electrodes placed close to the surface of the cell and capable of detecting ion currents generated by and sustaining the cell membrane potential; and (3) indirectly, by measuring the distribution of a charged organic ion or chloride ion that is passively distributed across the plasma membrane of the cell according to the membrane potential. Neutrophils are too small to be studied with microelectrodes, although the recent development of a technique referred to as patch recording may permit intracellular recordings in the future. To date, studies have been limited to use of charged organic ions (see Seligmann and Gallin, 1983*a*, for recent comparison of various available probes). We have used the cyanine dye di-O-C$_5$(3) for most of our studies. With this probe a depolarization of membrane potential causes a decrease in fluorescence while a hyperpolarization causes an increase in fluorescence. Probes of membrane potential distribute across all membrane compartments within complex cells. Therefore, it is important to recognize that the membrane potential of all intracellular compartments are monitored simultaneously with these probes.

1. Neutrophil Resting Membrane Potential

Numerous studies have characterized neutrophil resting membrane potential. Values ranging from -26 to -101 mV have been reported (Utsumi et al., 1977; Seligmann and Gallin, 1980; Whitin et al., 1980; Jones et al., 1980; Simchowitz et al., 1982; Mottola and Romeo, 1982). One cause for this wide range of values appears to be the method and length of storage of cells. However, all the reports indicate that the membrane potential of neutrophils can be depolarized by raising extracellular potassium or by treating cells with the sodium ionophore gramicidin. Neutrophil resting membrane potential can be hyperpolarized by addition of the potassium ionophore valinomycin (Utsumi et al., 1977; Seligmann et al., 1980; Whitin et al., 1980; Jones et al., 1980; Simchowitz et al., 1982; Mottola and Romeo, 1982).

There is considerable evidence that the Na-K-ATPase of resting neutrophils is electrogenic, thereby contributing to the membrane potential (Becker et al., 1978; Jones et al., 1980; Simchowitz et al., 1982). By means of an ion-selective electrode to study tetraphenylmethylphosphonium ion distribution in elicited guinea pig peritoneal neutrophils, it was demonstrated that ouabain, a specific inhibitor of the Na-K$^+$-ATPase, caused the membrane potential to gradually fall to the level attained by cells suspended in potassium-free medium, which also blocks pump activity (Kuroki et al., 1981; Jones et al., 1980). In a more comprehensive study, Simchowitz et al. (1982) demonstrated that the Na-K$^+$ pump contributed approximately 9 mV to the resting membrane potential of human neutrophils. Simchowitz et al. (1982) also observed that incubating the cells on ice in potassium-free medium for 3 hr led to sodium/potassium exchange and depolarization. In addition, resuspension at 37°C was observed to lead to rapid reestablishment of the normal intracellular potassium and sodium levels. Cells loaded with 70 mM sodium (similar to their condition on ice) exhibited a calculated membrane potential of -40 mV.

Since most investigators store cells on ice in calcium-free medium (to minimize calcium-promoted ion-exchange mechanisms) until use, the observations of sodium loading are quite relevant. Thus, if cells stored on ice are not incubated at 37°C for a sufficient length of time before assay, the ion gradients may not be restored, and anomalous results may be obtained.

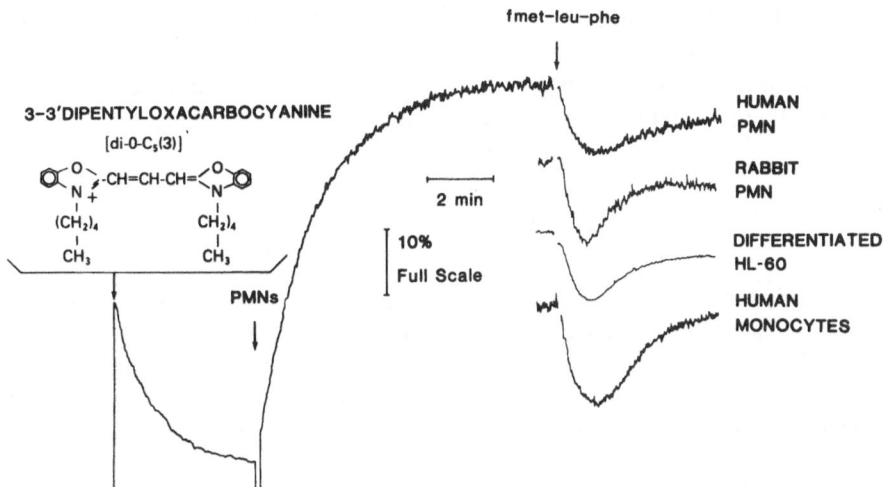

Figure 4. Membrane potential changes in human neutrophils as monitored with the cyanine dye di-0-C$_5$(3) shown at the left as described by Seligmann *et al.* (1980). Time and percentage of full-scale fluorescence are as indicated (center). The arrow indicates when the chemoattractant fMet-Leu-Phe (10^{-6} *M*) was added to cuvettes containing human, rabbit, phorbol ester-differentiated HL-60 cells or human monocytes, obtained by elutriation, all at 2.5 × 10^5 per ml.

fMet-Leu-Phe-induced membrane potential changes are the earliest events detected during activation of neutrophils. The differentiated HL-60 cell line and human monocytes exhibit similar membrane potential changes when stimulated (Fig. 4). The response shown by the differentiated cell line HL-60 is of particular interest, since undifferentiated cells, which do not exhibit phagocytic properties (Fontana *et al.*, 1980), do not exhibit the change in membrane potential. Studies using cyanine dyes (Gallin *et al.*, 1980) and microelectrodes (Gallin and Gallin, 1977) indicate that macrophages also produce these types of membrane potential changes in response to chemoattractants.

Ion substitution experiments could not clearly characterize the basis for the initial decrease in di-0-C$_5$(3) fluorescence induced by fMet-Leu-Phe (Seligmann *et al.*, 1980). The recovery was attributed to a stimulation of membrane permeability to potassium (efflux) and thus represented a repolarizing hyperpolarization. Recent studies using the fluorescent-activated cell sorter (see Section II.C) have indicated that the decrease in fluorescence represents a depolarization of 60%–80% of the neutrophil population (Seligmann and Gallin, 1983*b*).

At the moment it is difficult to relate the depolarization to cell function. The experiments discussed previously of Roberts and Gallin (1984), using increased potassium to modulate membrane potential, suggest an important role for depolarization in cell activation. However, until voltage-clamp studies are feasible, it will not be possible to conclude whether the alterations in neutrophil function induced by high potassium are a membrane potential effect or due to some other event induced by the high potassium.

IV. CONCLUSION

The dynamics of chemoattractant receptors is a field of investigation that has recently made major advances. The demonstration of receptors for fMet-Leu-Phe has led to studies indicating ligand and probably receptor internalization. It seems probable that there is either receptor recycling and/or a storage pool of receptors that provide a mechanism for replenishment of receptors at the cell surface.

Neutrophil responsiveness to fMet-Leu-Phe appears to involve several sensing mechanisms. Asymmetric distribution of the fMet-Leu-Phe receptors and affinity adaptation of the receptor through heterogeneity and/or negative cooperative interaction of the receptors are probably important. Assessment of neutrophil receptors assumes homogeneity of neutrophil populations. However, in recent studies assessing neutrophil functional responsiveness (elicited changes in membrane potential) as well as fMet-Leu-Phe binding, it has become clear that neutrophils are not homogeneous in terms of fMet-Leu-Phe receptor expression. Heterogeneity among neutrophils must therefore be considered when interpreting receptor studies on bulk cell preparations.

Less is known about the transduction mechanism than about fMet-Leu-Phe binding. There is some evidence to suggest that different affinity states of the receptor are important for different functions. A high-affinity state has been associated with transduction of chemotaxis and a low-affinity state with transduction of superoxide production and degranulation. The earliest measured event that follows chemoattractant binding is a change in membrane potential (depolarization). However, this has not yet been related to transduction of a signal. Recent studies have shown that incubation of neutrophils in high-potassium, conditions depolarizes the membrane, initiates shape changes and facilitates capping of the concanavalin A receptor. These potassium-induced events require extracellular calcium. The data suggest that a voltage-dependent calcium channel may be important in signal transduction.

Thus, studies with the fMet-Leu-Phe receptor have helped stimulate understanding of how neutrophils recognize, integrate, and process signals for the complex functions they carry out. In addition to refining our understanding of the dynamics of fMet-Leu-Phe receptors, future investigations comparing the formyl peptide receptors with other chemoattractant receptors are now indicated.

V. REFERENCES

Abramson, H. A., 1927, The mechanism of the inflammatory process. I. The electrophoresis of the blood cells of the horse and its relation to leukocyte emigration, *J. Exp. Med.* 46:987–1002.

Ambrose, E. S., and Forrester, J. A., 1968, Electrical phenomena associated with cell movements, *Symp. Soc. Biol.* 22:237–248.

Aswanikumar, S., Schiffmann, E., Corcoran, B. A., and Wahl, S. M., 1976, Role of a peptidase in phagocyte chemotaxis, *Proc. Natl. Acad. Sci. (USA)* 73:2439–2442.

Aswanikumar, S., Corcoran, B., Schiffmann, E., Day, A., Freer, R., Showell, H., and Becker, E., 1977, Demonstration of a receptor on rabbit neutrophils for chemotactic peptides, *Biochem. Biophys. Res. Commun.* 74:810–817.

Atkinson, J. P., Simchowitz, L., Mehta, J., and Steuison, W. F., 1982, 5,8,11,14-Eicosatetraynoic acid (ETYA) inhibits binding of N-formyl-methionyl-leucyl-phenylalanine (FMLP) to its receptor on human granulocytes: A note of caution, *Immunopharm.* 4:1–9.

Becker, E. L., 1979, A multifunctional receptor on the neutrophil for synthetic chemotactic oligopeptides, *J. Reticuloendothel. Soc.* 26:701–709.

Becker, E. L., Talley, J. V., Showell, H. J. Naccache, P. H., and Sha'afi, R. I., 1978, Activation of the rabbit polymorphonuclear leukocyte membrane "Na, K"-ATPase by chemotactic factor, *J. Cell Biol.* 77:329–333.

Becker, E. L., Sigman, M., and Oliver, J. M., 1979, Superoxide production induced in rabbit polymorphonuclear leukocytes by synthetic chemotactic peptides and A23187: The nature of the receptor and the requirement for Ca^{2+}, *Am J. Pathol.* 95:81–97.

Becker, E. L., Naccache, P. H., Showell, H. J., and Walenga, R. W., 1981, Early events in neutrophil activation: Receptor stimulation, ionic fluxes, and arachidonic acid metabolism, *Lymphokines* 4:297–334.

Boucek, M. M., and Snyderman, R., 1976, Calcium influx requirement for human neutrophil chemotaxis; Inhibition by lanthanum chloride, *Science* 194:905–907.

Chenoweth, D. E., and Hugli, T. E., 1978, Demonstration of specific C5a receptor on intact human polymorphonuclear leukocytes, *Proc. Natl. Acad. Sci. (USA)* 75:3943–3947.

Cividalli, G., and Nathan, D. G., 1974, Sodium and potassium concentration and transmembrane fluxes in leukocytes, *Blood* 43:861–869.

Clark, R. A. F., Gallin, J. I., and Fauci, A. S., 1979, Effect of in vivo prednisone on in vitro eosinophil and neutrophil adherence and chemotaxis, *Blood* 53:633–641.

Cramer, E. B., and Gallin, J. I., 1979, Localization of submembranous cations to the leading end of human neutrophils during chemotaxis, *J. Cell Biol.* 82:369–379.

Davis, B. H., Walter, R. J., Pearson, C. B., Becker, E. L., and Oliver, J. M., 1982, Membrane activity and topography of fMet-Leu-Phe treated polymorphonuclear leukocytes. Acute and sustained responses to chemotactic peptide, *Am. J. Pathol.* 108:206–216.

Donabedian, H., and Gallin, J. I., 1981, Deactivation of human neutrophil chemotaxis by chemoattractants: Effect on receptors for the chemotactic factor f-Met-Leu-Phe, *J. Immunol.* 127:839–844.

Fearon, D. T., and Collins, L. A., 1983, Increased expression of C3b receptors on polymorphonuclear leukocytes induced by purification procedures, *J. Immunol.* 130:370–375.

Fehr, J., and Grossman, H. C., 1979, Disparity between circulating and marginated neutrophils: Evidence from studies on the granulocyte alkaline phosphatase, a marker of cell maturity, *Am. J. Hematol.* 7:369–379.

Fletcher, M., and Gallin, J. I., 1980, Degranulating stimuli increase the availability of receptors on human neutrophils for the chemoattractant fMet-Leu-Phe, *J. Immunol.* **124:** 1585-1588.

Fletcher, M., and Gallin, J. I., 1983, Human neutrophils contain an intracellular pool of putative receptors for the chemoattractant fMet-Leu-Phe, *Blood* **62:**792-799.

Fletcher, M., Seligmann, B., and Gallin, J. I., 1982, Correlation of human neutrophil secretion, chemoattractant receptor mobilization, and enhanced functional capacity, *J. Immunol.* **128:**941-948.

Fontana, J. A., Wright, D. G., Schiffman, E., Corcoran, B. A., and Deisseroth, A. B., 1980, Development of chemotactic responsiveness in myeloid precursor cells. Studies with a human leukemia cell line, *Proc. Natl. Acad. Sci. (USA)* **77:**3664-3668.

Gallin, E. K., and Gallin, J. I., 1977, Interaction of chemotactic factors with human macrophages. Induction of transmembrane potential changes, *J. Cell Biol.* **75:**277-289.

Gallin, E. K., Seligmann, B., and Gallin, J. I., 1980, Alteration of macrophage and monocyte membrane potential by chemotactic factors, in: *Mononuclear Phagocytes* (R. van Furth, ed.), pp. 505-523, Martinus Nijhoff, The Hague.

Gallin, J. I., 1980, Degranulating stimuli decrease the negative surface charge and increase the adhesiveness of human neutrophils, *J. Clin. Invest.* **65:**298-306.

Gallin, J. I., 1982, The role of neutrophil lysosomal granules in the evaluation of the inflammatory response, in: *Phagocytosis—Past and Future* (M. L. Karnovsky and L. Bolis, eds.), pp. 519-541, Academic Press, New York.

Gallin, J. I., 1984, Neutrophil heterogeneity exists, but is it biologically relevant? *Blood* (in press).

Gallin, J. I., and Rosenthal, A. S., 1974, The regulatory role of divalent cations in human granulocyte chemotaxis: Evidence for an association between calcium exchanges and microtubule assembly, *J. Cell Biol.* **62:**594-609.

Gallin, J. I., Durocher, J. R., and Kaplan, A. P., 1975, Interaction of leukocyte chemotactic factors with the cell surface. I. Chemotactic factor-induced changes in human granulocyte surface charge, *J. Clin. Invest.* **551:**967-974.

Gallin, J. I., Wright, D. G., and Schiffmann, E., 1978, Role of secretory events in modulating human neutrophil chemotaxis, J. *Clin. Invest.* **62:**1364-1374.

Gallin, J., Gallin, E., and Schiffmann, E., 1979, Mechanism of leukocyte chemotaxis, in: *Advances in Inflammation Research,* Vol. 1 (G. Weissmann, B. Samuelsson, and R. Paoletti, eds.), pp. 123-138, Raven Press, New York.

Gallin, J. I., Fletcher, M. P., Seligman, B. E., Hoffstein, S., Cehrs, K., and Mounessa, N., 1982, Human neutrophil specific granule deficiency; a model to assess the role of neutrophil specific granules in the evolution of the inflammatory response, *Blood* **59:**1317-1329.

Gallin, J. I., Seligmann, B., and Fletcher, M., 1983, Dynamics of human neutrophil receptors for the chemoattractant fmet-leu-phe, in: *Leukocyte Locomotion and Chemotaxis. Agents and Actions Supplements* Vol. 12 (H. U. Keller, and G. O. Till, eds.), pp. 290-308, Birkhauser Verlag, Basel.

Gallin, J. I., Metcalf, J. A., Roos, D., Seligmann, B., and Friedman, M. M., 1984, Organelle-depleted human neutrophil cytoplasts used to study fMet-Leu-Phe receptor modulation and cell function, *J. Immunol.* (in press).

Goetzl, E., Foster, D., and Goldman, D., 1981, Isolation and partial characterization of human neutrophil receptors for chemotactic formylmethionyl peptides, *Biochemistry.* **20:**5717-5722.

Goetzl, E. J., Foster, D. W., and Goldman, D. W., 1982, Specific effects on human neutrophil of antibodies to a membrane protein constituent of neutrophil receptors for chemotactic formyl-methionyl peptides, *Immunology* **45:**249-256.

Hoffstein, S. T., Friedman, R. S., and Weissman, G., 1982, Degranulation membrane addition and shape change during chemotactic factor-induced aggregation of human neutrophils, *J. Cell Biol.* 95:234–241.

Jesaitis, A., Naemara, J. R., Painter, R. G., Sklar, L. A., and Cochrane, C. G., 1982, Intracellular localization of N-formyl chemotactic receptor and Mg^{2+} dependent ATPase in human granulocytes, *Biochem. Biophys. Acta* 719:556–568.

Jesaitis, A., Naemura, J. R., Painter, R. G., Sklar, L. A., and Cochrane, C. G., 1983, The fate of an N-formylated chemotactic peptide in stimulated human granulocytes. Subcellular fractionation studies, *J. Biol. Chem.* 258:1968–1977.

Jones, P. C. T., 1966, A contractile protein model for cell adhesion, *Nature* 212:365–369.

Jones, G. S., VanDyke, K., and Castranova, V., 1980, Purification of human granulocytes by centrifugal elutriation and measurement of transmembrane potential, *J. Cell Physiol.* 104:425–431.

Klempner, M. S., and Gallin, J. I., 1978, Separation and functional characterization of human neutrophil subpopulations, *Blood* 51:659–669.

Koo, C., and Snyderman, R., 1980, Chemotactic peptide protects against inhibition by cytochalasin B of peptide bonding on human polymorphonuclear leukocytes: A potential mechanism for enhanced gradient sensing, *Clin. Res.* 28:373A.

Koo, C., Lefkowitz, R., and Snyderman, R., 1982, The oligopeptide chemotactic factor receptor on human polymorphonuclear leukocyte membranes exists in two affinity in states, *Biochem. Biophys. Res. Commun.* 106:442–449.

Korchak, H. M., and Weissmann, G., 1978, Changes in membrane potential of human granulocytes antecede the metabolic responses to surface stimulation, *Proc. Natl. Acad. Sci. (USA)* 75:3818–3822.

Kuroki, M., Satoh, H., Kamo, N., and Kobatake, Y., 1981, Contribution to the membrane potential of the electrogenic Na^+, K^+ pump in guinea pig polymorphonuclear leukocytes, *FEBS Lett.* 123:177–180.

Lehmeyer, J. E., Snyderman, R., and Johnston, R. B., 1979, Stimulation of neutrophil oxidative metabolism by chemotactic peptides: Influence of calcium ion concentration and cytochalasin B and comparison with stimulation by phorbol myristate acetate, *Blood* 54:35–45.

Levin, G. E., Collinson, P., and Baron, D. N., 1976, The intracellular pH of human leukocytes in response to acid–base change *in vivo, Clin. Sci. Mol. Med.* 50:293–299.

Liao, C. S. and Freer, R. J., 1980, Cryptic receptors for chemotactic peptides in rabbit neutrophils, *Biochem. Biophys. Res. Commun.* 93:566–571.

Lichtman, M. A., and Weed, R. I., 1972, Alteration of the cell periphery during granulocyte maturation relationship to cell function, *Blood* 39:301–315.

Lohr, K. M., and Snyderman, R., 1982, Amphotericin B alters the affinity and functional activity of the oligopeptide chemotactic factor receptor on human polymorphonuclear leukocytes, *J. Immunol.* 129:1594–1599.

MacGregor, R. R., Spagnuolo, B. E., and Lentnek, A. L., 1974, Inhibition of granulocyte adherence by ethanol, prednisone, and aspirin, *N. Engl. J. Med.* 291:642–645.

Mackin, W. M., Huang, C., and Becker, E. L., 1982, The formylpeptide chemotactic receptor on rabbit peritoneal neutrophils. 1. Evidence for two binding sites with different affinities, *J. Immunol.* 129:1608–1611.

Marasco, W. A., and Becker, E. L., 1982, Antiidiotype as antibody against the formyl peptide chemotaxis receptor of the neutrophil, *J. Immunol.* 128:963–968.

Marasco, W. A., Showell, H. J., Freer, R. J., and Becker, E. L., 1982, Anti-fmet-leu-phe: Similarities in fine specificity with the formyl peptide chemotaxis receptor of the neutrophil, *J. Immunol.* 128:956–962.

Molski, T. F. P., Naccache, P. H., Volpi, M., Wolpert, L. M., and Sha'afi, R. I., 1980, Specific modulation of the intracellular pH or rabbit neutrophils by chemotactic factors, *Biochem. Biophys. Res. Commun.* 94:508–514.

Molski, T. F. P., Naccache, P. H., Borgest, P., and Sha'afi, R. I., 1981, Similarities in the mechanisms by which formyl-methionyl-leucyl-phenyl-alanine, arachidonic acid and leukotriene B_4 increase calcium and sodium influxes in rabbit neutrophils, *Biochem. Biophys. Res. Commun.* 103:227–232.

Mottola, C., and Romeo, D., 1982, Calcium movement and membrane potential changes in the early phase of neutrophil activation by phorbol myristate acetate: A study with ion-selective electrodes, *J. Cell Biol.* 93:129–134.

Naccache, P. H., Showell, H. J., Becker, E. L., and Sha'afi, R. I., 1977, Transport of sodium, potassium, and calcium across rabbit polymorphonuclear leukocyte membranes: Effect of chemotactic factor, *J. Cell Biol.* 73:428–444.

Niedel, J., 1981, Detergent solubilization of the formyl peptide chemotactic receptor. Strategy based on covalent affinity labeling, *J. Biol. Chem.* 256:9295–9299.

Niedel, J. E., and Dolmatch, B. L., 1983, Cellular processing of the formyl peptide receptor, in *Leukocyte Locomotion and Chemotaxis*. Agents and Actions Supplements Vol. 12 (H. U. Keller and G. O. Till, eds.), pp. 309–322, Birkhauser Verlag, Basel.

Niedel, J., Kahane, I., and Cuatrecasas, P., 1979a, Receptor-mediated internalization of fluorescent chemotactic peptide by human neutrophils, *Science* 205:1412–1414.

Niedel, J., Wilkinson, S., and Cuatrecasas, P., 1979b, Receptor-mediated uptake and degranulation of ^{125}I-chemotactic peptide by human neutrophils, *J. Biol. Chem.* 254: 10700–10706.

Niedel, J., Frothingham, R., and Cuatrecasas, P., 1980a, Inhibition of ^{125}I-chemotactic peptide uptake by protease inhibitors, *Biochem. Biophys. Res. Commun.*, 94:667–673.

Niedel, J., Kahane, I., Lachman, L., and Cuatrecasas, P., 1980b, A subpopulation of cultured human promyelocytic leukemia cells (HL-60) displays the formyl peptide chemotactic receptor, *Proc. Natl. Acad. Sci. (USA)* 77:1000–1004.

Nuccitelli, R., 1983, Transcellular ion currents: Signals and effectors of cell polarity, in: *Modern Cell Biology*, Vol. 2, *Spatial Organization of Eukaryotic Cells* (J. R. McIntosh, ed.), New York (in press).

Orida, N., and Feldman, J. D., 1982, Directional protrusive pseudopodial activity and motility in macrophages induced by extracellular electric fields, *Cell Motil.* 2:243–255.

Roberts, R. L., Mouuessa, N. L. and Gallin, J. I., 1984, Increasing extracellular potassium causes calcium-dependent shape change and facilitates concanavalin A capping in human neutrophils, *J. Immunol.* (in press).

Roos, D., Voetman, A. A., and Meerhof, L. J., 1983, Functional activity of enucleated human polymorphonuclear leukocytes, *J. Cell Biol.* 97:368–377.

Rossi, F., Della Bianca, V., and Davoli, A., 1981, A new way for inducing a respiratory burst in guinea pig neutrophils, *FEBS Lett.* 132:273–277.

Schaak, T. M., Takeuchi, A., Spilberg, I., and Persellin, R. H., 1980, Alteration of polymorphonuclear leukocyte surface charge by endogenous and exogenous chemotactic factors, *Inflammation* 4:37–44.

Schiffmann, E., and Gallin, J. I., 1979, Biochemistry of phagocyte chemotaxis, *Curr. Top. Cell Regul.* 15:203–261.

Schiffmann, E., Corcoran, B., Wahl, S., 1975, N-formylmethionyl peptides as chemoattractants for leukocytes, *Proc. Natl. Acad. Sci. (USA)* 72:1059–1062.

Schiffmann, E., Aswanikumas, S., Venkatasubramanian, K., Corcoran, B. A., Pert, C. B., Brown, J., Gross, E., Day, A. B., Freer, R. J., Showell, A. H., and Becker, E. L., 1980, Some characteristics of the neutrophil receptor for chemotactic peptides, *FEBS Lett.* 117:1–7.

Schmitt, M., Painter, P. G., Algirder, A. J., Preissner, K., Sklar, L. A., and Cochrane, C. G.,

1983, Photoaffinity labeling of the N-formyl peptide receptor binding site of intact human polymorphonuclear leukocytes, *J. Biol. Chem.* **258**:649–654.

Seligmann, B. E., and Gallin, J. I., 1980, Use of lipophilic probes of membrane potential to assess human neutrophil activation. Abnormality in chronic granulomatous disease, *J. Clin. Invest.* **66**:493–503.

Seligmann, B. E., and Gallin, J. I., 1983a, Comparison of indirect probes of membrane potential utilized in studies of human neutrophils, *J. Cell. Physiol.* **115**:105–115.

Seligmann, B., and Gallin, J. I., 1983b, Abnormality in elicited membrane potential changes in neutrophils from patients with chronic granulomatous disease, in: *Advances in Host Defense Mechanisms* (J. I. Gallin and A. S. Fauci, eds.), pp. 195–226, Raven Press, New York.

Seligmann, B. E., Gallin, E. K., Martin, W., Shain, W., and Gallin, J. I., 1980, Interaction of chemotactic factors with human polymorphonuclear leukocytes: Studies using a membrane potential sensitive cyanine dye, *J. Membr. Biol.* **52**:257–272.

Seligmann, B., Chused, T. M., and Gallin, J. I., 1981, Human neutrophil heterogeneity identified using flow microfluorometry to monitor membrane potential, *J. Clin. Invest.* **68**:1125–1131.

Seligmann, B. E., Chused, T. M., and Gallin, J. I., 1982a, Binding of fluoresceinated chemoattractant peptide to human neutrophils is heterogeneous and correlates with the heterogeneous stimulation of membrane potential changes, *J. Cell Biol.* **95**:444a.

Seligmann, B. E., Fletcher, M. P., and Gallin, J. I., 1982b, Adaptation of human neutrophil responsiveness to the chemoattractant *N*-formylmethionylleucylphenylalanine: Heterogeneity and/or negative cooperative interaction of receptors, *J. Biol. Chem.* **257**:6280–6286.

Sha'afi, R. I., Molski, T. F. P., and Naccache, P. H., 1981, Chemotactic factors activate differentiable permeation pathways for sodium and calcium in rabbit neutrophils. Effects of amiloride, *Biochem. Biophys. Res. Commun.* **99**:1271–1276.

Simchowitz, L., and Spilberg, I., 1979, Chemotactic factor-induced generation of superoxide radicals by human neutrophils: Evidence for the role of sodium, *J. Immunol.* **123**:2428–2435.

Simchowitz, L., Spilberg, I., and DeWeer, P., 1982, Sodium and potassium fluxes and membrane potential of human neutrophils, *J. Gen. Physiol.* **79**:453–479.

Sklar, L. A., Jesaitis, A. J., Painter, R. G., and Cochrane, C. G., 1981a, The kinetics of neutrophil activation. The response to chemotactic peptides depends upon whether ligand–receptor interaction is rate-limiting, *J. Biol. Chem.* **256**:9909–9914.

Sklar, L. A., Oades, Z. G., Jesaitis, A. J., Painter, R. G. and Cochrane, C. G., 1981b, Fluoresceinated chemotactic peptide and high-affinity antifluorescein antibody as a probe of the temporal characteristics of neutrophil stimulation, *Proc. Natl. Acad. Sci. (USA)* **78**:7540–7544.

Skubitz, K., Craddock, P., Hammerschmidt, D., and August, J., 1981, Corticosteroids block binding of chemotactic peptide to its receptor on granulocytes and causes disaggregation of granulocyte aggregates *in vitro*, *J. Clin. Invest.* **68**:13–20.

Spilberg, I., and Mehta, J., 1979, Demonstration of a specific neutrophil receptor for a cell-derived chemotactic factor, *J. Clin. Invest.* **63**:85–88.

Stossel, T., 1979, The mechanism of leukocyte locomotion, in: *Leukocyte Chemotaxis: Methods, Physiology and Clinical Implications* (J. I. Gallin and P. G. Quie, eds.), pp. 143–160, Raven Press, New York.

Sullivan, S., and Zigmond, S., 1980, Chemotactic peptide receptor modulation in polymorphonuclear leukocytes, *J. Cell Biol.* **85**:703–711.

Sullivan, S. J., and Zigmond, S. H., 1982, Asymmetric receptor distribution of PMNs, *J. Cell Biol.* **95**:418a.

Tsung, P., Showell, H., and Becker, E., 1980, Surface membrane enzyme chemotactic responsiveness of rabbit peripheral and peritoneal neutrophils, *Inflammation* **4**: 271–277.

Utsumi, K., Sugiyama, K., Miyahara, M., Naito, M., Awai, M., and Inoue, M., 1977, Effect of concanavalin A on membrane potential of polymorphonuclear leukocyte monitored by fluorescent dye, *Cell Struct. Function* **2**:203–209.

Van Epps, D., and Garcia, M., 1980, Enhancement of neutrophil function as a result of prior exposure to chemotactic factor, *J. Clin. Invest.* **66**:167–175.

Van Zwieten, R., Wever, R., Hamers, M. N., Weening, R. S., and Roos, D., 1981, Extracellular proton release by stimulated neutrophils, *J. Clin. Invest.* **68**:310–313.

Weissmann, G., Smolen, J. E., and Korchak, H. M., 1980, Release of inflammatory mediators from stimulated neutrophils, *N. Engl. J. Med.* **303**:27–34.

Weissmann, G., Serhan, C., Smolen, J., Radin, A., Goetzl, E. J., and Samuelsson, B., 1982, Leukotriene B_4 (LTB_4) as a mediator of inflammation: Human neutrophil (PMN) activation and calcium (Ca) ionophoresis, *Clin. Res.* **30**:573a.

Whitin, J. C., Capman, C. E., Simons, E. R., Chovaniec, M. E., and Cohen, H. J., 1980, Correlation between membrane potential changes and superoxide production in human granulocytes stimulated by phorbol myristate acetate, *J. Biol. Chem.* **255**:1874–1878.

Wilkinson, P. C., 1982, *Chemotaxis and Inflammation*, Churchill Livingston, Edinburgh.

Wilkinson, P. C., and Allan, R. B., 1981, Binders of protein chemotactic factors to the surfaces of neutrophil leukocytes and its modification with lipid specific bacterial toxins, *Mol. Cell Biochem.* **20**:25–40.

Williams, L., Snyderman, R., Pike, M., and Lefkowitz, R., 1977, Specific receptor sites for chemotactic peptides on human polymorphonuclear leukocytes, *Proc. Natl. Acad. Sci. (USA)* **74**:1204–1208.

Wright, D. G., and Gallin, J. I., 1979, Secretory responses of human neutrophils: exocytosis of specific (secondary) granules by human neutrophils during adherence *in vitro* and during exudation *in vivo*, *J. Immunol.* **123**:285–294.

Yuli, I., Tomonaga, A., and Snyderman, R., 1982, Chemoattractant receptor functions in human polymorphonuclear leukocytes are divergently altered by membrane fluidizers, *Proc. Natl. Acad. Sci. (USA)* **79**:5906–5910.

Zigmond, S. H., 1974, Mechanisms of sensing chemical gradients by polymorphonuclear leukocytes, *Nature* **29**:450–452.

Zigmond, S. H., 1981, Consequences of chemotactic peptide receptor modulation, *J. Cell Biol.* **88**:644–647.

Zigmond, S. H., and Sullivan, S. J., 1979, Sensory adaptation of leukocytes to chemotactic peptides, *J. Cell Biol.* **82**:517–527.

Zigmond, S., Sullivan, S., and Lauffenburger, D., 1982, Kinetic analysis of chemotactic peptide receptor modulation, *J. Cell Biol.* **92**:34–43.

Chapter 4

Mechanisms of Leukocyte Regulation by Complement-Derived Factors

Tony E. Hugli and Edward L. Morgan

Department of Immunology
Scripps Clinic and Research Foundation
La Jolla, California 92037

I. INTRODUCTION

As early as the mid-1960s it was recognized that factors derived from the blood complement system could stimulate leukocytes and promote directed leukocyte migration (Ward *et al.*, 1965, 1967; Shin *et al.*, 1968; Snyderman *et al.*, 1968). Shortly thereafter assignments were made that identified anaphylatoxins as the humoral chemotactic factors in question (Jensen *et al.*, 1969; Hill and Ward, 1969; Ward 1967, 1969; Cochrane and Müller-Eberhard, 1968; Fernandez *et al.*, 1978). Anaphylatoxins are low-molecular-weight fragments released from serum components C3, C4, and C5 when the complement cascade is activated; these fragments have been designated C3a, C4a, and C5a, respectively. Several recent reviews describe the properties of the anaphylatoxins in great detail (Hugli and Müller-Eberhard, 1978; Hugli, 1978, 1981, 1982). Before the anaphylatoxins were identified as chemotaxins, they were noted primarily for their spasmogenic and permeability-enhancing activities, mediated largely via vasoamines released from the mast cell (Johnson *et al.*, 1975). However, it was the recognition of neutrophil-anaphylatoxin interactions, using chemotaxis as an indicator of cellular activation, that prompted discovery of numerous other leukocyte responses mediated by these anaphylatoxins. The current status of our knowledge concerning the multiple effects of the anaphylatoxins on leukocyte function is the subject of this chapter.

Before the realization that components generated in blood were capable of attracting leukocytes to sites of inflammation, cellular sequestration events occurring without benefit of some external intervention or overt tissue injury seemingly defied rational explanation. Even today these types of inflammatory reactions (e.g., arthritis) are poorly understood in terms of the sequence of mediator involvement. The picture is further complicated by the fact that complex lipids called leukotrienes are manufactured by the chemotactic cells, and certain of these molecules are themselves chemotactic in nature (Ford-Hutchinson *et al.*, 1980; Malmsten *et al.*, 1980). Evidence that the humoral chemotactic factor C5a stimulates cellular release of leukotrienes, including the chemotactic product LTB_4 (Stimler *et al.*, 1982; Clancy *et al.*, 1983), may provide our first glimpse at the actual sequence of events leading to autoinflammatory responses.

Other phenomena associated with chemotaxis, including both cellular aggregation and adherence, are common responses caused by activators such as the formylated peptides (fMet-Leu-Phe) and C5a. Characteristic cellular unresponsiveness of leukocytes exposed to excessive levels of the anaphylatoxins has been described phenomenologically as desensitization. However, interpretation of desensitization at the cellular level is perhaps different from that proposed earlier at a phenomenologic level. We will examine the differences between cellular "activation" and the actual triggering of a cellular response.

Leukocyte responsiveness to the anaphylatoxins far exceeds just the chemotactic event. Recent evidence identifies specific ligand interactions that exist between anaphylatoxins and the neutrophils (Chenoweth and Hugli, 1978), the eosinophils (Kay *et al.*, 1973; Glovsky *et al.*, 1979), and the basophils (Siraganian and Hook, 1976; Glovsky *et al.*, 1979), each with its own characteristic activation profile. Far too little is known about the interplay between mediators released from these various cell types after activation has occurred. However, we know that the patterns of response to C3a are quite distinct from those to C5a for each of the different cell types. Indeed, our challenge for the future is to fully characterize responses of each individual cell type to the complement mediators and to interpret these effects in meaningful physiologic terms.

What has clearly been shown is that anaphylatoxins are important mediators in host-defense mechanisms involving the leukocyte. The role of these humoral factors appears to extend well beyond cell recruitment and activation phenomena. Anaphylatoxins may funcion at an even more complex level of cellular interplay involving networks of cell-derived mediators.

Until recently, lymphocytes were excluded from consideration as a cell type showing significant responsiveness to the anaphylatoxins. This oversight has been remedied by recent evidence of a potentially important role for factors C3a and C5a in immunoregulation. Current concepts of the role and mechanisms of anaphylatoxin involvement in the immune response are outlined in Section IV. The C3a anaphylatoxin elicits immune suppressive responses in *in vitro* assays, while C5a proves to enhance the cellular immune response. A physiologic equivalent to these recently discovered functions of anaphylatoxins in immune regulation is yet to be discerned.

A brief discussion of a unique complement-derived factor, called C3d-K, has been included. It has long been known that a fragment or fragments from C3 was capable of suppressing T-cell proliferative responses and that another fragment, called C3e, produces leukocytosis in a rabbit model. We propose that a single fragment, designated C3d-K, contains the molecular portion of C3 responsible for both activities and thereby identifies yet another factor derived from complement that regulates leukocyte function.

Consequently, these many activities for C3a, C5a, and other C3 fragments are undeniable evidence for signal mechanisms between complement and the immune system that have previously been unappreciated, uncharacterized, or have gone largely unrecognized. There promises to be a regulatory loop for modulating lymphocytic host-defense mechanisms controlled by these various products of the complement system. Consequently, elucidation of the physiologic role of complement must include an understanding of how these humoral factors are involved in immunomodulation.

II. NEUTROPHIL ACTIVATION EVENTS INDUCED BY THE ANAPHYLATOXINS

A. Chemotaxis and Chemokinesis

Various forms of cellular motility are described as locomotion. However, the specialized movement of leukocytes stimulated by external factors generally falls into one of two classes—either chemotaxis or chemokinesis—the distinction being that chemotaxis is directed or "smart" locomotion toward or away from a gradient, whereas chemokinesis is an enhanced rate of locomotion that lacks discernible purpose or direction. Since chemotactic factors stimulate directional locomotion, it does matter how they are presented to the cells. Factors may be chemokinetic and yet unable to elicit a chemotactic response. Other substances may induce both chemotactic and chemokinetic responses from the neutrophil. Numerous reviews on the subject now exist, including those by Wilkinson (1974), Ward and Becker (1976), Zigmond (1980), and Gallin and Quie (1978).

We will focus here on only the migratory behavior of the leukocytes and monocytes in response to the complement-derived factors C3a or C5a. One very basic aspect to motility of the white blood cell that must be emphasized is the fact that these cells crawl or glide over a surface during migration and are not free-swimming cells as are bacteria. In this respect, the usual substrate or surfaces over which these cells climb are other cells such as endothelial cells, epithelial cells, or basement membrane (Shaw *et al.*, 1980).

Several approaches have been developed to monitor cellular migration *in vitro* of which two have found general acceptance. One method relies on a two-chamber apparatus designed by Boyden (1962) and later adapted and modified by other investigators (Gallin *et al.*, 1973; Gallin and Quie, 1978). By adding the stimulant in one chamber and the cells in another separated by a porous filter, a gradient can be temporarily established, so that directed migration into or through the filter may be assessed. A second method was designed to measure the migration of cells over the surface of a petri dish or microscope slide using agarose as the template into which wells are punched to accommodate the cells and reagents. This method was first described in detail by Cutler (1974). Later adaptations by Nelson *et al.* (1975), Orr and Ward (1978), and Chenoweth *et al.* (1979) were added to improve the procedure operationally. Both methods of assessing chemotaxis suffer from limitations. Perhaps the two most serious problems are an inability to assess the proportion of cells responding and a failure of either approach to definitively distinguish chemotaxis from chemokinesis. The former effect can be determined using a technique that measures the distance that each cell migrates as devised by Maderazo and Woronich (1978). The latter deficiency is circumvented using the method of Zigmond and Hirsch (1973) to differentiate between directed migration and chemokinetic events.

Evidence that chemotactic factors are generated during activation of the complement system (Ward *et al.*, 1965, 1967) prompted an interest in complement products as factors governing cellular sequestration at inflammatory sites. Initially it was believed that the activation fragment C3a, from the third component of complement, possessed potent chemotactic activity originally observed in complement-activated serum (Ward, 1967; Bokisch *et al.*, 1969). Later, however, it became clear that the more potent chemotactic factor for neutrophils was the activation factor from C5, the C5a molecule. It was the observation of Shin *et al.* (1968), Snyderman *et al.* (1969), and Jensen *et al.* (1969), working with guinea pig components, that identified the anaphylatoxic fragment from C5 as chemotactic. Shortly thereafter, the corresponding chemotactic fragment from human C5 was described and partially characterized (Ward and Newman, 1969). Human and porcine C5a was first isolated from whole serum by Vallota and co-workers (Vallota and Müller-Eberhard, 1973; Vallota *et al.*, 1973) in quantities that permitted chemical analysis. He activated complement in fresh serum containing ε-aminocaproic acid (6-aminohexanoic acid), an inhibitor used for the purpose of generating intact anaphylatoxins by blocking an endogenous carboxypeptidase known as anaphylatoxin inactivator or serum carboxypeptidase N (Bokisch and Müller-Eberhard, 1970; Plummer and Hurwitz, 1978). Before this innovation was introduced to the field, intact anaphylatoxins could not be recovered directly from complement-activated serum, since the des Arg form of these molecules was rapidly formed by the endogenous carboxypeptidase. Using modifications of Vallota's isolation scheme, we later isolated the anaphylatoxins and elucidated the complete chemical structures of the human C5a (Fernandez and Hugli, 1976, 1978) and porcine C5a (Gerard and Hugli, 1979, 1980).

It was this chemical analysis of the chemotactic factors that led to an explanation of the significant functional differences between human $C5a_{des\ Arg}$ and the des Arg forms of C5a from certain experimental animals. The spasmogen activity of porcine $C5a_{des\ Arg}$ is 100 to 1000 times greater than that of human $C5a_{des\ Arg}$ (Gerard and Hugli, 1981). Since human C5a contains a bulky oligosaccharide group and C5a from such animals as rats and pigs is devoid of carbohydrate, we suspected that this structural variation might be responsible for observed differences in the spasmogenic and chemotactic behavior of human and animal C5a. Indeed we showed that removal of the complex oligosaccharide unit increased both the spasmogenic and chemotactic activities of human $C5a_{des\ Arg}$ (Gerard and Hugli, 1981; Gerard et al., 1981).

Purified human components C3a, C5a, and $C5a_{des\ Arg}$ have been assayed in the Boyden system using human neutrophils; C5a is active between the concentrations of 1×10^{-10} M to 4×10^{-8} M, while $C5a_{des\ Arg}$ is active between 2×10^{-9} M to 2×10^{-7} M. Under the same conditions, C3a fails to express activity at concentrations from 1×10^{-10} to 8×10^{-6} M. The C3a anaphylatoxin does not exhibit significant chemotactic activity at potential physiologic levels using the in vitro assay procedures. Although C5a is active in buffer alone, the des Arg form of C5a requires small quantities of fresh human serum to express activity. Similar behavior was reported earlier by Wissler et al. (1972) for porcine $C5a_{des\ Arg}$. In their report a cofactor was described called cocytotaxin, an 8500 M_r cationic polypeptide said to associate with the anaphylatoxin $C5a_{des\ Arg}$ to form an active binary complex. As in our results using the Boyden assay, Wissler claims that the anaphylatoxin by itself is not active. Unfortunately, chemical characterization of the "cocytotaxin" or "leukotactic helper factor" was not provided in sufficient detail to assess properly the merit of the extensive study by Wissler et al. Later attempts to isolate the chemotactic helper factor have been made, and recent evidence indicates that an anionic protein of 60,000 M_r serves this helper role (Perez et al., 1980).

Chemotaxis as monitored by the Boyden chamber assay gives a clear indication that serum is required for $C5a_{des\ Arg}$-induced chemotaxis. Alternatively, it has been shown that both C5a and $C5a_{des\ Arg}$ are potent chemotaxins in the absence of cofactors when assessed by the chemotaxis-under-agarose technique. This procedure was modified by Chenoweth et al. (1979) to use a microscope slide for the surface on which the stimulated cells may attach and crawl. In addition, gelatin was substituted for the serum, which presumably acts as a lubricant to decrease adherence between the cell and the surface so that the cells more readily detach and migrate. This observation does not prove that helper factor functions only to diminish neutrophil adherence in vivo. However, the fact is that under certain conditions $C5a_{des\ Arg}$ exhibits chemotactic activity in the absence of other serum proteins. This establishes that the physiologic des Arg form of the complement-derived chemotactic factor C5a is intrinsically active. The ability of $C5a_{des\ Arg}$ to promote neutrophil migration in vivo may indeed be facilitated or amplified by other components in serum; however, the chemo-tactic effector signal is mediated by the anaphylatoxin. Whether serum factor(s) potentiate(s) $C5a_{des\ Arg}$ activity by acting as a true cofactor, as Wissler *et al.* (1972) proposes, or by simply altering adherent behavior between the neutrophil and surfaces over which they crawl, is yet to be determined.

Without doubt there are modulatory molecules in serum that appear to in-fluence the functional expression of $C5a_{des\ Arg}$ as a chemotactic factor. Definition of the precise physicochemical nature of the helper factor(s) remains somewhat obscure, as does the means by which it enhances the chemoattractant capabilities of the $C5a_{des\ Arg}$. Indeed, the fact that intact C5a has no requirement for a helper factor in either of these *in vitro* assays remains an unexplained paradox.

The molecular entity C5a and derivatives of C5a have been characterized with respect to their ability to promote chemotaxis (Chenoweth and Hugli, 1980a). Using the chemotaxis-under-agarose method, a chemotactic index (CI) was determined for human C5a, $C5a_{des\ Arg}$, C5a 1-69, and the COOH-terminal pentapeptide of C5a, Met-Gln-Leu-Gly-Arg.* Table I summarizes the chemotactic

Table I. Chemotactic Response of Human Neutrophils to Human C5a and Selected C5a Derivatives

Materials	ED_{50}[a] (M)	CI[b]
Human C5a	$1-3 \times 10^{-9}$	2.3 ± 0.2
Human $C5a_{des\ Arg}$	$1-5 \times 10^{-8}$	3.1 ± 0.2
Human C5a (1-69)[c]	$>5 \times 10^{-6}$	0
Met-Gln-Leu-Gly-Arg[d] (70) (74)	$>5 \times 10^{-6}$	0

[a] ED_{50}, half-maximal neutrophil response.
[b] CI, chemotactic index is the quotion of directed migration divided by random migration.
[c] The derivative C5a (1-69) is a 69-residue enzymatic end product formed by digesting $C5a_{des\ Arg}$ with yeast carboxy-peptidase to remove residues 70-73.
[d] Met-Gln-Leu-Gly-Arg represents residues 70-74, the C-terminal pentapeptide from human C5a.

---

*Fragments of the anaphylatoxins or synthetic peptides based on the sequence of these natural factors are designated by identifying first the factor and then the numbers corre-sponding to residues within the linear sequence. For example, C3a 1-77 and C5a 1-74 represent the intact factors C3a and C5a anaphylatoxins.

responses of human neutrophils stimulated by these various factors. Human C5a and C5a$_{des\ Arg}$ were the only molecular forms that behaved as chemotaxins. The des Arg derivative of C5a actually stimulates cells to migrate over a greater distance, while C5a stimulates migration at a lower effective concentration. Both C5a and C5a$_{des\ Arg}$ desensitize neutrophils (e.g., inhibit migration) at elevated concentrations. However, the derivatives C5a 1-69 and the pentapeptide Met-Gln-Leu-Gly-Arg, either individually or in combination, fail to exhibit activity at concentrations 100- to 1000-fold higher than those required to induce migration by C5a or C5a$_{des\ Arg}$. We interpreted these results to indicate that an essential role is played by residues at the COOH-terminal end of the C5a molecule. Although arginine may be removed and 5%-10% of initial activity survives, removal of four additional residues apparently eliminates all activity of the chemotaxin. Since the COOH-terminal segment Met-Gln-Leu-Gly-Arg also fails to stimulate neutrophil migration, it is concluded that structural integrity of the C5a molecule dictates functional expression, but that the active center of the molecule is nevertheless located at the COOH-terminus.

A further complexity exists in understanding the chemotactic expression of the human C5a molecule, which involves the oligosaccharide unit. Unlike C5a from porcine, rat, and presumably other animal species, the human molecule is a glycopolypeptide. Removal of the oligosaccharide unit actually enhances activity of C5a$_{des\ Arg}$ as previously mentioned, but has no effect on C5a. Since the complex carbohydrate exerts its effect primarily on the spasmogenic activity of C5a$_{des\ Arg}$ rather than on chemotaxis, attachment of a sugar moiety can be considered as a post-translational modification that is advantageous to the host.

In order to summarize the status of the C5a chemotaxin in promoting neutrophil migratory behavior, one must consider a variety of mechanisms. Figure 1 presents a model illustrating the presently known influences of chemotaxins on neutrophil migration and modulators that act in concert with the humoral factor C5a. Upon complement activation the C5a is generated, and conversion to the des Arg form occurs within seconds by action of the endogenous carboxypeptidase. Under normal circumstances it is difficult to imagine that a gradient of the intact factor ever exists; however, a transient wave of C5a may suffice to stimulate migration of cells proximal to the site of activation. *In vitro*, C5a concentrations $> 10^{-8}$ *M* cause paralysis of the cells, a phenomenon often described as desensitization. It is unlikely that effective C5a concentrations $> 10^{-8}$ *M* would ever be attained *in vivo*. The predominant molecular species *in vivo* is believed to be C5a$_{des\ Arg}$, a form that is perhaps potentiated by a serum cofactor or helper factor to stimulate cellular migration. Since C5a$_{des\ Arg}$ fails to desensitize neutrophils *in vitro* at a maximal potential serum concentration of 3-5 $\times$ 10^{-7} *M*, desensitization may be largely a laboratory phenomenon experienced by cells in nature only under unusual pathologic conditions.

COMPLEMENT ACTIVATION

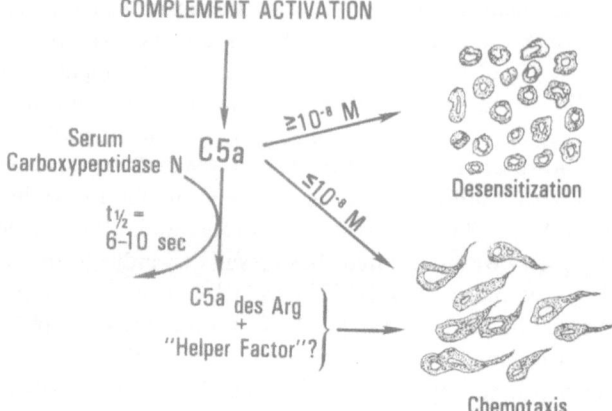

Figure 1. Schematic illustration showing influences of humoral chemotactic factor C5a on neutrophil migration. Complement activation leads to C5a formation. A competition then exists between the enzymatic conversion of C5a to C5a$_{des\ Arg}$ and binding of the C5a ligand to the leukocyte ($K_b \approx 10^{-8}\,M$). Exposure of leukocytes to C5a at concentrations $>10^{-8}\,M$ leads to immobilization, or desensitization. These immobilized cells are metabolically activated and undergo normal release reactions. The carboxypeptidase product C5a$_{des\ Arg}$, in association with a serum helper factor, is almost as potent a chemotactic factor *in vitro* as is C5a.

B. Aggregation and Release Phenomena

A prerequisite for neutrophil chemotaxis is adherence to a surface. Usually this surface would be vascular endothelium under normal *in vivo* conditions. The mechanisms that convert granulocytes from the usual circulating spheroid cells to irregular amoeboid-like cells having enhanced adhesive properties are not fully understood. What is clearly observed is that granulocytes exposed to either C5a or C5a$_{des\ Arg}$ undergo transformation from normal spheroid cells to activated cells that are especially sticky or adherent. These activated cells not only adhere to surfaces but readily aggregate into clumps (Craddock *et al.*, 1977a). Early work in the field was largely inferential concerning leukocyte aggregation induced by factor C5a. Reviews describing the adherent behavior of granulocytes induced as a consequence of complement activation, and more specifically as dependent on the component C5, have recently been written by Craddock *et al.* (1979) and by O'Flaherty and Ward (1978). A characteristic of C5a-induced aggregation of granulocytes is the reversibility of the phenomenon.

Methods currently used to monitor granulocyte aggregation include particle measurements with a Coulter counter to estimate changes in either particle concentration (Lackie, 1977) or particle volume (O'Flaherty *et al.*, 1977a). This approach can be misleading, since the chemotactic factor C5a causes the cells to adhere to the walls of the assay chamber and to the sampling chamber, resulting in overestimates of aggregation (e.g., underestimates of particle concentration due to adherent losses). Although volume changes or swelling of the cells are independent of aggregation phenomena, these two responses to stimuli have often been used interchangeably to indicate enhanced adherent behavior of the granulocytes.

A separate method of detecting granulocyte aggregation is to use the conventional platelet aggregometer. Increased light transmission through the cellular suspension is interpreted as aggregation (Craddock *et al.*, 1976, 1977*b*) and provides a facile *in vitro* test of altered cellular adhesiveness.

A number of variables influence the degree of granulocyte aggregation. One important variable appears to be species differences: the rabbit polymorphonuclear leukocyte (PMN) undergoes spontaneous aggregation more readily than does the human PMN (O'Flaherty and Ward, 1978). Methods of isolation can also alter PMN aggregating ability. For instance, PMNs isolated by Ficoll-Hypaque sedimentation are less readily aggregated by chemotactic stimuli than are cells obtained by dextran sedimentation (O'Flaherty *et al.*, 1978).

Temperature is an important variable, since the aggregation phenomenon is decreased if the temperature is reduced significantly below $37°C$. This response suggests a metabolic dependency on cell aggregation that is further supported by requirements for Mg^{2+} and Ca^{2+} or by the fact that inhibitors of glycolysis such as deoxyglucose or iodoacetate prevent chemotactic factor-induced aggregation (O'Flaherty *et al.*, 1977*b*). Numerous drugs affect granulocyte aggregation, of which perhaps the fungal metabolite cytochalasin B has been given the most attention. Unexpected results were obtained when cytochalasin B-treated granulocytes were stimulated by C5a. These cells do not develop pseudopods or undergo the usual swelling or amoeboid shape transformation; nevertheless, they do undergo aggregation. Moreover, the aggregation is more pronounced and, unlike that of untreated granulocytes, is irreversible (Craddock *et al.*, 1978).

Although blebs and plasma membrane invaginations are observed in cytochalasin B-treated granulocytes after stimulation by C5a, no dramatic increase in plasma membrane surface area is seen. Consequently, expansion of membrane surface alone does not appear to account for increased adhesiveness of the stimulated granulocyte. Other parameters such as surface charge have been reported to change when granulocytes are stimulated by C5a. Gallin *et al.* (1975) showed that the surface charge of stimulated granulocytes is less anionic than that of unstimulated cells, perhaps reducing the electrostatic repulsion between cells. Ultimately, the mechanism for cell adhesion in granulocytes must be reduced to an interaction between cellular constituents that are intrinsically sticky for surfaces or other cells. These substances may be secreted glycoproteins, such as fibronectins, or components in perturbed or disoriented plasma membrane, such

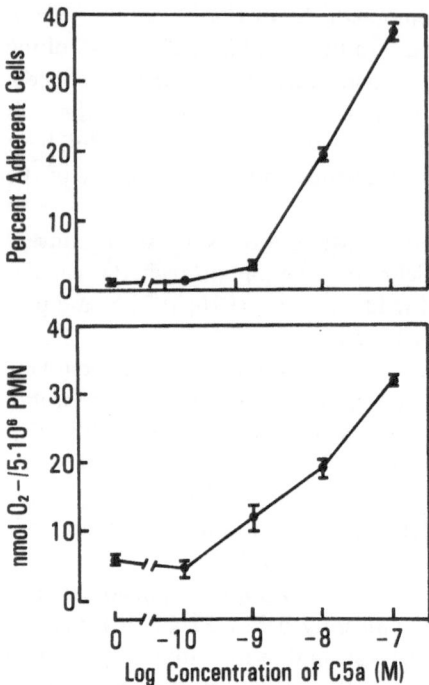

Figure 2. Evidence is given that C5a-induced adherence of neutrophils correlates with the release of superoxide ion from these cells. Adherence occurs in a dose-dependent manner when polymorphonuclear leukocytes (PMNs) are incubated in plastic Petri dishes for 40 min at 37°C after a pretreatment with various concentrations of C5a at 0°C. Superoxide production was measured as a function of C5a concentration using a separate fraction of the PMN. (Adapted from Dahinden et al., 1983.)

as lipoproteins. Both materials could meet the criteria for reversibility, one by dissociation from the cell surface and the other by local membrane reorganization.

Studies concerning C5a-induced granulocyte aggregation are extensive; however, none was performed with purified components so that the quantitative impact of the humoral chemotactic factor could be assessed. To the extent that cell–cell aggregation and cell–surface adherence correlate, a study has been performed to determine the dose response of cell adherence to C5a (Fig. 2). Human PMNs begin adhering to a plastic surface in the presence of 10^{-9} M C5a, and 40% of the cell population attaches to the surface as the C5a concentration approaches 10^{-7} M (Dahinden et al., 1983). Chemotaxis is promoted by C5a at approximately a 10-fold lower concentration than is adherence. In fact, maximal adhesiveness is observed at C5a concentrations that inhibit cellular migration. Although this phenomenon has been referred to as desensitization, it may actually result from cells attaching too tightly to the support to permit detachment and migration.

The phenomenon of complement-induced leukocyte aggregation has apparent clinical manifestations. Acute leukopenia is observed in patients undergoing hemodialysis; the cause associated with a transient disappearance of granulocytes from circulation was identified as C5a dependent (Craddock et al., 1977a, b). Similarly, other forms of extracorporeal blood treatment such as leukapheresis

(Hammerschmidt *et al.*, 1978) and exposure to materials in the pump oxygenator during cardiopulmonary bypass (Chenoweth *et al.*, 1981) lead to significant levels of complement activation. This extracorporeal activation of the complement cascade results in C5a formation, which in turn promotes neutropenia caused by a pulmonary-vascular leukostasis that occurs when the blood re-enters circulation.

Correspondingly, it is now believed that C5a exacerbates pulmonary dysfunction in some forms of acute respiratory distress (Hammerschmidt *et al.*, 1980). A major pathologic event in patients experiencing adult respiratory distress syndrome (ARDS) or "shock lung" is microvascular stasis caused by granulocyte aggregation. These pateients all have serious ongoing underlying disease processes such as sepsis or severe trauma that may predispose massive complement activation. The resultant damage transmitted to the lungs of persons whose neutrophil pool is activated by circulating C5a (C5a$_{des\ Arg}$) is far from characterized. However, one may suspect that the tissue damage caused by leukostasis is only a part of the injury mediated by the activated cells. The C5a-stimulated PMNs are also capable of releasing toxic oxygen products (Sacks *et al.*, 1978), numerous enzymes, and arachidonate metabolites (Stimler *et al.*, 1982) that contribute to both the extent and severity of tissue damage in these persons.

C. Receptors and Ligand Processing

Receptors for the anaphylatoxins on leukocytes remain poorly characterized. The neutrophil is the only cell type for which convincing evidence has been obtained that a specific and saturable receptor exists for the anaphylatoxins. The only ligand that has been examined carefully using human cells is the human C5a molecule (Chenoweth and Hugli, 1978). Other studies have demonstrated anaphylatoxin receptors on mast cells (ter Laan *et al.*, 1974; Johnson *et al.*, 1975), and a putative receptor for C3a was identified on vascular endothelial cells (Denny and Johnson, 1979).

Uptake studies using the radioligands [^{125}I]-C3a and [^{125}I]-C5a have implicated that differential binding patterns exist on leukocytes for these two complement factors (Glovsky *et al.*, 1979). The C3a ligand binds preferentially to eosinophils with moderate uptake by basophils, neutrophils, and monocytes, while C5a binds preferentially to neutrophils with lesser binding to eosinophils, basophils, and monocytes (Table II). The ligand uptake studies give little indication that a significant interaction may exist between the anaphylatoxins and lymphocytes. However, functional studies (see Section IV) now suggest that a select subpopulation of T cells may indeed have C3a and C5a receptors.

Structure–function studies of the anaphylatoxins have resulted in a seemingly valid conceptual model of the active center in C3a and a hypothetical model for the more complex C5a–receptor interaction. Conformational studies of C3a in-

Table II. Binding of Radiolabeled C3a and C5a to
Human Leukocytes[a]

Cell type	C3a (%)	C5a (%)
Eosinophils	99	66
Neutrophils	31	99
Basophils	45	36
Monocytes	19	35
Lymphocytes	2	2

[a] Binding was evaluated by autoradiography and the data represents an average from three individual donors. The percentage of each cell type containing >10 grains/cell were calculated from a total of 200–500 cells. (Adapted from Glovsky et al., 1979.)

dicate the molecular folding is important for optimal activity (Hugli et al., 1975). However, a series of investigations with synthetic peptides, based on the sequence of human C3a, have established that the active site is located in a linear C-terminal portion of the molecule (Caporale et al., 1980; Hugli and Erickson, 1977). More recent studies appear to explain the reason for these two seemingly divergent observations. Although the minimal active site of C3a is clearly represented by a simple pentapeptide, Leu-Gly-Leu-Ala-Arg, this pentapeptide is only 0.2% as active as native C3a. We initially proposed that in the native folded conformation of C3a the active site portion assumes a favorable configuration for interacting with the C3a receptor on cells. Conversely, the more flexible pentapeptide may spend relatively little time in the appropriate conformation for binding to the receptor and is therefore less effective on a molar basis. Since the C-terminal portion of C3a adjacent to the active site assumes an α-helical conformation, it may be this folding arrangement that dictates a favorable orientation of the pentapeptide side chains, thereby optimizing receptor binding. Keeping this hypothesis in mind, we examined the activity of a 21-residue synthetic C3a peptide (C3a 57–77, a peptide based on human C3a structure) that contains the α-helical portion of the C-terminal end of the molecule (Huber et al., 1980). The synthetic peptide C3a 57–77 was found to exhibit activity nearly equivalent to that of intact C3a for inducing smooth muscle contraction (Huey et al., 1984) and for suppressing the immune response (Morgan et al., 1983c). In addition, we found that the synthetic peptide C3a 57–77 was easily induced into a helical conformation by adding trifluoroethanol, an agent used to promote helix formation of polypeptides in aqueous solution (Fig. 3). Taken together, these data suggest that although the active site residues in C3a are contained in the linear sequence Leu-Gly-Leu-Ala-Arg, folding of the adjacent peptide sequence into an α-helix may direct side chain orientation in the acitve site and thereby promote receptor binding.

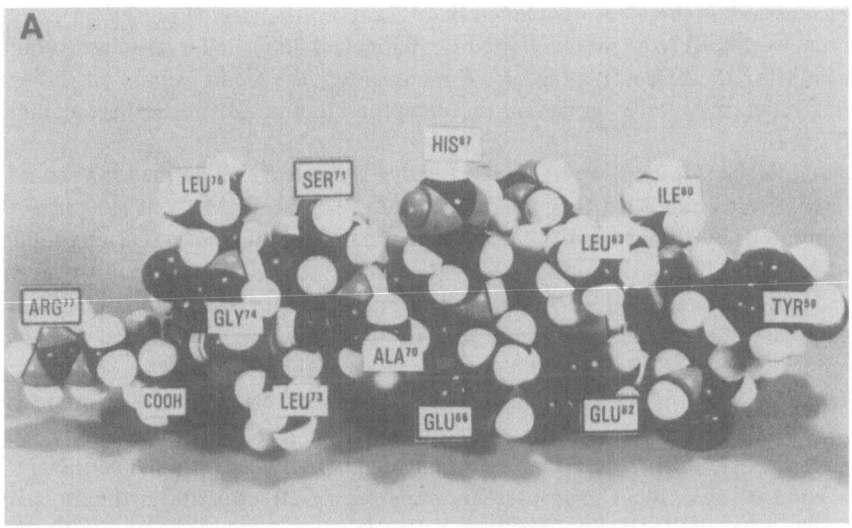

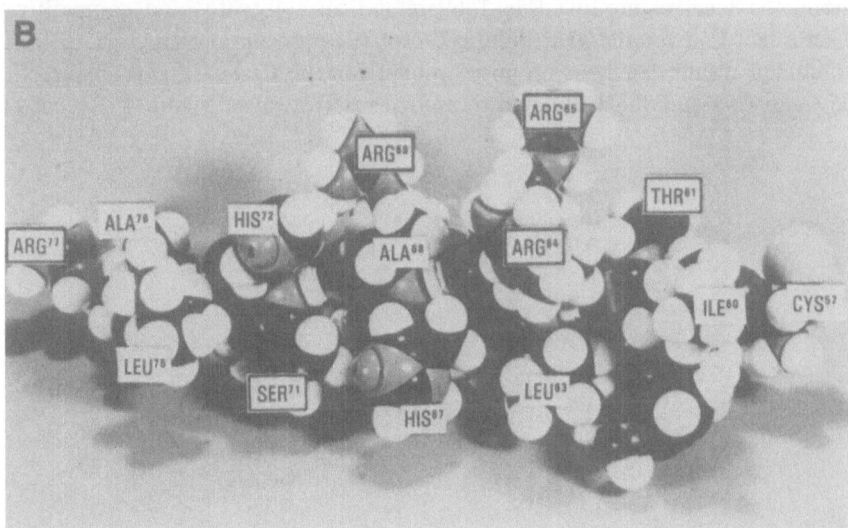

Figure 3. A space-filling model of the 21-residue peptide C3a 57–77. The peptide has been folded in an α-helical conformation with the C-terminus (Arg 77) to the left. (A) Orientation with a largely hydrophobic surface; (B) hydrophilic arginine cluster on the helical surface. The helical conformation of C3a 57–77 was based on the circular dichroism spectra of the peptide obtained in 12 percent trifluoroethanol and the X-ray structural analysis of crystalline human C3a. Hydrophilic residues are identified by black-bordered boxes.

The biological activity of the synthetic C3a analogue C3a 57–77 was measured in several assay systems, and activity was equivalent to that obtained with C3a in each case. It is therefore concluded that C3a receptors located on the various cell types examined (e.g., mast cells and lymphocytes) have similar structural requirements for the effector molecule. Consequently, the C3a receptor on different cell types may vary; however, the receptor binding site must share common features.

Molecular description of the C5a active site is less well defined than that for C3a. It was established that the active center of C5a, like C3a, is located at the C-terminus by studies utilizing carboxypeptidases to obtain degradation products from both human and porcine C5a (Gerard *et al.*, 1979). End-point digestion products human C5a 1–69 and porcine C5a 1–70 were recovered after carboxypeptidase Y treatment. Human C5a 1–69 was less than 1% as active as the 73-residue human $C5a_{des\,Arg}$ molecule for both chemotactic and spasmogenic behavior. In comparison, porcine C5a 1–70 was inactive as a spasmogen but retains 85% of the chemotactic activity exhibited by the 73-residue porcine $C5a_{des\,Arg}$ molecule. From these results it was concluded that the C-terminal pentapeptide portion of C5a, like C3a, represents the essential effector site in the molecule. Unlike C3a, the C-terminal arginine in C5a is not essential for activity. Furthermore, the inactive product C5a 1–69 retains an ability to bind competitively with intact C5a for the neutrophil receptor (Chenoweth and Hugli, 1978). The combined results led to a proposed model for the ligand–receptor interaction between C5a and the leukocyte receptor as portrayed in Figure 4. Recent evi-

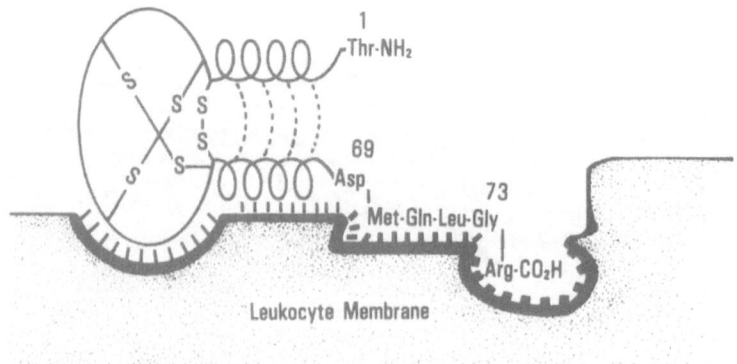

Figure 4. A proposed model for the C5a–receptor interaction on the leukocyte surface. Features include the arginine binding site adjacent to a binding site for the essential C-terminal residues Met-Gln-Leu-Gly. An additional ligand binding site is located amino terminal to Met 70 based on the competitive binding of C5a 1–69. Relative contribution of the various ligand interactions is portrayed by the intensity of the lines between the C5a molecule and the receptor surface. A weak interaction is suggested between the NH_2- and COOH-terminal helices and may explain the activity loss that accompanies removal of the amino terminal residues 1–20.

dence by Damerau *et al.* (1983) shows that removal of 18–20 residues from the NH_2-terminus of porcine C5a also inactivates the molecules. Although it is not believed that the effector site resides in the NH_2-terminal portion of this molecule, these data suggest that in the folded molecule the NH_2-terminal portion exerts an important influence on presentation of the COOH-terminal effector site to the receptor.

Events occurring after the anaphylatoxins interact with surface receptors have been studied in detail regarding cellular phenomenology; however, ligand processing has drawn less attention. One indirect study with C3a was reported using rat mast cells as the target (ter Laan *et al.*, 1974). When C3a was presented to rat mast cells producing degranulation, no C3a antigen was detected on the cell surface. However, if degranulation prevented by adding EDTA or disodium cromoglycate, then spots of C3a were detected on the cell surface by indirect immunofluorescence. The interpretation by the investigator was that degranulation leads to release of the ligand from the cellular surface. Unfortunately these experiments need to be repeated using radiolabeled ligands in order to appraise the fate of the receptor-bound effector molecule accurately.

A thorough study of the fate of C5a on the human neutrophil was performed by D. E. Chenoweth (unpublished results). These studies have shown that C5a is taken up by the neutrophil in a time-dependent and saturable manner. Binding of C5a maximizes in 5–10 min at 37°C. At 37°C the C5a binds and tends not to be released from the cells, but is transferred from the membrane to the cell cytosol. After 120-min exposure of the cells to $[^{125}I]$-C5a, more than 65% of the ligand has been internalized, degraded to low-molecular-weight material believed to be monoiodotyrosine, and expelled to the supernatant. This mobilization of ligand is an energy-dependent process and results in a transient downregulation of receptors, where 90–99% of the cell's capacity to bind C5a is lost after exposure to 10^{-7} M ligand.

It should be emphasized that processing subnanomolar quantities of C5a may occur efficiently *in vivo* without producing significant receptor downregulation due to the large neutrophil pool and the high affinity between C5a and the receptor. Correspondingly, neutrophils must be exposed to relatively larger quantities of the C5a$_{des Arg}$ ligand (e.g., 10^{-8} M) in order to cause comparable downregulation, since C5a$_{des Arg}$ binds to the neutrophil receptor with less affinity than does C5a. The ID_{50} for human C5a and C5a$_{des Arg}$ binding to human neutrophils is 1–3 nM and 420 nM, respectively, (Gerard *et al.*, 1981), and C5a$_{desArg}$ fails to exhibit detectable biological activity at concentrations of $<10^{-8}$ M. Consequently, we conclude that three parameters will influence downregulation of neutrophils by C5a *in vivo:* (1) the rate of C5 conversion, (2) the extent of conversion, and (3) the effective competition between C5a conversion to C5a$_{des Arg}$ by carboxypeptidase N and direct binding of C5a to the neutrophil. *In vitro* binding studies indicate that C5a$_{des Arg}$ should cause no more than 50% downregulation of neutrophils *in vivo* based on ED_{50} and ID_{50} values of 1–4×10^{-7} M and on a maximal serum C5a$_{des Arg}$ concentration in the same range. What is yet to be determined is the extent to which the transient, but more active, C5a influences receptor downregulation of neutrophils under *in vivo* conditions.

Finally, it must be recognized that downregulation is expressed at the receptor level by reduced ligand binding and at the behavioral level by a decrease in chemotactic responsiveness. These cells appear to be desensitized to the stimulant when measuring migrating activity. However, when these same cells come into contact with a surface, they behave metabolically like normal activated phagocytes releasing enzymes, arachidonate products, and toxic oxygen metabolites (Dahinden *et al.*, 1983).

D. Regulatory Mechanisms

Regulation of the effector function of anaphylatoxins can occur at three levels, according to current understanding of this humoral mediator system. The first level is the serum inactivator system, which involves enzymatic removal of an arginyl residue from the C-terminus of the respective anaphylatoxin molecule. This mechanism is highly efficient, since cleavage occurs in seconds and removal of a COOH-terminal arginine from either C3a or C4a irreversibly inactivates these factors. However, enzymatic cleavage of arginine from C5a by serum carboxypeptidase (carboxypeptidase N, EC 3.4.12.7) fails to eliminate activity. Removal of the COOH-terminal arginine from human C5a significantly reduces its ability to promote spasmogenic responses; however, the $C5a_{des\,Arg}$ retains the capacity to stimulate leukocyte function. Because $C5a_{des\,Arg}$ retains significant residual chemotactic activity, alternative regulatory mechanisms must exist to control this function of the anaphylatoxin.

The second level of regulation focuses on modulation of $C5a_{des\,Arg}$ activity, the putative physiologic species of C5a. This form of control is manifest at the cellular level as desensitization. It has long been recognized that at elevated concentrations the chemotactic factor C5a prevents leukocyte migration (Fernandez *et al.*, 1978). The mechanism appears simply to involve receptor saturation coupled with a downregulation of receptor expression. The resultant effect is to paralyze the cells for migration or to desensitize the cells to effector stimulation, a beautifully subtle means of damping the cellular response. Other leukocyte responses, such as enzyme release, oxygen radical production, and arachidonate metabolism, are not affected by desensitization. Therefore, a third mechanism of control is required to limit these inflammatory responses. The third control mechanism is also mediated at the cellular level and involves intracellular processing of the C5a molecule. It has been demonstrated that the C5a (or $C5a_{des\,Arg}$), once bound to the leukocyte receptor, can be internalized, degraded, and expelled

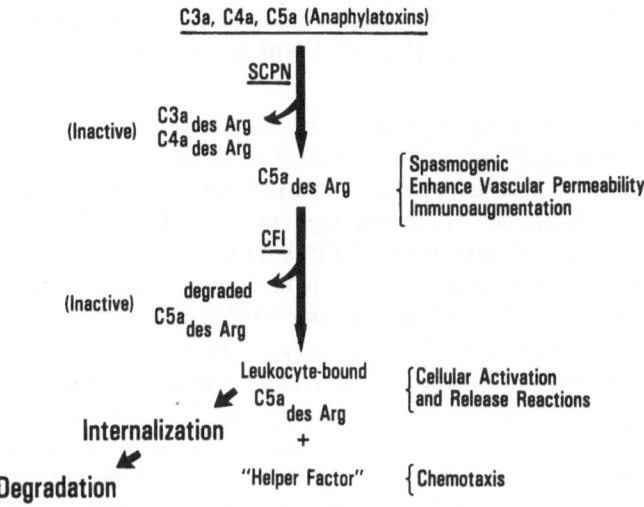

Figure 5. Various regulatory mechanisms believed to exert an influence on anaphylatoxin function *in vivo*. SCPN, serum carboxypeptidase N; CFI, chemotactic factor inactivator.

from the cell in an inactive form (Chenoweth and Hugli, 1980b). This control mechanism serves as an effective means of removing C5a or $C5a_{des\,Arg}$ from blood and preventing an accumulation of the stimulator *in vivo*.

Other mechanisms of control have been suggested that relate primarily to the chemotactic activity of the anaphylatoxin. Among these are modulatory plasma components such as the chemotactic factor inactivator (CFI) (Berenberg and Ward, 1973; Till and Ward, 1975). The inactivator CFI is believed to inactivate C5a by a proteolytic mechanism. This inactivator of C5a occurs in patients with pathological conditions such as Hodgkin's disease (Ward and Berenberg, 1974), hepatic cirrhosis (Maderazo et al., 1975), sarcoidosis (Maderazo et al, 1976), and lepromatous leprosy (Ward et al., 1976). However, the CFI in normal serum has no influence on the activity of $C5a_{des\,Arg}$ when measured in *in vitro* chemotactic assays.

A helper factor exists in plasma that modulates the chemotactic activity of the des Arg form of C5a by elevating it to a level comparable to that exhibited by intact C5a in a serum-free system. The helper factor is an anionic polypeptide that presumably complexes with the cationic C5a molecule (Beebe et al., 1980; Perez et al., 1980) and is potentially of major importance in the physiological expression of $C5a_{des\,Arg}$ chemotactic activity. Figure 5 summarizes the various regulatory mechanisms of the anaphylatoxins that are believed to be operative *in vivo*.

III. ANAPHYLATOXIN INTERACTIONS WITH EOSINOPHILS, BASOPHILS, AND MACROPHAGES

Studies characterizing interactions of the anaphylatoxins with cell types other than neutrophils are quite limited. Most of the evidence that a receptor-dependent interaction exists between anaphylatoxins and cells such as eosinophils, basophils, and monocytes is indirect. Our current evidence is based primarily on the ability of these effector molecules to bind to the cells in question (Glovsky *et al.*, 1979) and to elicit cell-specific chemotactic migration. For instance, the work of Kay *et al.* (1973) clearly demonstrated that C5a stimulates eosinophil chemotaxis. In addition, it was shown that a synergy exists between C5a and a low-molecular-weight eosinophil chemotactic factor (ECF-A) derived from ana-phylactic lung diffusate obtained from guinea pigs. At higher than normal physiologic ratios of eosinophils to neutrophils (e.g., >9%), C5a preferentially attracts the eosinophil, indicating that neutrophils may exert a negative influence on migration of the eosinophil. There is no convincing evidence that C3a is chemotactic for eosinophils; however, C3a does cause degranulation of these cells and, according to the binding studies of Glovsky *et al.* (1979), all eosinophils have receptors for C3a.

Human basophils respond chemotactically to C5a (Boetcher and Leonard, 1973; Ward *et al.*, 1975), this response is augmented by a chemotactic factor derived from mitogen-stimulated lymphocytes (LDCF). There is a possibility that the influence of C5a on lymphocytes (Morgan *et al.*, 1983*a*) may promote LDCF release and thereby amplify the effect of the humoral chemotactic factor on basophils *in vivo*. Basophilic histamine release by the anaphylatoxins has been reported by many investigators (Grant *et al.*, 1975; Hook *et al.*, 1975). Histamine release by C3a occurs over a concentration range of 1–10 μM, and C5a causes release within a range approximately one-tenth of this concentration. Both C3a and C5a bind to basophils (35%–40% of cells), and receptors on these cells are believed to correspond in specificity to those on other leukocytes. That is, C3a and C5a bind to distinct receptor populations. Furthermore, synthetic active site peptides of C3a mimic the biological effects of natural C3a on basophils, indicating that the C3a receptors on these cells recognize the same linear portion of the effector molecule as do other cell types and tissues.

Human mononuclear leukocytes appear to bind both C3a and C5a poorly; however, C5a has been documented to promote chemotaxis of these cells on a par with a chemotactic factor derived from mitogen-stimulated leukocytes (Snyderman *et al.*, 1972). It remains to be determined how the influence of these humoral mediators on the various cell types described here relate to cell-derived mediator function. One hypothesis is that cell-derived activators released from leukocytes, such as arachidonate products, aid in augmenting the primary effects of anaphylatoxins on target cells, thereby producing an amplification loop.

These activities are yet to be fully elucidated under actual physiological conditions, such as at an injury site. It has recently been shown that anaphylatoxin levels are markedly elevated during trauma (Heideman and Hugli, 1984); abnormal responsiveness of the cellular immune system in these patients may be attributed in part to effects that the humoral complement mediators impart on the phagocytic system.

IV. ROLE OF ANAPHYLATOXINS IN IMMUNOREGULATION

Regulation of the immune response by complement has been extensively investigated. The concept that complement may influence cellular immune responses first arose from the observation that leukocytes from several species possess receptors for various fragments of complement components (reviewed by Ross and Newman, 1984).

The third component of complement (C3) has been implicated in the regulation of humoral and cell-mediated immune responses (reviewed by Weiler *et al.*, 1982). However, the nature of this regulation remains controversial. Pepys (1976) first demonstrated that mice depleted of C3 by cobra venom factor (CVF) were refractory to stimulation by thymus-dependent (TD) antigens. Subsequent to this observation, C3 or fragments from C3 have been reported to be mitogenic for bone marrow-derived (B) and thymus-derived (T) cells (Hartmann and Bokisch, 1975; Dukor *et al.*, 1974; Hartmann, 1975), to induce lymphokine secretion (Mackler *et al.*, 1974; Wahl *et al.*, 1974; Koopman *et al.*, 1976), to enhance serum-induced mitogenesis (Payan *et al.*, 1982), to suppress TD antibody responses (Hobbs *et al.*, 1982; Morgan *et al.*, 1982; Pepys and Butterworth, 1974; Pepys *et al.*, 1976; Martinelli *et al.*, 1978; Romball *et al.*, 1980), and to inhibit mitogen- and antigen-induced lymphocyte proliferation (Schenkein and Genco, 1979; Burger and Schvach, 1979; Needleman *et al.*, 1981; Meuth *et al.*, 1983). Thus, there are many studies that contradict one another and provide no rational basis for interpreting the role of complement. Confusion over the role of complement in immunoregulation may be attributable to the lack of defined culture conditions and the use of ill-defined reagents.

To overcome the potential pitfalls, we chose to study the roles of two highly purified human complement fragments, C3a and C5a, in regulation of the immune response (Morgan *et al.*, 1982, 1983*a*). These complement fragments were assessed for effects in both proliferation and humoral immune response models under conditions in which the effects of serum on these fragments were negated.

A. Suppression of Polyclonal Antibody Responses by C3a

To study the effect of human C3a on polyclonal antibody responses we chose the Fc fragment-mediated polyclonal antibody response model. The Fc fragments derived from papain cleavage of human immunoglobulin (Ig) induce B cell proliferation (Morgan and Weigle, 1979, 1980a) and polyclonal antibody production (Morgan and Weigle, 1980b, 1981). Moreover, the cellular interactions required in order for Fc to stimulate lymphocytes are characterized.

Addition of purified C3a to cultures of human peripheral blood lymphocytes (PBLs) results in suppression of polyclonal antibody responses induced by Fc fragments (Fig. 6) (Morgan et al., 1982). Maximum suppression (80%) is achieved with 5 μM C3a. In contrast, C3a$_{des\ Arg}$ (C3a minus the carboxy-terminal arginine) at concentrations up to 20 μM is ineffective in suppressing this response. To measure C3a-mediated suppressive effects in serum-containing culture systems, we added 2-mercaptomethyl-5-guanidinopentanoic acid, a potent serum carboxypeptidase inhibitor (Ondetti et al., 1979). If the inhibitor is omitted, the endogenous carboxypeptidase N rapidly cleaves C3a to C3a$_{des\ Arg}$ (Ondetti et al., 1979), thus inactivating C3a (Table III). A requirement for the carboxy-terminal arginine in C3a-mediated suppression is consistent with other responses to C3a, such as the spasmogenic properties of C3a (Hugli, 1981), i.e., removal of the terminal arginine from C3a renders the molecule incapable of inducing smooth muscle contraction.

C3a was also assessed for its ability to suppress a murine polyclonal antibody response. C3a at a concentration of 5 μM suppresses the Fc fragment-mediated polyclonal antibody response by approximately 100% (Fig. 7). In contrast, addi-

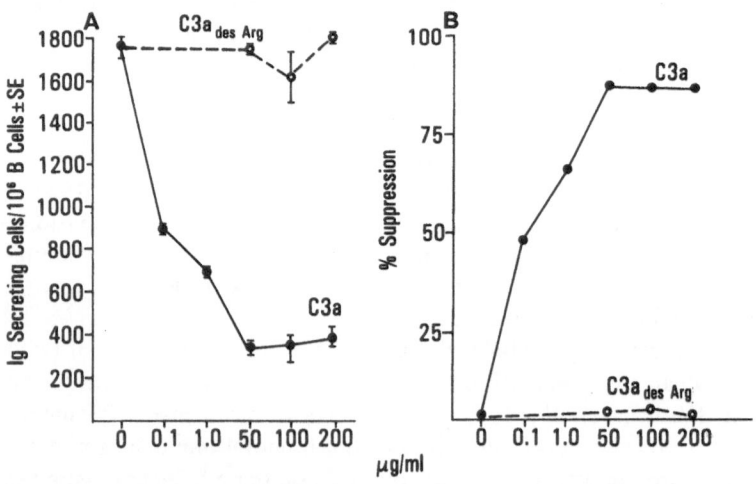

Figure 6. Human peripheral blood lymphocytes (PBLs) (1×10^5 B cells and 2×10^5 T cells) were cultured with 5 μg/ml of Fc fragments. Increasing amounts of C3a (●) or C3a$_{des\ Arg}$ (○) were added. One μg of C3a per milliliter is equal to 10^{-7} M. The polyclonal antibody response was measured on day 6 of culture. One mM 2-mercaptomethyl-5-guanidinopentanoic acid was present in all cultures to inhibit the serum carboxypeptidase. (A) Plot of actual data; (B) data expressed as percent of suppression.

**Table III. Requirement of a COOH-Terminal Arginine for C3a-Mediated
Suppression of the Fc Fragment-Mediated Polyclonal Antibody Response**

SCPN inhibitor[a]	Fc[b]	C3a[c]	C3a$_{des\,Arg}$	Ig-Secreting cells/ 10^6 B cells ± SE	Percent suppression
+	+	−	−	1721 ± 131	0
+	+	+	−	341 ± 71	80
+	+	−	+	1538 ± 174	10
−	+	−	−	1364 ± 96	0
−	+	+	−	1415 ± 69	0
−	+	−	+	1470 ± 74	0

[a] The serum carboxypeptidase (SCPN) inhibitor 2-mercaptomethlyl-5-guanidinopentanoic acid was used at a final concentration of 1 mM.
[b] The Fc concentration was 5 μg/ml.
[c] The C3a and C3a$_{des\,Arg}$ concentration was 50 μg/ml (5.5 μM).

tion of C3a$_{des\,Arg}$ to cultures produce little, if any, suppression of the polyclonal antibody response.

B. Suppression of Specific Antibody Responses by C3a

C3a is also capable of suppressing antigen specific *in vitro* antibody responses (Morgan *et al.*, 1982). Addition of C3a to cultures containing peripheral blood

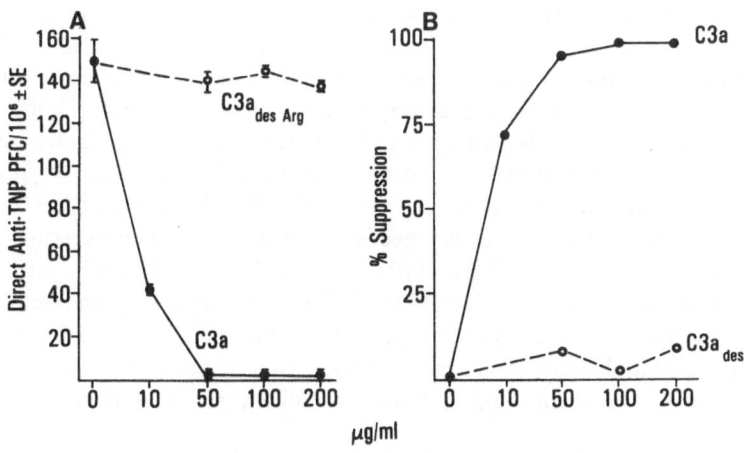

Figure 7. Murine splenic lymphocytes (6 × 10^5 cells) were cultured with 250 μg/ml of Fc fragments and increasing amounts of C3a (•) or C3a$_{des\,Arg}$ (○) were added. The polyclonal antibody response was measured on day 3 of culture. One mM 2-mercaptomethyl-5-guanidinopentanoic acid was present in all cultures. (A) Plot of actual data; (B) data expressed as percent of suppression.

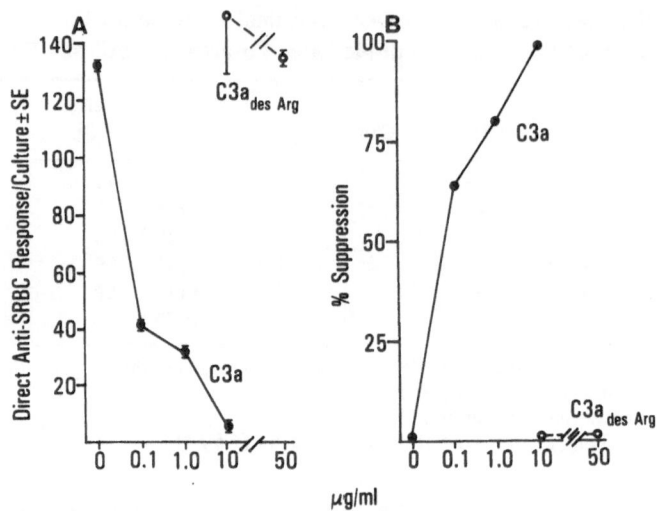

Figure 8. Human peripheral blood lymphocytes (PBLs) (5×10^6 cells) were cultured with 1×10^6 sheep erythrocytes (SRBC) and increasing amounts of C3a (•) or C3a$_{des\ Arg}$ (○). The direct anti-SRBC response was measured on day 11 of culture. One mM 2-mercapto-methyl-5-guanidinopentanoic acid was present in all cultures. (A) Plot of actual data; (B) data expressed as percent of suppression.

lymphocytes (PBLs) and sheep erythrocytes (SRBCs) results in complete suppression of the anti-SRBC response (Fig. 8). Maximal suppression (100%) is achieved with 1 μM C3a. When C3a$_{des\ Arg}$ is substituted for C3a no suppression is observed, indicating that the terminal arginine residue is essential for suppression. C3a also suppressed the murine anti-SRBC response in a dose-dependent manner, whereas C3a$_{des\ Arg}$ fails to suppress even at very high concentrations (Fig. 9). The main difference between the effect of C3a on the human and murine immune response is the concentration of human C3a needed to produce suppression. Suppression of the murine humoral immune response to the 50% level required ~100-fold greater quantities of C3a than are needed to achieve equal suppression of the human immune response (0.1 μg/ml (0.01 μM) vs 10 μg/ml (1 μM)). This difference may indicate better binding of human C3a to receptor sites on homologous versus heterologous cells. Another possibility is that there are more C3a reactive cells in the homologous model system. Such large species differences are not discerned from the spasmogenic activities of human, rat, or porcine C3a (Hugli, 1981).

To determine whether C3a suppresses antibody responses to antigens other than thymus-dependent (TD) antigens, we assessed the effects of C3a on responses elicited by the thymus-independent (TI) antigens, TNP-LPS and TNP-Ficoll. TNP-LPS is the prototype for the TI-1 class of antigens and stimulates the least

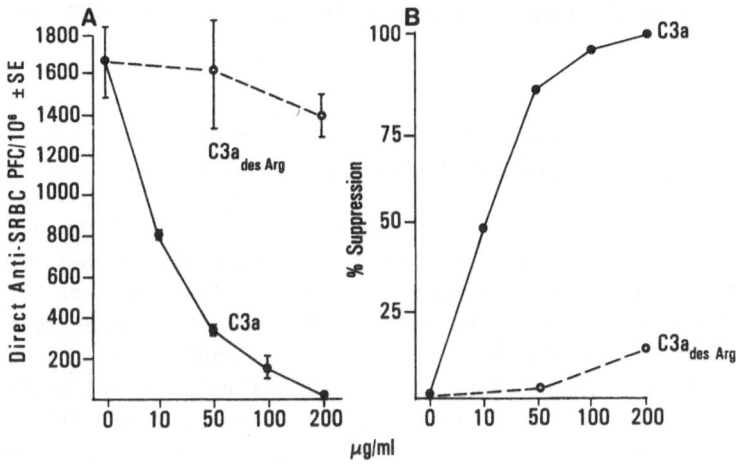

Figure 9. Murine splenic lymphocytes (6×10^5 cells) were cultured with 1×10^6 sheep erythrocytes (SRBC) and increasing amounts of C3a (•) or C3a$_{des\ Arg}$ (○). The direct anti-SRBC response was measured on day 4 of culture. One mM 2-mercaptomethyl-5-guanidinopentanoic acid was present in these cultures. (A) Plot of actual data; (B) data expressed as percent of suppression.

mature subpopulation of B cells (Scher *et al.*, 1975; Mosier *et al.*, 1976). TNP–Ficoll, a TI-2 antigen stimulates a more mature subpopulation of TNP-reactive B cells (Scher *et al.*, 1975; Mosier *et al.*, 1976). Addition of C3a at a concentration capable of inducing 100% suppression of TD antibody responses (5 μM) has no effect on either TI-1 or TI-2 antibody responses. These results are consistent with T cells being a component of C3a-mediated immunosuppression.

C. Inability of C3a to Suppress Proliferative Responses

The effect of C3a on antigen-specific T-cell-proliferative responses is assessed by coculturing human PBLs with tetanus toxoid and C3a. Addition of $\leqslant 5$ μM C3a to PBL cultures fails to suppress the tetanus toxoid-induced proliferative response. C3a has also been examined for an ability to suppress mitogen-induced proliferative responses. Neither C3a nor C3a$_{des\ Arg}$ is capable of suppressing the T-cell response to phytohemagglutinin (PHA) or the T- and B-cell-proliferative responses to pokeweed mitogen (PWM).

In addition to stimulating polyclonal antibody production, Fc fragments induce both murine (Morgan and Weigle, 1979, 1980*a*) and human (Morgan and Weigle, 1981) B cells to proliferate. When C3a is added along with Fc fragments to murine spleen cell cultures, the proliferative response is unaffected. These results show that B-cell proliferation in the human or murine system is unaffected by C3a.

D. Cellular Level of C3a-Mediated Suppression of Humoral Immune Responses

Experiments were designed to test whether C3a is capable of suppressing the Fc fragment-mediated polyclonal and antigen-specific TD antibody responses without affecting antibody responses to TI antigens. The Fc fragment-mediated polyclonal antibody response was chosen to dissect these cellular effects of C3a. Fc fragments activate B cells to secrete polyclonal antibody by a two-stage or signal process (Morgan and Weigle, 1980b, 1981). The first signal, a proliferative signal, is generated by the interaction of B cells with a 14,000–19,000-M_r Fc subfragments (Morgan and Weigle, 1980a,b, 1981). The Fc subfragment is generated by macrophage enzymatic cleavage of the Fc fragment. The Fc subfragment also stimulates T cells to secrete a T-cell-replacing factor, termed Fc-TRF (Thoman et al., 1980a,b, 1981; Morgan and Weigle, 1980b), which induces the proliferating B cells to differentiate into antibody-secreting cells (signal 2). Thus, the polyclonal antibody response requires the participation of both macrophages and T cells. Our results indicate that the site of C3a-mediated suppression of the polyclonal antibody response is not at the level of the proliferating B cell (Morgan et al., 1982). To ascertain whether C3a-mediated suppression occurs at the level of the macrophage, plasmin-derived Fc fragments (pFc) were used as the stimulating agent. It has been shown that the requirement for macrophages in the Fc-induced polyclonal antibody response can be bypassed with pFc fragments (Morgan and Weigle, 1980c). Addition of C3a and pFc to macrophage-depleted murine spleen cell cultures results in a marked suppression of the polyclonal antibody response (Table IV). These results indicate that the macrophage is not the target of C3a-mediated suppression.

Table IV. Ability of C3a to Suppress the pFc-Induced Polyclonal Antibody Response by Macrophage-Depleted Murine Lymphocytes

Spleen cells[a]	pFc[b]	C3a[c]	Direct anti-TNP PFC/10^6 ± SE
+	–	–	10 ± 1
+	+	–	112 ± 3
+	+	+	9 ± 1

[a] Spleen cells were depleted of macrophages by filtration through columns of Sephadex G10.
[b] p^1Fc 175 μg/ml.
[c] C3a was 50 μg/ml (5.5 μM).

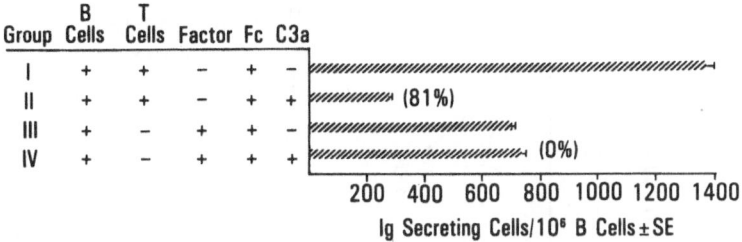

Figure 10. Human peripheral blood lymphocytes (PBLs) B cells (1×10^5 cells) were cultured with either 2×10^5 T cells or Sephadex G-100 purified, phytohemagglutinin (PHA)-induced T-cell factor (25 μl). Each culture was activated with 5 μg Fc/ml. C3a was added to group II and IV cultures at 5 μM. The polyclonal antibody response was measured on day 4 of culture. One mM 2-mercaptomethyl-5-guanidinopentanoic acid was present in these cultures.

The role of the T cell in C3a-mediated suppression was also examined using the Fc fragment-induced polyclonal antibody response model. It has been established that the T-cell requirement in this system can be replaced by a factor derived from either concanavalin A- (Thoman *et al.*, 1980*a*) or Fc fragment- (Thoman *et al.*, 1980*b*, 1981) stimulated Lyt 1^+2^- T cells. Since C3a may act at the level of the helper T cell, Fc-TRF was substituted for T cells and the Fc fragment-mediated polyclonal antibody response was measured. Addition of C3a to Fc-TRF-containing cultures fails to suppress the polyclonal antibody response (Fig. 10, group III). In contrast, addition of C3a to cultures containing T cells results in an 81% suppression of the polyclonal antibody response (Fig. 10, group IV). These results indicate that C3a-mediated suppression occurs at the level of the helper T-cell population.

E. C3a-Induced Suppressor T Cells

To determine whether immunosuppression occurs through the generation of suppressor T cells, we cultured human peripheral blood T cells with C3a for 24 hr and then added the T cells to PBL cultures from the same donor. The Fc polyclonal antibody response was measured, the results of which are shown in Figure 11. Incubation of human T cells with C3a results in the induction of cells capable of suppressing the polyclonal antibody response (Morgan *et al.*, 1984). The serum carboxypeptidase N was not inactivated; therefore, C3a carried over with the T cells was converted to the nonsuppressive C3a$_{\text{des Arg}}$ form.

F. Suppression of Humoral Immune Responses by Synthetic C3a Peptides

Six synthetic oligopeptides based on the COOH-terminal sequence of human C3a were assayed for their ability to suppress polyclonal antibody production by

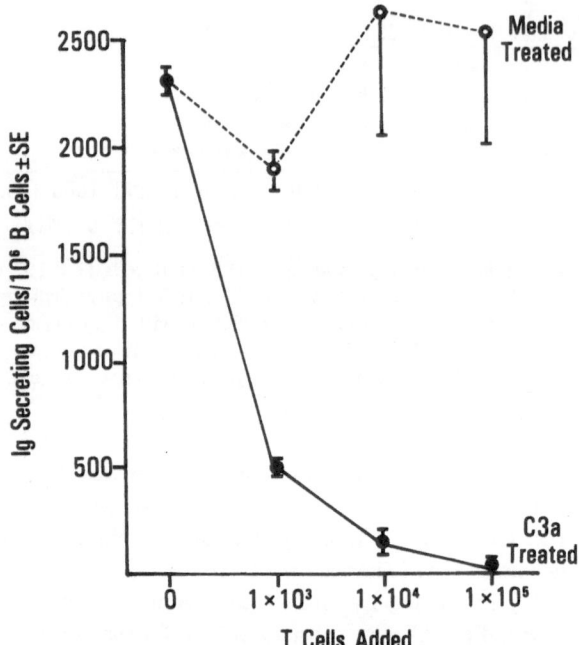

Figure 11. Purified blood-derived T cells (human) were incubated with media (⊚) or with 25 μg C3a/ml (●) for 24 hr. Treated T cells were titrated into human PBL cultures, and Ig was measured on day 6 of culture.

Table V. Relative Potency of Synthetic Analogue Peptides of C3a

Peptide	Percent relative activity[a]	M[b]
Native C3a (C3a 1–77)	100	4.4×10^{-8}
Native C3a$_{\text{des Arg}}$ (C3a 1–76)	0	NA[c]
C3a 57–77	44	9.9×10^{-8}
C3a 65–77	1	4.3×10^{-6}
C3a 70–77	0.3	1.4×10^{-6}
C3a 73–77	0.03	1.4×10^{-5}
C3a 65–77–glycine	0	NA

[a] Values represent the activity relative to native C3a.
[b] Concentration of each material required to suppress the Fc fragment-mediated polyclonal antibody response by human PBL to the 50% level.
[c] NA, not active.

human PBLs (Morgan *et al.*, 1983*b*). Table V compares the relative ability of C3a and the synthetic analogue peptides to suppress the Fc fragment-mediated polyclonal antibody response. The concentration of C3a needed to achieve 50% suppression (4.4×10^{-8} M) is set at 100%, and the activity of each peptide is compared with this value on a molar basis. Peptide C3a 57–77 showed approximately 44% the activity of C3a on a molar basis. The remaining peptides were <1% as active as C3a. Addition of a glycyl residue to the carboxy-terminal end of peptide C3a 65–77 rendered the peptide incapable of suppressing the polyclonal antibody response. These results appear to map the active site of C3a for immunosuppression at the carboxy-terminus of the molecule. These same synthetic C3a peptides exhibit spasmogenic properties like that of intact C3a (Hugli and Erickson, 1977). The synthetic peptides described are capable of inducing smooth muscle contraction and of enhancing vascular permeability (Hugli and Erickson, 1977) with quantitative efficacies similar to those described in Table V.

G. Enhancement of Polyclonal Antibody Responses by C5a

Introduction of either purified human C5a or C5a$_{des Arg}$ to cultures of human PBL results in an enhanced Fc fragment-mediated polyclonal antibody response (Table VI) (Morgan *et al.*, 1983*a*). The ability of C5a to augment *in vitro* responses in serum-containing media was also assessed in the presence of the serum carboxypeptidase inhibitor, 2-mercaptomethyl-5-guanodinopentanoic acid. Maximal enhancement with both C5a (5-fold) and C5a$_{des Arg}$ (3-fold) occurs at 1 μM. Neither C5a nor C5a$_{des Arg}$ alone induces polyclonal antibody responses.

Table VI. Ability of C5a and C5a$_{des Arg}$ to Augment the Fc Fragment-Mediated Polyclonal Antibody Response by Human Peripheral Blood Lymphocytes

PBL	Fc[a]	C5a[b] (μg/ml)	C5a$_{des Arg}$[b] (μg/ml)	Ig-Secreting cells/10^6 B cells ± SE
+	–	–	–	40 ± 2
+	+	–	–	341 ± 55
+	+	0.1	–	792 ± 42
+	+	1	–	1025 ± 142
+	+	10	–	1567 ± 236
+	+	–	0.1	417 ± 62
+	+	–	1	667 ± 49
+	+	–	10	1005 ± 78

[a] Fc was used at a final concentration of 1 μg/ml.
[b] 10 μg/ml = 1.2 μM.

Table VII. Ability of C5a to Augment the Primary *in Vitro*
Anti-SRBC Response by Human PBL

Stimulator	µg/ml	SRBC[a]	Direct anti-SRBC PFC/culture ± SE
–	–	–	30 ± 9
–	–	+	150 ± 15
C5a	0.1	+	551 ± 28
C5a	1.0	+	675 ± 52
C5a$_{des\,Arg}$	0.1	+	598 ± 31
C5a$_{des\,Arg}$	1.0	+	620 ± 15

[a] 1×10^6 sheep erythrocytes/culture.

H. Enhancement of Specific Antibody Responses by C5a

The effects of C5a on antigen-specific antibody responses have been assessed using the *in vitro* primary response of human PBL to SRBC as an assay system. As observed for the polyclonal antibody response (Table VI), both C5a and C5a$_{des\,Arg}$ have the capacity to enhance specific antibody responses (4–5-fold) (Table VII). In addition to augmenting antigen-specific human antibody responses, C5a$_{des\,Arg}$ have the capacity to enhance specific antibody responses (4- to 5-fold) approximately a 3-fold enhancement of the anti-SRBC response (Table VIII). These results are in agreement with those of Goodman *et al.* (1982), which show that *in vitro* murine anti-SRBC responses are enhanced in the presence of either human C5a or C5a$_{des\,Arg}$.

To determine whether C5a augments TI antibody responses, the effects of C5a$_{des\,Arg}$ on the antibody responses to TI-1 (TNP–LPS) and TI-2 (TNP–Ficoll) antigens were assessed. In contrast to enhancing antibody responses to TD antigens, C5a$_{des\,Arg}$ is unable to augment responses to TI antigens.

Table VIII. Ability of C5a to Augment the *in Vitro* Anti-SRBC
Response by Murine Spleen Cells

Spleen cells	SRBC[a]	C5a$_{des\,Arg}$[b]	Direct anti-SRBC PFC/10^6 ± SE
+	–	–	35 ± 1
+	+	–	143 ± 5
+	+	+	380 ± 30

[a] 1×10^5 sheep erythrocytes/culture.
[b] C5a$_{des\,Arg}$ was used at a final concentration of 10 µg/ml (1.2 µM).

I. Enhancement of Antigen-Induced Proliferative Responses by C5a

To determine the effect of C5a on antigen-specific T-cell proliferation, human PBLs are stimulated with tetanus toxoid in the presence or absence of $C5a_{des\,Arg}$. $C5a_{des\,Arg}$ is capable of potentiating the antigen-induced proliferative response (2-fold). Maximal enhancement occurred with the addition of 10 $\mu g/ml$ $C5a_{des\,Arg}$ to culture. Addition of $C5a_{des\,Arg}$ to culture, in the absence of tetanus toxoid, fails to produce a proliferative response.

The T-cell population affected by C5a, has a specific phenotype, characterized by monoclonal antibodies (OKT) directed against surface antigens. Most T cells bear the $OKT3^+$ phenotype, whereas helper T cells belong to the $OKT4^+$ subpopulation and suppressor-cytotoxic T to the $OKT8^+$ subpopulation. Depletion of either $OKT3^+$ or $OKT4^+$ T cells from the responding population abrogated the ability of $C5a_{des\,Arg}$ to enhance the response. In contrast, depletion of $OKT8^+$ cells has no effect on $C5a_{des\,Arg}$-mediated enhancement of the proliferative response (Morgan et al., 1983a). These results indicate that augmentation of the polyclonal antibody response by C5a requires the presence of an $OKT3^+4^+$ helper T cell.

To explore further the effects of C5a on T-cell proliferation, we assessed whether $C5a_{des\,Arg}$ could augment alloantigen-induced T-cell proliferation. The results reveal that addition of $C5a_{des\,Arg}$ to primary mixed lymphocyte cultures (MLCs) result in ~3-fold enhancement compared with the control response.

To determine whether $C5a_{des\,Arg}$ augments mitogen lymphocyte proliferation, $C5a_{des\,Arg}$ was added to cultures containing PHA or PWM. No effect on the proliferative response was observed. These results indicate that antigen nonspecific proliferative responses are not susceptible to the enhancing properties of $C5a_{des\,Arg}$. Moreover, substitution of C5a for $C5a_{des\,Arg}$ and introduction of the presence of carboxypeptidase inhibitor fails to augment the proliferative response (Morgan et al., 1983a).

J. Cellular Level of C5a-Mediated Enhancement
of Humoral Immune Responses

The role of the T cell in $C5a_{des\,Arg}$-mediated enhancement of the immune response was investigated using the Fc fragment-induced polyclonal antibody response model. When $C5a_{des\,Arg}$ is added to cultures of human PBLs depleted of T cells and Fc-TRF, it fails to enhance the Fc fragment-induced polyclonal antibody response (Fig. 12, groups IV and V). The ability of Fc-TRF to override the enhancing effect of C5a suggests that C5a acts through a T-cell-dependent mechanism. The role of macrophages in C5a-mediated enhancement was investigated using the polyclonal antibody response induced by a plasmin-digested IgG fragment (pFc). As mentioned previously, the putative role of the macrophage

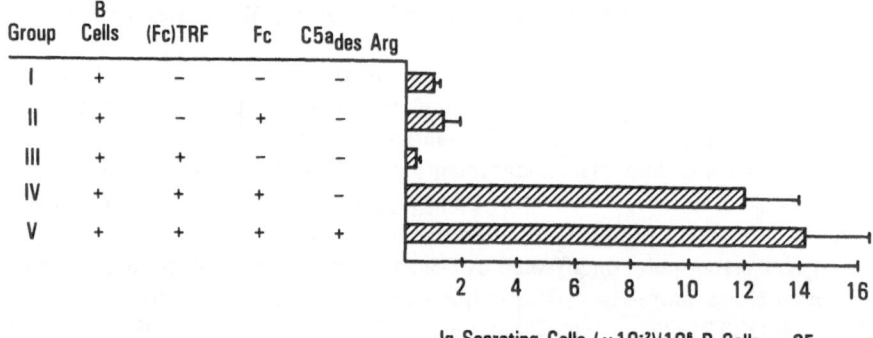

Figure 12. T-cell-depleted peripheral blood lymphocytes (PBLs) populations were cultured with T-cell replacing factor (Fc) (TRF) (10 μl) to determine whether $C5a_{des\ Arg}$ (1.2 μM) was capable of enhancing the Fc responses. A total of 3 μg/ml of Fc was employed and the response was measured on day 6 of culture. In the absence of T cells, no augmentation was observed.

in the polyclonal antibody response is to cleave the Fc fragment into biologically active subfragments (Morgan and Weigle, 1980b, 1981). Once the Fc subfragments are produced, macrophages are no longer needed for the response (Morgan and Weigle, 1980b). The pFc fragments behave like Fc subfragments in that they trigger polyclonal antibody production in the absence of macrophages (Morgan and Weigle, 1980c). Addition of $C5a_{des\ Arg}$ to monocyte-depleted cultures, previously stimulated with pFc, results in an enhanced polyclonal antibody response (4-fold) (Fig. 13). Thus, for C5a enhancement of Fc fragment-mediated polyclonal antibody responses, neither macrophages nor monocytes appear to be required.

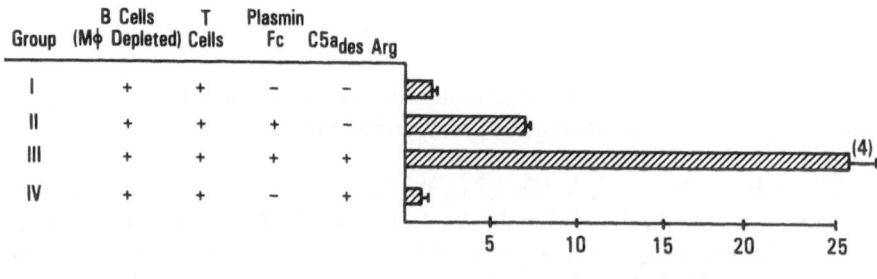

Figure 13. Monocyte-depleted peripheral blood lymphocytes (PBLs) (1×10^5 B cells and 2×10^5 T cells) were cultured with 3 μg/ml pFc and 1.2 μM $C5a_{des\ Arg}$. The polyclonal antibody response was measured on day 6 of culture, and significant augmentation by $C5a_{des\ Arg}$ was observed.

K. Immune Responses to Combinations of C3a and C5a

The dichotomy of opposing actions for C3a and C5a on humoral immune responses compelled us to ask whether enhancement or suppression would result if both factors were added to culture simultaneously. We have previously shown that both C3a (Morgan *et al.*, 1982) and C5a (Morgan *et al.*, 1983*a*) must be added to culture no later than day 1 to observe suppression or enhancement, respectively. These data suggest that C3a and C5a both act at an early phase of the immune response. When C3a and $C5a_{des\,Arg}$ are simultaneously added to human PBL cultures along with Fc fragments, the polyclonal antibody response is enhanced by approximately 3-fold. Addition of C5a alone results in a similar degree of enhancement, whereas C3a alone suppresses the polyclonal response by 55%. These results indicate that the immunopotentiating properties of C5a override the immunosuppressive effects of C3a.

L. Conclusions

The C3a molecule has the capacity to suppress both specific and nonspecific humoral immune responses. Addition of C3a to cultures of human PBL or murine splenic lymphocytes results in suppression of both the anti-SRBC response and the Fc fragment-mediated polyclonal antibody response. In contrast to these results, mitogen- and antigen-induced T- and B-cell-proliferative responses are not affected by C3a. Concentrations of C3a that are 10-fold greater than those required to suppress fully the anti-SRBC response have no effect on the proliferative response induced by tetanus toxoid. Similar concentrations of C3a fail to suppress the nonspecific proliferative responses to PHA or PWM. In addition, B cell proliferation induced by Fc fragments of LPS remain unaffected by C3a.

Immune suppression mediated by C3a occurs at an early phase in the antibody response. This conclusion came from our observation that when C3a is added on day 0, maximal suppression is achieved; however, when added on day 1, only marginal suppression is observed. In addition, interaction of purified T cells with C3a for as little as 30 min results in pronounced suppression. Moreover, the protective action of the carboxypeptidase inhibitor dictates that C3a must act relatively early in the response because the inhibitor acts by a competitive mechanism and C3a conversion to $C3a_{des\,Arg}$ occurs over several hours.

The carboxy-terminal arginine in C3a is essential. Immunosuppressive properties are lost if the arginine is removed. These results are consistent with the spasmogenic properties of C3a being dependent on the COOH-terminal arginine (Hugli, 1981). Taken together, our results indicate that the COOH-terminal portion of C3a is the active center for producing immunosuppressive actions. Therefore, the serum carboxypeptidase serves the same role in controlling the immunosuppressive activities of C3a as it does in restricting spasmogenic action. Data derived using synthetic C3a peptides based on the human C3a structure maps the active region of the molecule as the carboxy terminus.

T lymphocytes are concluded to be the target of C3a-mediated suppression of the immune response. Substitution of T cells by a soluble T-cell factor in the Fc polyclonal antibody response abrogates the suppressive response of C3a. Additional evidence for the T cell being the target of C3a-mediated suppression is drawn from the observation that incubation of purified T cells with C3a renders the T cells incapable of helping in the Fc-induced polyclonal antibody response. Moreover, C3a fails to suppress *in vitro* antibody responses to the T-cell-independent antigens, TNP-LPS and TNP-Ficoll. Interestingly, C3a is incapable of suppressing either antigen- or mitogen-induced T-cell proliferation. It is proposed that C3a interferes with the T-cell–macrophage interaction, a mechanism given to explain the action of other C3 cleavage products (Schenkein and Genco, 1979). This is presumably not the case here because C3a can suppress the macrophage-independent polyclonal antibody response.

C3a also fails to suppress the LPS- or Fc fragment-mediated proliferative responses. The Fc polyclonal antibody response results from the delivery of two signals to the B cell (Morgan and Weigle, 1980*b,c*; Thoman *et al.*, 1980*a,b*). The first is a proliferative signal that stimulates the B cells, and in the presence of a second T-cell-derived signal they differentiate to antibody-secreting cells. The B-cell proliferative phase is an integral part of the polyclonal response without which little or no antibody is produced. The inability of C3a to suppress the Fc proliferative response in the presence or absence of T cells gives further support to the hypothesis that C3a exerts its action at the level of the helper T cell.

Incubation of T cells with C3a results in the generation of suppressor T cells (Morgan *et al.*, 1984). The action of C3a-suppressor T cells is nonspecific in nature because these cells are capable of suppressing both anti-SRBC and Fc polyclonal antibody responses. The mechanism through which C3a acts is the generation of suppressor T cells. C3a-mediated suppression does not appear to involve an activation of existing suppressor T cells. Depletion of either Lyt 1^-2^+ or OKT4$^-$8$^+$ cells before C3a treatment has no effect on the level of suppression (Morgan *et al.*, 1982). Suppressor cells are generated in culture by C3a activation of an Lyt 1^+2^- or OKT4$^+$8$^-$ suppressor inducer that then activates a suppressor population (Morgan *et al.*, 1984). Once activated, the suppressor cell population interferes with the action of helper T cells.

The quantity of human C3a needed to suppress human PBL responses is 100-fold lower than that needed to suppress murine immune responses. It is not currently known whether species differences are expressions of receptor specificity or of true variations in sensitivity between human and murine helper T cells. It is clear that the level of C3a required to suppress the antibody response falls well within the physiologic concentration range in humans. Significant suppression of human PBL responses is observed at C3a concentrations of 0.1–1 μg/ml, levels well below the potential 50–60 $\mu g/ml$ of C3a generated by maximal human C3 conversion.

In addition to the immunosuppressive properties of C3a described here, C3a has recently been shown to reduce generation of leukocyte inhibitory factor (LIF) by human T cells cultured with mitogens or antigens (Payan et al., 1982). Moreover, a synthetic C3a octapeptide, C3a 70–77, was found to reduce LIF levels. Reduction of LIF production by C3a is not mediated through a reduction in T-cell proliferation. Neither C3a nor C3a 70–77 altered the [^{3}H]-TdR uptake by human T cells exposed to mitogen or antigen (Payan et al., 1982).

Human C5a has the ability to potentiate both antigen specific and mitogen-induced immune responses in vitro in either human or murine systems (Morgan et al., 1983a). Addition of either C5a or the des Arg form of the molecule to human PBL cultures results in enhancement of both the anti-SRBC response and the Fc fragment-mediated polyclonal antibody response. These results are in agreement with the report of Goodman et al. (1982) who showed that the murine anti-SRBC response is enhanced by human C5a and C5a$_{des\ Arg}$. The specific T-cell proliferative response to tetanus toxoid is also augmented by C5a$_{des\ Arg}$. These results are in contrast to those obtained with mitogen-induced proliferative responses. Concentrations of C5a$_{des\ Arg}$ capable of augmenting antigen-induced proliferation have no effect on the PHA- or PWM-induced proliferative responses.

The C-terminal arginine in C5a is not essential for it to exhibit immunopotentiating properties. Removal of the terminal arginine by serum carboxypeptidase N (Morgan et al., 1983a) exerts only a minor effect on the ability of the molecule to augment nonspecific or specific immune responses. These results are consistent with the findings that when C5a is converted to C5a$_{des\ Arg}$, the spasmogen action is lost but C5a$_{des\ Arg}$ retains the ability to promote neutrophil chemotaxis and degranulation (Webster et al., 1980). Both C5a and C5a$_{des\ Arg}$ appear to be equally effective as augmentors of specific and nonspecific humoral immune responses. In contrast, C5a$_{des\ Arg}$ was found to be 10- to 30-fold less active than C5a when assessed for neutrophil chemotactic activity as observed by ourself and others (Webster et al., 1980).

T lymphocytes are involved in C5a-mediated enhancement of the human immune response. Replacement of T cells by a soluble human T-cell factor, Fc-TRF, in the Fc polyclonal antibody response abrogates the enhancing properties of C5a$_{des\ Arg}$. The action of C5a on T cells could be through T-cell–macrophage interaction and the reason mitogen-induced proliferative responses are not enhanced is that their macrophage requirements are different from antigen-induced responses. In addition, C5a is unable to augment in vitro antibody responses to either TI-1 or TI-2 antigens.

Immunopotentiation of the Fc fragment-induced polyclonal antibody response by C5a does not appear to require macrophages or monocytes. This finding is in contrast to the results of Goodman et al. (1982), who showed that preincubation of macrophages with C5a and their subsequent addition to culture is sufficient to cause enhancement of the murine anti-SRBC response. It was also observed that culture supernates obtained from splenic adherent cells or macrophage-like cell lines treated with C5a enhance murine anti-SRBC responses and contain interleukin-1 (IL-1)-like activity (Goodman *et al.*, 1983). These workers postulated that C5a enhances antibody responses by inducing IL-1 secretion by macrophages. Thus, there appears to be more than one potential pathway for C5a to augment humoral immune responses.

The physiologic significance of C3a- and C5a-mediated immunoregulation is a matter of speculation. Regulation of immune responses by complement components may form an *in vivo* nonspecific immunoregulatory network. Produc-

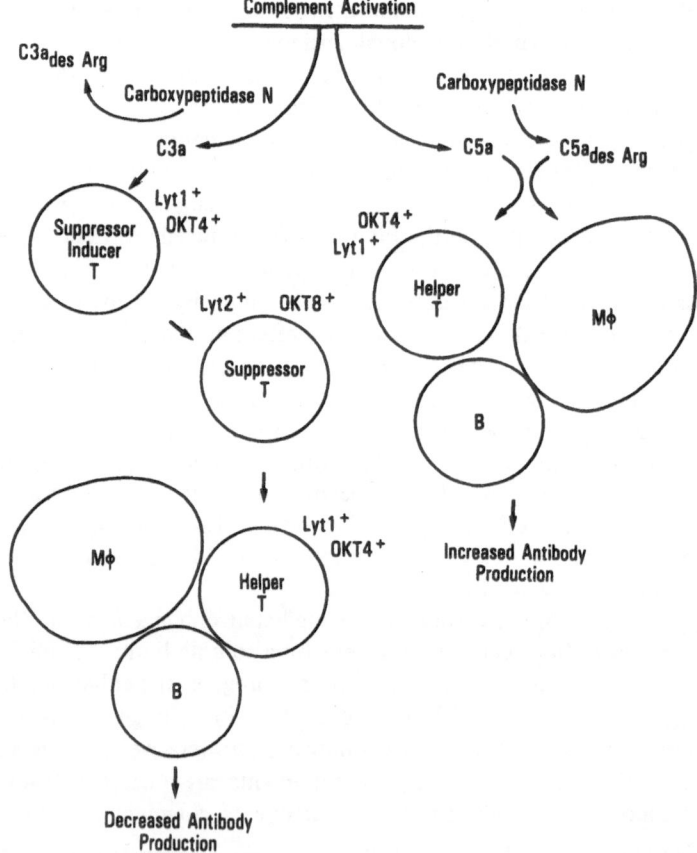

Figure 14. Models for regulation of the immune response by C3a and C5a. C3a is inactivated by the serum carboxypeptidase when converted to C3a$_{des\ Arg}$. Intact C3a interacts with an Lyt 1$^+$ T-cell subpopulation believed to be a suppressor–inducer cell that in turn inhibits T-helper cell function by a suppressor mechanism. Both C5a and C5a$_{des\ Arg}$ appear to augment the immune response at the level of the T helper cell.

tion of C3a *in vivo* by either the classical or alternate pathway of complement activation could potentiate a nonspecific suppressor circuit capable of reducing both ongoing humoral and T-cell-mediated responses (Fig. 14). Although C3a is relatively short-lived in circulation, the fact that suppression is mediated by a C3a-induced suppressor cell lends validity to its potential action *in vivo*. The presence of serum carboxypeptidase N could act as a control mechanism for C3a suppressive action. Production of relatively high concentrations of C3a in a microenvironment of interacting T cells, B cells and accessory cells could lead to activation of suppressor T cells before the C3a is inactivated by the carboxypeptidase. In contrast, generation of C5a may activate a potent nonspecific enhancement network which not only affects antibody responses to TD antigens but overrides the suppressive effects of C3a (Fig. 14). Thus there appears to be a complex interplay between complement peptides and various cellular components in regulating immune responses.

V. ROLE OF C3 FRAGMENTS (C3d-K) IN LEUKOCYTE REGULATION

A. Immunoregulatory Responses of C3d-K

In addition to the anaphylatoxins, other fragments of C3 have been shown to be involved in immunoregulation (Hobbs *et al.*, 1982; Meuth *et al.*, 1983; Schenkien and Genco, 1979).

Treatment of iC3b with kallikrein isolated from human plasma results in the generation of a fragment, C3d-K, which is capable of suppressing T-cell proliferative response (Meuth *et al.*, 1983). Addition of C3d-K to human PBL cultures results in a pronounced suppression of PHA-induced proliferation (Fig. 15). The suppressive effects of C3d-K on antigen-specific proliferative responses have been assessed. Addition of C3d-K to human spleen cell cultures along with tetanus toxiod results in a pronounced suppression of the proliferative response. In the antigen-induced proliferative studies 50% suppression is attained with quantities equivalent to conversion of 0.2% of the circulating C3 concentration to C3d-K. Taken together, the results of the mitogen- and antigen-induced proliferative studies indicate C3d-K is capable of suppressing both nonspecific and specific T-cell proliferative responses. Suppression of antibody responses by fragments of C3 have also recently been reported (Hobbs *et al.*, 1982). These investigators found that a small molecular weight fragment of human C3 was capable of inhibiting both thymus-dependent and -independent *in vitro* antibody responses in the rat.

B. Leukocytosis Induced by C3d-K

Intravenous injection of C3d-K but not C3, C3a, C3b, or C3c-K results in a 2- to 3-fold increase in the total number of circulating leukocytes in both rabbits

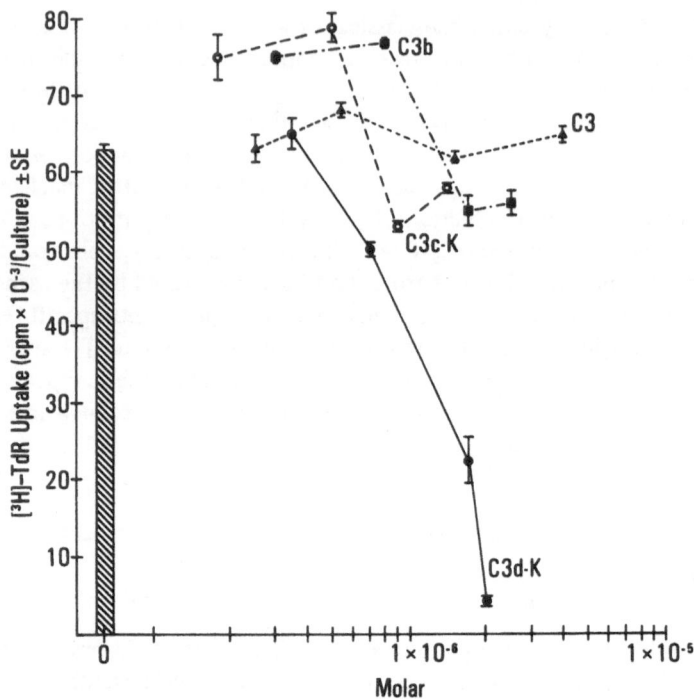

Figure 15. Mitogen-induced T-cell proliferation is inhibited by the fragment C3d-K. Human peripheral blood lymphocytes (2.5×10^5) were cultured with 1% phytohemagglutinin (PHA) and then exposed to C3 (▲), C3b (■), C3c-K (o), or C3d-K (•) over a concentration range of 8×10^{-7} to 5×10^{-6} M. The mitogen response was assayed on day 4 of culture and only C3d-K exhibited a dose-dependent inhibition. The hashed bar at the left indicates the control level of PHA-stimulated proliferation. (Adapted from Meuth et al., 1983.)

and mice (Fig. 16) (Meuth et al., 1983). Identification of a C3-derived fragment capable of inducing leukocytosis in rabbits is similar to the work of Rother (1972) and Ghebrehiwet and Müller-Eberhard (1979). These latter workers reported that a 10,000-M_r acidic peptide termed C3e was able to induce leukocytosis in rabbits. Since C3d-K and C3e induce leukocytosis, we conclude that C3d-K contains both the active site of C3e and the effector site for immune suppression.

VI. SUMMARY

Progress over the past five years has drawn attention to the fact that the anaplylatoxins are important factors in both leukocyte activation and regulation events. The C5 anaphylatoxin has been proposed to play major role in leukocyte

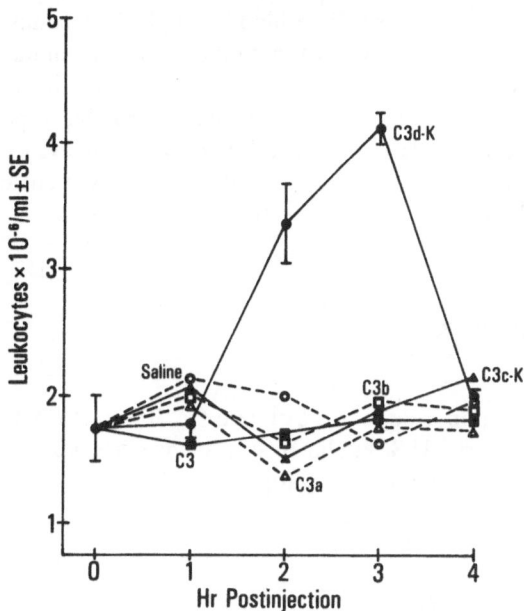

Figure 16. Leukocytosis was induced in mice by C3d-K. When C3 (■), C3a (△), C3b (□), C3c-K (▲), or C3d-K (●) are injected IV into mice at a level of 1 nmole/kg of body weight only C3d-K stimulated leukocytosis. The mice were bled at hourly intervals and the leukocytes determined by counting nucleated cells. (Adapted from Meuth *et al.*, 1983.)

aggregation and adherence phenomenon. Influences of C5a on the leukocyte may lead to clinical manifestations such as respiratory distress syndrome after trauma or postpump syndrome after cardiopulmonary bypass, both effects derived from leukocyte sequestration. Many other clinical conditions involving repeated transient sequestration of leukocytes, particularly in the pulmonary vasculature, may eventually be recognized as a complication of systemic complement activation. Dramatic pathologic changes observed in the lungs of animals exposed to either C3a or C5a emphasizes the potential damage that these factors may exert via cellular activation mechanisms (Huey *et al.*, 1983).

More recent evidence that the anaphylatoxins are potent immunoregulatory factors under *in vitro* conditions suggests a physiologic role for these humoral factors in nonspecific modulation of the immune response. It is an attractive hypothesis to suggest that once activated, complement is capable of relaying information to the cellular immune system via the anaphylatoxins. Other components of the complement system have long been known to exert regulatory influences on the immune system, and perhaps molecular description of such entities as the C3d-K fragment will serve to unravel this seemingly more complex effector system. In any case, as our understanding of both the chemical and biologic nature of factors derived from blood complement components advances, it has become apparent that a major function of complement may be to modulate the immune response. We have already demonstrated that these factors are selective both for cell type and for eliciting a variety of cellular responses. From this, one can infer that manipulation of the cellular events will eventually be possible. Hence a therapeutic value may be realized once involvement of these complement factors under *in vivo* conditions is better characterized.

ACKNOWLEDGMENTS

This work was supported in part by grants CA 3064, AI/CA 19723, HL 16411, and AI 17354 from the U.S. Public Health Service. We wish to thank Ms. Alice Bruce Kay and Ellye Lukaschewsky for their able assistance in the preparation of this manuscript.

VII. REFERENCES

Beebe, D. P., Ward, P. A., and Spitznagel, S. K., 1980, Isolation and characterization of acidic chemotactic factor from complement activated human serum, *Clin. Immunol. Immunopathol.* 15:88–105.

Berenberg, J. L., and Ward, P. A., (1973), The chemotactic factor inactivator in normal human serum, *J. Clin Invest.* 52:1200–1206.

Boetcher, D. A., and Leonard, E. J., 1973, Basophil chemotaxis: Augmentation by a factor from stimulated lymphocyte cultures, *Immunol. Commun.* 2(4):421–429.

Bokisch, V. A., and Müller-Eberhard, H. J., 1970, Anaphylatoxin inactivator of human plasma: Its isolation and characterization as a carboxypeptidase, *J. Clin. Invest.* 49:2427–2436.

Bokisch, V. A., Müller-Eberhard, H. J., and Cochrane, C. G., 1969, Isolation of a fragment (C3a) of the third component of human complement containing anaphylatoxin and chemotactic activity and description of an anaphylatoxin inactivator of human serum, *J. Exp. Med.* 129:1109–1130.

Boyden, S., 1962, The chemotactic effect of mixtures of antibody and antigen on polymorphonuclear leukocytes, *J. Exp. Med.* 115:453–466.

Burger, R., and Schvach, E. M., 1979, Evaluation of the role of C4 in the cellular immune response in vitro, *J. Immunol.* 122:2388–2394.

Caporale, L. H., Tippett, P. S., Erickson, B. W., and Hugli, T. E., 1980, The active site of C3a anaphylatoxin, *J. Biol. Chem.* 255:10758–10763.

Chenoweth, D., and Hugli, T. E., 1978, Demonstration of specific C5a receptor on intact human polymorphonuclear leukocytes, *Proc. Natl. Acad. Sci. USA* 75:3943–3947.

Chenoweth, D. E., and Hugli, T. E., 1980a, Human C5a and C5a analogs as probes of the neutrophil C5a receptor, *Mol. Immunol.* 17:151–161.

Chenoweth, D. E., and Hugli, T. E., 1980b, Binding, internalization and degradation of human C5a by human neutrophils, *Fed. Proc.* 39:1049.

Chenoweth, D. E., Rowe, J. B., and Hugli, T. E., 1979, A modified method for chemotaxis under agarose, *J. Immunol. Methods* 25:337–353.

Chenoweth, D. E., Cooper, S. W., Hugli, T. E., Stewart, R. W., Blackstone, E. H., and Kirklin, J. W., 1981, Complement activation during cardiopulmonary bypass, *N. Engl. J. Med.* 304:497–503.

Clancy, R. M., Dahinden, C. A., and Hugli, T. E., 1983, Arachidonate metabolism by human polymorphonuclear leukocytes stimulated by N-formyl peptide or C5a is independent of phopholipase activation, *Proc. Natl. Aca. Sci.* 80:7200–7204.

Cochrane, C. G., and Müller-Eberhard, H. J., 1968, The derivation of two distinct anaphylatoxin activities from the third and fifth components of human complement, *J. Exp. Med.* 127:371–386.

Craddock, P. R., Hammerschmidt, D. E., White, J. G., and Jacob, H. S., 1976, Granulocyte (PMN) aggregometry–a new technique for the study of complement and C5a effects upon PMNs and their plasma membranes, *Blood* 48:961–966.

Craddock, P. R., Hammerschmidt, D., White, J. G., Dalmasso, A. P., and Jacob, H. S., 1977a, Complement (C5a)-induced granulocyte aggregation in vitro. A possible mechanism of complement-mediated leukostasis and leukopenia, *J. Clin. Invest.* 60:260–264.

Craddock, P. R., Fehr, J., Brigham, K. L., Kronenberg, R., and Jacob, H. S., 1977b, Complement and leukocyte-mediated pulmonary dysfunction in hemodialysis, *N. Engl. J. Med.* 296:769–776.

Craddock, P. R., White, J. G., and Jacob, H. S., 1978, Potentiation of complement (C5a)-induced granulocyte aggregation by cytochalasin B, *J. Lab. Clin. Med.* 91:490–496.

Craddock, P. R., Hammerschmidt, D. E., Moldow, C. F., Yamada, O., and Jacob, H. S., 1979, Granulocyte aggregation as a manifestation of membrane interactions with complement: Possible role in leukocyte margination, micro-vascular occulsion, and endothelial damage, *Semin Hematol.* 16:140–194.

Cutler, J. E., 1974, A simple in vitro method for studies on chemotaxis, *Proc. Soc. Exp. Biol. Med.* 147:471–474.

Dahinden, C. A., Fehr, J., and Hugli, T. E., 1983, Role of cell surface contact on the kinetics of superoxide production by granulocytes, *J. Clin. Invest.* 72:113–121.

Damerau, B., Zimmerman, B., Wustefeld, H., Czorniak, K., and Vogt, W., 1983, Involvement of the N terminus of HOG C3a, C5a, and C5a-desArg in their biological activities, *Immunobiology* 164(3/4):229 (abst).

Denny, J. B., and Johnson, A. R., 1979, Uptake of ^{125}I-labeled C3a by cultured human endothelial cells, *Immunology* 36:169–177.

Dukor, P., Schumann, G., Gisler, R. H., Dierich, M., Konig, W., Hadding, U., and Bitter-Suermann, D., 1974, Complement dependent B-cell activation by cobra venom factor and other mitogens, *J. Exp. Med.* 139:337–354.

Fernandez, H. N., and Hugli, T. E., 1976, Partial characterization of human C5a anaphylatoxin. I. Chemical description of the carbohydrate and polypeptide portions of human C5a, *J. Immunol.* 117:1688–1694.

Fernandez, H. N., and Hugli, T. E., 1978, Primary structural analysis of the polypeptide portion of human C5a anaphylatoxin. I. Polypeptide sequence determination and assignment of the oligosaccharide attachment site in C5a, *J. Biol. Chem.* 253:6955–6964.

Fernandez, H. N., Henson, P. M., Otani, A., and Hugli, T. E., 1978, Chemotaxis response to human C3a and C5a anaphylatoxins. I. Evaluations of C3a and C5a leukotaxis in vitro and under simulated in vivo conditions, *J. Immunol.* 120:109–115.

Ford-Hutchinson, A. W., Bray, M. A., Doing, M. V., Shipley, M. E., and Smith, J. H., 1980, Leukotriene B, a potent chemokinetic and aggregating substance released from polymorphonuclear leukocytes, *Nature* 286:264–265.

Gallin, J. I., and Quie, P. G. (eds.), 1978, in: *Leukocyte Chemotaxis: Methods, Physiology and Clinical Implications*, Raven Press, New York.

Gallin, J. I., Clark, R. A., and Kimbal, H. R., 1973, Granulocytes chemotaxis: An improved in vitro assay employing ^{51}Cr-labeled granulocytes, *J. Immunol.* 110:233–240.

Gallin, J. I., Durocher, J. R., and Kaplan, A. P., 1975, Interaction of leukocyte chemotactic factors with the cell surface. I. Chemotactic factor-induced changes in human granulocyte surface change, *J. Clin. Invest.* 55:967–974.

Gerard, C., and Hugli, T. E., 1979, Anaphylatoxin from the fifth component of porcine complement. I. Purification and partial chemical characterization, *J. Biol. Chem.* 254: 6346–6351.

Gerard, C., and Hugli, T. E., 1980, Amino acid sequence of the anaphylatoxin from the fifth component of porcine complement, *J. Biol. Chem.* 255:4710–4715.

Gerard, C., and Hugli, T. E., 1981, Identification of the classical anaphylatoxins C5a$_{des Arg}$: Evidence of a modulator role for the oligosaccharide unit in human C5a, *Proc. Natl. Acad Sci. USA* 78:1833–1837.

Gerard, C., Chenoweth, D. E., and Hugli, T. E., 1979, Molecular aspects of the serum chemotactic factors, *J. Reticuloendothel. Soc.* 26:711–718.

Gerard, C., Chenoweth, D. E., and Hugli, T. E., 1981, Response of human neutrophils to C5a: A role of the oligosaccharide moiety of human C5a$_{des Arg-74}$ but not of C5a in biological activity, *J. Immunol.* 127:1978–1982.

Ghebrehiwet, B., and Müller-Eberhard, H. J., 1979, C3e: An acidic fragment of human C3 with leucocytosis inducing activity, *J. Immunol.* 123:616–621.

Glovsky, M. M., Hugli, T. E., Ishizaka, T., Lichtenstein, L. M., and Erickson, B. W., 1979, Anaphylatoxin-induced histamine release with human leukocytes: Studies of C3a leukocyte binding and histamine release, *J. Clin. Invest.* 64:804–811.

Goodman, M. G., Chenoweth, D. E., and Weigle, W. O., 1982, Potentiation of the primary humoral immune response in vitro by C5a anaphylatoxins, *J. Immunol.* 129:70–75.

Goodman, M. G., Chenoweth, D. E., and Weigle, W. O., 1983, Induction of interleukin-1 secretion and enhancement of humoral immunity by binding of human C5a to macrophage surface C5a receptors, *J. Exp. Med.* 156:912–917.

Grant, J. A., Dupree, E., Goldman, A. S., Schultz, D. R., and Jackson, A. L., 1975, Complement mediated release of histamine from human leukocytes, *J. Immunol.* 114: 1101–1106.

Hammerschmidt, D. E., Craddock, P. R., McCullough, J., Kronenberg, R. S., Dalmasso, A. P., and Jacob, J. S., 1978, Complement activation and pulmonary leukostasis during nylon fiber filtration leukopheresis, *Blood* 51:721–730.

Hammerschmidt, D. E., Weaver, L. J., Hudson, L. D., Craddock, P. R., and Jacob, H. S., 1980, Association of complement activation and elevated plasma-C5a with adult respiratory distress syndrome: Pathophysiological relevance and possible prognostic value, *Lancet* 1:947–949.

Hartmann, F. U., 1975, Possible involvement of C3 during stimulation of B lymphocytes, *Transplant. Rev.* 23:98–103.

Hartmann, K. U., and Bokisch, H., 1975, Stimulation of murine B lymphocyte in isolated C3b, *J. Exp. Med.* 142:600–610.

Heideman, M., and Hugli, T. E., 1984, Anaphylatoxin generation in multisystem organ failure, *Trauma* (in press).

Hill, J. H., and Ward, P. A., 1969, C3 leukotactic factors produced by a tissue protease, *J. Exp. Med.* 130:505–518.

Hobbs, M. V., Feldbush, T. L., Needleman, B. W., and Weiler, M. J., 1982, Inhibition of secondary in vitro antibody responses by the third component of complement, *J. Immunol.* 128:1470–1475.

Hook, W. A., Siraganian, R. P., Wahl, S. M., 1975, Complement induced histamine release from human basophils. Generation of activity in human serum, *J. Immunol.* 114: 1185–1190.

Huber, R., Scholze, H., Paques, E. P., and Deisenhofer, J., 1980, Crystal structure analysis and molecular model of human C3a anaphylatoxin, *Hoppe Seylers Z. Physiol. Chem.* 361:1389-1399.

Huey, R., Bloor, C. M., Kawahara, M. S., and Hugli, T. E., 1983, Potentiation of the anaphlytoxins *in vivo* using an inhibitor of serum carboxypeptidase N (SCPN). I. Lethality and effects on pulmonary tissue. *Am. J. Pathol.* 112:48-60.

Huey, R., Erickson, B. W., Bloor, C. W., and Hugli, T. E., 1984, Contraction of guinea pig lung by synthetic oligopeptides related to human C3a, *Immunopharmacology* (submitted).

Hugli, T. E., 1978, Chemical aspects of the serum anaphylatoxins, in: *Contemporary Topics in Molecular Immunology*, Vol. 7 (R. A. Reisfeld and F. Inman, eds.), pp. 181-214, Plenum Press, New York.

Hugli, T. E., 1981, The structural basis for anaphylatoxin and chemotactic functions of C3a, C4a, and C5a, in: *Critical Reviews in Immunology*, I, 4, pp. 321-366, CRC Press Review, Boca Raton, Florida.

Hugli, T. E., 1982, Bioactive factors of the blood complement system in: *Proteins in Biology and Medicine*, (R. A. Bradshaw, R. L. Hill, and J. Tang, eds.), pp. 91-117, Proceedings of P.R.C.-USA Conference in Shanghai, China, Academic Press.

Hugli, T. E., and Erickson, B. W., 1977, Synthetic peptides with the biological activities and specificity of human C3a anaphylatoxin, *Proc. Natl. Acad. Sci. USA* 74:1826-1830.

Hugli, T. E., and Müller-Eberhard, H. J., 1978, Anaphylatoxins: C3a and C5a, *Adv. Immunol.* 26:1-48.

Hugli, T. E., Morgan, W. T., and Müller-Eberhard, H. J., 1975, Circular dichroism of C3a anaphylatoxin: Effects of pH, heat, guanidinium and chloride and mercaptoethanol on conformation and function, *J. Biol. Chem.* 250:1479-1483.

Jensen, J. A., Snyderman, R., and Mergenhagen, S. E., 1969, Chemotactic activity, a property of guinea pig C5-anaphylatoxins, in: *Cellular and Humoral Mechanisms in Anaphlaxis and Allergy* (H. Z. Movat, ed.), pp. 265-278, S. Karger, New York.

Johnson, A. R., Hugli, T. E., and Müller-Eberhard, H. J., 1975, Release of histamine from rat mast cells by the complement peptides C3a and C5a, *Immunology* 28:1067-1080.

Kay, A. B., Shin, H. S., and Austen, K. F., 1973, Selective attraction of eosinophils and synergism between eosinophil chemotactic factor of anaphylaxis (ECF-A) and a fragment cleaved from the fifth component of complement (C5a), *Immunology* 24:969-976.

Koopman, W. J., Sandberg, A. L., Wahl, S. M., and Mergenhagen, S. E., 1976, Interaction of soluble C3 fragments with guinea pig lymphocytes. Comparison of effects of C3a, C3b, C3c, and C3d on lymphokine production and lymphocyte proliferation, *J. Immunol.* 117:331-336.

ter Laan, B., Molenaar, J. L., Feltkamp-Vroom, T. M., and Pondman, K. W., 1974, Interaction of human anaphylatoxin C3a with rat mast cells demonstrated by immunofluorescence, *Eur. J. Immunol.* 4:393-395.

Lackie, J. M., 1977, The aggregation of rabbit polymorphonuclear leukocytes (PMNs): Effects of agents which affect the acute inflammatory response and correlation with secretory activity, *Inflammation* 2:1-15.

Mackler, B. F., Altman, L. C., Rosenstreich, D. L., and Oppenheim, J. J., 1974, Induction of lymphokine production by EAC and of blastogenesis by soluble mitogens during human B-cell activation, *Nature* 249:834-837.

Maderazo, E. G., and Woronich, C. L., 1978, Micropore filter assay of human granulocyte locomotion: Problems and solutions, *Clin. Immunol. Immunopathol.* 11:196-211.

Maderazo, E. G., Ward, P. A., and Quintilliani, R., 1975, Defective regulation of chemotaxis in cirrhosis, *J. Lab. Clin. Med.* 85:621-624.

Maderazo, E. G., Ward, P. A., Woronick, C. L., Kubik, J., and DeGraff, A. C., 1976, Leukotactic dysfunction in sarcoidosis, *Ann Intern. Med.* 84:414-417.

Malmsten, C. L., Palmblad, J., Uden, A.-M., Radmark, O., Engstedt, L., and Samuelsson, B.

1980, Leukotriene B$_4$: A highly potent and stereospecific factor stimulating migration of polymophonuclear leukocytes, *Acta Physiol. Scand.* 110:449-451.

Martinelli, G. P., Matsuda, T., and Osler, A. G., 1978, Studies on immunosuppression by cobra venom factor. I. An early IgG and IgM response to sheep erythrocyte and DNP-protein conjugates, *J. Immunol.* 121:2043-2047.

Meuth, J. L., Morgan, E. L., DiScipio, R. G., and Hugli, T. E., 1983, Suppression of T lymphocyte functions by human C3 fragments. I. Inhibition of human T cell proliferative responses by a kallikrein cleavage fragment of human iC3b, *J. Immunol.* 130: 2605-2611.

Morgan, E. L., and Weigle, W. O., 1979, Macrophage requirement in the Fc fragment-induced proliferative response of murine spleen cells, *J. Exp. Med.* 150:256-266.

Morgan, E. L., and Weigle, W. O., 1980a, Regulation of Fc fragment-induced murine spleen cell proliferation, *J. Exp. Med.* 151:1-11.

Morgan, E. L., and Weigle, W. O., 1980b, Polyclonal activation of murine B lymphocytes by Fc fragments. I. The requirement for two signals in the generation of the polyclonal antibody response induced by Fc fragments, *J. Immunol.* 124:1330-1335.

Morgan, E. L., and Weigle, W. O., 1980c, Regulation of B lymphocyte activation by the Fc portion of immunoglobulin, *J. Supramol. Struct.* 14:201-208.

Morgan, E. L., and Weigle, W. O., 1981, Polyclonal activation of human B lymphocytes by Fc fragments for Fc fragment-mediated polyclonal antibody secretion by human peripheral blood lymphocytes, *J. Exp. Med.* 154:778-790.

Morgan, E. L., Weigle, W. O., and Hugli, T. E., 1982, Anaphylatoxin mediated regulation of the immune response. I. C3a-mediated suppression of human and murine humoral immune responses, *J. Exp. Med.* 155:1412-1426.

Morgan, E. L., Thoman, M. L., Weigle, W. O., and Hugli, T. E., 1983a, Anaphylatoxin-mediated regulation of the immune response. II. C5a-mediated enhancement of human humoral and T cell-mediated immune responses, *J. Immunol.* 130:1257-1266.

Morgan, E. L., Weigle, W. O., Erickson, B. W., Fok, K-F, and Hugli, T. E., 1983b, Suppression of humoral immune responses by synthetic C3a peptides, *J. Immunol.* 131: 2258-2261.

Morgan, E. L., Thoman, M. L., Weigle, W. O., and Hugli, T. E., 1984. Human C3a-mediated suppression of the immune response. I. Suppression of human and murine *in vitro* antibody response occurs through the generation of nonspecific suppressor T cells. *J. Immunol.* (submitted).

Mosier, D. E., Scher, I., and Paul, W. E., 1976, In vitro responses of CBA/N mice: Spleen cells of mice with an X-linked defect that precludes immune responses to several thymus-independent antigens can respond to TNP-lipopolysaccharide, *J. Immunol.* 117:1363-1369.

Needleman, B. M., Weiler, J. M., and Feldbush, T. L., 1981, The third component of complement inhibits human lymphocyte blastogenesis, *J. Immunol.* 125:1586-1589.

Nelson, R. D., Quie, P. G., and Simons, R. L., 1975, Chemotaxis under agarose: A new and simple method for measuring chemotaxis and spontaneous migration of human polymorphonuclear leukocytes and monocytes, *J. Immunol.* 115:1650-1656.

O'Flaherty, J. T., and Ward, P. A., 1978, Leukocyte aggregation induced by chemotactic factors, *Inflammation* 3:177-194.

O'Flaherty, J. T., Kreutzer, D. L., and Ward, P. A., 1977a, Neutrophil aggregation and swelling induced by chemotactic agents, *J. Immunol.* 119:232-239.

O'Flaherty, J. T., Kreutzer, D. L., Showell, H. J., and Ward, P. A., 1977b, Influence of inhibitors of cellular function on chemotactic factor induced neutrophil aggregation, *J. Immunol.* 119:1751-1756.

O'Flaherty, J. T., Kreutzer, D. L., and Ward, P. A., 1978, Chemotactic factor influences on the aggregation, swelling and foreign surface adhesiveness of human leukocytes, *Am. J. Pathol.* 90:537-550.

Ondetti, M. A., Condon, M. E., Reid, J., Sabo, E. F., Cheung, H. S., and Cushman, D. W., 1979, Design of potent and specific inhibitors of carboxypeptidases A and B, *Biochemistry* 18:1427–1430.

Orr, W., and Ward, P. A., 1978, Quantitation of leukotaxis in agarose by three different methods, *J. Immunol. Methods* 20:95–107.

Payan, D. G., Trentham, D. E., and Goetzl, E. J., 1982, Modulation of human lymphocyte function by C3a and C3a (70–77), *J. Exp. Med.* 156:756–765.

Pepys, M. D., and Butterworth, A. F., 1974, Inhibitions by C3 fragments of C3-dependent rosette formation and antigen-induced lymphocyte transformation, *Clin. Exp. Immunol.* 18:273–280.

Pepys, M. B., 1976, Role of complement in the induction of immunological responses, *Transplant. Rev.* 32:93.

Pepys, M. B., Mujah, D. D., and Dash, A. C., 1976, Immunosuppression by cobra venom factor: Distribution, antigen-induced blast transformation and trapping of lymphocyte during in vivo complement depletion, *Cell. Immunol.* 21:327–336.

Perez, H. D., Goldstein, I. M., Chernoff, D., Webster, R. O., and Henson, P. M., 1980, Chemotactic activity of $C5a_{des Arg}$: Evidence of a requirement for an anionic peptide "Helper factor" and inhibition by a cationic protein in serum from patients with systemic lupus erythematous, *Mol. Immunol.* 17:163–169.

Plummer, T. H., and Hurwitz, N. Y., 1978, Human plasma carboxypeptidase N, *J. Biol. Chem.* 253:3907–3912.

Reinherz, E. L., Kung, P. C., Goldstein, G., and Schlossman, S. F., 1979, Further characterization of the human inducer T cell subset defined by monoclonal antibody, *J. Immunol.* 123:2894–2896.

Romball, C. G., Ulevitch, R. J., and Weigle, W. O., 1980, role of C3 in the regulation of a splenic PFC response in rabbits, *J. Immunol.* 124:151–155.

Ross, G. D., and Newman, S. L., 1984, Macrophage function by complement, complement receptor, and IgG-Fc receptors, in: *The Reticuloendothelial System: A Comprehensive Treatise*, Vol. 6 (J. A. Bellanti and H. D. Herscowitz, eds.), pp. 87–112, Plenum Press, New York.

Rother, K., 1972, Leukocyte mobilizing factor: A new biological activity derived from the third component of complement, *Eur. J. Immunol.* 2:550–558.

Sacks, T., Moldow, C. F., Craddock, P. R., Bowers, T. K., and Jacob, H. S., 1978, Oxygen radicals mediate endothelial damage by complement-stimulated granulocytes: An in vitro model of immune vascular damage, *J. Clin. Invest.* 61:1161–1167.

Schenkein, H. A., and Genco, R. H., 1979, Inhibition of lymphocyte blastogenesis by C3c and C3d, *J. Immunol.* 122:1126–1133.

Scher, I., Steinberg, A. D., Benning, A. K., and Paul, W. E., 1975, X-linked B-lymphocyte immune defect in CBA/N mice. II. Studies of the mechanisms underlying the immune defect, *J. Exp. Med.* 142:637–650.

Shaw, J. O., Henson, P. M., Henson, J., and Webster, R. O., 1980, Lung inflammation induced by complement-derived chemotactic fragments in the alveolus, *Lab. Invest.* 42:547–558.

Shin, H. S., Snyderman, R., Friedman, E., Mellors, A., and Mayer, M. M., 1968, Chemotactic and anaphylatoxic fragment cleaved from the fifth component of guinea pig, *Science* 162:361–363.

Siraganian, R. P., and Hook, W. A., 1976, Complement induced histamine release from human basophils. II. Mechanisms of the histamine reaction, *J. Immunol.* 116:639–646.

Snyderman, R., Gewruz, H., and Mergenhagen, S. E., 1968, Interactions of the complement system with endotoxic lipopolysaccharide, *J. Exp. Med.* 128:259–275.

Snyderman, R., Shin, H. S., Phillips, J. K., Gewruz, H., and Mergenhagen, S. E., 1969, A neutrophil chemotactic factor derived from C'5 upon interaction of guinea pig serum with endotoxin, *J. Immunol.* 103:413–422.

Snyderman, R., Altman, L. C., Hausman, M. S., and Mergenhagen, S. E., 1972, Human mononuclear leukocyte chemotaxis: A quantitative assay for humoral and cellular chemotactic factors, *J. Immunol.* 108:857–860.

Stimler, N. P., Bach, M. K., Bloor, C. M., and Hügli, T. E., 1982, Release of leukotrienes from guinea pig lung stimulated by C5a$_{des\,Arg}$ anaphylatoxin, *J. Immunol.* 128: 2247–2252.

Thoman, M. L., Morgan, E. L., and Weigle, W. O., 1980a, Activation of T lymphocytes by the Fc position of immunoglobulin, *J. Supramol. Struct.* 13:479–486.

Thoman, M. L., Morgan, E. L., and Weigle, W. O., 1980b, Polyclonal activation of murine B lymphocytes by Fc fragments. II. Replacement of T cells by a soluble helper T cell-replacing factor (TRF), *J. Immunol.* 125:1630–1633.

Thoman, M. L., Morgan, E. L., and Weigle, W. O., 1981, Fc fragment activation of T lymphocyte. I. Fc fragments trigger Lyti 2^{+}3^{-} T lymphocytes to release a helper T cell-replacing factor, *J. Immunol.* 126:632–635.

Till, G., and Ward, P. A., 1975, Two distinct chemotactic factor inactivators in human serum, *J. Immunol.* 114:834–847.

Vallota, E. H., and Müller-Eberhard, H. J., 1973, Formation of C3a and C5a anaphylatoxins in whole human serum after inhibition of the anaphylatoxin inactivator, *J. Exp. Med.* 137:1109–1123.

Vallota, E. H., Hugli, T. E., and Müller-Eberhard, H. J., 1973, Isolation and characterization of a new and highly active form of C5a anaphylatoxin from epsilon-aminocaproic acid-containing porcine serum, *J. Immunol.* 111:294 (abst).

Wahl, S. M., Iverson, G. M., and Oppenheim, J. J., 1974, Induction of guinea pig B-cell lymphokine synthesis by mitogenic and nonmitogenic signals to Fc, Ig, and C3 receptors, *J. Exp. Med.* 140:1631–1645.

Ward, P. A., 1967, A plasmin-split fragment of C'3 as a new chemotactic factor, *J. Exp. Med.* 126:189–206.

Ward, P. A., 1969, The heterogeneity of chemotactic factors for neutrophils generated from the complement system, in: *Cellular and Humoral Mechanisms in Anaphylaxis and Allergy* (N. Movat, ed.), pp. 279–310, S. Karger, Basel, New York.

Ward, P. A., and Becker, E. L., 1976, Biology of Leukotaxis, *Rev. Physiol. Biochem. Pharmacol.* 77:125–148.

Ward, P. A., and Berenberg, J. L., 1974, Defective regulation of inflammatory mediators in Hodgkin's disease. Supernormal levels of chemotactic factor inactivator, *N. Engl. J. Med.* 290:76–78.

Ward, P. A., and Newman, L. J., 1969, A neutrophil chemotactic factor from Human C5, *J. Immunol.* 102:93–99.

Ward, P. A., Cochrane, C. G., and Müller-Eberhard, H. J., 1965, The role of serum complement of chemotaxis pf PMNs, *J. Exp. Med.* 122:327–346.

Ward, P. A., Cochrane, C. G., and Müller-Eberhard, H. J., 1967, Further studies on the chemotactic factor of complement and its formation in vivo, *Immunology* 11:141–153.

Ward, P. A., Dvorak, H. F., Cohen, S., Yoshida, T., Data, R., and Selvaggio, S. S., 1975, Chemotaxis of basophils by lymphocyte-dependent and lymphocyte-independent mechanisms, *J. Immunol.* 114:1523–1531.

Ward, P. A., Goralnick, S., and Bullock, W. E., 1976, Defective leukotaxis in patients with lepromatous leprosy, *J. Lab. Clin. Med.* 87:1025–1029.

Webster, R. O., Hong, S. R., Johnston Jr., R. B., and Henson, P. M., 1980, Biological effects of the human complement fragments C5a and C5a$_{des\,Arg}$ on neutrophil function, *Immunopharmacology* 2:201–219.

Weiler, J. M., Ballas, Z. B., Needleman, B. W., Hobbs, M. W., and Feldbush, T. L., 1982, Complement fragments suppress lymphocyte immune responses, *Immunol. Today* **3**: 738–743.

Wilkinson, P. C., 1974, *Chemotaxis and Inflammation*, Churchill-Livingstone, Edinburgh, Scotland.

Wissler, J. H., Stecher, V. J., and Sorkin, E., 1972, Biochemistry and biology of a leucotactic binary serum peptide system related to anaphylatoxin, *Int. Arch. Allergy Appl. Immunol.* 42:722–728.

Zigmond, S. H., 1980, Polymorphonuclear leucocyte chemotaxis: Detection of the gradient and development of cell polarity, *Ciba Found. Symp.* 71:299–311.

Zigmond, S. H., and Hirsch, H. G., 1973, Leukocyte locomotion and chemotaxis: New methods for evaluation, and demonstration of a cell-derived chemotactic factor, *J. Exp. Med.* 137:387–410.

Chapter 5

Regulation of Human Leukocyte Function by Lipoxygenase Products of Arachidonic Acid

Frank H. Valone

Cancer Research Institute
University of California School of Medicine
San Francisco, California 94143

I. GENERATION OF LIPOXYGENASE PRODUCTS OF ARACHIDONIC ACID IN LEUKOCYTES

Arachidonic acid released from membrane phospholipids undergoes oxygenation by two distinct pathways that differ in terms of both their products and their susceptibility to regulation by biological and pharmacological agents (Fig. 1). The cyclooxygenase pathway yields unstable endoperoxide intermediates that undergo spontaneous or enzymatic conversion to a variety of products including prostaglandins, prostacyclin, and thromboxanes. Oxygenation of arachidonic acid by the lipoxygenase pathway generates a series of unstable hydroperoxy-eicosatetraenoic acids (OOHETES or HPETES), of which 5-OOHETE is quantitatively predominant in several types of leukocytes, 12-OOHETE is the major product in platelets, and 11-OOHETE and 5-OOHETE in rabbit alveolar macrophages (Borgeat and Samuelsson, 1979a; Goetzl and Sun, 1979; Valone *et al.*, 1980).

The OOHETES serve not only as the biosynthetic precursors of monohydroxy-eicosatetraenoic acid (mono-HETES), but are critical intermediates in the generation of a family of complex HETES, termed leukotrienes, that contain additional polar substituents and three conjugated double bonds (Samuelsson, 1981, 1982). The leukotrienes have been the objects of intensive investigation because of the observations that some leukotrienes derived from 5-OOHETE are potent mediators of leukocyte function and other leukotrienes comprise the slow-

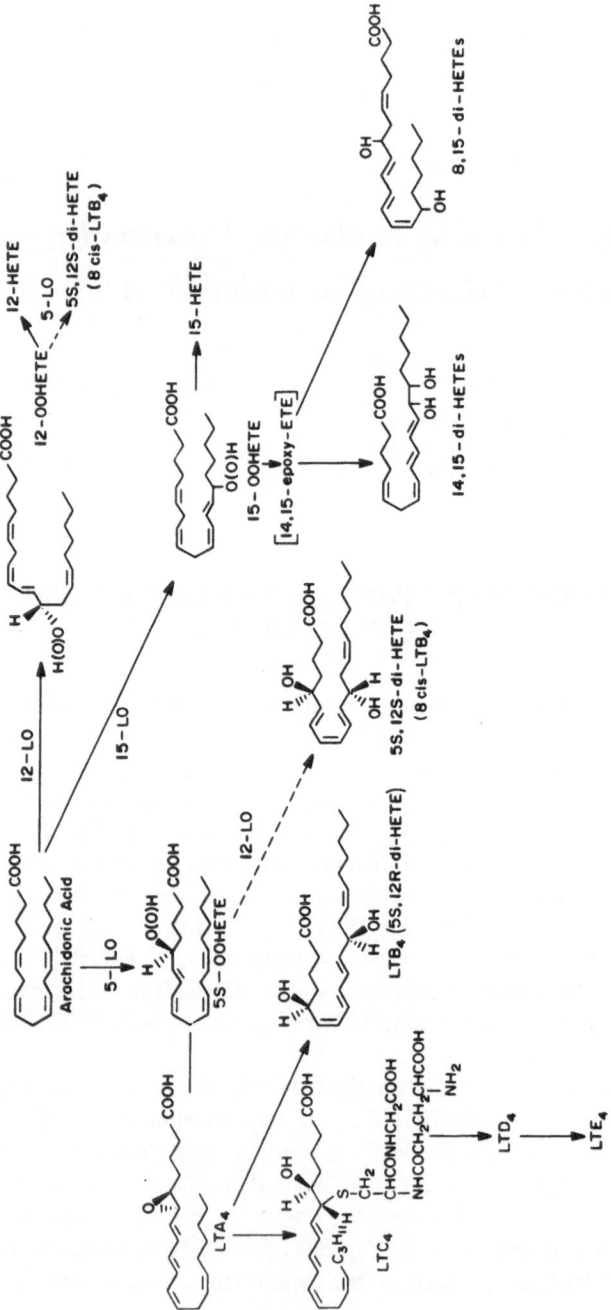

Figure 1. Lipoxygenase pathway of arachidonic acid oxygenation.

reacting substance of anaphylaxis. Elimination of the hydroxyl anion from the hydroperoxy group of 5-OOHETE and abstraction of a proton at C-10 yields the highly reactive 5,6-epoxy-eicosa-7,9,11,14-tetraenoic acid termed leukotriene A_4 (LTA_4), where the subscript 4 indicates the total number of double bonds in the molecule (Borgeat and Samuelsson, 1979b). LTA_4 is hydrated enzymatically to form 5(S),12(R)-dihydroxy-eicosa-6,14-cis-8,10-$trans$-tetraenoic acid (LTB_4) (Samuelsson, 1982), which is a potent stimulus of leukocyte chemotaxis and other functions in $vivo$ and in $vitro$ (Ford-Hutchinson et $al.$, 1980; Palmer et $al.$, 1980; Goetzl and Pickett, 1980; Goetzl and Sun, 1981). Nonenyzmatic hydrolysis of the epoxide at C-6 and C-12 through a mechanism involving a carbonium ion yields isomeric 5,12- and 5,6-dihydroxy acids, which also contain the stable conjugated triene structure (Borgeat and Samuelsson, 1979c). The analogue of LTB_4, 5(S),12(S)-dihydroxy-6-$trans$, 8-cis, 10-$trans$, 14-cis-eicosatetraenoic acid [5(S),12(S)-di-HETE] is formed by double oxygenation of arachidonic acid rather than from the epoxide LTA_4 (Borgeat et $al.$, 1982). The observation that the polymorphonuclear leukocyte (PMN) C-5 lipoxygenase can form 5(S),12(S)-di-HETE from platelet-derived 12-HETE is a novel example of cell–cell cooperation in the biogenesis of an immunological mediator. In this system 12-HETE competes with arachidonic acid for the 5-lipoxygenase and thereby limits the generation of leukotrienes. LTA_4 can also combine enzymatrically with γ-glutamylcysteinylglycine (glutathione) to yield 5-hydroxy-6-sulfido-glutathionyl-ETE (LTC_4) (Murphy et $al.$, 1979). LTC_4 is converted peptidolytically by a γ-glutamyl transpeptidase to 5(S)-hydroxy-6(R)-(S)-cysteinyl-glycine-7,9-$trans$-11, 14-cis-eicosatetraenoic acid (LTD_4) and then by cysteinyl-glycinase to 5(S)-hydroxy-6-sulfido-cysteine-ETE (LTE_4) (Orning and Hammarstrom, 1980). LTC_4, LTD_4, and LTE_4 are potent vasoactive and contractile factors that represent the principal active components of the slow-reacting substance of anaphylaxis (SRS-A), which is released by in $vitro$ and in $vivo$ immunological stimulation of human lung and other tissues (Murphy et $al.$, 1979; Samuelsson, 1981). The products of the C-15 lipoxygenase constitute an additional family of leukotrienes, which are formed by unique mechanisms. C-5 and C-15 are located symmetrically with respect to the C-10 methylene group and the two diene structures of arachidonic acid. Thus the carbons in the 5- and 15-positions could undergo similar reactions. However, the epoxide LTA_4 is oxygenated by a hydrolytic mechanism, whereas the epoxide derived from the 15-lipoxygenase 14,15(S)-oxido-5,8,10,12-eicosatetraenoic acid (14,15-LTA_4) is oxygenated by insertion of an oxygen radical to yield two isomers of 14,15-dihydroxy-5,8,10, 12-eicosatetraenoic acid (14,15-LTB_4) (Borgeat and Samuelsson, 1979b; Samuelsson, 1981; Maas et $al.$, 1981, 1982; Radmark et $al.$, 1982). A similar mechanism of insertion of an oxygen radical into 14,15-LTA_4 may account for the formation of the two isomers of 8,15-dihydroxy-5,9,11,13-eicosatetraenoic acid. The observation that generation of these dihydroxy-derivatives of 14,15-LTA_4 is diminished in broken cells suggests that the oxygen radicals that react with

14,15-LTA$_4$ derive from nonlipoxygenase pathways such as the superoxide generating pathway. Although 12-OOHETE may be as reactive as 15-OOHETE and 5-OOHETE, the only complex products that have been identified definitively are several trihydroxy-eicosatetraenoic acids.

Analysis of the lipoxygenase products of different leukocytes has required the addition of exogenous radiolabeled or nonradiolabeled arachidonic acid in order to obtain quantities of each metabolite sufficient for accurate quantitation by optical or radiochemical methods. Recently, sensitive radioimmunoassays have been developed for specific lipoxygenase products (Levine *et al.*, 1980; Salmon *et al.*, 1982; Aehringhaus *et al.*, 1982) that may permit reliable assessment of the quantities of mediators in the absence of exogenous arachidonic acid. It is apparent, however, from studies of the lipoxygenase products of exogenously supplied arachidonic acid that the predominant products of lipoxygenation of arachidonic acid differ with both the class of leukocytes and the species of origin. Human granulocytes all produce a substantial quantity of 5-HETE, which is the major mono-HETE of neutrophils and basophils (Borgeat *et al.*, 1976; Goetzl and Sun, 1979). In contrast, human and murine eosinophils (Turk *et al.*, 1982) and human peripheral blood T lymphocytes (Goetzl, 1981) generate more 15-HETE than 5-HETE and 12-HETE. 11-HETE is the most predominant mono-HETE product of murine mixed spleen cells, rabbit alveolar macrophages, and canine mastocytoma cells (Valone *et al.*, 1980; Payan *et al.*, 1983*b*). Similar differences are apparent with respect to the leukotriene products. LTB$_4$ is the predominant product of human neutrophils and T lymphocytes and of murine mixed spleen cells (Borgeat and Samuelsson, 1979*a*; Goetzl, 1981). In contrast, approximately equal amounts of LTB$_4$ and the C-6 peptide leukotrienes are generated by rabbit alveolar macrophages, dog mastocytoma cells, and human basophils (Payan *et al.*, 1983*b*). Stimulation of most leukocytes by specific and nonspecific stimuli has in general increased the quantity of each lipoxygenase product generated without substantially altering the ratios of the products (Valone *et al.*, 1980, 1983). However, the relative distribution of lipoxygenase products may differ substantially between resting and stimulated macrophages (Scott *et al.*, 1982*a,b*). Resident murine peritoneal macrophages spontaneously produce mono-HETEs, 6-keto PGF$_{1\alpha}$ (the stable metabolic product of prostacyclin), and PGE$_2$ in a ratio of $67:24:9$, whereas the ratio changes considerably in response to a phagocytic stimulus (HETEs:6-keto PGF$_{1\alpha}$:PGE$_2$: LTC$_4$,$15:25:40:15$-20). Substantial differences are also noted in the arachidonic acid oxygenation products of resident and elicited peritoneal macrophages. Compared with resident peritoneal macrophages *Corynebacterium parvum* elicited macrophages demonstrated reduced mobilization of arachidonic acid upon stimulation of phagocytosis and the cyclooxygenase products constituted a greater proportion of the arachidonic acid metabolites. Furthermore, the activated macrophages displayed greatly reduced synthesis of prostacyclin and LTC$_4$ compared with other metabolites. It thus appears that *in vivo* activation of murine macrophages leads to alterations in the activity of inducible phospholi-pases and synthetic enzymes for specific oxygenated products. Different results were obtained by analyses of the lipoxygenase products of human peripheral blood monocytes activated by incubation with lymphokines for 18 hr *in vitro* (Obrist *et al.*, 1983). In these studies, activated and nonactivated macrophages demonstrated the same capacity to lipoxygenate arachidonic acid and the relative distribution of the lipoxygenase products after stimulation by incuba-tion with tumor target cells was similar for both groups of macrophages.

II. REGULATION OF THE GENERATION AND ACTIVITIES OF LIPOXYGENASE PRODUCTS OF ARACHIDONIC ACID

The natural mechanisms for the control of biosynthesis and degradation of oxygenated metabolites of arachidonic acid have been elucidated only partially in platelets, leukocytes, and other cellular elements of hypersensitivity and inflammatory reactions. Both products of the lipoxygenation pathways and other normal intracellular constituents may enhance, inhibit, or irreversibly inactivate the catalytic functions of specific enzymes. 12-OOHETE augments the capacity of platelet lipoxygenase to generate 12-OOHETE and concurrently suppresses the catalytic activity of platelet cyclooxygenase, while 15-OOHETE inactivates prostacyclin synthetase, but not thromboxane A_2 synthetase. 15-OOHETE has the apparently unique and selective capacity to block the 12-lipoxygenase of platelets and the 5-lipoxygenase of PMNs and human and mouse T lymphocytes, without altering cyclooxygenase activity (Vanderhoek *et al.*, 1980*a,b*; Goetzl, 1981).

In contrast, 15-HETE enhances the rate of 5-lipoxygenation in basophils and mast cells of some species. Physiological concentrations of vitamin E *in vitro* enhance the production of 5-HETE and LTB_4 by human neutrophils (Goetzl, 1980), whereas at higher concentrations vitamin E inhibits the activity of plate-let cyclooxygenase and of the lipoxygenases of platelets, human neutrophils, and human T lymphocytes (Goetzl, 1980; Ali *et al.*, 1980).

A consideration of the numerous pharmacological inhibitors of the lipoxy-genation of arachidonic acid reveals that in general these inhibitors suppress the lipoxygenase pathway without significant selectivity for individual lipoxygenase products. Inhibitors of phospholipase function including corticosteroids and agents that elevate intracellular levels of cyclic $3',5'$-adenosine monophosphate (cAMP) block the mobilization of arachidonic acid from membrane phospho-lipids and thereby impair the oxygenation of arachidonic acid by both the lipoxygenase and cyclooxygenase pathways. Several types of compounds in-cluding indomethacin suppress lipoxygenation by blocking the transformation of OOHETEs to HETEs. However, the concentrations required to block the transformation exceed those attainable *in vivo*, and these reports remain to be confirmed with isolated enzyme systems (Siegel *et al.*, 1980*a,b*). The acetylenic class of reversible inhibitors has been studied intensively. 5,8,11-Eicosatriynoic acid inhibits the 12-lipoxygenase of platelets more than 10 times as effectively as the cyclooxygenase, in contrast to 5,8,11,14-eicosatetraynoic acid (ETYA), which inhibits both pathways with approximately equal potency, and 9,12-octadecadiynoic acid (DYA), which inhibits the cyclooxygenase preferentially (Vanderhoek and Lands, 1973; Sams *et al.*, 1982). Recently, purified 4,7,10,13-icosatetraynoic acid and 4,8,11,14-henicosatetraynoic acid have been shown to express a 100- to 200-fold preference for the lipoxygenase over the cyclooxygenase (Wilhelm *et al.*, 1981). Other pharmacological inhibitors, including nordihydroguaiaretic acid (NDGA) (Obrist *et al.*, 1983) and benoxaprofen (Walker and Dawson, 1979), inhibit both pathways of oxygenation of arachidonic acid with a slight degree of selectivity for lipoxygenase activities in some types of cells.

III. MODULATION OF PMN LEUKOCYTE FUNCTION BY LIPOXYGENASE PRODUCTS OF ARACHIDONIC ACID

The results of the earliest investigations of the *in vitro* leukocyte-directed activities of the lipoxygenase products of arachidonic acid demonstrated that mono-HETEs stimulate the chemotaxis of human eosinophils and neutrophils and, to a lesser extent, human monocytes, in modified Boyden Micropore filter chambers (Goetzl *et al.*, 1977). A rank order of potency is manifested in the series of mono-HETEs, such that 5-HETE $\gg$ 8-HETE = 9-HETE > 11-HETE = 12-HETE $\gg$ 15-HETE (Goetzl *et al.*, 1980*b*). Studies of the complex lipoxygenase products that are sufficiently stable to be purified indicated that LTB_4 is by far the most potent lipid chemotactic factor for human PMN's, while trihydroxyeicosatetraenoic acids from platelets and LTC_4 are essentially inactive in this respect (Goetzel *et al.*, 1981). LTB_4 evokes neutrophil and eosinophil chemotactic responses equal in magnitude to the maximal responses to C5a and the *N*-formyl-methionyl peptides (Ford-Hutchinson *et al.*, 1980; Goetzl and Pickett, 1980; Palmer *et al.*, 1980). Microgram quantities of 12-HETE, a fraction of a microgram of 5-HETE and 10–30 ng of LTB_4 elicited a rapid accumulation of eosinophils and a later influx of neutrophils in the guinea pig peritoneal cavity. LTB_4 but not LTC_4, LTD_4, 5-HETE, or 12-HETE elicited the accumulation of leukocytes following injection into the anterior chamber of the rabbit eye (Bhattacherjee *et al.*, 1981). Similarly, intradermal injection of LTB_4 but not of 5-OOHETE promoted the accumulation of PMNs in rabbit skin (Carr *et al.*, 1981).

The *in vitro* and *in vivo* chemotactic activities of the mono-HETEs are eliminated by methylation of the free fatty acids (Goetzl *et al.*, 1979*a*). The methyl esters are specific competitive inhibitors of the PMN chemotactic responses to parent stimuli but have no effect on the leukocyte responses to *N*-formyl-methionyl peptides or to chemotactic fragments of the fifth component of complement. Acetylation of the hydroxyl-groups or alterations in the double bonds of the triene portion of LTB_4 reduce the chemotactic potency for PMNs (Goetzl and Pickett, 1980) indicating that both the free hydroxyl-groups and the sequence of conjugated double bonds are functionally critical determinants. The PMN chemotactic potency of LTB_4 also exceeds by several fold the potency of the leukotrienes generated by the 15-lipoxygenase pathway (Jubiz et al., 1981). Omega-oxidation of LTB_4 to yield the 20-OH and 20-COOH derivatives significantly reduces the chemotactic potency of LTB_4, suggesting that further oxidation of LTB_4 represents a mechanism for inactivation of LTB_4 (Samuelsson, 1982).

At concentrations approximately 3- to 10-fold higher than those required to stimulate maximal chemotaxis, LTB_4 evokes a wide range of PMN responses independent of migration (Fig. 2). LTB_4 induces lysosomal degranulation of PMNs; the maximal enzyme release by LTB_4, however, is only 25%–30% of that achieved by N-fMet-Leu-Phe and the phospholipid platelet-activating factor, 1-O-hexadecyl-2-acetyl-SN-glycero-3phosphorylcholine (AGEPC) (Table I). Neutrophil adherence to columns of Sephadex G-25 is increased 1- to 2-fold by LTB_4, LTC_4, and LTD_4 in a concentration-dependent manner (Goetzl et al., 1983). The cyclooxygenase product thromboxane A_2 mediates the enhanced neutrophil adherence by LTC_4 and LTD_4, whereas LTB_4 enhances PMN adherence primarily by a direct mechanism (Fig. 2). LTB_4 also elicits PMN aggregation, as assessed by standard platelet aggregometry techniques (Ford-Hutchinson et al., 1982). LTB_4 and 5-HETE, but not LTC_4, LTD_4, or 15-HETE, enhance the expression of C3b receptors on human neutrophils (Goetzl et al., 1980a) and eosinophils (Nagy et al., 1982) in vitro, with lesser increases in IgG-Fc receptors as assessed by rosetting techniques.

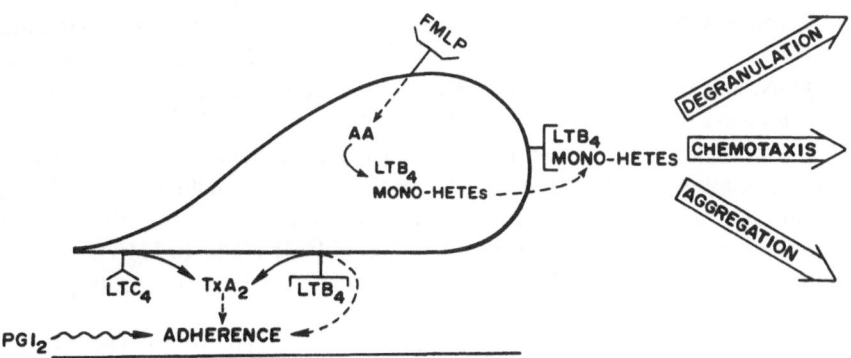

Figure 2. Modulation of polymorphonuclear leukocyte (PMN) function by lipoxygenase and cyclo-oxygenase products of arachidonic acid ($\longrightarrow$) Generation, ($-\rightarrow$) stimulation, ($\rightsquigarrow$) suppression. LTB_4/LTC_4, leukotriene B_4/C_4; TXA_2, thromboxane; AA, arachidonic acid; FMLP, fMet-Leu-Phe.

Table I. Specific Desensitization of PMN Leukocyte Degranulation by LTB₄, AGEPC, and N-fMet-Leu-Phe

Deactivating agent[a]	Degranulating stimulus		
	LTB₄ (5 ng/ml)	AGEPC (0.2 μM)	N-fMet-Leu-Phe (0.3 μM)
Hank's buffer	8.3 ± 1.9[b]	26.9 ± 8.1	34.4 ± 7.7
LTB₄ (5 ng/ml)	0.6 ± 0.2	19.9 ± 6.4	31.8 ± 9.2
AGEPC (0.2 μM)	7.2 ± 2.1	10.6 ± 4.3	39.1 ± 6.5
N-fMet-Leu-Phe (0.3 μM)	6.3 ± 0.5	18.9 ± 4.4	11.4 ± 3.8

Abbreviations: AGEPC, 1-O-alkyl-2-acetyl-SN-glycero-3-phosphorylcholine; LTB₄, leukotriene B₄; PMN, polymorphonuclear leukocyte.

[a] 3×10^6 PMN leukocytes were incubated with the indicated deactivating agent for 30 min at 37°C and washed three times with Hank's buffer. The release of β-glucuronidase after incubation with the homologous factor or with different factors was then assessed (Valone and Goetzl, 1983).

[b] Mean (± SD), net percentage release of β-glucuronidase (N = 3).

The preincubation of suspensions of PMNs with maximally chemotactic or degranulating concentrations of LTB₄ at 37°C induces a stimulus-specific state of reduced responsiveness, termed deactivation. That is, cells exposed to LTB₄ under nonactivating conditions and then washed demonstrate significantly reduced degranulating (Table I) and chemotactic (Goetzl and Pickett, 1980) responses to stimulation by LTB₄ while retaining nearly complete responses to stimulation by other agents such as N-fMet-Leu-Phe and AGEPC. The capacity to induce specific functional deactivation is similar to that of other stimuli (Table I) and has been attributed to changes in membrane receptors for the specific stimulus (Zigmond and Sullivan, 1979; Donabedian and Gallin, 1981; Valone and Goetzl, 1983).

Recently a distinct subset of PMN receptors for LTB₄ was defined (Goldman and Goetzl, 1982). LTB₄ is bound stereospecifically by 26,000–40,000 receptors per PMN, and the receptors have a K_D of 10.8–13.9 nM. Analyses of competitive inhibition of the binding of [³H]-LTB₄ to PMN leukocytes by analogues of LTB₄ revealed a close correlation between the chemotactic potency of related 5-lipoxygenase products and their capacity to inhibit the binding of [³H]-LTB₄. In contrast, maximally chemotactic concentrations of C5a and N-formyl-methionyl peptides do not inhibit the binding of [³H]-LTB₄ to PMNs. Analyses of the subcellular distribution of PMN receptors for LTB₄ by density gradient centrifugation techniques reveal that the LTB₄ receptor is preferentially recovered in the membrane fraction (Goldman and Goetzl, 1983). This observation supports the suggestion that LTB₄ may function both as an intracellular intermediate in leukocyte activation by other agents and as an extracellular mediator of leukocyte function (Fig. 2).

Numerous studies have demonstrated that LTB_4 and mono-HETEs modify a wide range of biochemical events in neutrophils and eosinophils. LTB_4 and 5-HETE stimulate the influx of calcium and the uptake of hexose into PMNs, while only LTB_4 triggers the mobilization of calcium from intracellular stores (Naccache et al., 1981). The latter effect of LTB_4 has been attributed to its capacity to function directly as a calcium ionophore (Serhan et al., 1982). Concentrations of LTB_4, which are 100- to 1000-fold greater than those that maximally stimulate cellular function selectively, increase the permeability of liposomes to calcium. Other lipoxygenase products including the all-*trans* isomer of LTB_4 do not promote calcium entry into liposomes. Further delineation of the potential role of LTB_4 as an endogenous ionophore however will require careful analysis of the temporal relationship between the generation of LTB_4 and the mobilization of calcium as well as studies of the blockade of each pathway in intact cells. At concentrations lower than those required to evoke an optimal chemotactic response, some HETEs increase the level of cyclic $3',5'$-guanosine monophosphate (cGMP) in PMNs (Goetzl et al., 1980a). These effects may be part of the biochemical sequence of leukocyte activation, but neither the mechanisms of coupling to activation nor the order of events has been elucidated.

IV. INTERACTIONS OF LIPOXYGENASE AND CYCLOOXYGENASE PRODUCTS OF ARACHIDONIC ACID IN THE MODULATION OF PMN LEUKOCYTE FUNCTION

Initial studies suggested that prostaglandins are potent mediators of PMN function. Subsequent analyses, however, indicated that these effects resulted from oxidative products of the prostaglandins and that the primary effects of cyclo-oxygenase products on PMN function are limited to stimulation of chemokinesis and alterations in adherence to surfaces (Goetzl et al., 1979b; Spagnuolo et al., 1980; Boxer et al., 1980; Valone, 1982). In addition, both prostaglandins and thromboxane A_2 mediate and modulate the effects of leukotrienes and mono-HETEs on PMN function. Nanomolar concentrations of PGD_2 and PGE_2 evoke chemokinesis and enhance the chemotactic responses to LTB_4 (Goetzl et al., 1979b), while higher concentrations of each prostaglandin inhibit chemotaxis in association with elevation of the intraleukocyte level of cyclic adenosine $3',5'$-monophosphate (cAMP). The inhibition of chemotaxis by high concentrations of PGE_2 and PGD_2 may result from diminished adherence of the PMNs: PGI_2 inhibits PMN adherence to foreign surfaces in part by elevating the intraleukocyte level of cAMP (Boxer et al., 1980). The chemotactic responses of neutrophils and eosinophils to LTB_4, but not to other stimuli, are inhibited by equimolar concentrations of LTC_4 and LTD_4 (Pickett et al., 1983). However, optimally inhibitory concentrations of LTC_4 do not interfere with the binding of LTB_4 to PMNs, suggesting that the functional consequences of the interaction of LTC_4 with PMNs are mediated by a subset of recognition sites independent of the LTB_4 receptor.

Thromboxane A_2 is a potent promoter of PMN adherence (Spagnuolo et al., 1980) and mediates the enhanced adherence induced by LTC_4, but not by LTB_4 (Fig. 2). Both LTB_4 and LTC_4 increase PMN adherence to Sephadex G-25 with maximal 1- to 2-fold increases occurring within 1 min. LTC_4 also stimulates by 1- to 2-fold the generation of thromboxane A_2 by PMNs as assessed by radioimmunoassay of the stable metabolite thromboxane B_2, whereas concentrations of LTB_4 that maximally stimulate adherence did not increase the generation of thromboxane A_2 (Goetzl et al., 1983). Indomethacin at a concentration of 10 μM suppressed the enhanced adherence by LTC_4 by 90% while suppressing enhanced adherence by LTB_4 by less than 50%. Thus LTB_4 increases PMN adherence predominantly by a direct effect, whereas LTC_4 stimulates the generation of thromboxane A_2, which accounts for most of the effect of LTC_4 on adherence.

V. LIPOXYGENASE PRODUCTS OF ARACHIDONIC ACID AS MEDIATORS OF T-LYMPHOCYTE FUNCTION

Initial studies revealed the presence of the 5-lipoxygenase pathway in human peripheral blood lymphocytes (Kelly and Parker, 1979). Subsequent studies revealed that purified unstimulated human T lymphocytes lipoxygenate arachidonic acid to 15-HETE, 12-HETE, 11-HETE, 5-HETE, LTB_4, and several structural isomers of LTB_4 (Goetzl, 1981). Stimulation of the T lymphocytes by the addition of 10 μM calcium ionophore A23187 or of 2–10 ng/ml of the tumor promoter 12-O-tetradecanoylphorbol-13-acetate (TPA) increased the concentrations of the mono-HETEs by 7- to 11-fold and of the di-HETEs by 12- to 20-fold. The simultaneous addition of optimal doses of A23187, concanavalin A, or TPA further increased the concentrations of all products, suggesting that these agents stimulate the lipoxygenase pathway by different mechanisms. Analysis of the modulation of the lipoxygenase pathway revealed that concentrations of 15-HETE and 15-OOHETE similar to those achieved in stimulated lymphocytes noncytolytically inhibited the increases in content of LTB_4 and 5-HETE but not of 11-HETE or prostaglandin E_2 (Goetzl, 1981; Bailey et al., 1982). The capacity of 15-HETE to suppress the 5-lipoxygenase of PMNs (Vanderhoek et al., 1980b) and the 12-lipoxygenase of platelets (Vanderhoek et al., 1980a) has also been demonstrated.

The pattern of migration of lymphocytes is fundamentally different from the pattern of migration of PMNs. The T-lymphocyte response to stimulation by a variety of agents is characterized by enhanced random migration, or chemokinesis, rather than by directed migration, or chemotaxis (Payan and Goetzl,

Table II. Modulation of Human T-Lymphocyte Function by Lipoxygenase and Cyclooxygenase Products of Arachidonic Acid[a]

Modulator	Lymphocyte chemokinesis	Generation of lymphokines	Lymphocyte transformation
LTB_4	↑	↓	↓
LTC_4	0	↓	0
15-HETE	↓	0	0
5-HETE	↑	0	0
PGD_2/PGE_2	0	↓	↓

Abbreviations: LTB_4, leukotriene B_4; LTC_4, leukotriene C_4; 5-HETE, 5(S)-hydroxy-6,8, 11,14-eicosatetraenoic acid; 15-HETE, 15(S)-hydroxy-5,8,11,13-eicosatetraenoic acid; PGD_2/PGE_2, prostaglandins D_2 and E.
[a]Enhancement, ↑; inhibition, ↓; no effect, 0.

1981). LTB_4 elicits a maximal 2- to 4-fold increase in T-lymphocyte chemokinesis at concentrations of 3–30 ng/ml, whereas 5-HETE, concanavalin A, and TPA elicit lesser chemokinetic responses at concentrations 100- to 1000-fold higher than for LTB_4. 11-HETE, LTC_4, and LTD_4 have no effect on T-lymphocyte migration (Table II). Lipoxygenase products of arachidonic acid may also mediate enhanced T lymphocyte chemokinesis by other stimuli. 15-HETE suppressed the chemokinetic responses of human T lymphocytes to concanavalin A, α-thioglycerol, and TPA. Dose–response studies indicated that 15-OOHETE and 15-hydroxy-eicosatrienoic acid were more potent than 15-HETE in inhibiting T-lymphocyte migration and that for each compound the concentration dependence of the inhibition of migration was similar to that observed for the suppression of T-lymphocyte 5-lipoxygenase activity. Thus the 5-lipoxygenation of arachidonic acid may be a critical intermediate step in stimulating T-lymphocyte chemokinesis.

The effects of lipoxygenase products of arachidonic acid on lymphocyte function have also been assessed in terms of both transformation and the generation of the lymphokine designated leukocyte-inhibitory factor (LIF) (Payan et al., 1982). The elaboration of LIF by T lymphocytes stimulated with phytohemagglutinin (PHA) is inhibited in a concentration-dependent manner by 10^{-9} to 10^{-6} M LTB_4. LTC_4 also inhibited lymphokine generation, although the maximal inhibition achieved was one-half that of LTB_4. Prostaglandins E_2 and D_2 and human C3a are also potent inhibitors of lymphokine generation, whereas mono-HETEs such as 15-HETE and leukotrienes such as 5(S),12(S)LTB_4 do not affect the elaboration of lymphokines (Table II).

Distinct products of both the cyclooxygenase and lipoxygenase pathways suppress the proliferation of PHA-stimulated T lymphocytes. LTB_4 inhibits significantly the proliferation of T lymphocytes (Payan et al., 1982), and this effect has been attributed to the induction of a subset of T-suppressor cells

(Rola-Pleszcznski *et al.*, 1982; Payan *et al.*, 1983*a*). Prostaglandins E_2 and D_2 exert a similar suppressive effect on proliferation, although the mechanisms of suppression have not been elucidated. In contrast, LTC_4, 15-HETE, and human C3a have no effect on stimulated proliferation. Thus, LTC_4, 15-HETE, and human C3a exert a selective inhibitory effect on the generation of LIF, whereas LTB_4, PGE_2, and PGD_2 inhibit both the generation of lymphokine and proliferation (Payan *et al.*, 1982). The accumulated observations of the specific regulation of human T-lymphocyte function by concentrations of mast cell and macrophage products of the oxygenation of arachidonic acid *in vitro* suggest that immunoregulation may be one of the major *in vivo* roles of lipid mediators of immediate hypersensitivity reactions.

VI. SUMMARY

Oxygenation of arachidonic acid via the 5- and 15-lipoxygenase pathways yields a variety of products, including monohydroxyeicosatetraenoic acids (HETEs) and more complex products termed leukotrienes. Of these products leukotriene B_4 (LTB_4) is the most potent modulator of PMN function. Nanomolar concentrations of LTB_4 elicit PMN chemotaxis both *in vitro* and *in vivo*, and 3- to 10-fold higher concentrations of LTB_4 promote lysosomal degranulation, PMN leukocyte aggregation, and adherence, in addition to enhancing the expression of neutrophil and eosinphil C3b receptors. The PMN-directed effects of LTB_4 are mediated by binding to a distinct subset of PMN receptors. LTB_4 is bound stereospecifically by 26,000–40,000 receptors per PMN, and the receptors have a K_D of 10.8–13.9 nM. The receptor for LTB_4 may also mediate PMN activation by other 5-lipoxygenase products, as the capacity of these products to activate PMN leukocyte function correlates with their capacity to compete with LTB_4 for binding by the receptor. Several observations suggest that LTB_4 may function both as an extracellular mediator of PMN function and as a critical intracellular intermediate in cellular activation by other agents. These observations include the localization of the LTB_4 receptor in neutrophil granules, the dependence of PMN activation by different stimuli on the lipoxygenation of arachidonic acid, and the capacity of LTB_4 to promote calcium flux in liposomes. Arachidonic acid oxygenation products have complex effects on T-lymphocyte function. LTB_4 enhances T-lymphocyte chemokinesis and inhibits the generation of lymphokines and cellular transformation. LTC_4 inhibits the generation of lymphokines without affecting transformation or chemokinesis. 5-HETE enhances and 15-HETE inhibits chemokinesis, whereas these products have no effects on the other lymphocyte functions. Thus, the lipoxygenase products of arachidonic acid are potent modulators of T-lymphocyte and PMN-function; these products may function both as extracellular mediators and as intracellular intermediates in cellular activation.

VII. REFERENCES

Aehringhaus, V., Wolbling, R. H., Konig, W., Partono, C., Peskar, B. M., and Peskar, B. A., 1982, Release of leukotriene C_4 from human polymorphonuclear leukocytes as determined by radioimmunoassay, *FEBS Lett.* **146**:111.

Ali, M., Gudbranson, C. G., and McDonald, J. W. P., 1980, Inhibition of human platelet cyclooxygenase by alpha-tocopherol, *Prostaglandins Med.* **4**:79.

Bailey, J. M., Bryant, R. W., Low, C. E., Pupillo, M. B., and Vanderhoek, J. Y., 1982, Role of lipoxygenases in regulation of PHA and phorbol ester-induced mitogenesis, in: *Leukotrienes and Other Lipoxygenase Products* (B. Samuelsson and R. Paoletti, eds.), pp. 341–353, Raven Press, New York.

Bhattacherjee, P., Eakins, K. E., and Hammond, B., 1981, Chemotactic activity of arachidonic acid lipoxygenase products in the rabbit eye, *Br. J. Pharmacol.* **73**:254.

Borgeat, P., and Samuelsson, B., 1979*a*, Metabolism of arachidonic acid in polymorphonuclear leukocytes: Structural analysis of novel hydroxylated compounds, *J. Biol. Chem.* **254**:7865.

Borgeat, P., and Samuelsson, B., 1979*b*, Arachidonic acid metabolism in polymorphonuclear leukocytes: Unstable intermediate in formation of dihydroxy acids, *Proc. Natl. Acad. Sci. (USA)* **76**:3213.

Borgeat, P., and Samuelsson, B., 1979*c*, Transformation of arachidonic acid by rabbit polymorphonuclear leukocytes, *J. Biol. Chem.* **254**:2643.

Borgeat, P., Hamberg, M., and Samuelsson, B., 1976, Transformation of arachidonic acid and homo-γ-linolenic acid by rabbit polymorphonuclear leukocytes. Monohydroxy acids from novel lipoxygenases, *J. Biol. Chem.* **251**:7816.

Borgeat, P., Fruteaude Laclos, B., Pickard, S., Vallerand, P., and Sirois, P., 1982, Double dioxygenation of arachidonic acid in leukocytes by lipoxygenases, in: *Leukotrienes and Other Lipoxygenase Products* (B. Samuelsson and R. Paoletti, eds.), pp. 45–51, Raven Press, New York.

Boxer, L. A., Allen, J. M., Schmidt, M., Yoder, M., and Baehner, R. L., 1980, Inhibition of polymorphonuclear leukocyte adherence by prostacyclin, *J. Lab. Clin. Med.* **95**:672.

Carr, S. C., Higgs, G. A., Salmon, J. A., and Spayne, J. A., 1981, The effects of arachidonate lipoxygenase products on leukocyte migration in rabbit skin, *Br. J. Pharmacol.* **73**:253.

Donabedian, H., and Gallin, J. I., 1981, Deactivation of human neutrophil chemotaxis by chemoattractants: Effect on receptors for the chemotactic factor fMet-Leu-Phe, *J. Immunol.* **127**:839.

Ford-Hutchinson, A. W., Bray, M. A., Doig, M. V., Shipley, M. E., and Smith, M. J. H., 1980, Leukotriene B, a potent chemokinetic and aggregating substance released from polymorphonuclear leukocytes, *Nature* **286**:264.

Ford-Hutchinson, A. W., Packham, A., Zamboni, R., Rokach, J., and Roy, S., 1982, Leukotriene B_4 and neutrophil function: A review, *J. R. Soc. Med.* **74**:831.

Goetzl, E. J., 1980, Vitamin E modulates the lipoxygenation of arachidonic acid in leukocytes, *Nature* **288**:183.

Goetzl, E. J., 1981, Selective feed-back inhibition of the 5-lipoxygenation of arachidonic acid in human T-lymphocytes, *Biochem. Biophys. Res. Commun.* **101**:344.

Goetzl, E. J., and Pickett, W. C., 1980, The human PMN leukocyte chemotactic activity of complex hydroxy-eicosatetraenoic acids (HETEs), *J. Immunol.* **125**:1789.

Goetzl, E. J., and Sun, F. F., 1979, Generation of unique mono-hydroxyeicosatetraenoic acids from arachidonic acid by human neutrophils, *J. Exp. Med.* **150**:406.

Goetzl, E. J., and Sun, F. F., 1981, Generation of unique mono-hydroxyeicosatetraenoic acids from arachidonic acid by neutrophils, *J. Exp. Med.* **150**:406.

Goetzl, E. J., Woods, J. M., and Gorman, R. R., 1977, Stimulation of human eosinophil

168   Frank H. Valone

and neutrophil polymorphonuclear leukocyte chemotaxis and random migration by 12-L-hydroxy-5,8,10,14-eicosatetraenoic acid (HETE), *J. Clin. Invest.* **59**:179.

Goetzl, E. J., Valone, F. H., Reinhold, V. N., and Gorman, R. R., 1979a, Specific inhibition of the polymorphonuclear leukocyte chemotactic response to hydroxy-fatty acid by methyl ester derivatives, *J. Clin. Invest.* **63**:1181.

Goetzl, E. J., Weller, P. F., and Valone, F. H., 1979b, Biochemical and functional bases of the regulatory and protective roles of the human eosinophil, in: *Advances in Inflammation Research*, Vol. I (G. Weissman, B. Samuelsson, and R. Paoletti, eds.), pp. 157–167, Raven Press, New York.

Goetzl, E. J., Hill, H. R., and Gorman, R. R., 1980a, Unique aspects of the modulation of human neutrophil function by 12-L-hydroperoxy-5,8,10,14-eicosatetraenoic acid, *Prostaglandins* **19**:71.

Goetzl, E. J., Brash, A. R., Tauber, A. I, Oates, J. A., and Hubbard, W. C., 1980b, Modulation of human neutrophil function by monohydroxyeicosatetraenoic acids, *Immunology* **39**:491.

Goetzl, E. J., Goldman, D. W., and Valone, F. H., 1981, Lipid mediators of leukocyte function in immediate-type hypersensitivity reactions, in: *Biochemistry of the Acute Allergic Reactions, Fourth International Symposium* (E. L. Becker, A. S. Simon, and K. F. Austen, eds.), pp. 169–182, Alan R. Liss, New York.

Goetzl, E. J., Brindley, L. L., and Goldman, D. W., 1983, Enhancement of human neutrophil adherence by synthetic leukotriene constituents of the slow-reacting substance of anaphylaxis, *Immunology* **50**:35.

Goldman, D. W., and Goetzl, E. J., 1982, Specific binding of leukotriene B_4 to receptors on human polymorphonuclear leukocytes, *J. Immunol.* **129**:1600.

Goldman, D. W., and Goetzl, E. J., 1983, Subcellular distribution of human neutrophil receptors for leukotriene B_4, *Fed. Proc.* **42**:894.

Jubiz, W., Radmark, O., Lindgren, J. A., Malmsten, C., and Samuelsson, B., 1981, Novel leukotrienes: Products formed by initial oxygenation of arachidonic acid at C-15, *Biochem. Biophys. Res. Commun.* **99**:976.

Kelly, J. P., and Parker, C. W., 1979, Effects of arachidonic acid and other unsaturated fatty acids on mitogenesis in human lymphocytes, *J. Immunol.* **122**:1556.

Levine, L., Alam, I., Gjika, H., Carty, T. J., and Goetzl, E. J., 1980, The development of a radioimmunoassay for 12-L-hydroxyeicosatetraenoic acid, *Prostaglandins* **20**:923.

Maas, R. L., Brash, A. R., and Oates, J. A., 1981, A second pathway of leukotriene biosynthesis in porcine leukocytes, *Proc. Natl. Acad. Sci. (USA)* **78**:5523.

Maas, R. L., Brash, A. R., and Oates, J. A., 1982, Novel leukotrienes and lipoxygenase products from arachidonic acid, in: *Leukotrienes and Other Lipoxygenase Products* (B. Samuelsson and R. Paoletti, eds.), pp. 29–51, Raven Press, New York.

Murphy, R. C., Hammarstrom, S., and Samuelsson, B., 1979, Leukotriene C: A slow reacting substance from murine mastocytoma cells, *Proc. Natl. Acad. Sci. (USA)* **76**:4275.

Naccache, P. H., Sha'afi, R. I., Borgeat, P., and Goetzl, E. J., 1981, Mono- and di-hydroxyeicosatetraenoic acid alter calcium homeostasis in rabbit neutrophils, *J. Clin. Invest.* **67**:1584.

Nagy, L., Lee, T. H., Goetzl, E. J., Pickett, W. C., and Kay, A. B., 1982, Complement receptor enhancement and chemotaxis of human neutrophils and eosinophils by leukotrienes and other lipoxygenase products, *Clin. Exp. Immunol.* **47**:541.

Obrist, R., Valone, F., Knapp, R. C., and Bast, R. C., 1983, Inhibitors of arachidonic acid oxygenation enhance lymphokine mediated activation of human monocytes, *Proc. Am. Assoc. Can. Res.* **24**:215.

Orning, L., and Hammarstrom, S., 1980, Inhibition of leukotriene C and leukotriene D biosynthesis, *J. Biol. Chem.* **255**:8023.

Palmer, R. M. J., Steprey, R. J., Higgs, G. A., and Eakins, K. E., 1980, Chemotactic acitvity of arachidonic acid lipoxygenase products in leukocytes from different species, *Prostaglandins* 20:411.

Payan, D. G., and Goetzl, E. J., 1981, The dependence of human T-lymphocyte migration on the 5-lipoxygenation of endogenous arachidonic acid, *J. Clin. Immunol.* 1:266.

Payan, D. G., Trentham, D. E., and Goetzl, E. J., 1982, Modulation of human lymphocyte function by C3a and C3a (70–77), *J. Exp. Med.* 156:756.

Payan, D. G., Valone, F. H., and Goetzl, E. J., 1983a, Leukotriene modulation of human T-lymphocyte function, *Fed. Res.* 42:444.

Payan, D. G., Goldman, D. W., and Goetzl, E. J., 1983b, Biochemical and cellular characteristics of the regulation of human leukocyte function by lipoxygenase products of arachidonic acid, in: *The Chemistry and Biology of Leukotrienes and Related Substances* (L. W. Chakrin and D. M. Bailey, eds.), Academic Press, New York.

Pickett, W. C., Goldman, D. W., and Goetzl, E. J., 1983, Characteristics of human leukocyte receptors for leukotrienes, *Life Sci.* (in press).

Radmark, O., Lundberg, U., Jubiz, W., Malmsten, C., and Samuelsson, B., 1982, New group of leukotrienes formed by initial oxygenation at C-15, in: *Leukotrienes and Other Lipoxygenase Products* (B. Samuelsson and R. Paoletti, eds.), pp. 61–70, Raven Press, New York.

Rola-Pleszczynski, M., Borgeat, P., and Sirois, P., 1982, Leukotriene B_4 induces human suppressor lymphocytes, *Biochem. Biophys. Res. Commun.* 108:1531.

Salmon, J. A., Simmons, P. M., Palmer, R. M. J., 1982, Synthesis and metabolism of leukotriene B_4 in human neutrophils measured by specific radioimmunoassay, *FEBS Lett.* 146:18.

Sams, A. R., Sprecher, H., Sankarappa, S. K., and Needleman, P., 1982, Selective inhibitors of platelet arachidonic acid metabolism: Aggregation independent of lipoxygenase, in: *Leukotrienes and Other Lipoxygenase Products* (B. Samuelsson and R. Paoletti, eds.), pp. 19–28, Raven Press, New York.

Samuelsson, B., 1981, Oxidative products of arachidonic acid: Leukotrienes, a new group of compounds, including slow-reacting substance of anaphylaxis, in: *Biochemistry of the Acute Allergic Reaction, Fourth International Symposium* (E. L. Becker, A. S. Simon, and K. F. Austen, eds.), pp. 1–12, Alan R. Liss, New York.

Samuelsson, B., 1982, The Leukotrienes: An introduction, in: *Leukotrienes and Other Lipoxygenase Products* (B. Samuelsson and R. Paoletti, eds.), pp. 1–27, Raven Press, New York.

Scott, W. A., Pawlowski, N. A., Andreach, M., and Cohn, Z. A., 1982a, Resting macrophages produce metabolites from exogenous arachidonic acid, *J. Exp. Med.* 155:535.

Scott, W. A., Pawlowski, N. A., Murray, H. W., Andreach, M., Zrike, J., and Cohn, Z. A., 1982b, Regulation of arachidonic acid metabolism by macrophage activation, *J. Exp. Med.* 155:1148.

Serhan, C. N., Fridovich, J., Goetzl, E. J., Dunham, P. B., and Weissman, G., 1982, LTB_4 and phosphatidic acid are calcium ionophores, *J. Biol. Chem.* 257:4746.

Siegel, M. I., McConnell, R. T., Porter, N. A., and Cuatrecasas, P., 1980a, Arachidonate metabolism via lipoxygenase and 12-L-hydroperoxy-5,8,10,14-icosatetraenoic acid peroxidase sensitive to anti-inflammatory drugs, *Proc. Natl. Acad. Sci. (USA)* 77:308.

Siegel, M. I., McConnell, R. T., Porter, N. A., Selph, J. L., Truax, J. F., Vinegar, R., and Cuatrecasas, P., 1980b, Aspirin-like drugs inhibit arachidonic acid metabolism via lipoxygenase and cyclo-oxygenase in rat neutrophils from carrageenan pleural exudates, *Biochem. Biophys. Res. Commun.* 92:688.

Spagnuolo, P. J., Ellner, J. J., Hassid, A., and Dunn, M. J., 1980, Thromboxane A_2 mediates augmented polymorphonuclear leukocyte adhesiveness, *J. Clin. Invest.* 66:406.

Turk, J., Maas, R. L., Brash, A. R., Roberts, L. J., and Oates, J. A., 1982, Arachidonic acid 15-lipoxygenase products from human eosinophils, *J. Biol. Chem.* **257**:7068.

Valone, F. H., 1982, Polymorphonuclear leukocyte chemotaxis: Lipid chemotactic factors, in: *Immunopharmacology and the Regulation of Leukocyte Function* (D. R. Webb, ed.), pp. 93–104, Marcel Dekker, New York.

Valone, F. H., and Goetzl, E. J., 1983, Specific binding by human polymorphonuclear leukocytes of the immunological mediator 1-*O*-hexadexyl/octadecyl-2-acetyl-*SN*-glycero-3-phosphoryl-choline, *Immunology* **48**:141.

Valone, F. H., Franklin, M., Sun, F. F., and Goetzl, E. J., 1980, Alveolar macrophage lipoxygenase products of arachidonic acid. Isolation and recognition as the predominant constituents of the neutrophil chemotactic activity elaborated by alveolar macrophages, *Cell. Immunol.* **54**:390.

Valone, F. H., Obrist, R., Tarlin, N., and Bast, R. C., 1983, Enhanced arachidonic acid lipoxygenation by K562 cells stimulated with 12-0-tetradecanoylphorbol-13-acetate, *Cancer Res.* **43**:197.

Vanderhoek, J. Y., and Lands, W. E. M., 1973, The inhibition of the fatty acid oxygenase of sheep vesicular gland by antioxidants, *Biochim. Biophys. Acta* **296**:374.

Vanderhoek, J. Y., Bryant, R. W., and Bailey, J. M., 1980a, 15-hydroxy-5,8,11,13-eicosatetraenoic acid. A potent and selective inhibitor of platelet lipoxygenase, *J. Biol. Chem.* **255**:5996.

Vanderhoek, J. Y., Bryant, R. W., and Bailey, J. M., 1980b, Inhibition of leukotriene biosynthesis by the leukocyte product 15-hydroxy-5,8,11,13-eicosatetraenoic acid, *J. Biol. Chem.* **255**:10064.

Walker, J. R., and Dawson, W., 1979, Inhibition of rabbit PMN lipoxygenase activity by benoxaprofen, *J. Pharm. Pharmacol* **31**:778.

Wilhelm, T. E., Sankarappa, S. K., VanRollins, M., and Sprecher, H., 1981, Selective inhibitors of platelet lipoxygenase: 4,7,10,13-icosatetraynoic acid and 5,8,11,14-henicosatetraynoic acid, *Prostaglandins* **21**:323.

Zigmond, S., and Sullivan, S., 1979, Sensory adaptation of leukocytes to chemotactic peptides, *J. Cell. Biol.* **82**:517.

Chapter 6

Structure and Modulation of Fc and Complement Receptors

Jay C. Unkeless and Samuel D. Wright

Department of Cellular Physiology and Immunology
Rockefeller University
New York, New York 10021

I. INTRODUCTION

A striking feature of the professional phagocytes first observed by Metchnikoff (1887) is their ability to bind and ingest foreign particles. In carrying out this vital task, the polymorphonuclear leukocyte (PMN) or macrophage must first recognize the intruder. The mechanism by which cells accomplish this recognition is, for many particles such as Latex or carbon, not well understood, and may not proceed through interaction of the particle with a receptor. On the other hand, many highly dangerous particles, such as bacteria and yeast, are recognized with the aid of opsonins—proteins that bind specifically to the intruder as a signal for phagocytosis (Griffin, 1977). Ingestion of these opsonin-coated particles is triggered by interaction with specific glycoprotein receptors on the cell plasma membrane. This chapter addresses exclusively receptor-mediated phagocytosis.

II. RECEPTOR-MEDIATED PHAGOCYTOSIS

When a macrophage or neutrophil comes in contact with an opsonized particle, receptors in the plasma membrane bind to the opsonins, and a number of intracellular processes are coordinately activated. Most obvious is the elaboration of pseudopods in the general direction of the particle. The pseudopods appear

to result from local changes in the polymerization and crosslinking of actin filaments since a large feltwork of actin forms near the zone of contact with the
particle (Reaven and Axline, 1973) and since pseudopods are not extended in
the presence of cytochalasins (Axline and Reaven, 1974), which are drugs that
inhibit the polymerization of actin. The advancing pseudopod makes very close
contact with the target particle (Wright and Silverstein, 1982a), and this allows
further interaction of receptors with opsonins and further generation of pseudopods. When the target is completely surrounded, opposing pseudopods fuse to
pinch off a sealed phagosome into the cytoplasmic compartment.

The response of the cell to a phagocytic challenge appears to be by nature a
highly localized event, since macrophages can ingest opsonized *Pneumococcus*,
whereas unopsonized red cells attached to adjacent segments of the phagocytosing plasma membrane are not eaten, i.e., bystander particles are not ingested
(Griffin and Silverstein, 1974). Furthermore, when macrophages are presented
with a hemispherically opsonized particle, pseudopods advance around only as
far as the opsonins, and closed phagosomes never result. It thus appears that the
advancing pseudopods must be directed at each step by interaction with new
opsonic ligands. This observation embodies the so-called zipper hypothesis of
phagocytosis (Griffin *et al.*, 1975).

Opsonin–receptor complexes on the phagocyte plasma membrane surface appear to generate an interacellular second message to which the cytoplasm responds; since the phagocytic response is so highly localized, the second message
must also be highly localized in the cytoplasm. The phenomenon of phagocytosis
thus provides an inviting opportunity to examine the mechanisms by which
specific receptors control localized movements of the cytoplasm. The identity
of the second message(s) sent by phagocytosis-promoting receptors is still not
clear, but recent work on the structure of isolated receptor proteins is providing
critical insight into this and other functions of these receptors. Here we review
current knowledge of the structure of the receptors that promote phagocytosis
and consider evidence for possible second messages the receptors send. Our discussion is restricted to receptors for the predominant opsonic ligands of mammals:
IgG and the third component of complement, C3.

III. HETEROGENEITY OF Fc RECEPTORS

The existence of receptors specific for the Fc domain of immunoglobulin,
FcR, was first reported by Berken and Benacerraf (1966), who used the method
of rosette formation with sensitized erythrocyes to demonstrate the receptors on
macrophages. Rosette formation is still an invaluable method for qualitative
analysis of FcR, although for quantitation of the number and avidity of receptors,
the binding of labeled ligands is a more satisfactory method. The analysis of Fc

receptors has been complicated by the existence of a variety of receptors specific for different classes and subclasses of immunoglobulin. Low-avidity receptors for IgE, present on lymphocytes (Gonzalez-Molina and Spiegelberg, 1978; Yodoi and Ishizaka, 1979a,b) and on macrophages (Capron et al., 1975; Anderson and Spiegelberg, 1981), as well as high-avidity IgE Fc receptors on basophils (Metzger, 1978), have been reported. In addition, there are lymphocyte Fc recptors specific for IgA (Gebel et al., 1979), and IgM (Dickler, 1976). Fc receptors specific for IgA have also been described on human neutrophils and monocytes (Fanger et al., 1980).

Many studies have employed competitive inhibition experiments to distinguish between receptors for different subclasses of IgG. In general, when competition experiments using monomeric immunoglobulins are performed, all subclasses of IgG will compete, given a high enough concentration (Segal and Titus, 1978; Haeffner-Cavaillon et al., 1979). However, several groups have found evidence for lack of competition between different IgG subclasses when immune complexes or aggregated IgG subclasses are tested. Results from such experiments indicate that guinea pig macrophages have separate receptors specific for the two subclasses of guinea pig IgG (Leslie and Cohen, 1977), and mouse macrophages have separate Fc receptors for murine IgG2a, IgG1 and IgG2b, and IgG3 (Walker, 1976; Diamond et al., 1978; Diamond and Scharff, 1980; Diamond and Yelton, 1981). These receptors are referred to as $Fc_{\gamma 2a}R$, $Fc_{\gamma 2b/\gamma 1}R$, and $Fc_{\gamma 3}R$, respectively. Similar experiments on rat macrophages provide evidence that rat macrophages have one type of receptor for rat IgG2a, another for both rat IgG1 and IgG2b, and a third receptor specific for IgE (Boltz-Nitulescu et al., 1981).

Other lines of evidence for receptor multiplicity include differential inactivation by proteases and phospholipases. The mouse $Fc_{\gamma 2a}R$, for example, is sensitive to trypsin, while the mouse $Fc_{\gamma 2a/\gamma 1}R$ is trypsin resistant (Unkeless and Eisen, 1975; Anderson and Grey, 1978). Detergent-solubilized mouse $Fc_{\gamma 2a}R$ is inactivated by phospholipase C, whereas the mouse $Fc_{\gamma 2b/\gamma 1}R$ is resistant (Anderson and Grey, 1978). The independence of the IgG2a and IgG2b/IgG1 FcR values can also be demonstrated by capping or modulation experiments, as demonstrated by Michl et al. (1979).

Another independent line of evidence on Fc receptor multiplicity comes from studies with monoclonal anti-Fc receptor antibodies. This approach has the advantage that the antibodies, by definition, react with unique determinants and can be used for analysis of functional sites. The Fab fragment of the rat monoclonal antibody 2.4G2 (Unkeless, 1979; Mellman and Unkeless, 1980) inhibits the binding of IgG2b and IgG1 immune complexes to cells of the J774 mouse macrophage cell line, but has minimal effect on the binding of IgG2a monomer or complexes. This suggests that IgG2b and IgG1 share the same Fc receptor binding site, an obervation confirmed by Diamond and Scharff (1980). In a similar application of monoclonal technology, Fleit et al. (1982) have characterized a mouse monoclonal antibody, 3G8, directed against the huamn Fc receptor for

IgG complexes, and demonstrated that the antibody does not crossreact with blood monocytes or the human cell lines HL-60 or U937. These cell lines and monocytes have high-avidity human IgG1 Fc receptors. Further differences between the neutrophil and monocyte IgG Fc receptors were found by Kurlander and Batker (1982), who found 100- to 1000-fold lower binding avidity of IgG1 dimers and trimers to neutrophils compared with monocytes.

IV. PURIFICATION OF Fc RECEPTORS

Considerable effort has been expended to characterize Fc receptors biochemically; these experiments have proceeded along two lines—the use of affinity chromatography on IgG aggregates or complexes and the use of monoclonal antibodies as affinity reagents. The use of affinity chromatography to purity Fc receptor has been most notably successful for the IgE Fc receptor of mast cells and basophils. This receptor, which has an avidity for IgE on the order of 10^9 M^{-1} (Metzger, 1978), has been purified to homogeneity (Kannellopoulos et al., 1979) and is a glycoprotein of 50,000 M_r that runs with broad mobility on SDS-polyacrylamide gel electrophoresis (PAGE). The 50,000 M_r IgE-binding protein is associated with a 30,000-M_r protein that can be labeled by the photoactivatible lipid-soluble probe (Holowka et al., 1980; Holowka and Metzger, 1982).

Similar use of affinity chromatography to isolate Fc receptors for IgG has not been as successful perhaps because of the lower avidity of IgG Fc receptors for the ligands. When applied to the isolation of labeled plasma membrane proteins, however, affinity chromatography has given useful results. Despite imperfect agreement between different groups on the structure of Fc receptors for IgG, a consensus of sorts is emerging in the published reports on characterization of the proteins. Loube et al. (1978) isolated a 57,000-M_r protein from P388D$_1$ cells, and Loube and Dorrington (1980) later isolated biosynthetically labeled FcR binding material shed into the supernatant medium from the same cells that exibited two peptides of 62,000 and 58,000 M_r. These results are very similar to those of Schneider et al. (1981), who isolated proteins of 50,000–65,000 M_r from P388D$_1$ and J774.2 mouse macrophage cell lines.

Monoclonal anti-Fc receptor antibodies have been used for purification of receptors from both mouse Fc receptor-bearing cells (Mellman and Unkeless, 1980) and human neutrophils (Fleit et al., 1982). Affinity chromatography of nonionic detergent lysates of J774 cells on a 2.4G2 Fab–Sepharose column resulted in a 5000-fold purification of the IgG2b/IgG1-specific Fc receptor, which exhibited two poorly resolved peptides of 47,000 and 60,000 M_r. The purified receptor retained binding activity for IgG complexes and, in the presence of nonionic detergent, bound with specificity to IgG2b and IgG1 complexes (I. S. Mellman and J. C. Unkeless, unpublished results). Lane and Cooper (1982) found that ^{125}I-labeled macrophage surface proteins isolated by affinity chromatography on 2.4G2 were similar to proteins isolated after passage over an IgG2b column. However, labeled protein from an IgG2a column differed slightly in isoelectric point (pI = 3.8–4.7) from the IgG2b or 2.4G2-isolated protein, which had an isoelectric point range of 4.7–5.8. The IgG2b-purified protein had a M_r of 65,000, whereas the IgG2a-purified material consisted of two peptides: 60,000 and 70,000 M_r. There thus appear to be small but consistent differences between the two receptors.

Fc receptors have been purified from the U937 human monocyte cell line by Anderson (1982), who reported the isolation from lysates of iodinated cells of two molecules of M_r 72,000 and 40,000–43,000 by affinity chromatography on IgG-Sepharose columns. The human neutrophil Fc receptor has been purified by affinity chromatography on 3G8 Fab Sepharose and consists of two poorly resolved peptides centered at 53,000 and 66,000 M_r (Fleit et al., 1982). Although there is no crossreactivity between the monoclonal antibodies directed against the human neutrophil and mouse macrophage Fc receptors, the two proteins are strikingly similar upon SDS-PAGE, suggesting that there may be a family of related receptors.

V. MODULATION OF Fc RECEPTOR PHAGOCYTOSIS AND EXPRESSION

Phagocytosis is clearly a complicated event that can be modulated at numerous levels, either at the level of the second signal(s) or at the level of receptor expression. It is apparent that both types of control exist. The number of $Fc_{\gamma 2a}R$ can be increased by treatment of mouse macrophages (Hamburg et al., 1980) or the RAW 309Cr.1 macrophage cell line (Yoshie et al., 1982) with interferon. Hamburg et al. (1980) reported no increase in $Fc_{\gamma 2b/\gamma 1}R$, as measured by 2.4G2 IgG binding, but Yoshie et al. (1982) reported an increase in both receptors upon α or β interferon treatment. Similar results have been obtained by Vogel et al. (1983), who analyzed receptor induction by β-interferon on C3H/HeJ macrophages. Echoing these results, Guyre et al. (1981) found a dramatic increase in FcR on monocytes, HL-60 cells, and U937 cells after treatment with mixed lymphocyte culture (MLC)-conditioned media. The increase in FcR expression on these lines and on monocytes has been shown to be due to the effect of γ-interferon (Guyre et al., 1983). Of great interest is the observation that receptors on lymphocytes can be induced by the ligand to which they are directed, which has been demonstrated for IgE (Yodoi and Ishizaka, 1979) and for IgA (Hoover and Lynch, 1980). Another clear case of induction of FcR is reported by Fleit et al. (1982), who find that the low-avidity neutrophil FcR identified by the monoclonal antibody 3G8 appears on monocytes, which are initially negative, after in vitro culture for 7 days.

It is also apparent that Fc receptors specific for IgG2a and IgG2b/IgG1 are inserted into the membrane and/or cytoskeleton of the cell in different fashion and may be regulated independently as well. Anderson and Grey (1978) reported different association of the IgG2a- and IgG2b-specific FcR values with lipid, as judged by isopyknic centrifugation. The $Fc_{\gamma 2a}R$ is largely inactive with respect to rosette formation at 4°C and is relatively insensitive to cytochalasin B (Diamond et al., 1978). Cyclic nucleotides play a role in receptor modulation of phagocytosis as demonstrated by Muschel et al. (1977), who found that variants of J774 cells defective in phagocytosis of EIgG could be corrected to varying degrees by cyclic adenosine monophosphate (cAMP) analogues. The variant cell lines were not impaired in phagocytosis of Latex, which suggests that the phagocytic defect of the cells was specific to the FcR. Using a novel Trojan horse selection procedure, Diamond and Scharff (1980) isolated variants of J774 cells capable of binding, but not ingesting, IgG2a-opsonized erythrocytes. The adherence and phagocytosis of IgG2b-opsonized erythrocytes was normal.

With the multiplicity of FcR values reported in the literature one's attention naturally focuses on the possible role played by the different receptors in macrophage, neutrophil, and lymphocyte physiology. Walker (1977) reported that IgG2a antibody mediated phagocytosis, whereas IgG2b mediated lysis of chicken erythrocytes by IC-21, a mouse macrophage cell line. However, in studies using monoclonal anti-sheep erythrocyte antibodies, Ralph et al. (1980) report that all classes of mouse IgG mediate phagocytosis and lysis by mouse peritoneal exudate macrophages. It is not necessarily correct to extrapolate from an erythrocyte model to the in vivo activity of immunoglobulin subclasses. Results of Matthews et al. (1981) and Langlois et al. (1981) demonstrate potent capacity of anti-adenocarcinoma 755a serum of the IgG2a subclass to mediate macrophage antibody-dependent cellular cytotoxicity and to protect mice against challenge with the tumor. Further studies are clearly necessary to clarify this area.

Patients with diseases characterized by large numbers of circulating immune complexes often exhibit defects in clearance of IgG-sensitized erythrocytes (Frank et al., 1983). This defect might well be secondary to saturation and subsequent clearance of Fc receptors from the cell surface. The process of internalization and degradation of macrophage Fc receptors has been carefully studied using monoclonal and polyvalent anti-Fc receptor sera (Mellman et al., 1980, 1983). Using a method to label pinosomes with ^{125}I after ingestion of lactoperoxidase, Mellman et al. (1980) were able to demonstrate that, in the absence of ligand, pinocytic vesicles were found to have a collection of proteins representative of those found on the plasma membrane, with the possible exception of a low-M_r protein identified by monoclonal 2.6, which was enriched in the labeled pinosome proteins. However, the fate of Fc receptors internalized after ingestion of IgG-opsonized erythrocyte ghosts was quite different. The Fc receptors internalized after interaction with immune complexes were rapidly and specifically degraded. The normal half-life of receptor turnover was 10 hr; after phagocytosis, the rate of degradation of internalized receptor increased to a half-life of < 2 hr.

The rate of degradation of unrelated antigens was not altered. Furthermore, recovery of normal levels of FcR assayable at the cell surface (measured by binding of monoclonal antibodies) was very slow, probably reflecting the time needed for resynthesis.

VI. MECHANISM OF Fc RECEPTOR SIGNALING

Suzuki *et al.* (1982) have reported the isolation of Fc-receptor specific for IgG2b from P388D$_1$ cells by affinity chromatography over phosphatidyl choline analogue coupled to Sepharose (PC-Sepharose), and of IgG2a-specific Fc receptor by affinity chromatography over heat-aggregated IgG on Sepharose. The isolated Fc$_{\gamma 2b}$R, which constituted about 2% of total cell protein, had a sharp isoelectric point of 5.8, as well as two major peptides, of M_r 40,000 and 80,000. The IgG-binding protein likewise constituted about 2% of total cell protein and had peptides of M_r 50,000 and 25,000. The Fc-binding protein inhibited the binding of IgG2b-coated erythrocytes, whereas the IgG-binding protein inhibited the binding of IgG2a-coated erthrocytes. The protein isolated from the PC-Sepharose column exhibited a Ca^{2+}-dependent phospholipase A$_2$ activity, which was stimulated 4-fold by incubation with aggregated IgG2b. These exciting results are clouded somewhat be uncertainty about the identification of these proteins as Fc receptors, since these proteins alleged to be Fc receptors are major cell proteins with a largely intracellular disposition. Nitta and Suzuki (1982) have demonstrated that the synthesis of cAMP by P388D$_1$ cells in response to binding of erythrocytes coated with IgG2a or IgG2b differs. Indomethacin and p-bromophenacybromide block cAMP synthesis stimulated by EIgG2b, while these drugs stimulate cAMP synthesis by EIgG2a. The relationship of these results to the cAMP stimulation of phagocytosis demonstrated in phagocytosis-deficient variants by Muschel *et al.* (1977) are clearly of interest with regard to cell physiology and cyclase regulation.

Young *et al.* (1983*a*) have used the membrane-permeant cation, tetraphenyl phosphonium ion (TPP$^+$), as a probe of membrane potential and have studied the response of the macrophage cell line J774 to monoclonal antibody against the Fc$_{\gamma 2b/\gamma 1}$R or immune complexes. These workers hypothesize the Fc$_{\gamma 2b/\gamma 1}$R acts as a ligand-dependent channel for monovalent cations, since addition of immune complexes to J774 cells results in a Na$^+$-dependent depolarization, the magnitude and duration of which is dependent on the degree of receptor cross-linking. TPP$^+$ has also been used to study the ion flux in plasma membrane vesicles prepared from J774 cells. When vesicles equilibrated with either Na$^+$ or K$^+$ were diluted into sucrose with [^{3}H]-TPP$^+$ and either immune complexes or 2.4G2 IgG, there was a rapid efflux of cation, reflected by the accumulation of TPP$^+$. Three other monoclonal antibodies directed against major J774 plasma membrane proteins, 1.21J, 2D2C, and 2E2A (Mellman *et al.*, 1980) had little or no effect. In addition, phospholipid vesicles reconstituted with purified Fc$_{\gamma 2b/\gamma 1}$R displayed the same TPP$^+$ uptake in the presence of 2.4G2 IgG as the plasma membrane vesicles, demonstrating that the changes in cation permeability are mediated by the receptor independent of other plasma membrane proteins (Young et al., 1983b). Finally, reconstitution of purified Fc$_{\gamma 2b/\gamma 1}$R into black lipid films resulted in the appearance of ligand-dependent cation specific ion channels with a conductance of 60 ± 5 pS, demonstrating that the receptor functions as an ion channel rather than merely altering permeability (Young et al., 1983c).

VII. RECEPTORS FOR C3 ON PHAGOCYTES

Complement was recognized in 1888 as an agent that could lyse bacteria (Nuttal, 1888), but it was not until 1903 that the opsonic activity of complement was delineated (Wright and Douglas, 1903). Since then it has become clear that opsonization is a vital primary function of complement. Patients with deficiencies of opsonic complement components suffer recurrent pyogenic infections despite normal levels of immunoglobulins, while those with deficiencies of the lytic complement components are usually healthy (Day et al., 1977). Essentially all the opsonic activity of complement resides in the pivotal component, C3. C3 is the most abundant complement protein in serum (1.3 mg/ml), and it can be deposited on target particles by either of two pathways: the "classical pathway," which is activated by prior binding of immune IgG or IgM to the target, or through the alternative pathway, which is antibody independent. Both pathways initiate a remarkable reaction that causes C3 to bind covalently to the target (Law and Levine, 1977). Upon proteolytic activation, an internal thioester bond in C3 is rearranged to yield (1) a free sulfhydryl group on C3 (Tack et al., 1980) and (2) an ester link between C3 and an hydroxyl functionality on the target (Law et al., 1979). The resulting covalently bound molecule is termed C3b.

For many years it was believed that C3b is the principal opsonic form of complement. It has recently been appreciated, however, that this view is oversimplified. Serum contains a highly specific enzyme (C3b inactivator, or simply, I) that cleaves C3b at one or more closely spaced sites on the alpha polypeptide (Law et al., 1979a; Ross et al., 1982). The resulting molecule, termed C3bi (also called C3b'), resists further degradation by serum enzymes; as complement action proceeds, C3bi becomes the predominant species attached to the target. Since phagocytic leukocytes bear separate receptors for C3b and C3bi (see below), one must carefully control the complement enzymes in order to be certain which C3 receptor is being studied. Unfortunately, the methodologies employed by many early investigators yielded a mixture of C3b and C3bi on experimental target particles, and the resulting data are difficult to interpret. We will concentrate here on recent work in which the contributions of the two complement receptors is clearly defined.

Evidence for separate receptors for C3b and C3bi comes from several sources. First, their cellular distribution is different, i.e., primate erythrocytes have receptors for C3b but not for C3bi (Carlo *et al.*, 1979). The receptors are also antigenically different. Antibodies against the C3b receptor do not inhibit the C3bi receptor (Fearon, 1980), and antibodies against the C3bi receptor do not inhibit the C3b receptor (Beller *et al.*, 1982; Wright *et al.*, 1983a,b). Furthermore the two C3 receptors are independently mobile in the plane of the membrane (Wright and Silverstein, 1982b). When human macrophages are permitted to spread on a C3b-coated surface, their C3b receptors disappear from the apical surface, while the C3bi receptors remain in place. Conversely, when macrophages spread on a C3bi-bearing surface, C3bi receptors disappear from the nonattached portion of the macrophage, while C3b receptors remain in place. (The ligand-specific down modulation of receptors results from random lateral diffusion in the plane of the membrane and subsequent binding to ligands on the culture surface (Michl *et al.*, 1983). Finally, the two C3 receptors have different cation dependence: the C3bi receptor requires both Ca and Mg for optimal activity, while the C3b receptor has no requirement for divalent cations (Wright and Silverstein, 1982b).

VIII. STRUCTURE OF THE COMPLEMENT RECEPTORS

Fearon (1980) has characterized the human C3b receptor as a 205,000-M_r membrane glycoprotein. The receptor protein appears identical when isolated from monocytes, polymorphonuclear leukocytes, lymphocytes, or erythrocytes. Interestingly, the C3b receptor can promote not only phagocytosis, but absorptive endocytosis in coated vesicles (Fearon *et al.*, 1981).

The C3bi receptor has been identified on mouse and human macrophages with monoclonal antibodies (Beller *et al.*, 1982; Wright *et al.*, 1983a,b). In both species, the receptor consists of two polypeptide chains: an alpha chain of M_r 180,000, and a beta chain of M_r 100,000. The cellular distribution of the C3bi receptor is essentially identical to that of the C3b receptor, with the exception of the absence of the C3bi receptor from erythrocytes. C3bi receptors are found on all monocytes, macrophages, and polymorphonuclear leukocytes, as well as on a subset of lymphocytes (Springer *et al.*, 1979; Wright *et al.*, 1983a). The C3bi receptor appears to be a member of a family of two-chain leukocyte antigens (Springer *et al.*, 1982; Trowbridge and Omary, 1981; Wright *et al.*, 1983b). In this family, the beta chain appears to be invariant, but the alpha chains are structurally and functionally distinct. The murine antigen, LFA-1, which appears to be involved in T-cell-mediated cytolytic reactions, is a member of this family (Davignon *et al.*, 1981). LFA-1, which is distributed primarily on lymphocytes, has a beta chain indistinguishable from that of the C3bi receptor but an antigenically distinct alpha chain.

IX. MODULATION OF C3 RECEPTOR FUNCTION

Although both Fc and C3 receptors promote phagocytosis, their activities differ in numerous other respects. From a physiological point of view, the most striking difference between C3 and Fc receptors is that while the FcR is constitutively capable of promoting phagocytosis, the phagocytosis-promoting capability of the C3 receptors can be modulated. Macrophages harvested from the peritoneal cavity of healthy mice can bind complement-coated particles but cannot ingest them. In contrast, thioglycollate broth-elicited macrophages can readily bind and ingest complement-coated particles (Bianco et al., 1975). Human macrophages behave in a similar fashion. Resting macrophages bind but do not ingest either C3b- or C3bi-coated particles but, after a brief (< 20-min) stimulation with the tumor promoter, PMA, the macrophages readily eat both C3b- and C3bi-bearing particles (Wright and Silverstein, 1982b). It thus appears that the C3 receptors can exist either as inactive molecules that can bind C3 but cannot generate an intracellular signal for phagocytosis, or as active receptors capable of generating an effective intracellular signal.

J. A. Griffin and Griffin (1979) have discovered that T lymphocytes can elaborate a protein that acts on macrophages to make them capable of phagocytosis via their complement receptors. The action of this factor on macrophages is rapid (within 2 min) and occurs in the absence of protein synthesis. The factor appears to operate by binding to a receptor on the macrophage, which then activates the complement receptors. The factor is secreted or released after incubation of the T cells with macrophages that have ingested immune complexes, presumably at a locale and time at which enhanced phagocytic activity would be beneficial. Additional factors may also control C3 receptor activity. Tuftsin and substance P have been reported to enhance the phagocytic capacity of macrophages (Bar-Shavit et al., 1980), and complement-mediated phagocytosis can also be modulated by the level of intracellular cyclic nucleotides (Lehmeyer and Johnston, 1978; S. D. Wright and S. C. Silverstein, unpublished observations).

The structural basis for the activation of C3 receptors is not yet clear. F. M. Griffin and Mullinax (1981) have described a strong correlation between the activity of murine C3 receptors and the ability of these receptors to diffuse in the plane of the membrane. When macrophages with active C3 receptors settle on a C3-coated surface, the C3 receptors disappear from the apical surface of the macrophages, apparently through simple diffusion in the plane of the membrane and subsequent trapping on the ventral surface. By contrast, macrophages with inactive C3 receptors fail to exhibit downmodulation on a C3-coated surface. When macrophages are activated with the T cell factor, the C3 receptors are mobilized with a time course consistent with the time course of acquisition of phagocytic activity. Thus, inactive C3 receptors appear anchored in the membrane, and mobilization is a prerequisite for their activity. The correlation between receptor mobility and phagocytosis-promoting ability is not maintained, however, by human macrophages. Resting human macrophages have mobile C3 receptors that are not capable of promoting phagocytosis (Wright and Silverstein, 1982b). Thus, receptor mobility may be a necessary condition for activity, but it is not a sufficient condition.

The physiologic usefulness of receptors whose phagocytosis-promoting capacity can be modulated is not altogether clear. Perhaps the inactive state prevents macrophages from damaging host cells adventitiously coated with complement while preserving the destructive potential of the macrophage for ready deployment. It should be noted in this regard that complement receptors that are inactive with respect to the promotion of phagocytosis may yet have other activities. The inactive C3b receptor can function as a cofactor in the enzymic degradation of C3b by I (Iida and Nussenzweig, 1981). Furthermore, inactive C3b receptors markedly enhance the phagocytosis of particles coated with C3b and limited quantities of IgG (Ehlenberger and Nussenzweig, 1977). This amplification of Fc-mediated phagocytosis may represent a primary role for C3 receptors, since the deposition of C3 is often initiated by the prior binding of immune IgG to the target.

X. INTRACELLULAR SIGNALS GENERATED BY C3 AND Fc RECEPTORS

There is no evidence in the literature that suggests the biochemical nature of the second signal generated by C3 receptors. Certain data, however, suggest that the second message employed by C3 receptors is different from that of the Fc receptor. C3- and Fc-mediated phagocytosis are morphologically distinct, both by scanning (Kaplan, 1977) and by transmission electron microscopy (Lawrence et al., 1981; S. D. Wright and S. C. Silverstein, unpublished observations). C3- and Fc-mediated phagocytosis have different sequellae: ligation of Fc receptors leads to the secretion of superoxide and peroxide, but ligation of C3 receptors does not (K. Yamamoto and R. B. Johnston, personal communication; Wright and Silverstein, 1983). Furthermore, antibodies against the Fc receptor of J774 macrophages cause marked depolarization of the cell, while antibodies against the C3bi receptor do not (J.-D. E. Young and J. C. Unkeless, unpublished observations). These data, in concert with the previously mentioned differences in the physiology of the Fc and C3 receptors, suggest that they generate biochemically distinct intracellular second signals. This hypothesis is further supported by the observation that Fc and C3 receptors show marked synergy in the promotion of phagocytosis (Ehlenberger and Nussenzweig, 1977).

The apparently different function of C3 and Fc receptors is in keeping with their different molecular structures. Fc receptors are $\sim M_r$ 50,000, while C3 receptors are M_r 200,000–280,000. It is our hope and belief that current work on isolated receptor proteins will lead to a biochemical understanding of the function of phagocytosis-promoting receptors.

XI. SUMMARY

Recent experiments have revealed the structure of some phagocytosis-promoting receptors. The C3b receptor is a single-chain membrane glycoprotein of M_r 205,000, while the C3bi receptor is composed of two surface glycoprotein chains, of M_r 180,000 and 100,000. Fc receptors all appear to be single-chain glycoproteins of $\sim M_r$ 50,000. Despite this structural similarity, Fc receptors display a broad range of heterogeneity with respect to ligand specificity. One type of Fc receptor ($Fc_{\gamma 2b/\gamma 1}R$) appears to function as a ligand-dependent ion channel; the ion flux initiated by the ligation of this receptor may represent the proximal signal sent by this Fc receptor. The second signal sent by other Fc receptors and by the C3 receptors is uncharacterized, except for the observation that the second signal generated by C3 receptors is distinct from that of $Fc_{\gamma 2b/\gamma 1}R$.

ACKNOWLEDGMENT

This work was supported by grants AI-14603 and CA-30198 from the U.S. Public Health Service. J. C. U. is an American Cancer Society Research Scholar.

XII. REFERENCES

Anderson, C. L., 1982, isolation of the receptor for IgG from a human monocyte cell line (U937) and from human peripheral blood monocytes, *J. Exp. Med.* 156:1794.

Anderson, C. L., and Grey, H. M., 1978, Physicochemical separation of two distinct Fc receptors on murine macrophage-like cell lines, *J. Immunol.* 121:648.

Anderson, C. L., and Spiegelberg, H. L., 1981, Macrophage receptors for IgE: binding of IgE to specific IgE receptors on a human macrophage cell line U 937, *J. Immunol.* 126:2470.

Azline, S. G., and Reaven, E. P., 1974, Inhibition of phagocytosis and plasma membrane mobility of the cultivated macrophage by cytochalasin b. Role of subplasmalemmal microfilaments, *J. Cell Biol.* 62:647.

Bar-Shavit, Z., Goldman, R., Stabinsky, Y., Gottlieb, P., Fridkin, M., Teichberg, V. I., and Blumberg, S., 1980, Enhancement of phagocytosis—a newly found activity of Substance P residing in its N-terminal tetrapeptide sequence, *Biochem. Biophys. Res. Commun.* 94:1445.

Beller, D. I., Springer, T. A., and Schreiber, R. D., 1982, Anti-Mac-1 selectively inhibits the mouse and human type three complement receptor, *J. Exp. Med.* 156:1000.

Berken, A., and Benacerraf, B., 1966, Properties of antibodies cytophilic for macrophages, *J. Exp. Med.* 123:119.

Bianco, C., Griffin, F. M., and Silverstein, S. C., 1975, Studies of the macrophage complement receptor. Alteration of receptor function upon macrophage activation. *J. Exp. Med.* 141:1278.

Boltz-Nitulescu, G., Bazin, H., and Spiegelberg, H. L., 1981, Specificity of Fc receptors for IgG2a, IgG1/IgG2b, and IgE in rat macrophages, *J. Exp. Med.* 154:374.

Capron, A., Dessaint, J.-P., Capron, M., and Bazin, H., 1975, Specific IgE antibodies in immune adherence of normal macrophages to *Schistosoma mansoni* schistosomules, *Nature* 253:747.

Carlo, J. R., Ruddy, S., Studer, E. J., and Conrad, D. H., 1979, Complement receptor binding of C3b-coated cells treated with C3b inactivator, beta 1H globulin and trypsin, *J. Immunol.* 123:523.

Davignon, D., Martz, E., Reynolds, T., Kurzinger, K., and Springer, T. A., 1981, Lymphocyte function-associated antigen 1 (LFA-1): A surface antigen distinct from Lyt-2,3 that participates in T lymphocyte-mediated killing, *Proc. Natl. Acad. Sci. (USA)* 78:4535.

Day, N. K., Moncada, B., and Good, R. A., 1977, Inherited deficiencies of the complement system, in: *Comprehensive Immunology*, Vol. 2: *Biological Amplification Systems in Immunology* (N. K. Day and R. A. Good, eds.), pp. 229–245, Plenum, New York.

Diamond, B., and Scharff, M. D., 1980, IgG1 and IgG2b share the Fc receptor on mouse macrophages, *J. Immunol.* 125:631.

Diamond, B., and Yelton, D. E., 1981, A new Fc receptor on mouse macrophages binding IgG3, *J. Exp. Med.* 153:514.

Diamond, B., Bloom, E. R., and Scharff, M. D., 1978, The Fc receptors of primary and cultured phagocytic cells studied with homogeneous antibodies, *J. Immunol.* 121:1978.

Dickler, H. B., 1976, Lymphocyte receptors for immunoglobulin, *Adv. Immunol.* 24:167.

Ehlenberger, A. G., and Nussenzweig, V., 1977, The role of membrane receptors for C3b and C3d in phagocytosis, *J. Exp. Med.* 145:357.

Fanger, M. W., Shen, L., Pugh, J., and Bernier, G. M., 1980, Subpopulations of human peripheral granulocytes and monocytes express receptors for IgA, *Proc. Natl. Acad. Sci. (USA)* 77:3640.

Fearon, D. T., 1980, Identification of the membrane glycoprotein that is the C3b receptor of the human erythrocyte, polymorphonuclear leukocyte, and monocyte, *J. Exp. Med.* 152:20.

Fearon, D. T., Kaneko, I., and Thomson, G. G., 1981, Membrane distribution and adsorptive endocytosis by C3b receptors on human polymorphonuclear leukocytes, *J. Exp. Med.* 153:1615.

Fleit, H. B., Wright, S. D., and Unkeless, J. C., 1982, Human neutrophil Fc receptor distribution and structure, *Proc. Natl. Acad. Sci. (USA)* 79:3275.

Frank, M. M., moderator, Lawley, T. J., Hamburger, M. I., and Brown, E. J., discussants, 1983, Immunoglobulin G Fc receptor-mediated clearance in autoimmune diseases, *Ann. Intern. Med.* 98:206.

Gebel, H., Hoover, R. G., and Lynch, R. G., 1979, Lymphocyte surface membrane immunoglobulin in myeloma. I. M315-bearing T lymphocytes in mice with MOPC-315, *J. Immunol.* 123:1110.

Gonzalez-Molina, A., and Spiegelberg, H. L., 1978, A subpopulation of normal human periphaeral B lymphocytes that bind IgE, *J. Clin. Invest.* 59:616.

Griffin, F. M., Jr., 1977, Opsonization, in: *Comprehensive Immunology,* Vol. 2: *Biological Amplification Systems in Immunology* (N. K. Day and R. A. Good, eds.), pp. 85–113, Plenum, New York.

Griffin, J. A., and Griffin, F. M., Jr., 1979, Augmentation of macrophage complement receptor function *in vitro*. I. Characterization of the cellular interactions required for the generation of a T-lymphocyte product that enhances macrophage complement receptor function, *J. Exp. Med.* 150:653.

Griffin, F. M., Jr., and Mullinax, P. J., 1981, Augmentation of macrophage complement receptor function *in vitro*. III. C3b receptors that promote phagocytosis migrate within the plane of the macrophage membrane, *J. Exp. Med.* 154:291.

Griffin, F. M., Jr., and Silverstein, S. C., 1974, Segmental response of the macrophage plasma membrane to a phagocytic stimulus, *J. Exp. Med.* 139:323.

Griffin, F. M., Jr., Griffin, J. A., Leider, J. E., and Silverstein, S. C., 1975, Studies on the mechanism of phagocytosis. I. Requirements for circumferential attachment of particle-bound ligands to specific receptors of the macrophage plasma membrane. *J. Exp. Med.* 142:1263.

Guyre, P. M., Crabtree, G. R., Bodwell, J. E., and Munck, A., 1981, MLC-conditioned media stimulate an increase in Fc receptors on human macrophages, *J. Immunol.* 126:666.

Guyre, P. M., Morganelli, P. M., and Miller, R., 1983, Recombinant immune interferon increases IgG Fc receptors on cultured human mononuclear phagocytes, *J. Clin. Invest.* 72:393.

Haeffner-Cavaillon, N., Klein, M., and Dorrington, K. J., 1979, Studies on the Fc gamma receptor of the murine macrophage-like cell line P388D1. I. The binding of homologous and heterologous immunoglobulin G, *J. Immunol.* 123:1905.

Hamburg, S. I., Fleit, H. B., Unkeless, J. C., and Rabinovitch, M., 1980, Mononuclear phagocytes: Responders to and producers of interferon, *Ann. NY Acad. Sci.* 350:72.

Holowka, D., and Metzger, H., 1982, Further characterization of the B-component of the receptor for immunoglobulin E, *Mol. Immunol.* 19:219.

Holowka, D., Hartmann, H., Kanellopoulos, J., and Metzger, H., 1980, Association of the receptor for immunoglobulin E with an endogenous polypeptide in rat basophilic leukemia cells, *J. Recept. Res.* 1:41.

Hoover, R. G., and Lynch, R. G., 1980, Lymphocyte surface membrane immunoglobulin in myeloma II. T cells with IgA-Fc receptors are markedly increased in mice with IgA plasmacytomas, *J. Immunol.* 125:1280.

Iida, K., and Nussenzweig, V., 1981, Complement receptor is an inhibitor of the complement cascade, *J. Exp. Med.* 153:1138.

Kanellopoulos, J., Rossi, G., and Metzger, H., 1979, Preparative isolation of the cell receptor for immunoglobulin E, *J. Biol. Chem.* 254:7691.

Kaplan, G., 1977, Differences in the mode of phagocytosis with Fc and C3 receptors in macrophages, *Scand. J. Immunol.* 6:797.

Kurlander, R. J., and Batker, J., 1982, The binding of human immunoglobulin G1 monomer and small cross-linked polymers of immunoglobulin G1 to human peripheral blood monocytes and polymorphonuclear leukocytes, *J. Clin. Invest.* 69:1.

Langlois, A. J., Matthews, T., Roloson, G. J., Thiel, H.-J., Collins, J. J., and Bolognesi, D. P., 1981, Immunologic control of the ascites form of murine adenocarcinoma 755. V. Antibody-directed macrophages mediate tumor cell destruction, *J. Immunol.* 126:2337.

Lane, B. C., and Cooper, S. M., 1982, Fc receptors of mouse cell lines. I. Distinct proteins mediate the IgG subclass-specific Fc binding activities of macrophages, *J. Immunol.* 128:1819.

Law, S. K., and Levine, R. P., 1977, Interaction between the third complement protein and cell surface macromolecules, *Proc. Natl. Acad. Sci. (USA)* 74:2701.

Law, S. K., Fearon, D. T., and Levine, R. P., 1979a, Action of the C3b-inactivator on cell-bound C3b, *J. Immunol.* 122:759.

Law, S. K., Lichtenberg, N. A., and Levine, R. P., 1979b, Evidence for an ester linkage between the labile binding site of C3b and receptive surfaces, *J. Immunol.* 123:1388.

Lawrence, W. D., Packman, C. H., Rowe, C. H., and Lichtman, M. A., 1981, Attachment of particle-bound IgG and complement to human neutrophils, *Blood* 58:772.

Lehmeyer, J. E., and Johnston, R. B., Jr., 1978, Effect of anti-inflammatory drugs and agents that elevate intracellular cyclic AMP on the release of toxic oxygen metabolites by phagocytes: Studies in a model of tissue-bound IgG, *Clin. Immunol. Immunopathol.* 9:482.

Leslie, R. G. Q., and Cohen, S., 1977, Comparison of the cytophilic activities of guinea pig IgG1 and IgG2 antibodies, *Eur. J. Immunol.* 6:848.

Loube, S. R., and Dorrington, K. J., 1980, Isolation of biosynthetically-labeled Fc-binding proteins from detergent lysates and spent culture fluid of a macrophage-like cell line (P388D$_1$), *J. Immunol.* 125:970.

Loube, S. R., McNabb, T. C., and Dorrington, K. J., 1978, Isolation of an Fc-binding protein from the cell membrane of a macrophage-like cell line (P388D$_1$) after detergent solubilization, *J. Immunol.* 120:709.

Matthews, T. J., Collins, J. J., Roloson, G. J., Thiel, H.-J., and Bolognesi, D. P., 1981, Immunologic control of the ascites form of murine adenocarcinoma 755. IV. Characterization of the protective antibody in hyperimmune serum, *J. Immunol.* 126:2332.

Mellman, I. S., and Unkeless, J. C., 1980, Purification of a functional mouse Fc receptor through the use of a monoclonal antibody, *J. Exp. Med.* 152:580.

Mellman, I. S., Steinman, R. M., Unkeless, J. C., and Cohn, Z. A., 1980, Selective iodination and polypeptide composition of pinocytic vesicles, *J. Cell. Biol.* 86:712.

Mellman, I. S., Plutner, H., Steinman, R. M., Unkeless, J. C., and Cohn, Z. A., 1983, Internalization and degradation of macrophage Fc receptors during receptor-mediated phagocytosis, *J. Cell. Biol.* 96:887.

Metchnikoff, E., 1887, Sur la lutta des cellules de l'organismes centre l'invasion des microbes, *Ann. Inst. Pasteur* 1:321.

Metzger, H., 1978, The IgE–mast cell system as a paradigm for the study of antibody mechanisms, *Immunol. Rev.* 41:186.

Michl, J., Pieczonka, M. M., Unkeless, J. C., and Silverstein, S. C., 1979, Effects of immobilized immune complexes on Fc- and complement-receptor function in resident and thioglycollate-elicited mouse peritoneal macrophages, *J. Exp. Med.* 150:607.

Michl, J., Unkeless, J. C., Pieczonka, M. M., and Silverstein, S. C., 1983, Modulation of Fc receptors of mononuclear phagocytes by immobilized antigen–antibody complexes. Quantitative analysis of the relationship between ligand concentration and Fc receptor response, *J. Exp. Med.* 157:1746.

Muschel, R. J., Rosen, N., and Bloom, B. R., 1977, Isolation of variants in phagocytosis of a macrophage-like continuous cell line, *J. Exp. Med.* 145:175.

Nitta, T., and Suzuki, T., 1982, Biochemical signals transmitted by Fc receptors: Triggering mechanisms of the increased synthesis of adenosine-3′,5′-cyclic monophosphate mediated by Fc$_{\gamma 2a}$ and Fc$_{\gamma 2b}$ receptors of a murine macrophage-like cell line (P388D$_1$), *J. Immunol.* 129:2708.

Nuttal, G., 1888, Experimente uber die bacterienfeindlichen Einflusse des thierischen Korpers, *Z. Hyg. IngektKr.* 4:353.

Ralph, P., Nakoinz, I., Diamond, B., and Yelton, D., 1980, All classes of murine IgG antibody mediate macrophage phagocytosis and lysis of erythrocytes, *J. Immunol.* 125:1885.

Reaven, E. P., and Axline, S. G., 1973, Subplasmalemmal microfilaments and microtubules in resting and phagocytizing cultivated macrophages, *J. Cell Biol.* 59:12.

Ross, G. D., Lambris, J. D., Cain, J. A., and Newman, S. L., 1982, Generation of three different fragments of bound C3 with purified factor I or serum. I. Requirements for Factor H *vs* CR1 cofactor activity, *J. Immunol.* 129:2051.

Schneider, R. J., Atkinson, J. P., Krause, V., and Kulczycki, 1981, Characterization of ligand-binding activity of isolated murine Fc receptor, *J. Immunol.* 126:735.

Segal, D. M., and Titus, J. A., 1978, The subclass specificity for the binding of murine myeloma proteins to macrophage and lymphocyte cell lines and to normal spleen cells, *J. Immunol.* **120:**1395.

Springer, T. A., Galfre, G., Secher, D. S., and Milstein, C., 1979, Mac-1: A macrophage differentiation antigen identified by monoclonal antibody, *Eur. J. Immunol.* **9:**301.

Springer, T. A., Davignon, D., Ho, M.-K., Kurzinger, K., Martz, E., and Sanches-Madrid, F., 1982, LFA-1 and Lyt-2,3, molecules associated with T lymphocyte-mediated killing; and Mac-1, an LFA-1 homologue associated with complement receptor functions, *Immunol. Rev.* **68:**171.

Suzuki, T., Tatsuo, S-T., and Nitta, T., 1982, Biochemical signal transmitted by Fc receptors: Phospholipase A_2 activity of Fc 2b receptor of murine macrophage cell line $P388D_1$, *Proc. Natl. Acad. Sci. (USA)* **79:**591.

Tack, B. F., Harrison, R. A., Janatova, J., Thomas, M. L., and Prahl, J. W., 1980, Evidence for presence of an internal thiolester bond in third component of human complement, *Proc. Natl. Acad. Sci. (USA)* **77:**5764.

Trowbridge, I. S., and Omary, M. B., 1981, Molecular complexity of leukocyte surface glycoproteins related to the macrophage differentiation antigen, Mac-1, *J. Exp. Med.* **154:**1517.

Unkeless, J. C., 1979, Characterization of a monoclonal antibody directed against the mouse macrophage and lymphocyte Fc receptor, *J. Exp. Med.* **150:**580.

Unkeless, J. C., and Eisen, H. N., 1975, Binding of monomeric immunoglobulins to Fc receptors of mouse macrophages, *J. Exp. Med.* **142:**1520.

Vogel, S. N., Finbloom, D. S., English, D. L., Rosenstreich, D. L., and Langreth, S. G., 1983, Interferon-induced enhancement of macrophage Fc receptor expression: B interferon treatment of C3H/HeJ macrophages results in increased numbers and density of Fc receptors, *J. Immunol.* **130:**1210.

Walker, W. S., 1976, Separate Fc receptors for Immunoglobulins IgG2a and IgG2b on an established cell line of mouse macrophages, *J. Immunol.* **116:**911.

Walker, W. S., 1977, Mediation of macrophage cytolytic and phagocytic activities by antibodies of different classes and class-specific Fc receptors, *J. Immunol.* **119:**367.

Wright, A. E., and Douglas, S. R., 1903, An experimental investigation of the role of the body fluids in connection with phagocytosis, *Proc. R. Soc. (Lond)* **72:**357.

Wright, S. D., and Silverstein, S. C., 1982a, Phagocytosiing macrophages exclude soluble macromolecules from the zone of contact with ligand-coated targets, *J. Cell Biol.* **95:** 433a.

Wright, S. D., and Silverstein, S. C., 1982b, Tumor-promoting phorbol esters stimulate C3b and C3b' receptor-mediated phagocytosis in cultured human monocytes, *J. Exp. Med.* **156:**1149.

Wright, S. D., and Silverstein, S. C., 1983, Receptors for C3b and C3bi promote phagocytosis but not the release of toxic oxygen from human phagocytes, *J. Exp. Med.* **158:** 2016.

Wright, S. D., Van Voorhis, W. C., and Silverstein, S. C., 1983a, Identification of the C3b' receptor on human leukocytes using a monoclonal antibody, *Fed. Proc.* **42:**1079.

Wright, S. D., Rao, P. E., Van Voorhis, W. C., Iida, K., Craigmyle, L. S., Goldstein, G., and Silverstein, S. C., 1983b, Identification of the C3bi receptor of human monocytes and macrophages with monoclonal antibodies, *Proc. Natl. Acad. Sci. (USA)* **80:**5099.

Yodoi, J., and Ishizaka, K., 1979a, Lymphocytes bearing Fc receptors for IgE. I. Presence of human and rat T lymphocytes with Fc_e receptors, *J. Immunol.* **122:**2577.

Yodoi, J., and Ishizaka, K., 1979b, Lymphocytes bearing receptors for IgE. III. Transition of Fc R (+) cells to Fc_eR (+) cells by IgE, *J. Immunol.* **123:**2004.

Yoshie, O., Mellman, I., Broeze, R. J., Garcia-Blanco, M., and Lengyel, P., 1982, Interferon action: Effect of of mouse a and B interferons on rosette formation, phagocytosis, and surface antigen expression of cell of the macrophage type cell line RAW 309 Cr. 1, *Cell. Immunol.* **73**:128.

Young, J. D.-E., Unkeless, J. C., Kaback, H. R., and Cohn, Z. A., 1983a, Macrophage membrane potential changes associated with 2b/1 Fc receptor-ligand binding, *Proc. Natl. Acad. Sci. (USA)* **80**:1357.

Young, J. D.-E., Unkeless, J. C., Kaback, H. R., and Cohn, Z. A., 1983b, Mouse macrophage Fc receptor for IgG 2b/1 in artificial and plasma membrane vesicles functions as a ligand-dependent ionophore, *Proc. Natl. Acad. Sci. (USA)* **80**:1636.

Young, J. D.-E., Unkeless, J. C., Young, T. M., Mauro, A., and Cohn, Z. A., 1983c, Role for mouse macrophage IgG Fc receptor as ligand-dependent ion channel, *Nature* **306**:186.

Chapter 7

Neutrophil Degranulation

Ira M. Goldstein

Rosalind Russell Arthritis Research Laboratory
Medical Service
San Francisco General Hospital
Department of Medicine
University of California
San Francisco, California 94110

I. INTRODUCTION

Metchnikoff (1883) is credited with formulating the concept that acute inflammation in virtually all multicellular organisms occurs largely as a consequence of a coordinated series of events whereby phagocytic cells attempt to defend the host against foreign invaders. This concept and Metchnikoff's remarkable insight are illustrated by the following quotation (Metchnikoff, 1905):

> But it is not micro-organisms only which set up this inflammatory reaction accompanied by the emigration and accumulation of leucocytes. The introduction of inert bodies and of aseptic fluids brings about the same result. The phagocytes are, as a matter of fact, endowed with a special susceptibility, which enables them to perceive exceedingly small changes in the chemical or physical composition of the medium that surrounds them.
>
> The leucocytes, having arrived at the spot where the intruders are found, seize them after the manner of the *Amoebae* and within their bodies subject them to intracellular digestion. This digestion takes place in the vacuoles in which usually is a weakly acid fluid which contains digestive ferments; of these a very considerable number are now recognised.

In man, as in most higher organisms, it is the polymorphonuclear leukocyte (or neutrophil) that is primarily responsible for seeking out and destroying most foreign invaders. Central to the roles played by neutrophils in maintaining normal host defenses and in mediating inflammatory reactions are the substances, i.e., the "cytases" referred to above, sequestered within their cytoplasmic granules, or lysosomes. The nature of these substances, the mechanisms by which they are released from lysosomes, and factors that regulate their release are the subjects of this review.

II. THE LYSOSOMAL SYSTEM OF NEUTROPHILS

Originally described in rat liver (de Duve *et al.*, 1955), lysosomes are a class of subcellular organelles that contain various hydrolytic enzymes, predominantly with acid pH optima, bound in latent form within a relatively impermeable membrane. The isolation and characterization of lysosomal granules from rabbit (Cohn and Hirsch, 1960*a*) and human (Hirschhorn and Weissmann, 1965) neutrophils opened an era of intensive research during which the origin, composition, and function of these organelles were elucidated.

A. Origin and Content of Neutrophil Lysosomal Granules

Bainton *et al.* (1971) were among the first to examine human neutrophils and their precursors in blood and bone marrow by histochemical staining and by electron microscopy. On the basis of morphology and staining characteristics, these investigators identified two major types of neutrophil cytoplasmic granules: azurophils and specifics. Azurophil granules, containing peroxidase and other lysosomal hydrolases, appeared in the cytoplasm during the promyelocyte stage of development and were observed to arise from the concave surface of the Golgi complex. Specific granules, on the other hand, were formed from the convex face of the Golgi complex during the myelocyte stage of maturation and contained predominantly alkaline phosphatase and basic proteins. These observations were analogous to those made previously in studies of rabbit neutrophils by Bainton and Farquhar (1966, 1968*a,b*) and supported the findings of Olsson (1969), who separated human neutrophil granules on density gradients into two major subfractions: a dense granule fraction containing acid phosphatase, β-galactosidase, and β-glucuronidase (i.e., acid hydrolases) and a heterogeneous lighter granule fraction containing all of the alkaline phosphatase.

Other investigators have reported even greater heterogeneity than that described above among granules isolated from human and rabbit neutrophils. Welsh and Spitznagel (1971), for example, found at least three, or possibly four, types of lysosomes in subcellular fractions prepared by differential centrifugation of human neutrophil homogenates. In a subsequent study, Spitznagel *et al.* (1974) used velocity centrifugation to resolve homogenates of highly purified human neutrophils into three well-separated bands. Specific granules made up predominantly of lysozyme and lactoferrin as well as azurophil granules containing acid hydrolases, constituted bands II and III, respectively. Band I consisted primarily of "empty" vesicles, but nevertheless contained 85% of biochemically measurable alkaline phosphatase. It is clear now that alkaline phosphatase in human neutrophils is not a granule-associated enzyme, but is associated only with the plasma membrane (Bretz and Baggiolini, 1974; West et al., 1974; Dewald et al., 1982). In rabbit neutrophils, however, 90% of total cellular alkaline phosphatase sediments with specific granules (Baggiolini et al., 1969; Zeya and Spitznagel, 1971).

Zonal sedimentation, velocity sedimentation, and isopyknic equilibration techniques have enabled investigators to localize more precisely most of the granule-associated enzymes of human neutrophils. It has been established, for example, that azurophil granules contain all the myeloperoxidase and β-glucuronidase found in human neutorphils (Bretz and Baggiolini, 1974; West et al., 1974; Dewald et al., 1982). Azurophil granules also contain all the elastase and cathepsin G (Folds et al., 1972), the bulk of other acid glycosidases (Dewald et al., 1982), and approximately 50% of the lysozyme in these cells (Leffell and Spitznagel, 1972; West et al., 1974). Specific granules, on the other hand, contain all the lactoferrin in human neutrophils and the remainder of their lysozyme (Leffell and Spitznagel, 1972; West et al., 1974). Specific granules also contain latent collagenase (Murphy et al., 1980) and vitamin B_{12}-binding protein (Kane and Peters, 1975). Less well-defined human neutrophil granules contain N-acetyl-β-glucosaminidase and a latent, neutral gelatinase (Bretz and Baggiolini, 1974; Dewald et al., 1982). Thus human neutrophils contain granule-associated enzymes capable of hydrolyzing a wide variety of both natural and synthetic substrates, including simple and complex polysaccharides, oligopeptides, polypeptides, and phosphate esters. The roles played by these enzymes in maintaining normal host defense and in mediating inflammation have been the subject of several reviews (Goldstein, 1973, 1976; Babior, 1978; Weissmann et al., 1980; Weissmann, 1982).

B. Functions of Neutrophil Lysosomal Granules

Lysosomes constitute the vacuolar system, or internal digestive system, of phagocytic cells. Lysosomes that have not participated in acts of digestion (i.e., membrane-bound structures containing newly synthesized acid hydrolases) have been termed primary lysosomes or storage granules (Novikoff et al., 1964). When foreign material enters a cell as a consequence of either phagocytosis, endocytosis, or pinocytosis, it is engulfed within a vacuole formed from an invagination of the cell membrane. This vacuole, laden with potential substrate, has been referred to as a phagosome (Straus, 1964). Shortly after this structure is formed, lysosomal hydrolases are introduced by merger, i.e., by membrane fusion, of the phagosome with a primary lysosome (Cohn and Hirsch, 1960b).

The resultant structure has been called a phagolysosome (Straus, 1964), phagocytic vacuole (Cohn and Fedorko, 1969), or digestive vacuole (de Duve and Wattiaux, 1966). Phagolysosomes therefore contain not only acid hydrolases, but substrate as well. In phagocytic cells that encounter and engulf microorganisms, formation of phagolysosomes is crucial to normal host defense (Densen and Mandell, 1978). For example, when microorganisms are engulfed by neutrophils, the cells degranulate, i.e., cytoplasmic granules fuse with, and discharge their contents into, newly formed phagosomes. It is within the phagolysosomes formed by this process that killing and digestion take place (Hirsch and Cohn, 1960; Cohn and Hirsch, 1960b; Zucker-Franklin and Hirsch, 1964). Stossel *et al.* (1971) isolated phagolysosomes from human and guinea pig neutrophils and confirmed biochemically that degranulation occurs coincidentally with ingestion. On the basis of the kinetics of particle uptake and translocation of granule constituents into phagolysosomes, these investigators concluded that the triggering mechanisms for both phagocytosis and degranulation may be similar or identical.

Degranulation of neutrophils is not a uniform process. Azurophil and specific granules discharge their contents at different rates during phagocytosis (Stossel *et al.,* 1971; Leffell and Spitznagel, 1974). Bainton (1973) found that specific granules of rabbit neutrophils fuse with phagosomes and discharge their contents more rapidly than do azurophil granules. In addition, although azurophil and specific granules discharge their contents during phagocytosis, specific granule constituents appear to be more accessible for extracellular release (Leffell and Spitznagel, 1974, 1975; Bentwood and Henson, 1980). Finally, based on the responses of neutrophils to mechanical and other nonphagocytic stimuli, it has been suggested that specific granules actually may be secretory granules and that their contents function extracellularly rather than intracellularly (Leffell and Spitznagel, 1975; Wright *et al.,* 1977; Wright and Gallin, 1979). The precise mechanism whereby specific granules fuse so readily with portions of the neutrophil plasma membrane has not been elucidated. Nevertheless, it has been found that azurophil and specific granules differ not only with respect to their contents, but in other respects as well. Nachman *et al.* (1972), for example, observed that membranes prepared from rabbit azurophil and specific granules had similar ultrastructural appearances, but differed with respect to their content of cholesterol, phospholipid, and protein.

III. EXTRACELLULAR RELEASE OF NEUTROPHIL GRANULE CONSTITUENTS

Whereas the contents of neutrophil granules are most often discharged intracellularly into phagosomes, under certain circumstances they can be released extracellularly. Four major mechanisms have been described whereby granule constituents are extruded from neutrophils.

A. Cell Death

One mechanism whereby granule constituents are extruded from neutrophils is simply cell death. When neutrophils are exposed to a variety of toxins, injury to the plasma membrane is an early consequence, and ultimately, all intracellular materials are released from the injured cells, including those ordinarily sequestered within azurophil and specific granules. Biologic detergents, for example, such as the amphipath mellitin, act in this manner to induce primary lysis of cell membranes and, only subsequently, disruption of cytoplasmic granules (Weissmann *et al.*, 1969). Under these circumstances, cytoplasmic enzymes and other cellular constituents, in addition to lysosomal hydrolases, are released into the medium surrounding dead and dying neutrophils.

B. Perforation from Within

Another mechanism by which lysosomal constituents can be released from neutrophils conforms to the suicide sac hypothesis proposed by de Duve and Wattiaux (1966). Under some circumstances, materials gain access to the interior of the cells' vacuolar system wherein they cause membranes of lysosomes to rupture. Such damage to lysosomal membranes subsequently leads to release from neutrophils of cytoplasmic enzymes and other intracellular constituents as the cells die as a consequence of perforation from within of their vacuolar system (Weissmann *et al.*, 1971a, 1972). Crystalline substances, such as monosodium urate and silica, act on neutrophils—and other phagocytic cells—in this fashion (Weissmann *et al.*, 1971a; Weissmann and Rita, 1972; Schumacher and Phelps, 1971; Allison *et al.*, 1968).

C. Regurgitation During Feeding

After the demonstration by Cohn and Hirsch (1960b) that neutrophil granule contents are discharged into phagosomes, it was suggested that intense endocytosis might lead to release of acid hydrolases from newly formed phagolysosomes (Weissmann and Uhr, 1968). Several studies subsequently demonstrated that a portion of the contents of neutrophil lysosomes is discharged into the medium surrounding intact, viable cells engaging in phagocytosis. This release is not accompanied by leakage of cytoplasmic enzymes and appears to be attributable to the extrusion of lysosomal granule contents from incompletely sealed phagosomes, open at their external borders to the extracellular space but already joined at their internal borders by lysosomal granules actively discharging their contents. The cell engaging in phagocytosis remains viable, but its released lysosomal enzymes are free to act extracellularly. This is probably a common mechanism whereby neutrophils provoke tissue injury in a variety of disease states (Goldstein, 1976; Weissmann, 1982). Biochemical and morphologic evidence for this mechanism, termed regurgitation during feeding by Weissmann *et al.* (1971*a*, 1972), has been presented for several experimental systems involving particle ingestion by neutrophils (Hawkins, 1972; Henson, 1971*a*, 1972; Henson *et al.*, 1972; Henson and Oades, 1975; Weissmann *et al.*, 1971*a*, 1972; Wright and Malawista, 1972; Zurier *et al.*, 1973*a*).

Phagocytosis per se is not an absolute prerequisite for degranulation by neutrophils. In fact, a substantial amount of evidence has been accumulated indicating that degranulation of neutrophils can be provoked not only by appropriate ligand–surface membrane receptor interactions, but also by nonspecific membrane perturbation. Degranulation of neutrophils under these circumstances appears to occur by reverse endocytosis.

D. Reverse Endocytosis

When neutrophils encounter either immune complexes or aggregated immunoglobulins deposited on solid surfaces, such as Micropore filters (Henson, 1971*a,b*; Henson *et al.*, 1972; Henson and Oades, 1975; Johnston and Lehmeyer, 1976; Weissmann *et al.*, 1972; Zurier *et al.*, 1973*a*) and collagen membranes (Hawkins, 1971, 1972), the cells adhere to these surfaces and selectively release a portion of their granule contents. A similar phenomenon occurs when adherent cells encounter some soluble stimuli, such as the complement component, C5a (Becker *et al.*, 1974). Under these conditions, lysosomal enzyme release occurs by a process of reverse endocytosis (Weissmann *et al.*, 1972) or frustrated phagocytosis (Henson, 1971*b*), during which merger of granules with the plasma membrane results in discharge of granule constituents directly to the outside of cells as though into phagosomes. Phagocytosis per se does not occur, and the viability of adherent cells is not altered. The process is basically one in which material previously stored within lysosomal granules is exported to the external milieu as a consequence of cell surface membrane stimulation. This mechanism of granule constituent release from neutrophils very likely is relevant to the pathogenesis of tissue injury in a variety of diseases in which immune complexes are deposited on cell surfaces or extracellular structures, such as vascular basement membranes and articular cartilage (Goldstein, 1976; Weissmann, 1982).

1. Cytochalasin B-Treated Neutrophils

Lysosomal enzyme release from neutrophils by the mechanism of reverse endocytosis is facilitated greatly when cells are treated with the fungal metabolite, cytochalasin B. Cytochalasin B interferes with the function of cytoplasmic microfilaments and inhibits membrane transport of sugars and nucleosides in cultured cells (Carter, 1967; Hartwig and Stossel, 1976; Plagemann and Estensen, 1972; Zigmond and Hirsch, 1972). Cytochalasin B-treated neutrophils are unable to ingest particles, but nevertheless release or secrete lysosomal but not cyto-plasmic constituents (i.e., degranulate) when appropriate particles or soluble stimuli come into contact with their surfaces (Becker *et al.*, 1974; Becker, 1976; Davis *et al.*, 1971; Goldstein *et al.*, 1973*a,b*, 1975*a;* Hawkins, 1973; Zigmond and Hirsch, 1972; Zurier *et al.*, 1973*a,b*, 1974). With some soluble stimuli (e.g., complement-derived and synthetic peptide chemotactic factors), treatment of neutrophils with cytochalasin B is an absolute prerequisite for maximal degranu-lation (Goldstein *et al.*, 1973*a,b;* Becker, 1976; Showell *et al.*, 1976). Ultrastruc-tural studies of cytochalasin B-treated neutrophils have revealed membrane fusion between lysosomal granules and the plasma membrane as the morpholog-ical accompaniment of biochemically measurable enzyme release (Zurier *et al.*, 1973*b;* Goldstein *et al.*, 1973*b*). Cytochalasin B therefore converts neutrophils from phagocytic cells into model secretory cells, making it possible to monitor extracellularly (after fusion of lysosomes with plasma membranes) those pro-cesses that ordinarily occur intracellularly, (i.e., fusion of lysosomes with phago-somes.) The precise mechanism whereby cytochalasin B facilitates fusion between lysosomal membranes and the plasma membranes of stimulated neutrophils leading to the discharge of granule contents is unknown.

2. Degranulation of Neutrophils in Response to Soluble Stimuli

As indicated above, cytochalasin B-treated neutrophils degranulate when exposed to the soluble, low-molecular-weight complement component, C5a (Goldstein *et al.*, 1973*a,b;* Becker *et al.*, 1974). Such cells respond similarly to other chemotactic factors, e.g., products of bacteria, synthetic peptides, and oxygenation products of arachidonic acid (Becker *et al.*, 1974; Becker, 1976; Showell *et al.*, 1976; Stenson and Parker, 1980; O'Flaherty *et al.*, 1981). Yet other soluble stimuli are capable of provoking degranulation of normal neu-trophils: (1) the tumor-promoting agent, phorbol myristate acetate (PMA) (specific granules only) (Estensen *et al.*, 1974; Goldstein *et al.*, 1975*b*); (2) calcium ions with or without the ionophore A23187 (azurophil and/or specific granules) (Goldstein *et al.*, 1974, 1975*c;* Zabucchi and Romeo, 1976); and (3) the cell surface-reactive lectin concanavalin A (Con A) (specific granules only) (Hoffstein *et al.*, 1976; Goldstein *et al.*, 1977*a;* Romeo *et al.*, 1973). De-granulation of neutrophils in response to these soluble stimuli occurs in the absence of cytochalasin B, particles, or adherence to surfaces, and is not associ-ated with any alterations of cell viability. The mechanism by which specific granule constituents (e.g., lysozyme) are selectively released from neutrophils exposed to PMA, calcium, and Con A is unknown. Some data, however, sug-gest that the limiting membranes of specific granules have unique physical and/or chemical properties that facilitate fusion with the neutrophil plasma membrane (Nachman *et al.*, 1972; Avila and Convit, 1973).

IV. RELATIONSHIP BETWEEN DEGRANULATION AND OTHER RESPONSES OF NEUTROPHILS TO STIMULATION

A. Enhanced Oxidative Metabolism

Marked changes in oxidative metabolism ordinarily accompany ingestion by neutrophils of a variety of particles (Karnovsky, 1968; DeChatelet, 1975, 1978; Babior, 1978). The cells consume increased amounts of oxygen, by a mechanism that is insensitive to cyanide, to produce hydrogen peroxide (Root et al., 1975) and several highly reactive unstable intermediates, such as superoxide anion radicals (Babior et al., 1973; Curnutte and Babior, 1974; Goldstein et al., 1975a; Weening et al., 1975), hydroxyl radicals (Tauber and Babior, 1977), and probably singlet oxygen (Krinsky, 1974). Concomitantly, there is stimulation of the hexose monophosphate shunt pathway of glucose oxidation and iodination of protein mediated by the granule enzyme, myeloperoxidase (Klebanoff, 1967; Root and Stossel, 1974). The importance of these metabolic events in relationship to microbial killing by neutrophils has been reviewed extensively (DeChatelet, 1975, 1978; Babior, 1978).

As is the case with degranulation, there is considerable evidence that these metabolic events can be stimulated in the absence of phagocytosis. For example, normal human neutrophils adherent to nonphagocytosable surfaces increase their oxidative metabolism, particularly if the surfaces are coated with immune reactants such as aggregated IgG (Henson and Oades, 1975; Johnston and Lehmeyer, 1976) or the opsonic fragment of the third component of complement (C3b) (Tedesco et al., 1975; Goldstein et al., 1976a). Similarly, neutrophils rendered incapable of ingesting particles by treatment with cytochalasin B exhibit enhanced oxidative metabolism when exposed to appropriate stimuli (Curnutte and Babior, 1975; Goldstein et al., 1975a, 1977a; Roos et al., 1976; Root and Metcalf, 1977). Finally, neutrophils exposed to certain soluble stimuli, in the absence of cytochalasin B or adherence to surfaces, increase their oxygen uptake, production of superoxide anion, and hexose monophosphate shunt activity. These soluble stimuli include immune reactants, such as aggregated IgG (Henson and Oades, 1975) and chemotactic peptides (Goetzl and Austen, 1974; Goldstein et al., 1975a,d), as well as a variety of nonimmune, surface-reactive compounds such as phospholipase c (Kaplan et al., 1972), PMA (Goldstein et al., 1975a; DeChatelet et al., 1976; Repine et al., 1974), Con A (Romeo et al., 1973; Goldstein et al., 1977a), and digitonin (Cohen and Chovaniec, 1978). The metabolic responses of neutrophils to these soluble stimuli require intact viable cells and closely resemble those observed during phagocytosis.

Cell-surface stimulation of neutrophils in the absence of phagocytosis is therefore sufficient to provoke degranulation and the burst of oxidative metabolism that ordinarily accompany ingestion of particles. What is the relationship between these two responses of neutrophils to stimulation? Whereas it is true that when normal neutrophils are allowed to ingest particles the two responses appear to be inseparable, studies with nonphagocytic stimuli indicate that they can occur independently. For example, it has been demonstrated (Goldstein *et al.*, 1975*a*) that there is no significant correlation between the ability of various stimuli to provoke lysosomal enzyme release from neutrophils (i.e., degranulation) and their ability to enhance generation of superoxide anion radicals. This finding suggests (1) that these two phenomena are mediated by independent membrane signals, (2) that fusion of granule membranes with plasma or phagosomal membranes is not a prerequisite for superoxide generation, and (3) that release of superoxide is not coincidentally linked to extrusion of lysosomal constituents.

Additional evidence that neutrophil functions are determined by cell surface recognition of, and stimulation by, specific ligands has been provided by studies of the independent effects on these cells of IgG and complement (C3b). For example, several investigators have demonstrated that the neutrophil C3b receptor is primarily involved in recognition and attachment and that it only inefficiently promotes ingestion of bound or adherent particles. In contrast, particle binding through the neutrophil IgG receptor, although less efficient, appears to be necessary for the induction of optimal phagocytosis (Mantovani, 1975; Scribner and Fahrney, 1976; Ehlenberger and Nussenzweig, 1977). In order to determine the influence of these specific ligand–surface membrane interactions on other neutrophil functions, nonphagocytosable particles, i.e., serum-treated Sepharose beads, coated with fragments of C3 and/or IgG were used to investigate whether these provide a sufficient stimulus for the metabolic changes and degranulation that ordinarily accompany phagocytosis (Tedesco *et al.*, 1975; Goldstein *et al.*, 1976*a*). It was demonstrated that normal human neutrophils recognize and adhere to Sepharose beads coated with fragments of C3 and that they consequently increase their oxidative metabolism, measured as superoxide anion generation. This neutrophil response occurred in the absence of IgG but could be amplified if this immunoglobulin was also present on the bead surfaces. In contrast to metabolic stimulation, degranulation, i.e., selective extracellular release of lysosomal constitutents, was observed only when neutrophils encountered both C3 fragments and IgG on the beads. These results indicate further that cell-surface stimulation of human neutrophils is not an all-or-none phenomenon and that certain vital functions of these cells, namely degranulation and increased oxidative metabolism, may be mediated or modulated independently.

B. Changes in Membrane Fluidity and Apparent Membrane Potential

The phenomenon of stimulus–response coupling in neutrophils is throught to involve a complex series of events that occur on and within the plasma membrane. Several investigators have provided evidence of conformational changes in the plasma membranes of neutrophils after stimulation (Berlin and Fera, 1977; Ingraham et al., 1981; Romeo et al., 1970). Berlin and Fera (1977), for example, demonstrated a reorganization of neutrophil membrane lipids that occurred as a consequence of phagocytosis. Using fluorescence depolarization techniques, these workers were able to demonstrate a marked decrease in rabbit neutrophil plasma membrane microviscosity that paralleled the extent of phagocytosis of either polystyrene Latex beads or paraffin oil droplets. Similar changes in microviscosity were demonstrated in liposomes prepared from extracts of membrane lipids, suggesting that the alterations of microviscosity were due, in part, to changes in lipid composition. Additional evidence that phagocytosis provokes alterations in the microviscosity (or fluidity) of neutrophil plasma membranes has been provided by studies using electron spin resonance (ESR) spectroscopy. Ingraham et al. (1981) used this technique to demonstrate that human neutrophil plasma membrane fluidity is increased when cells are exposed to opsonized zymosan particles. Interestingly, neutrophils from patients with chronic granulomatous disease failed to exhibit phagocytosis-induced changes in membrane fluidity. These cells are unable to generate superoxide radicals but appear to degranulate normally when appropriately stimulated (Baehner et al., 1969). Consequently it cannot be concluded that changes in membrane fluidity are an absolute prerequisite for degranulation. Indeed, Haak et al. (1979) found that neutrophils from patients with the Chediak–Higashi syndrome, which do not degranulate normally (Gallin et al., 1974), possess membranes that are more fluid than those of controls.

In addition to altered fluidity, plasma membranes of stimulated neutrophils exhibit other changes. Gallin et al. (1975), for example, demonstrated that the negative surface charge of human neutrophils is diminished after incubation with chemotactic factors, but not after incubation with other nonchemotactic proteins. This phenomenon could not be attributed simply to masking of negatively charged membrane sites, but appeared to be attributable to effects of chemoattractants on membrane transport of cations. There is ample evidence that changes in calcium, sodium, and potassium ion fluxes accompany neutrophil stimulation (see Section V.A). There also is evidence that these changes in ion fluxes are associated with apparent changes in neutrophil membrane potential.

After the studies by Gallin and Gallin (1977), which directly demonstrated membrane potential changes in human macrophages exposed to chemotactic stimuli, several investigators have documented that similar changes occur in human neutrophils. Since neutrophils are too small for direct intracellular measurements of membrane potential by means of microelectrodes, a number of indirect methods were used in these studies. In experiments using one indirect probe, i.e., radiolabeled triphenylmethylphosphonium ion, Korchak and Weissmann (1978) found that changes in the apparent membrane potential of human neutrophils antecede the metabolic responses of these cells to surface stimulation with Con A and immune complexes. Utsumi et al. (1977), using the cyanine dye,

3-3'-dipropylthiocarbocyanine iodide, also found evidence that concanavalin A provokes changes in neutrophils compatible with a small membrane hyperpolarization followed by a large depolarization. In studies using yet another membrane potential-sensitive cyanine dye (i.e., 3,3'-dipentyloxacarbocyanine), Seligmann et al. (1980) described changes in fluorescence after stimulation of neutrophils with chemotactic factors compatible with a rapid depolarization of the plasma membrane followed by a prolonged hyperpolarization. The ability of various synthetic peptides to provoke changes in fluorescence corresponded to their relative potency as chemoattractants. On the basis of these findings, it has been suggested that changes in neutrophil membrane potential are very early, and possibly necessary, events in stimulus–response coupling (Korchak and Weissmann, 1978). Support for this suggestion was provided recently by several studies demonstrating that neutrophils incapable of generating superoxide anion radicals, i.e., cells from patients with chronic granulomatous disease, also do not exhibit changes in membrane potential when appropriately stimulated (Whitin et al., 1980; Seligmann and Gallin, 1980; Seligmann et al., 1981; Castranova et al., 1981). Since neutrophils from patients with chronic granulomatous disease are capable of migrating in a directed fashion (Seligmann and Gallin, 1980) and of degranulating (Baehner et al., 1969), it appears that neutrophil membrane potential changes may not, in fact, be necessary events in the pathways leading from cell surface stimulation to these neutrophil responses. Indeed, the relationships among chemotactic factor-induced neutrophil membrane potential changes, chemotaxis, and degranulation remain to be established.

C. Arachidonic Acid Metabolism

Under conditions in which neutrophils are stimulated to release lysosomal constitutents, they simultaneously synthesize and release various products of arachidonic acid. Zurier and Sayadoff (1975), for example, found that human neutrophils released prostaglandins of the E and F series to the surrounding medium when exposed to opsonized zymosan particles. Prostaglandin E (PGE) was found in the highest concentration in the medium, and the PGE:PGF ratio was ~3:1. Human neutrophils exposed to opsonized zymosan particles also are stimulated to generate thromboxane B_2, the stable end product of thromboxane A_2, in a time- and concentration-dependent fashion (Goldstein et al., 1978). Conversion by stimulated neutrophils of [^{14}C]arachidonic acid to [^{14}C]thromboxane B_2 was confirmed by thin-layer radiochromatography, radio-gas chromatography, and mass spectromety. Generation of thromboxane B_2 was independent of platelet contamination and could be prevented by the cyclooxygenase inhibitor indomethacin.

It is now well established that neutrophils respond to a number of particulate and soluble stimuli, e.g., opsonized bacteria, the calcium ionophore A23187, and chemotactic peptides, by converting arachidonic acid (through the cyclo-oxygenase pathway) to stable prostaglandins and thromboxanes (Wentzell and Epand, 1978; Higgs *et al.*, 1976; Stenson and Parker, 1979). Although neutrophils respond to these same stimuli by releasing lysosomal constituents (including phospholipases) (Traynor and Authi, 1981), the precise relationship between degranulation and metabolism of arachidonic acid by the cyclooxygenase pathway is unclear. Indeed, it is somewhat paradoxical that some products of neutrophil arachidonic acid metabolism, e.g., prostaglandin E, actually can inhibit degranulation (see Section V.B).

A great deal of attention has been directed recently toward the lipoxygenase pathways of neutrophils. These pathways lead to the formation by stimulated cells of a variety of monohydroxy- and dihydroxy-eicosatetraenoic acids—HETEs, diHETEs, and leukotrienes (Borgeat *et al.*, 1976; Borgeat and Samuelsson, 1979a,b; Goetzl and Sun, 1979; Stenson and Parker, 1979; Bokoch and Reed, 1980; Walsh *et al.*, 1981). Interestingly, a number of lipoxygenase products, e.g., 5-HETE, 12-HETE, and leukotriene B_4, have been found capable of provoking degranulation of cytochalasin B-treated neutrophils (Stenson and Parker, 1980; Goetzl and Pickett, 1980; Bokoch and Reed, 1981; O'Flaherty *et al.*, 1981; Showell *et al.*, 1982, Serhan *et al.*, 1982). Cytochalasin B-treated neutrophils from some species, such as rabbits, even degranulate in response to unaltered arachidonic acid (Naccache *et al.*, 1979a; Walenga *et al.*, 1980). In general, however, high concentrations of these compounds are required to provoke degranulation. In addition, the extent to which neutrophils degranulate in response to even the most potent lipoxygenase products is quite modest as compared with the extent to which they degranulate in response to other soluble stimuli (e.g., chemotactic peptides) (Stenson and Parker, 1980; Goetzl and Pickett, 1980). Nevertheless, several observations have led to the suggestion that metabolites of arachidonic acid, particularly those formed by the 5-lipoxygenase pathway, play a physiological role in regulating degranulation of neutrophils exposed to diverse particulate and soluble stimuli. A number of investigators, for example, have found that inhibitors of arachidonic acid metabolism, such as nordihydroguaiaretic acid (NDGA), 5,8,11,14-eicosatetraynoic acid (ETYA), and certain nonsteroidal anti-inflammatory agents, inhibit degranulation of neutrophils provoked by arachidonic acid, the calcium ionophore A23187, peptide chemotactic factors, and opsonized zymosan particles (Smith, 1977, 1978, 1979; Naccache *et al.*, 1979a; O'Flaherty *et al.*, 1979; Smolen and Weissmann, 1980; Walenga *et al.*, 1980). In addition, it has been observed that NDGA inhibits transport of calcium into rabbit neutrophils exposed to arachidonic acid (Volpi *et al.*, 1980) and chemotactic peptides (Nacchache *et al.*, 1979a). These observations, as well as the findings that lipoxygenase products per se (particularly leukotriene B_4) stimulate calcium uptake by neutrophils (Naccache *et al.*, 1981) and translocation of intracellular calcium (Sha'afi *et al.*, 1981; Serhan *et al.*, 1982), have led to the suggestion that arachidonic acid metabolism by neutrophils is linked to the changes in calcium metabolism that appear to be involved in stimulus–response coupling (see Section V.A).

Despite the observations summarized above, the precise relationship between arachidonic acid metabolism by the 5-lipoxygenase pathway and neutrophil degranulation remains unclear. One reason for this is the uncertain specificity of the inhibitors used in most studies. For example, it was recently demonstrated that the nonsteroidal anti-inflammatory agents, indomethacin and piroxicam, as well as NDGA, inhibit binding of synthetic chemotactic peptides to human neutrophils (Cost *et al.*, 1981; Edelson *et al.*, 1982; Atkinson *et al.*, 1982). These compounds may also affect neutrophil phospholipase A_2 activity (Kaplan *et al.*, 1978), cyclic nucleotide metabolism (Mikulikova and Trnavsky, 1982), cation fluxes (Smith *et al.*, 1981*a*), and membrane lipid composition (Stenson and Parker, 1980; Rubin *et al.*, 1981) independently of any effects they may have on the formation of products of arachidonic acid by either the cyclooxygenase or lipoxygenase pathways. It is interesting in this respect that ETYA, NDGA, and indomethacin have been found capable to inhibiting degranulation of neutrophils provoked by leukotriene B_4 (O'Flaherty *et al.*, 1981). These observations are inconsistent with the suggestion that leukotriene B_4 is a physiologically important endogenous mediator of degranulation. Finally, Smith *et al.* (1981*a*) found that ETYA and other putative inhibitors of 5-lipoxygenase activity were capable of inhibiting degranulation of neutrophils at concentrations that did not inhibit production of 5-HETE. Conversely, some phenylhydrazone derivatives were found capable of inhibiting production of 5-HETE, but not degranulation. It is obvious that much more work is required to establish the relationship, if any, between arachidonic acid metabolism by lipoxygenases and neutrophil degranulation.

V. REGULATION OF NEUTROPHIL DEGRANULATION

The shuttle and flow of lysosomes in stimulated phagocytes resembles the type of intracellular traffic involving similar organelles observed in secretory cells. Constituents within neutrophil lysosomes are destined to pass into vacuoles that are essentially "outside" the cytoplasm, in much the same way that exocrine or endocrine products are discharged from true secretory cells. It is not surprising, therefore, that substances that regulate the flow of stored and exportable proteins in such tissues as pancreas, salivary gland, and thyroid also act to regulate granule flow and fusion in neutrophils. These substances are discussed in the following sections.

A. Extracellular Ions

The selective extracellular release of granule-associated (i.e., lysosomal) enzymes from intact, viable neutrophils exposed to particulate and soluble stimuli is dependent on the translocation of granules to the cell periphery and membrane fusion between granule membranes and the plasma membrane. Like secretory processes in other cells, the effects of extracellular ions on the release of lysosomal constituents from neutrophils have been studied extensively. For the most part, however, it has been difficult to distinguish between the effects of extracellular cations and anions on the stimuli that provoke secretion from neutrophils versus their effects on the secretory process per se. For example, early reports of the effects of divalent cations on lysosomal enzyme release from neutrophils were based on studies of experimental systems in which enzyme release required either adherence of cells to nonphagocytosable surfaces (Becker and Showell, 1974; Henson, 1972; Ignarro, 1974a) or phagocytosis of particles (Ignarro and George, 1974a). Since both adherence and phagocytosis are cation-dependent processes (Bryant et al., 1966; Stossel, 1973), conclusions concerning the cation requirements for degranulation in these experimental systems were open to question.

One approach used to examine effects of divalent cations on neutrophil degranulation has been to perform studies with cytochalasin B-treated cells and soluble stimuli. The complement component C5a, for example, provokes selective release of granule-associated enzymes from intact, cytochalasin B-treated human neutrophils in the absence of phagocytosis or cellular adherence to surfaces (Goldstein et al., 1973b). Consequently, in this experimental system the influence of divalent cations on phagocytosis and adherence could be disregarded and their effects on enzyme secretion studied directly.

Goldstein et al. (1975c) found that cytochalasin B-treated human neutrophils exposed to C5a in calcium- and magnesium-free media consistently secreted significant amounts of the granule-associated enzymes, β-glucuronidase, and lysozyme. This basal secretory response was not diminished in cells preincubated with 5.0 mM ethylenediamine tetraacetic acid (EDTA), nor was it influenced if 2.0 mM EDTA was present in the reaction mixtures. The addition of calcium ($\leqslant$1.5–2.0 mM) produced a concentration-dependent enhancement of C5a-induced β-glucuronidase release, whereas increasing amounts of calcium ($>$2.0 mM) inhibited secretion of this enzyme. Lysozyme release also was enhanced by the addition of calcium, but inhibition with high concentrations was not observed. Calcium per se, in the absence of C5a, provoked only the release of lysozyme from neutrophils. Magnesium (0.5–5.0 mM) had no effect on C5a-mediated β-glucuronidase release either in the presence or absence of calcium. These studies documented that release of granule-associated enzymes from cytochalasin B-treated human neutrophils exposed to C5a can proceed in the absence of extracellular calcium. Optimal secretion of β-glucuronidase, however, required the presence of rather specific concentrations of calcium. Furthermore, calcium per se was capable of provoking secretion of lysozyme. It appears, therefore, that calcium (but not magnesium) plays a role in stimulus–secretion coupling in human neutrophils and that exocytosis of various granule populations in human neutrophils is regulated by independent mechanisms involving calcium.

Despite reports demonstrating uptake of calcium by stimulated neutrophils (Smith and Ignarro, 1975; Showell *et al.*, 1977; Naccache *et al.*, 1977; Petroski *et al.*, 1979), it is now generally agreed that extracellular calcium is not obligatory for degranulation to occur (Roos *et al.*, 1981; Smith *et al.*, 1981*b*; Smolen *et al.*, 1981). Indeed, there is evidence that some stimuli actually provoke an efflux of calcium from neutrophils (Gallin and Rosenthal, 1974; Barthélemy *et al.*, 1977). In fact, results of some very recent studies suggest that release of calcium from plasma membrane storage sites into the cytosol of neutrophils is crucial for degranulation (and other) responses to soluble and insoluble stimuli. For example, several investigators have demonstrated that neutrophils labeled with chlortetracycline (which forms fluorescent complexes with membrane-bound calcium and magnesium) rapidly lose fluorescence when exposed to a variety of soluble stimuli (Naccache *et al.*, 1979*b,c*; Takeshige *et al.*, 1980; Smolen and Weissmann, 1982). These findings have been interpreted as indicating translocation of calcium in stimulated neutrophils from membrane sites to the cytoplasm. Evidence supporting this interpretation was provided by Hoffstein (1979), who demonstrated histochemically that membrane-associated divalent cations are lost from human neutrophils exposed to both particulate and soluble stimuli. Interestingly, Hoffstein observed segmental loss of divalent cations from those portions of the plasmalemma in contact with particles *vs.* circumferential loss in response to soluble stimuli.

Additional evidence that release of membrane-bound calcium into the cytosol of neutrophils is an essential step in stimulus–response coupling has been provided by results of experiments using pharmacological antagonists. Several investigators, for example, have found that inhibitors (e.g., trifluoperazine) of the calcium-binding regulatory protein, calmodulin (Levin and Weiss, 1977) inhibit neutrophil degranulation responses to a variety of stimuli (Ochs and Reed, 1981; Smith *et al.*, 1981*b*; Smolen *et al.*, 1981). Similar inhibition was observed in experiments in which an antagonist of the mobilization of intracellular calcium (i.e., TMB-8) was used (Smith and Iden, 1979; Smith *et al.*, 1980; Smolen *et al.*, 1981). Problems of specificity notwithstanding, results of experiments with these inhibitors support the suggestion that degranulation of neutrophils may be triggered by transient changes in the concentration of cytosolic calcium.

Other ions influence degranulation responses of neutrophils as well. Korchak *et al.* (1980), for example, found that anion channel-blocking agents (e.g., stilbene derivatives and pyridoxal phosphate), at concentrations that inhibit sulfate fluxes, significantly inhibit lysosomal enzyme release from cytochalasin B-treated human neutrophils stimulated with immune complexes. Ultrastructural studies revealed evidence that these agents specifically inhibit fusion of lysosomes with the neutrophil plasma membrane. Optimal release of granule-associated enzymes from stimulated neutrophils also is inhibited by removing sodium and potassium from the media in which the cells are suspended (Showell et al., 1977; Korchak and Weissmann, 1980). An influx of sodium into neutrophils has been demonstrated as a response to a variety of stimuli (Naccache et al., 1977; Simchowitz and Spilberg, 1979).

B. Cyclic Nucleotides and Agents That Affect Microtubules

Among the substances known to regulate secretory events in nonphagocytic cells are those that influence accumulation within these cells of the cyclic nucleotides, cyclic 3',5'-adenosine monophosphate (cAMP) and cyclic 3',5'-guanosine monophosphate (cGMP), and those that affect the state of assembly of cytoplasmic microtubules. Studies during the past decade of the effects of such substances on neutrophils have yielded a great deal of information concerning the complex mechanisms regulating the intracellular flow of neutrophil lysosomal granules and fusion of these organelles with the plasma membrane.

Microtubules, found in a wide variety of plant and animal cells, are considered important in stabilizing cellular form, in controlling cellular motility, and in regulating intracellular granule flow. Although microtubules are in a dynamic state of assembly and disassembly, it is probably in their aggregated (or assembled) state that microtubules exert their influence on cell mechanics (Weisenberg et al., 1968; Olmsted and Borisy, 1973).

As would be expected, neither cyclic nucleotides nor microtubule-active agents influence release of neutrophil granule constituents induced by mechanisms involving cell death or perforation from within. They do, however, influence the selective discharge of neutrophil lysosomal enzymes that occurs as a consequence of either regurgitation during feeding or reverse endocytosis. In both instances, exogenous cAMP (plus the phosphodiesterase inhibitor, theophylline) and agents (e.g., isoproterenol, prostaglandins) that elevate cellular levels of cAMP reduce lysosomal enzyme release from stimulated neutrophils. In contrast, exogenous cGMP and agents (e.g., carbamylcholine) that elevate cellular levels of cGMP enhance lysosomal enzyme release (Weissmann et al., 1971a,b, 1972; Zurier et al., 1973a,b, 1974; Ignarro, 1974a,b; Ignarro and George, 1974a,b; Ignarro et al., 1974; Smith, 1977; Atkinson et al., 1977; Marone et al., 1980). Similarly, agents such as colchicine and vinblastine that promote disassembly of cytoplasmic microtubules reduce, and agents such as deuterium oxide that promote microtubule assembly enhance lysosomal enzyme release (Zurier et al., 1973a,b, 1974).

The concordance of these results with the observations of others concerning effects of these same agents on antigen-induced release of histamine and slow-reacting substance of anaphylaxis from sensitized basophils (Gillespie and Lichtenstein, 1972) and lung tissue (Kaliner *et al.*, 1972) has led to the suggestion that release from cells of a variety of mediators of inflammation is subject to pharmacological control at the level of cyclic nucleotide–tubulin interactions (Weissmann *et al.*, 1975*a*,*b*). Inhibition of neutrophil lysosomal enzyme release by colchicine and cAMP has been considered to be due to the direct or indirect effects of these agents on cytoplasmic microtubules (to cause disassembly) (Weissmann *et al.*, 1975*a*,*b*; Zurier *et al.*, 1973*a*,*b*, 1974). In contrast, stimulation of lysosomal enzyme release by cGMP, as in other systems (Kaliner *et al.*, 1972; Oliver, 1976; Oliver and Zurier, 1976), is mimicked by deuterium oxide, an agent that promotes assembly of microtubules (Gillespie and Lichtenstein, 1972). It should be noted, however, that definitive evidence is lacking to support the conclusion that cAMP and cGMP regulate secretion of neutrophil lysosomal enzymes simply by affecting the state of assembly of microtubules.

Hoffstein *et al.* (1977) reevaluated the role of microtubule assembly in lysosomal enzyme secretion from human neutrophils and found that microtubule numbers in both cytochalasin B-treated and -untreated neutrophils were increased by stimulation (with C5a and immune complexes) and depressed below resting levels in a dose–response fashion by colchicine concentrations above 10^{-7} M. These concentrations of colchicine also inhibited lysosomal enzyme release in a dose–response fashion, although inhibition of microtubule assembly was proportionately greater than inhibition of enzyme release. In fact, concentrations of colchicine that completely inhibited assembly of microtubules reduced enzyme release by only 40%. Morphological studies suggested that translocation of phagosomes within the cytoplasm of neutrophils was modulated by microtubule assembly rather than fusion itself and that correlations between microtubule assembly and disassembly and enhanced or diminished enzyme release (Weissmann *et al.*, 1975*a*,*b*) probably reflected events that took place earlier in the secretory process. Microtubules, therefore, appear to be involved in maintaining the internal organization of neutrophils and topological relationships between their organelles and the plasma membrane. Assembly may enhance, or disassembly diminish, the chances for contact between neutrophil granules and stimulated areas of the plasma membrane. Other structures, perhaps contractile proteins, may play a more direct role in permitting fusion of granules with either phagosomes or the plasma membrane.

A number of alternative possibilities could explain the effects of microtubule-active agents and cyclic nucleotides on neutrophil degranulation. For example, although colchicine is known to affect microtubules, it also can potentiate the increase in cellular levels of cAMP observed when neutrophils are exposed to either isoproterenol or prostaglandin E_1 (Rudolph *et al.*, 1977). Colchicine also has been reported to be capable of altering the fluidity of biomembranes (Wunderlich *et al.*, 1973). Effects on membrane fluidity may account for the ability of colchicine to retard the selective release of lysosomal enzymes from stimulated neutrophils.

Similarly, cyclic nucleotides may have direct or indirect effects on membranes to alter their stability (Kaliner and Austen, 1974; Ignarro and Colombo, 1973) and, consequently, either inhibit or enhance membrane fusion. Finally, these agents may act simply by influencing the manner by which various stimuli interact with the neutrophil cell surface to generate "signals" that provoke microtubule assembly and/or exocytosis. For example, Sajnani et al. (1976) found a relationship between degranulation of neutrophils provoked by aggregated IgG and redistribution of surface membrane receptors for this immunoglobulin. Receptor redistribution appeared to be a prerequisite, i.e., signal, for degranulation. Compounds such as colchicine and cAMP (plus theophylline), which inhibit release of lysosomal enzymes from neutrophils, also inhibited redistribution of surface IgG receptors. Cytochalasin B, on the other hand, increased receptor redistribution in accord with its ability to enhance exocytosis. Thus, the possibility remains that changes in intracellular levels of cyclic nucleotides and of the state of assembly of microtubules, while apparently associated with alterations in the extent of lysosomal enzyme release from stimulated neutrophils, are unrelated phenomena and play a very indirect physiological role in regulating degranulation.

As indicated above, there is ample evidence that exogenous cAMP and agents that elevate intracellular levels of cAMP inhibit neutrophil degranulation. It is somewhat paradoxical, therefore, that neutrophils respond to a variety of particulate and soluble stimuli, including opsonized zymosan particles, polystyrene Latex beads, immune complexes, complement-derived and synthetic chemoattractants, and A23187, with transient increments in levels of total cellular cAMP (Herlin et al., 1978; Jackowski and Sha'afi, 1979; Simchowitz et al., 1980; Smolen et al., 1980; Smolen and Weissmann, 1981; Stolc, 1981). Despite some reports to the contrary (Ignarro and George, 1974b; Hatch et al., 1977), however, most investigators have not observed changes in cellular levels of cGMP.

Maximally increased levels of neutrophil cAMP have been observed within 10–45 sec after stimulation (Simchowitz et al., 1980; Smolen et al., 1980). Levels decline by 1 min and reach baseline by 5 min. Because the small increments in cAMP antecede degranulation by stimulated neutrophils, it has been suggested that activation of adenylate cyclase is an early, perhaps necessary, event in stimulus–response coupling (Simchowitz et al., 1980). However, the precise role played by cAMP in the sequence of events leading to activation of neutrophils has not been determined.

Interestingly, neutrophils pretreated with agents that inhibit degranulation, e.g., prostaglandin E_1 and prostaglandin I_2, respond to surface stimulation with very marked increments in cellular levels of cAMP, sustained for several minutes (Smolen et al., 1980). It is therefore possible that the very modest and transient elevations of cAMP observed after exposure of neutrophils to secretagogues are insufficient to cause inhibition of degranulation. In contrast, inhibition of degranulation very likely occurs only when increments in cellular levels of cAMP are large and sustained.

C. Miscellaneous Agents

In addition to cyclic nucleotides and microtubule-active agents, a variety of other compounds have been found capable of influencing degranulation by stimulated neutrophils. For example, despite their apparent inability to alter the integrity of isolated neutrophil lysosomes *in vitro* (Persellin and Ku, 1974), adrenal corticosteroids do retard release of lysosomal constitutents from intact cells exposed to particles and nonphagocytosable stimuli (Wright and Malawista, 1973; Hawkins, 1974; Goldstein *et al.*, 1976b). One explanation for these findings is that corticosteroids act primarily at the level of the neutrophil surface membrane to modulate stimulus–membrane interactions. A direct action on membranes probably also accounts for the reduction of lysosomal enzyme release from neutrophils treated with local anesthetics, such as lidocaine and tetracaine (Goldstein *et al.*, 1977b). Alternative mechanisms by which these compounds may suppress neutrophil degranulation involve (1) inhibition by corticosteroids of phospholipase A_2 activity (Hirata *et al.*, 1980), (2) enhancement by corticosteroids of adenylate cyclase activity (Marone *et al.*, 1980), and (3) effects of local anesthetics on calmodulin (Tanaka and Hidaka, 1981).

It must be reemphasized that the effects of pharmacologic agents on specific events that occur in stimulated neutrophils often cannot be distinguished from effects on the stimulus–surface membrane interactions that provide the signals for these specific events. Such is the case with the effects on neutrophil degranulation of colchicine, cyclic nucleotides, corticosteroids, and other agents. Until it can be determined with certainty that these compounds do not influence the manner by which specific stimuli interact with neutrophils to provoke degranulation (i.e., exocytosis), no firm conclusions can be drawn concerning the precise mechanisms by which they act. It remains possible, for example, that these diverse pharmacological agents influence neutrophil functions by acting primarily at the level of the surface membrane.

VI. CONCLUSIONS

It should be apparent from the information summarized that considerable progress has been made during the past decade in deciphering what Weissmann *et al.* (1979) have termed the secretory code of the neutrophil. We must not forget, however, that the foundation of our current body of knowledge concerning events that occur in stimulated neutrophils was provided nearly a century

ago by Metchnikoff (1883). His original observations as well as recent developments in the fields of immunology, biochemistry, and cell biology have helped
teach us a great deal about the phenomenon of stimulus–response coupling in
neutrophils. It is reasonable to assume that future developments in the basic
sciences will help elucidate further the mechanisms whereby neutrophils dispose
of invading microorganisms and promote inflammation.

VII. REFERENCES

Allison, A. C., Harrington, J. S., and Birbeck, M., 1968, An examination of the cytotoxic
    effects of silica on macrophages, *J. Exp. Med.* **124**:141.
Atkinson, J. P., Sullivan, T. J., Kelly, J. P., and Parker, C. W., 1977, Stimulation by alcohols
    of cyclic AMP metabolism in human leukocytes. Possible role of cyclic AMP in the anti-
    inflammatory effects of ethanol, *J. Clin. Invest.* **60**:284.
Atkinson, J. P., Simchowitz, L., Mehta, J., and Stenson, W. F., 1982, 5,8,11,14-eicosatetray-
    noic acid (ETYA) inhibits binding of *N*-formyl-methionyl-leucyl-phenylalanine (FMLP)
    to its receptor on human granulocytes. A note of caution, *Immunopharmacology* **4**:1.
Avila, J. L., and Convit, J., 1973, Studies on human polymorphonuclear leukocyte enzymes.
    II. Comparative study of the physical properties of primary and specific granules, *Bio-
    chim. Biophys. Acta* **293**:409.
Babior, B. M., 1978, Oxygen-dependent microbial killing by phagocytes, *N. Engl. J. Med.*
    298:659.
Babior, B. M., Kipnes, R. S., and Curnutte, J. T., 1973, Biological defense mechanisms: The
    production by leukocytes of superoxide, a potential bactericidal agent, *J. Clin. Invest.*
    52:741.
Baehner, R. L., Karnovsky, M. J., and Karnovsky, M. L, 1969, Degranulation of leukocytes
    in chronic granulomatous disease, *J. Clin. Invest.* **48**:187.
Baggiolini, M., Hirsch, J. G., and de Duve, C., 1969, Resolution of granules from rabbit
    heterophil leukocytes into distinct populations by zonal sedimentation, *J. Cell. Biol.*
    40:529.
Bainton, D. F., 1973, Sequential degranulation of the two types of polymorphonuclear
    leukocyte granules during phagocytosis of microorganisms, *J. Cell. Biol.* **58**:249.
Bainton, D. F., and Farquhar, M. G., 1966, Origin of granules in polymorphonuclear leuko-
    cytes: Two types derived from opposite faces of the Golgi complex in developing granu-
    locytes, *J. Cell. Biol.* **28**:277.
Bainton, D. F., and Farquhar, M. G., 1968a, Differences in enzyme content of azurophil and
    specific granules of polymorphonuclear leukocytes. I. Histochemical staining of bone
    marrow smears, *J. Cell. Biol.* **39**:286.
Bainton, D. F., and Farquhar, M. G., 1968b, Differences in enzyme content of azurophil
    and specific granules of polymorphonuclear leukocytes. II. Cytochemistry and electron
    microscopy of bone marrow cells, *J. Cell. Biol.* **39**:299.
Bainton, D. F., Ullyot, J. L., and Farquhar, M. G., 1971, The development of neutrophilic
    polymorphonuclear leukocytes in human bone marrow. Origin and content of azurophil
    and specific granules, *J. Exp. Med.* **134**:907.
Barthélemy, A., Paridaens, R., and Schell-Frederick, E., 1977, Phagocytosis-induced [45] cal-
    cium efflux in polymorphonuclear leucocytes, *FEBS Lett.* **82**:283.
Becker, E. L., 1976, Some interrelationships of neutrophil chemotaxis, lysosomal enzyme
    secretion, and phagocytosis as revealed by synthetic peptides, *Am. J. Pathol.* **85**:385.

Becker, E. L., and Showell, H. J., 1974, The ability of chemotactic factors to induce lysosomal enzyme release. II. The mechanism of release, *J. Immunol.* **112**:2055.

Becker, E. L., Showell, H. J., Henson, P. M., and Hsu, L. S., 1974, The ability of chemotactic factors to induce lysosomal enzyme release. I. The characteristics of the release, the importance of surfaces and the relation of enzyme release to chemotactic responsiveness, *J. Immunol.* **112**:2047.

Bentwood, B. J., and Henson, P. M., 1980, The sequential release of granule constituents from human neutrophils, *J. Immunol.* **124**:855.

Berlin, R. D., and Fera, J. P., 1977, Changes in membrane microviscosity associated with phagocytosis: Effects of colchicine, *Proc. Natl. Acad. Sci (USA)* **74**:1072.

Bokoch, G. M., and Reed, P. W., 1980, Stimulation of arachidonic acid metabolism in the polymorphonuclear leukocyte by an *N*-formylated peptide. Comparison with ionophore A23187, *J. Biol. Chem.* **255**:10223.

Bokoch, G. M., and Reed, P. W., 1981, Effect of various lipoxygenase metabolites of arachidonic acid on degranulation of polymorphonuclear leukocytes, *J. Biol. Chem.* **256**:5317.

Borgeat, P., and Samuelsson, B., 1979*a*, Transformation of arachidonic acid by rabbit polymorphonuclear leukocytes. Formation of a novel dihydroxyeicosatetraenoic acid, *J. Biol. Chem.* **254**:2643.

Borgeat, P., and Samuelsson, B., 1979*b*, Arachidonic acid metabolism in polymorphonuclear leukocytes: Unstable intermediate in formation of a dihydroxy acids, *Proc. Natl. Acad. Sci. (USA)* **76**:3213.

Borgeat, P., Hamberg, M., and Samuelsson, B., 1976, Transformation of arachidonic acid and homo-γ-linolenic acid by rabbit polymorphonuclear leukocytes. Monohydroxy acids from novel lipoxygenases, *J. Biol. Chem.* **251**:7816.

Bretz, U., and Baggiolini, M., 1974, Biochemical and morphological characterization of azurophil and specific granules of human polymorphonuclear leukocytes, *J. Cell. Biol.* **63**:251.

Bryant, R. E., DesPrez, R. M., VanWay, M. H., and Rogers, D. E., 1966, Studies on human leucocyte motility. I. Effects of alterations in pH, electrolyte concentration, and phagocytosis on leucocyte migration, adhesiveness, and aggregation, *J. Exp. Med.* **124**:483.

Carter, S. B., 1967, Effects of cytochalasin on mammalian cells, *Nature* **213**:261.

Castranova, V., Jones, G. S., Phillips, R. M., Peden, D., and Vandyke, K., 1981, Abnormal responses of granulocytes in chronic granulomatous disease, *Biochim. Biophys. Acta* **645**:49.

Cohen, H. J., and Chovaniec, M. E., 1978, Superoxide generation by digitonin-stimulated guinea pig granulocytes. A basis for a continuous assay for monitoring superoxide production for the study of the activation of the generating system, *J. Clin. Invest.* **61**:1081.

Cohn, Z. A., and Fedorko, M. E., 1969, The formation and fate of lysosomes, in: *Lysosomes in Biology and Pathology*, Vol. 1 (J. Dingle and H. Fell, eds.), pp. 43–63, North-Holland, Amsterdam.

Cohn, Z. A., and Hirsch, J. G., 1960*a*, The isolation and properties of the specific cytoplasmic granules of rabbit polymorphonuclear leukocytes, *J. Exp. Med.* **112**:983.

Cohn, Z. A., and Hirsch, J. G., 1960*b*, The influence of phagocytosis on the intracellular distribution of granule-associated components of polymorphonuclear leucocytes, *J. Exp. Med.* **112**:1015.

Cost, H., Gespach, C., and Abita, J.-P., 1981, Effect of indomethacin on the binding of the chemotactic peptide formyl-met-leu-phe on human polymorphonuclear leukocytes, *FEBS Lett.* **132**:85.

Curnutte, J. T., and Babior, B. M., 1974, Biological defense mechanisms. The effect of bacteria and serum on superoxide production by granulocytes, *J. Clin. Invest.* **53**:1662.

Curnutte, J. T., and Babior, B. M., 1975, Effects of anaerobiosis and inhibitors on O_2^- production by human granulocytes, *Blood* **45**:851.

Davis, A. T., Estensen, R., and Quie, P. G., 1971, Cytochalasin B. III. Inhibition of human polymorphonuclear leukocyte phagocytosis, *Proc. Soc. Exp. Biol. Med.* **137**:161.

DeChatelet, L. R., 1975, Oxidative bactericidal mechanisms of polymorphonuclear leukocytes, *J. Infect. Dis.* **131**:295.

DeChatelet, L. R., 1978, Initiation of the respiratory burst in human polymorphonuclear neutrophils: A critical review, *J. Reticuloendothel. Soc.* **24**:73.

DeChatelet, L. R., Shirley, P. S., and Johnston, R. B., Jr., 1976, Effect of phorbol myristate acetate on the oxidative metabolism of human polymorphonuclear leukocytes, *Blood* **47**:545.

de Duve, C., and Wattiaux, R., 1966, Functions of lysosomes, *Annu. Rev. Physiol.* **28**:435.

de Duve, C., Pressman, B. C., Gianetto, R., Wattiaux, R., and Applemans, F., 1955, Tissue fractionation studies, 6. Intracellular distribution patterns of enzymes in rat liver tissue, *Biochem. J.* **60**:604.

Densen, P., and Mandell, G. L., 1978, Gonococcal interactions with polymorphonuclear neutrophils. Importance of the phagosome for bactericidal activity, *J. Clin. Invest.* **62**:1161.

Dewald, B., Bretz, U., and Baggiolini, M., 1982, Release of gelatinase from a novel secretory compartment of human neutrophils, *J. Clin. Invest.* **70**:518.

Edelson, H. S., Kaplan, H. B., Korchak, H. M., Smolen, J. E., and Weissmann, G., 1982, Dissociation by piroxicam of degranulation and superoxide anion generation from decrements in chlortetracycline fluorescence of activated human neutrophils, *Biochem. Biophys. Res. Commun.* **104**:247.

Ehlenberger, A. G., and Nussenzweig, V., 1977, The role of membrane receptors for C3b and C3d in phagocytosis, *J. Exp. Med.* **145**:357.

Estensen, R. D., White, J. G., and Holmes, B., 1974, Specific degranulation of human polymorphonuclear leukocytes, *Nature* **248**:347.

Folds, J. D., Welsh, I. R. H., and Spitznagel, J. K., 1972, Neutral proteases confined to one class of lysosomes of human polymorphonuclear leukocytes, *Proc. Soc. Exp. Biol. Med.* **139**:461.

Gallin, E. K., and Gallin, J. I., 1977, Interaction of chemotactic factors with human macrophages. Induction of transmembrane potential changes, *J. Cell. Biol.* **75**:277.

Gallin, J. I., and Rosenthal, A. S., 1974, The regulatory role of divalent cations in human granulocyte chemotaxis. Evidence of an association between calcium exchanges and microtubule assembly, *J. Cell. Biol.* **62**:594.

Gallin, J. I., Bujak, J. S., Patten, E., and Wolff, S. M., 1974, Granulocyte function in Chediak–Higashi syndrome of mice, *Blood* **43**:201.

Gallin, J., Durocher, J., and Kaplan, A., 1975, Interaction of leukocyte chemotactic factors with the cell surface. I. Chemotactic factor-induced changes in human granulocyte surface charge, *J. Clin. Invest.* **55**:967.

Gillespie, E., and Lichtenstein, L. M., 1972, Histamine release from human leukocytes: Studies with deuterium oxide, colchicine and cytochalasin B, *Br. J. Clin. Invest.* **51**:2941.

Goetzl, E. J., and Austen, K. F., 1974, Stimulation of human neutrophil leukocyte aerobic glucose metabolism by purified chemotactic factors, *J. Clin. Invest.* **53**:591.

Goetzl, E. J., and Pickett, W. C., 1980, The human PMN leukocyte chemotactic activity of complex hydroxy-eicosatetraenoic acids (HETEs), *J. Immunol.* **125**:1789.

Goetzl, E. J., and Sun, F. F., 1979, Generation of unique monohydroxy-eicosatetraenoic acids from arachidonic acid by human neutrophils, *J. Exp. Med.* **150**:406.

Goldstein, I. M., 1973, Lysosomal hydrolases and inflammatory materials, in: *Mediators of Inflammation* (G. Weissmann, ed.), pp. 51–84, Plenum Press, New York.

Goldstein, I. M., 1976, Polymorphonuclear leukocyte lysosomes and immune tissue injury, *Prog. Allergy* **20**:301.

Goldstein, I. M., Brai, M., Osler, A. G., and Weissmann, G., 1973*a*, Lysosomal enzyme release from human leukocytes: Mediation by the alternate pathway of complement activation, *J. Immunol.* **111**:33.

Goldstein, I., Hoffstein, S., Gallin, J., and Weissmann, G., 1973*b*, Mechanisms of lysosomal enzyme release from human leukocytes: Microtubule assembly and membrane fusion induced by a component of complement, *Proc. Natl. Acad, Sci. (USA)* **70**:2916.

Goldstein, I. M., Horn, J. K., Kaplan, H. B., and Weissmann, G., 1974, Calcium-induced lysozyme secretion from human polymorphonuclear leukocytes, *Biochem. Biophys. Res. Commun.* **60**:807.

Goldstein, I. M., Roos, D., Weissmann, G., and Kaplan, H., 1975*a*, Complement and immunoglobulins stimulate superoxide production by human leukocytes independently of phagocytosis, *J. Clin. Invest.* **56**:1155.

Goldstein, I. M., Hoffstein, S. T., and Weissmann, G., 1975*b*, Mechanisms of lysosomal enzyme release from human polymorphonuclear leukocytes. Effects of phorbol myristate acetate, *J. Cell. Biol.* **66**:647.

Goldstein, I. M., Hoffstein, S. T., and Weissmann, G., 1975*c*, Influence of divalent cations upon complement-mediated enzyme release from human polymorphonuclear leukocytes, *J. Immunol.* **115**:665.

Goldstein, I. M., Feit, F., and Weissmann, G., 1975*d*, Enhancement of nitroblue tetrazolium dye reduction by leukocytes exposed to a component of complement in the absence of phagocytosis, *J. Immunol.* **114**:516.

Goldstein, I. M., Kaplan, H. B., Radin, A., and Frosch, M., 1976*a*, Independent effects of IgG and complement upon human polymorphonuclear leukocyte function, *J. Immunol.* **117**:1282.

Goldstein, I. M., Roos, D., Weissmann, G., and Kaplan, H. B., 1976*b*, Influence of corticosteroids on human polymorphonuclear leukocyte function *in vitro*. Reduction of lysosomal enzyme release and superoxide production, *Inflammation* **1**:305.

Goldstein, I. M., Cerqueira, M., Lind, S., and Kaplan, H. B., 1977*a*, Evidence that the superoxide generating system of human leukocytes is associated with the cell surface, *J. Clin. Invest.* **59**:249.

Goldstein, I. M., Lind, S., Hoffstein, S. T., and Weissmann, G., 1977*b*, Influence of local anesthetics upon human polymorphonuclear leukocyte function *in vitro*. Reduction of lysosomal enzyme release and superoxide anion production, *J. Exp. Med.* **146**:483.

Goldstein, I. M., Malmsten, C. L., Kindahl, H., Kaplan, H. B., Radmark, O., Samuelsson, B., and Weissmann, G., 1978, Thromboxane generation by human peripheral blood polymorphonuclear leukocytes, *J. Exp. Med.* **148**:787.

Haak, R. A., Ingraham, L. M., Baehner, R. L., and Boxer, L. A., 1979, Membrane fluidity in human and mouse Chediak–Higashi leukocytes, *J. Clin. Invest.* **64**:138.

Hartwig, J. H., and Stossel, T. P., 1976, Interactions of actin, myosin, and an actin-binding protein of rabbit pulmonary macrophages, III. Effects of cytochalasin B, *J. Cell. Biol.* **71**:295.

Hatch, G. E., Nichols, W. K., and Hill, H. R., 1977, Cyclic nucleotide changes in human neutrophils induced by chemoattractants and chemotactic modulators, *J. Immunol.* **119**:450.

Hawkins, D., 1971, Biopolymer membrane. A model system for the study of the neutrophilic leukocyte response to immune complexes, *J. Immunol.* **107**:344.

Hawkins, D., 1972, Neutrophilic leukocytes in immunological reactions. Evidence for the selective release of lysosomal constituents, *J. Immunol.* **108**:310.

Hawkins, D., 1973, Neutrophilic leukocytes in immunologic reactions *in vitro*. Effect of cytochalasin B, *J. Immunol.* **110**:294.

Hawkins, D., 1974, Neutrophilic leukocytes in immunologic reactions *in vitro*. III. Pharmacologic modulation of lysosomal enzyme release, *Clin. Immunol. Immunopathol.* 2:141.

Henson, P. M., 1971*a*, Interaction of cells with immune complexes. Adherence, release of constituents, and tissue injury, *J. Exp. Med.* 134:114s.

Henson, P. M., 1971*b*, The immunologic release of constitutents from neutrophil leukocytes. I. The role of antibody and complement on nonphagocytosable surfaces or phagocytosable particles, *J. Immunol.* 107:1535.

Henson, P. M., 1972, Pathologic mechanisms in neutrophil-mediated injury, *Am. J. Pathol.* 68:593.

Henson, P. M., and Oades, Z. G., 1975, Stimulation of human neutrophils by soluble and insoluble immunoglobulin aggregates. Secretion of granule constituents and increased oxidation of glucose, *J. Clin. Invest.* 56:1053.

Henson, P. M., Johnson, H. B., and Spiegelberg, H. L., 1972, The release of granule enzymes from human neutrophils stimulated by aggregated immunoglobulins of different classes and subclasses, *J. Immunol.* 109:1182.

Herlin, T., Petersen, C. S., and Esmann, V., 1978, The role of calcium and cyclic adenosine 3′,5′-monophosphate in the regulation of glycogen metabolism in phagocytizing human polymorphonuclear leukocytes, *Biochim. Biophys. Acta* 542:63.

Higgs, G. A., Bunting, S., Moncada, S., and Vane, J. R., 1976, Polymorphonuclear leukocytes produce thromboxane A_2-like activity during phagocytosis, *Prostaglandins* 12:749.

Hirata, F., Schiffmann, E., Venkatasubramanian, K., Salomon, D., and Axelrod, J., 1980, A phospholipase A_2 inhibitory protein in rabbit neutrophils induced by glucocorticoids, *Proc. Natl. Acad. Sci. (USA)* 77:2533.

Hirsch, J. G., and Cohn, Z. A., 1960, Degranulation of polymorphonuclear leukocytes following phagocytosis of microorganisms, *J. Exp. Med.* 112:1005.

Hirschhorn, R., and Weissmann, G., 1965, Isolation and properties of human leukocyte lysosomes *in vitro*, *Proc. Soc. Exp. Biol. Med.* 119:36.

Hoffstein, S. T., 1979, Ultrastructural demonstration of calcium loss from local regions of the plasma membrane of surface-stimulated human granulocytes, *J. Immunol.* 123:1395.

Hoffstein, S., Soberman, R., Goldstein, I., and Weissmann, G., 1976, Concanavalin A induces microtubule assembly and specific granule discharge in human polymorphonuclear leukocytes, *J. Cell. Biol.* 68:781.

Hoffstein, S., Goldstein, I. M., and Weissmann, G., 1977, Role of microtubule assembly in lysosomal enzyme secretion from human polymorphonuclear leukocytes. A reevaluation, *J. Cell. Biol.* 73:242.

Ignarro, L. J., 1974*a*, Nonphagocytic release of neutral protease and β-glucuronidase from human neutrophils. Regulation by autonomic neurohormones in cyclic nucleotides, *Arthritis Rheum.* 17:25.

Ignarro, L. J., 1974*b*, Stimulation of phagocytic release of neutral protease from human neutrophils by cholinergic amines and cyclic 3′,5′-guanosine monophosphate, *J. Immunol.* 112:210.

Ignarro, L. J., and Colombo, C., 1973, Enzyme release from polymorphonuclear leukocyte lysosomes, *Science* 180:1181.

Ignarro, L. J., and George, W. J., 1974*a*, Mediation of immunologic discharge of lysosomal enzymes from human neutrophils by guanosine 3′,5′-monophosphate. Requirement of calcium, and inhibition by adenosine 3′,5′-monophosphate, *J. Exp. Med.* 140:225.

Ignarro, L. J., and George, W. J., 1974*b*, Hormonal control of lysosomal enzyme release from human neutrophils, elevation of cyclic nucleotide levels by autonomic neurohormones, *Proc. Natl. Acad. Sci. (USA)* 71:2027.

Ignarro, L. J., Lint, T. F., and George, W. J., 1974, Hormonal control of lysosomal enzyme release from human neutrophils. Effects of autonomic agents on enzyme release, phagocytosis, and cyclic nucleotide levels, *J. Exp. Med.* 139:1395.

Ingraham, L. M., Boxer, L. A., Haak, R. A., and Baehner, R. L., 1981, Membrane fluidity change accompanying phagocytosis in normal and in chronic granulomatous disease polymorphonuclear leukocytes, *Blood* **58**:830.

Jackowski, S., and Sha'afi, R. I., 1979, Response of adenosine cyclic 3', 5'-monophosphate level in rabbit neutrophils to the chemotactic peptide formyl-methionyl-leucyl-phenylalanine, *Mol. Pharmacol.* **16**:473.

Johnston, R. B., Jr., and Lehmeyer, J. E., 1976, Elaboration of toxic oxygen byproducts by neutrophils in a model of immune complex disease, *J. Clin. Invest.* **57**:836.

Kaliner, M., and Austen, K. F., 1974, Adenosine 3',5'-monophosphate: Inhibition of complement-mediated cell lysis, *Science* **183**:659.

Kaliner, M., Orange, R. P., and Austen, K. F., 1972, Immunologic release of histamine and slow reacting substance of anaphylaxis from human lung. IV. Enhancement by cholinergic and alpha adrenegic stimulation, *J. Exp. Med.* **136**:556.

Kane, S. P., and Peters, T. J., 1975, Analytical subcellular fractionation of human granulocytes with reference to the localization of vitamin B_{12}-binding proteins, *Clin. Sci. Mol. Med.* **49**:171.

Kaplan, L., Weiss, J., and Elsbach, P., 1978, Low concentrations of indomethacin inhibit phospholipase A_2 of rabbit polymorphonuclear leukocytes, *Proc. Natl. Acad. Sci. (USA)* **75**:2955.

Kaplan, S. S., Finch, S. C., and Basford, R. E., 1972, Polymorphonuclear leukocyte activation: Effects of phospholipase *c*, *Proc. Soc. Exp. Biol. Med.* **140**:540.

Karnovsky, M. L, 1968, The metabolism of leukocytes, *Semin. Hematol.* **5**:156.

Klebanoff, S. J., 1967, Iodination of bacteria: A bactericidal mechanism, *J. Exp. Med.* **126**:1063.

Korchak, H. M., and Weissmann, G., 1978, Changes in membrane potential of human granulocytes antecede the metabolic responses to surface stimulation, *Proc. Natl. Acad. Sci. (USA)* **75**:3818.

Korchak, H. M., and Weissmann, G., 1980, Stimulus–response coupling in the human neutrophil: Transmembrane potential and the role of extracellular Na^+, *Biochim. Biophys. Acta* **601**:180.

Korchak, H. M., Eisenstat, B. A., Hoffstein, S. T., Dunham, P. B., and Weissmann, G., 1980, Anion channel blockers inhibit lysosomal enzyme secretion from human neutrophils without affecting generation of superoxide anion, *Proc. Natl. Acad. Sci. (USA)* **77**:2721.

Krinsky, N. I., 1974, Singlet excited oxygen as a mediator of the antibacterial action of leukocytes, *Science* **186**:363.

Leffell, M. S., and Spitznagel, J. K., 1972, Association of lactoferrin with lysozyme in granules of human polymorphonuclear leukocytes. *Infect. Immun.* **6**:761.

Leffell, M. S., and Spitznagel, J. K., 1974, Intracellular and extracellular degranulation of human polymorphonuclear azurophil and specific granules induced by immune complexes, *Infect. Immun.* **10**:1241.

Leffell, M. S., and Spitznagel, J. K., 1975, Fate of human lactoferrin and myeloperoxidase in phagocytizing human neutrophils: Effects of immunoglobulin G subclasses and immune complexes coated on latex beads, *Infect. Immun.* **12**:813.

Levin, R. M., and Weiss, B., 1977, Binding of trifluoperazine to the calcium-dependent activator of cyclic nucleotides phosphodiesterase, *Mol. Pharmacol.* **13**:690.

Mantovani, B., 1975, Different roles of IgG and complement receptors in phagocytosis by polymorphonuclear leukocytes, *J. Immunol.* **115**:15.

Marone, G., Thomas, L. L, and Lichtenstein, L. M., 1980, The role of agonists that activate adenylate cyclase in the control of cAMP metabolism and enzyme release by human polymorphonuclear leukocytes, *J. Immunol.* **125**:2277.

Metchnikoff, E., 1883, Untersuchungen über die intracellular Verdauung bie wirbellosen Thieren, *Arb. Zool. Inst. Univ. Wein* **5**:141.

214   Ira M. Goldstein

Metchnikoff, E., 1905, *Immunity in Infective Diseases*, p. 572, Cambridge University Press, Cambridge, England.

Mikulikova, D., and Trnavsky, K., 1982, The effect of indomethacin and its ester on lysosomal enzyme release from polymorphonuclear leukocytes and intracellular levels of cAMP and cGMP after phagocytosis of urate crystals, *Biochem. Pharmacol.* 31:460.

Murphy, G., Bretz, U., Baggiolini, M., and Reynolds, J. J., 1980, The latent collagenase and gelatinase of human polymorphonuclear neutrophil leukocytes, *Biochem. J.* 192:517.

Naccache, P. H., Showell, H. J., Becker, E. L., and Sha'afi, R. I., 1977, Changes in ionic movements across rabbit polymorphonuclear leukocyte membranes during lysosomal enzyme release. Possible ionic basis for lysosomal enzyme release, *J. Cell. Biol.* 75:635.

Naccache, P. J., Showell, H. J., Becker, E. L, and Sha'afi, R. I., 1979a, Arachidonic acid induced degranulation of rabbit peritoneal neutrophils, *Biochem. Biophys. Res. Commun.* 87:292.

Naccache, P. H., Volpi, M., Showell, H. J., Becker, E. L., and Sha'afi, R. I., 1979b, Chemotactic factor-induced release of membrane calcium in rabbit neutrophils, *Science* 203:461.

Naccache, P. H., Showell, H. J., Becker, E. L., and Sha'afi, R. I., 1979c, Involvement of membrane calcium in the response of rabbit neutrophils to chemotactic factors as evidenced by the fluorescence of chlortetracycline, *J. Cell. Biol.* 83:179.

Naccache, P. H., Sha'afi, R. I., Borgeat, P., and Goetzl, E. J., 1981, Mono- and dihydroxyeicosatetraenoic acids alter calcium homeostasis in rabbit neutrophils, *J. Clin. Invest.* 67:1584.

Nachman, R., Hirsch, J. G., and Baggiolini, M., 1972, Studies on isolated membranes of azurophil and specific granules from rabbit polymorphonuclear leukocytes, *J. Cell. Biol.* 54:133.

Novikoff, A. B., Essner, E., and Quintana, N., 1964, Golgi apparatus and lysosomes, *Fed. Proc.* 23:1010.

Ochs, D. L., and Reed, P. W., 1981, Inhibition of the neutrophil oxidative burst and degranulation by phenothiazines, *Biochem. Biophys. Res. Commun.* 102:958.

O'Flaherty, J. T., Showell, H. J., Ward, P. A., and Becker, E. L., 1979, A possible role of arachidonic acid in human neutrophil aggregation and degranulation, *Am. J. Pathol.* 96:799.

O'Flaherty, J. T., Wykle, R. L., Lees, C. J., Shewmake, T., McCall, C. E., and Thomas, M. J., 1981, Neutrophil degranulating action of 5,12-dihydroxy-6,8,10,14-eicosatetraenoic acid and 1-O-alkyl-2-O-acetyl-sn-glycero-3-phosphocholine, *Am. J. Pathol.* 105:264.

Oliver, J. M., 1976, Impaired microtubule function correctable by cyclic GMP and cholinergic agonists in the Chediak–Higashi syndrome, *Am. J. Pathol.* 85:395.

Oliver, J. M., and Zurier, R. B., 1976, Correction of characteristic abnormalities of microtubule function and granule morphology in Chediak–Higashi syndrome with cholinergic agonists. Studies *in vitro* in man and *in vivo* in the beige mouse, *J. Clin. Invest.* 57:1239.

Olmstead, J. B., and Borisy, G. G., 1973, Microtubules, *Annu. Rev. Biochem.* 42:507.

Olsson, I., 1969, Isolation of human leukocyte granules using colloidal silica-polysaccharide density gradients, *Exp. Cell. Res.* 54:325.

Persellin, R. H., and Ku, L. C., 1974, Effects of steroid hormones on human polymorphonuclear leukocyte lysosomes, *J. Clin. Invest.* 54:919.

Petroski, R. J., Naccache, P. H., Becker, E. L., and Sha'afi, R. I., 1979, Effect of the chemotactic factor formyl-methionyl-leucyl-phenylalanine and cytochalasin B on the cellular levels of calcium in rabbit neutrophils, *FEBS Lett.* 100:161.

Plagemann, P. G. W., and Estensen, R. D., 1972, Cytochalasin B. VI. Competitive inhibition of nucleotide transport by cultured Novikoff rat hepatoma cells, *J. Cell. Biol.* 55:179.

Repine, J. E., White, J. G., Clawson, C. C., and Holmes, B. W., 1974, The influence of phorbol myristate acetate on oxygen consumption by polymorphonuclear leukocytes, *J. Lab. Clin. Med.* **83**:911.

Romeo, P., Cramer, R., and Rossi, F., 1970, Use of 1-anilino-8-naphthalene sulfonate to study structural transitions in cell membranes of PMN leucocytes, *Biochem. Biophys. Res. Commun.* **41**:582.

Romeo, D., Zabucchi, G., and Rossi, F., 1973, Reversible metabolic stimulation of polymorphonuclear leukocytes and macrophages by concanavalin A, *Nature (New Biol.)* **243**:111.

Roos, D. Homan-Müller, J. W. T., and Weening, R. S., 1976, Effect of cytochalasin B on the oxidative metabolism of human peripheral blood granulocytes, *Biochem. Biophys. Res. Commun.* **68**:43.

Roos, D., Bot, A. A. M., van Schaik, M. L. J., de Boer, M., and Daha, M. R., 1981, Interaction between human neutrophils and zymosan particles: The role of opsonins and divalent cations, *J. Immunol.* **126**:433.

Root, R. K., and Metcalf, J. A., 1977, H_2O_2 release from human granulocytes during phagocytosis. Relationship to superoxide anion formation and cellular catabolism of H_2O_2: Studies with normal and cytochalasin B-treated cells, *J. Clin. Invest.* **60**:1266.

Root, R. K., and Stossel, T. P., 1974, Myeloperoxidase-mediated iodination by granulocytes. Intracellular site of operation and some regulating factors, *J. Clin. Invest.* **53**:1207.

Root, R. K., Metcalf, J., Oshino, N., and Chance, B., 1975, H_2O_2 release from human granulocytes during phagocytosis. I. Documentation, quantitation, and some regulating factors, *J. Clin. Invest.* **55**:945.

Rubin, R. P., Sink, L. E., and Freer, R. J., 1981, On the relationship between formylmethionyl-leucyl-phenylalanine stimulation of arachidonyl phosphatidylinositol turnover and lysosomal enzyme secretion by rabbit neutrophils, *Mol. Pharmacol.* **19**:31.

Rudolph, S. A., Greengard, P., and Malawista, S. E., 1977, Effects of colchicine on cyclic AMP levels in human leukocytes, *Proc. Natl. Acad. Sci. (USA)* **74**:3404.

Sajnani, A. N., Ranadive, N. S., and Movat, H. Z., 1976, Redistribution of immunoglobulin receptors on human neutrophils and its relationship to the release of lysosomal enzymes, *Lab. Invest.* **35**:143.

Schumacher, H. R., and Phelps, P., 1971, Sequential changes in human polymorphonuclear leukocytes after urate crystal phagocytosis. An electron microscopic study, *Arthritis Rheum.* **14**:513.

Scribner, D. J., and Fahrney, D., 1976, Neutrophil receptors for IgG and complement: Their roles in the attachment and ingestion phases of phagocytosis, *J. Immunol.* **116**:892.

Seligmann, B. E., and Gallin, J. I., 1980, Use of lipophilic probes of membrane potential to assess human neutrophil activation. Abnormality in chronic granulomatous disease, *J. Clin. Invest.* **66**:493.

Seligmann, B. E., Gallin, E. K., Martin, D. L., Shain, W., and Gallin, J. I., 1980, Interaction of chemotactic factors with human polymorphonuclear leukocytes: Studies using a membrane potential sensitive dye, *J. Membr. Biol.* **52**:257.

Seligmann, B., Chused, T. M., and Gallin, J. I., 1981, Human neutrophil heterogeneity identified using flow microfluorometry to monitor membrane potential, *J. Clin. Invest.* **68**:1125.

Serhan, C. N., Radin, A., Smolen, J. E., Korchak, H., Samuelsson, B., and Weissmann, G., 1982, Leukotriene B_4 is a complete secretagogue in human neutrophils: A kinetic analysis, *Biochem. Biophys. Res. Commun.* **107**:1006.

Sha'afi, R. I., Naccache, P. H., Molski, T. F. P., Borgeat, P., and Goetzl, E. J., 1981, Cellular regulatory role of leukotriene B_4: Its effects on cation homeostasis in rabbit neutrophils, *J. Cell. Physiol.* **108**:401.

Showell, H. J., Freer, R. J., Zigmond, S. H., Schiffmann, E., Aswanikumar, S., Corcoran,

B., and Becker, E. L., 1976, The structure–activity relations of synthetic peptides as chemotactic factors and inducers of lysosomal enzyme secretion for neutrophils, *J. Exp. Med.* **143**:1154.

Showell, H. J., Naccache, P. H., Sha'afi, R. I., and Becker, E. L., 1977, The effects of extracellular K^+, Na^+ and Ca^{++} on lysosomal enzyme secretion from polymorphonuclear leukocytes, *J. Immunol.* **119**:804.

Showell, H. J., Naccache, P. H., Borgeat, P., Picard, S., Vallerand, P., Becker, E. L., and Sha'afi, R. I., 1982, Characterization of the secretory activity of leukotriene B_4 toward rabbit neutrophils, *J. Immunol.* **128**:811.

Simchowitz, L., and Spilberg, I., 1979, Generation of superoxide radicals by human peripheral neutrophils activated by chemotactic factor. Evidence for the role of calcium, *J. Lab. Clin. Med.* **93**:583.

Simchowitz, L., Fischbein, L. C., Spilberg, I., and Atkinson, J. P., 1980, Induction of a transient elevation in intracellular levels of adenosine-3′,5′-cyclic monophosphate by chemotactic factors: An early event in human neutrophil activation, *J. Immunol.* **124**:1482.

Smith, R. J., 1977, Modulation of phagocytosis by and lysosomal enzyme secretion from guinea-pig neutrophils: Effect of non-steroid anti-inflammatory agents and prostaglandins, *J. Pharmacol. Exp. Ther.* **200**:647.

Smith, R. J., 1978, Nonsteroid anti-inflammatory agents: Regulators of the phagocyte secretion of lysosomal enzymes from guinea-pig neutrophils, *J. Pharmacol. Exp. Ther.* **207**:618.

Smith, R. J., 1979, The guinea pig neutrophil calcium-dependent lysosomal enzyme secretory process. Inhibition by nonsteroid anti-inflammatory agents, *Biochem. Pharmacol.* **28**:2739.

Smith, R. J., and Iden, S. S., 1979, Phorbol myristate acetate-induced release of granule enzymes from human neutrophils: Inhibition by the calcium antagonist, 8-(N,N-diethylamino)-octyl-3,4,5-trimethoxybenzoate hydrochloride, *Biochem. Biophys. Res. Commun.* **91**:263.

Smith, R. J., and Ignarro, L. J., 1975, Bioregulation of lysosomal enzyme secretion from human neutrophils: Roles of guanosine 3′,5′-monophosphate and calcium in stimulus-secretion coupling, *Proc. Natl. Acad. Sci. (USA)* **72**:108.

Smith, R. J., Wierenga, W., and Iden, S. S., 1980, Characteristics of N-formyl-methionyl-leucyl-phenylalanine as an inducer of lysosomal enzyme release from human neutrophils, *Inflammation* **4**:73.

Smith, R. J., Sun, F. F., Iden, S. S., Bowman, B. J., Sprecher, H., and McGuire, J. G., 1981a, An evaluation of the relationship between arachiodonic acid lipoxygenation and human neutrophil degranulation, *Clin. Immunol. Immunopathol.* **20**:157.

Smith, R. J., Bowman, B. J., and Iden, S. S., 1981b, Effects of trifluoperazine on human neutrophil function, *Immunology* **44**:677.

Smolen, J. E., and Weissmann, G., 1980, The effects of indomethacin, 5,8,11,14-eicosatetraynoic acid, and p-bromophenacyl bromide on lysosomal enzyme release and superoxide anion generation by human polymorphonuclear leukocytes, *Biochem. Pharmacol.* **29**:533.

Smolen, J. E., and Weissmann, G., 1981, Stimuli which provoke secretion of azurophil enzymes from human neutrophils induce increments in adenosine cycle 3′,5′-monophosphate, *Biochim. Biophys. Acta* **672**:197.

Smolen, J. E., and Weissmann, G., 1982, The effect of various stimuli and calcium antagonists on the fluorescence response of chlortetracycline-loaded human neutrophils, *Biochim. Biophys. Acta* **720**:172.

Smolen, J. E., Korchak, H. M., and Weissmann, G., 1980, Increased levels of cyclic adenosine-3′,5′-monophosphate in human polymorphonuclear leukocytes after surface stimulation, *J. Clin. Invest.* **65**:1077.

Smolen, J. E., Korchak, H. M., and Weissmann, G., 1981, The roles of extracellular and intracellular calcium in lysosomal enzyme release and superoxide anion generation by human neutrophils, *Biochim. Biophys. Acta* **677**:512.

Spitznagel, J. K., Dalldorf, M. G., Leffell, M. S., Folds, J. D., Welsh, I. R. H., Cooney, M. H., and Martin, L. E., 1974, Character of azurophil and specific granules purified from human polymorphonuclear leukocytes, *Lab. Invest.* **30**:774.

Stenson, W. F., and Parker, C. W., 1979, Metabolism of arachidonic acid in ionophore-stimulated neutrophils. Esterification of a hydroxylated metabolite into phospholipids, *J. Clin. Invest.* **64**:1457.

Stenson, W. F., and Parker, C. W., 1980, Monohydroxyeicosatetraenoic acids (HETEs) induce degranulation of human neutrophils, *J. Immunol.* **124**:2100.

Stolc, V., 1981, Stimulatory effect of latex and zymosan particles on cyclic adenosine 3′,5′-monophosphate content in human granulocytes, *Mol. Immunol.* **18**:773.

Stossel, T. P., 1973, Quantitative studies of phagocytosis. Kinetic effects of cations and heat-labile opsonin, *J. Cell. Biol.* **58**:346.

Stossel, T. P., Pollard, T. D., Mason, R. J., and Vaughan, M., 1971, Isolation and properties of phagocytic vesicles from polymorphonuclear leukocytes, *J. Clin. Invest.* **50**:1745.

Straus, W., 1964, Occurrence of phagosomes and phagolysosomes in different segments of the nephron in relation to the reabsorption, transport, digestion, and extrusion of intravenously injected horseradish peroxidase, *J. Cell. Biol.* **21**:295.

Takeshige, K., Nabi, Z. F., Tatscheck, B., and Minakami, S., 1980, Release of calcium from membranes and its relation to phagocytic metabolic changes: A fluorescence study on leukocytes loaded with chloretetracycline, *Biochem. Biophys. Res. Commun.* **95**: 410.

Tanaka, T., and Hidaka, H., 1981, Interaction of local anesthetics with calmodulin, *Biochem. Biophys. Res. Commun.* **101**:447.

Tauber, A. I., and Babior, B. M., 1977, Evidence for hydroxyl radical production by human neutrophils, *J. Clin. Invest.* **60**:374.

Tedesco, F. S., Trani, S., Soranzo, M. R., and Patriarca, P., 1975, Stimulation of glucose oxidation in human polymorphonuclear leukocytes by C3-Sepharose and soluble C567, *FEBS Lett.* **51**:232.

Traynor, J. R., and Authi, K. S., 1981, Phospholipase A_2 activity of lysosomal origin secreted by polymorphonuclear leukocytes during phagocytosis or on treatment with calcium, *Biochim. Biophys. Acta* **665**:571.

Utsumi, K., Sugiyama, K., Miyahara, M., Naito, M., Auai, M., and Inoue, M., 1977, Effect of concanavalin A on membrane potential of polymorphonuclear leukocytes monitored by fluorescent dye, *Cell. Struct. Funct.* **2**:203.

Volpi, M., Naccache, P. H., and Sha'afi, R. I., 1980, Arachidonic metabolite(s) increase the permeability of the plasma membrane of the neutrophils to calcium, *Biochem. Biophys. Res. Commun.* **92**:1231.

Walenga, R. W., Showell, H. J., Feinstein, M. B., and Becker, E. L., 1980, Parallel inhibition of neutrophil arachidonic acid metabolism and lysosomal enzyme secretion by nordihydroguaiaretic acid, *Life Sci.* **27**:1047.

Walsh, C. E., Waite, B. M., Thomas, M. J., and DeChatelet, L. R., 1981, Release and metabolism of arachidonic acid in human neutrophils, *J. Biol. Chem.* **256**:7228.

Weening, R. S., Wever, R., and Roos, D., 1975, Quantitative aspects of the production of superoxide radicals by phagocytizing human granulocytes, *J. Lab. Clin. Med.* **85**:245.

Weisenberg, R. C., Borisy, G. G., and Taylor, E. W., 1968, The colchicine-binding protein of mammalian brain and its relation to microtubules, *Biochemistry* **7**:4466.

Weissmann, G., 1982, Activation of neutrophils and the lesions of rheumatoid arthritis, *J. Lab. Clin. Med.* **100**:322.

Weissmann, G., and Rita, G. A., 1972, Molecular basis of qouty inflammation: Interaction of monosodium urate crystals with lysosomes and liposomes, *Nature (New Biol.)* **240**:167.

Weissmann, G., and Uhr, J. W., 1968, Studies on lysosomes, IX. Localization of bacteriophages and thorotrast and their inflammatory properties, *Biochem. Pharmacol.* **17**: (Suppl.)5.

Weissmann, G., Hirschhorn, R., and Krakauer, K., 1969, Effect of mellitin upon cellular and lysosomal membranes, *Biochem. Pharmacol.* **18**:1771.

Weissmann, G., Zurier, R. B., Spieler, P. J., and Goldstein, I. M., 1971a, Mechanisms of lysosomal enzyme release from leukocytes exposed to immune complexes and other particles, *J. Exp. Med.* **134**:149s.

Weissmann, G., Dukor, P., and Zurier, R. B., 1971b, Effect of cyclic AMP on release of lysosomal enzymes from phagocytes, *Nature (New Biol.)* **231**:131.

Weissmann, G., Zurier, R. B., and Hoffstein, S., 1972, Leukocytic proteases and the immunologic release of lysosomal enzymes, *Am. J. Pathol.* **68**:539.

Weissmann, G., Goldstein, I., Hoffstein, S., Chauvet, G., and Robineaux, R., 1975a, Yin/ Yang modulation of lysosomal enzyme release from polymorphonuclear leukocytes by cyclic nucleotides, *Ann. NY Acad. Sci.* **256**:222.

Weissmann, G., Goldstein, I., Hoffstein, S., and Tsung, P-K., 1975b, Reciprocal effects of cAMP and cGMP on microtubule-dependent release of lysosomal enzymes, *Ann. NY Acad. Sci.* **253**:750.

Weissmann, G., Korchak, H. M., Perez, H. D., Smolen, J. E., Goldstein, I. M., and Hoffstein, S. T., 1979, The secretory code of the neutrophil, *J. Reticuloendothel. Soc.* **26**:687.

Weissmann, G., Smolen, J. E., and Korchak, H. M., 1980, Release of inflammatory mediators from stimulated neutrophils, *N. Engl. J. Med.* **303**:27.

Welsh, I. R. H., and Spitznagel, J. K., 1971, Distribution of lysosomal enzymes, cationic proteins, and bactericidal substances in subcellular fractions of human polymorphonuclear leukocytes, *Infect. Immun.* **4**:97.

Wentzell, B., and Epand, R. M., 1978, Stimulation of the release of prostaglandins from polymorphonuclear leukocytes by the calcium ionophore A23187, *FEBS Lett.* **86**:255.

West, B. C., Rosenthal, A. S., Gelb, N. A., and Kimball, H. R., 1974, Separation and characterization of human neutrophil granules, *Am. J. Pathol.* **77**:41.

Whitin, J. C., Chapman, C. E., Simons, E. R., Chovaniec, M. E., and Cohen, H. J., 1980, Correlation between membrane potential changes and superoxide production in human granulocytes stimulated by phorbol myristate acetate. Evidence for defective activation in chronic granulomatous disease, *J. Biol. Chem.* **255**:1874.

Wright, D. G., and Gallin, J. I., 1979, Secretory responses of human neutrophils: Exocytosis of specific (secondary) granules by human neutrophils during adherence *in vitro* and during exudation *in vivo, J. Immunol.* **123**:285.

Wright, D. G., and Malawista, S. E., 1972, The mobilization and extracellular release of granular enzymes from human leukocytes during phagocytosis, *J. Cell. Biol.* **53**:788.

Wright, D. G., and Malawista, S. E., 1973, Mobilization and extracellular release of granular enzymes from human leukocytes during phagocytosis. Inhibition by colchicine and cortisol but not by salicylate, *Arthritis Rheum.* **16**:749.

Wright, D. G., Bralove, D. A., and Gallin, J. I., 1977, The differential mobilization of human neutrophil granules. Effects of phorbol myristate acetate and ionophore A23187, *Am. J. Pathol.* **87**:273.

Wunderlich, F., Muller, R., and Speth, V., 1973, Direct evidence for a colchicine-induced impairment in the mobility of membrane components, *Science* **182**:1136.

Zabucchi, G., and Romeo, D., 1976, The dissociation of exocytosis and respiratory stimulation in leucocytes by ionophores, *Biochem. J.* **156**:209.

Zeya, H. I., and Spitznagel, J. K., 1971, Characterization of cationic protein-bearing granules of polymorphonuclear leukocytes, *Lab. Invest.* **24**:229.

Zigmond, S. H., and Hirsch, J. G., 1972, Effects of cytochalasin B on polymorphonuclear leukocyte locomotion, phagocytosis, and glycolysis, *Exp. Cell. Res.* **73**:383.

Zucker-Franklin, D., and Hirsch, J. G., 1964, Electron microscope studies on the degranulation of rabbit peritoneal leukocytes during phagocytosis, *J. Exp. Med.* **120**:569.

Zurier, R. B., and Sayadoff, D. M., 1975, Release of prostaglandins from human polymorphonuclear leukocytes, *Inflammation* **1**:93.

Zurier, R. B., Hoffstein, S., and Weissmann, G., 1973*a*, Mechanisms of lysosomal enzyme release from leukocytes. I. Effect of cyclic nucleotides and colchicine, *J. Cell. Biol.* **58**:27.

Zurier, R. B., Hoffstein, S., and Weissmann, G., 1973*b*, Cytochalasin B. Effect on lysosomal enzyme release from human leucocytes, *Proc. Natl. Acad. Sci. (USA)* **70**:844.

Zurier, R. B., Weissmann, G., Hoffstein, S., Kammerman, S., and Tai, H.-H., 1974, Mechanisims of lysosomal enzyme release from leukocytes. II. Effects of cAMP and cGMP, autonomic agonists, and agents which affect microtubule function, *J. Clin. Invest.* **53**:297.

Chapter 8

Exocytosis by Neutrophils

Marco Baggiolini* and Beatrice Dewald*

Research Institute Wander
A Sandoz Research Unit
Wander Ltd.
CH-3001 Berne, Switzerland

I. INTRODUCTION

Neutrophils are short-lived, highly specialized phagocytes. Their main function is to defend the host organism against invading microbes. The properties required to perform this function are chemotactic responsiveness, mobility, and the ability to phagocytose. Microorganisms are sensed through the chemotactic signals they emit or induce; are approached by the neutrophils, which move actively toward the source of these signals; and are engulfed and killed within the phagocytic vacuoles. Killing depends on the activation of the respiratory burst, which generates microbicidal oxygen metabolites, and on the release of enzymes and other proteins stored in the granules.

Neutrophil function is intimately linked to inflammation. An inflammatory reaction always accompanies infections; its magnitude usually depends on the extent of neutrophil infiltration. Inflammation in this case is linked to the release of neutrophil products—superoxide and congeners, arachidonic acid oxygenation metabolites, and lytic enzymes—into the pericellular environment.

The release of neutrophil products is involved both in preventing and inducing disease, i.e., in preventing infection and inducing inflammation. Knowledge of the mechanisms is therefore important. A distant but not altogether unrealistic goal is to find means to modulate these processes with therapeutic agents. This chapter describes the release of macromolecules—mostly enzymes—from

*Present address: Theodor Kocher Institute, University of Berne, CH-3000 Berne 9, Switzerland.

the different intracellular storage compartments of human neutrophils. Since active release is always induced by a selective stimulation of the cells, the interrelationship of release with other responses, i.e., the respiratory burst and the liberation and metabolism of arachidonic acid, will also be considered.

II. PATHWAYS OF EXOCYTOSIS

The active release of enzymes and other macromolecules from intracellular stores may be termed export from the cell, or exocytosis. This event requires fusion of the subcellular storage organelles with the plasma membrane. Since the neutrophil is a phagocyte, two pathways of exocytosis must be distinguished: (1) the release into phagocytic vacuoles by fusion of storage organelles with portions of the plasmalemma, which are committed to form or have already formed phagocytic vacuoles, and (2) phagocytosis-independent release by fusion of storage organelles with areas of the plasma membrane that are not involved in phagocytic uptake. The latter pathway is properly termed secretion. As will be seen, the differentiation between release into phagosomes and secretion is justified by the distinct kinetics of exocytosis from different subcellular storage compartments. However, if one looks at the appearance of storage enzymes in the cell-free suspending medium, the differentiation of the two mechanisms of exocytosis might appear unnecessary.

Enzyme release from neutrophils also occurs in a nonselective manner after membrane breakdown. Many neutrophils die at the site of infection. Rupture of the plasmalemma and of intracellular membranes results in this case in the indiscriminate release of all cellular enzymes, those of the cytosol as well as those confined to structured subcellular compartments. An alternative mechanism of nonselective liberation of enzymes is brought about by toxic lysosomotropic agents (see review by de Duve *et al.*, 1974, for a definition of lysosomotropism). Particulate or soluble agents that accumulate in the vacuolar (lysosomal) compartment after endocytosis or by diffusion may rupture the lysosomal membranes from within (Weissmann, 1971) and lead to cytolysis and loss of enzymes.

III. SUBCELLULAR STORAGE COMPARTMENTS OF THE NEUTROPHIL

A. Rabbit Heterophil Leukocytes

The identification and separation of two types of granules in neutrophils was achieved more than 10 years ago; hence the brief description that follows may be regarded as indulging in reminiscences. Rabbit heterophils, which are obtained in large numbers and in high purity in peritoneal exudates induced with glycogen, have been the accepted model since Cohn and Hirsch (1960a) first separated a granule fraction by differential centrifugation. A distinction between azurophil (or primary) and specific (or secondary) granules was first made by electron microscopic investigation of maturing rabbit heterophils. Bainton and Farquhar (1966) and Wetzel et al. (1967) described independently that a first population of granules is formed in the promyelocytes and a second one in the myelocytes. The choice of the species turned out to be fortunate: in rabbit heterophil leukocytes, the two types of granules differ sufficiently to permit their identification by conventional electron microscopy, and the Golgi apparatus where they are formed is particularly well developed. Rabbit heterophils were the obvious choice for subcellular fractionation. Since azurophil granules are both larger and denser than the specific granules, it was possible to resolve the two populations on the basis of either sedimentation or isopyknic equilibration (Baggiolini et al., 1969, 1970b). These experiments opened the way to the analysis of the biochemical composition of the two granules (Baggiolini et al., 1969, 1970a, b) and a reevaluation of the biochemical data already available (Baggiolini, 1972). Within a few years, the combination of electron microscopy and subcellular fractionation established firmly that the granules of neutrophils belong to two distinct populations of storage organelles that are formed at separate stages of cell maturation and that differ almost completely in their biochemical composition. On this basis, several groups of investigators began to work on human neutrophils, which were investigated thoroughly.

B. Human Neutrophil Granules

The maturation of human neutrophils was described by Bainton et al. (1971), who adopted the cytochemical staining technique for peroxidase to distinguish clearly between the azurophil granules, which contain this enzyme, and the specific granules, which lack it. The maturation process is similar to that first described in the rabbit. The use of peroxidase cytochemistry permitted exploration of the process of granule production in greater detail. In the promyelocytes, which form the azurophil granules, peroxidase is detectable throughout the endoplasmic reticulum and the Golgi apparatus, suggesting that during granule formation the whole machinery for synthesis and packaging of export enzymes is actively engaged.

Figures 1 and 2 represent sedimentation and isopyknic equilibration profiles of lysozyme and peroxidase, the two enzymes originally used as markers for the granules of human neutrophils (Bretz and Baggiolini, 1974). Fractionation techniques adopted for the studies of rabbit cells yielded virtually the same degree of resolution between azurophil and specific granules. Data presented in the same year by Spitznagel et al. (1974) and by West et al. (1974) were in keeping with our results: peroxidase, the characteristic constituent of azurophil gran-

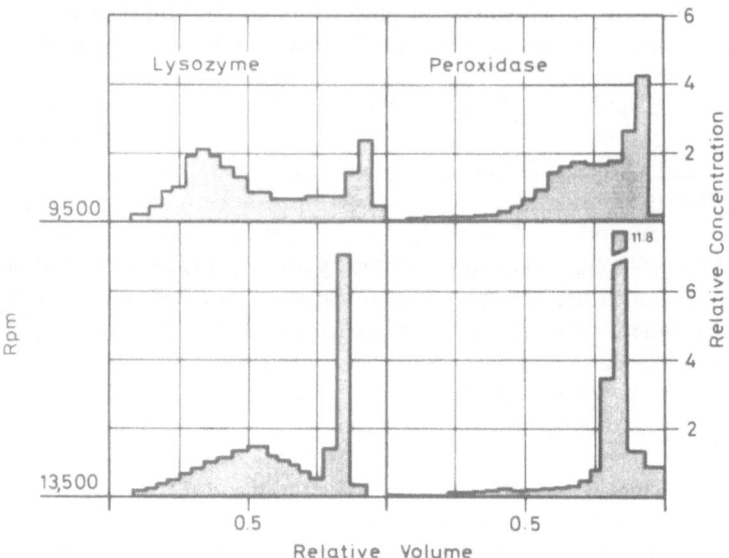

Figure 1. Resolution of azurophil and specific granules from human neutrophils by zonal differential sedimentation, showing the distribution profiles of lysozyme, which is localized in both granules, and of myeloperoxidase, which is present in the azurophil granules only. Results were obtained by a 15-min centrifugation at the angular velocities indicated. The azurophil granules sediment about four times faster than the specific granules and reach the outer limit of the gradient (right-hand side of histogram) in both experiments. (From Bretz and Baggiolini, 1974.)

ules, showed a unimodal profile and lysozyme, which is present in both granules, a bimodal profile. By zonal centrifugation in sucrose gradients of relatively high density, Spitznagel et al. (1974) and West et al. (1974) obtained data that suggested the existence of two subpopulations of azurophil granules differing somewhat in biochemical composition. Similar data were later reported by Wright et al. (1977).

Since 1974, numerous subcellular fractionation studies have helped identify many of the proteins stored in the granules, an updated list of which is presented in Table I. It can be readily seen that a great deal is known about the contents of the azurophil granules, while the information on the specific granules remains limited. The azurophil granules contain many acid hydrolases commonly found in lysosomes. Acid β-glycerophosphatase, several acid glycosidases, and two acid cathepsins were directly shown to be localized in the azurophil granules by fractionation experiments, such as those by Bretz and Baggiolini (1974), Spitznagel et al. (1974), West et al. (1974), and Baggiolini et al. (1978). In addition, many enzymes of this kind, i.e., acid ribonuclease (Cohn and Hirsch, 1960a), addi-

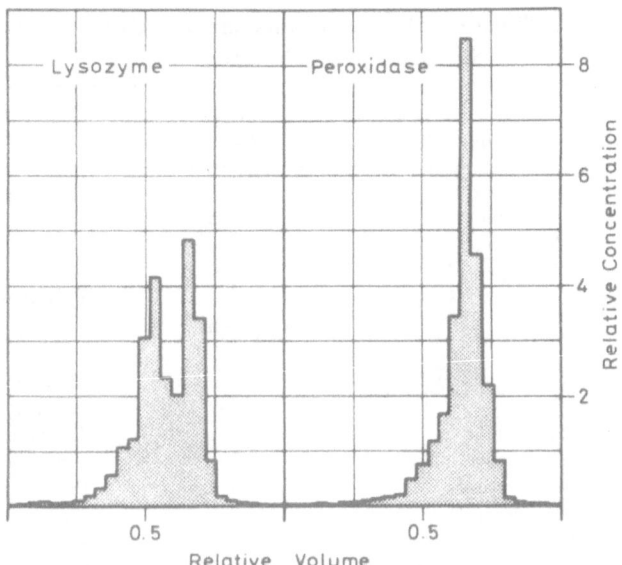

Figure 2. Resolution of azurophil and specific granules from human blood neutrophils by isopyknic equilibration in a sucrose gradient. The average densities of the specific and azurophil granules are 1.20 and 1.23 g/ml, respectively. (From Bretz and Baggiolini, 1974.)

tional acid glycosidases (Baggiolini, 1972; Avila and Convit, 1973), and aryl sulfatase (Bainton and Farquhar, 1968) were identified in whole granule preparations or neutrophil lysates or were demonstrated by cytochemistry. Taken together, these observations indicated that the azurophil granules have the complete enzymatic equipment of lysosomes (de Duve and Wattiaux, 1966). These granules, however, have a number of major consituents not normally found in lysosomes, i.e., myeloperoxidase (Bretz and Baggiolini, 1974; Spitznagel *et al.*, 1974), lysozyme (Bretz and Baggiolini, 1974; Spitznagel *et al.*, 1974), and neutral serine proteinases (Dewald *et al.*, 1975). With this outfit, azurophil granules appear perfectly suited to fulfil the main function of neutrophils in host defense, namely killing and digestion of phagocytosed microorganisms. The specific granules share lysozyme with the azurophils (Bretz and Baggiolini, 1974; Spitznagel *et al.*, 1974) and contain in addition a specific collagenase (Murphy *et al.*, 1977, 1980), lactoferrin (Leffell and Spitznagel, 1972), and vitamin B_{12}-binding protein (Kane and Peters, 1975). The function of these constituents is not self-evident, and an insight into the role of specific granules in the pathophysiology of the neutrophil will depend on further information on their biochemical composition.

Table I. Subcellular Localization of Enzymes and Other Constituents
Stored in Human Neutrophils[a]

Class of constituents	Azurophil granules	Specific granules	Smaller storage organelles[b]
Microbicidal enzymes	Myeloperoxidase		
	Lysozyme	Lysozyme	
Neutral proteinases	Elastase		
	Cathepsin G		
	Proteinase 3		Proteinase 3
		Collagenase	
			Gelatinase
			Plasminogen activator (?)
Acid hydrolases	N-Acetyl-β-glucosaminidase		N-Acetyl-β-glucosaminidase
	Cathepsin B		Cathepsin B
	Cathepsin D		Cathepsin D
	β-Glucuronidase		β-Glucuronidase
	β-Glycerophosphatase		β-Glycerophosphatase
	α-Mannosidase		α-Mannosidase
Other		Lactoferrin	
		Vitamin B_{12}-binding proteins	

[a]Attributions that are still uncertain are followed by a questionmark (?).
[b]Heterogeneous population of organelles including the C particles and secretory vesicles, which are postulated as the carrier of gelatinase.

C. Smaller Storage Organelles

In our first fractionation studies, we described a minor population of smaller organelles containing acid hydrolases, which were termed C particles (Baggiolini et al., 1969, 1970b; Bretz and Baggiolini, 1974). Unlike the granules, the C particles were never identified by electron microscopy either in intact cells or in subcellular fractions. Zonal differential sedimentation, however, clearly reveals their presence as a population of structures, possibly heterogeneous in composition, which are considerably smaller than the specific granules. Later work showed that structures of this type contain large proportions of cathepsin B and D and of a still ill-defined serine proteinase, distinct from elastase and cathepsin G, which we call proteinase 3 (Baggiolini et al., 1978).

Most recently we found that gelatinase, a metalloproteinase discovered in neutrophils by Sopata and Dancewicz (1974), is localized exclusively in such small organelles (Murphy et al., 1980; Dewald et al., 1982). Figure 3 shows the resolution of the gelatinase-containing particles from the granules and the membrane fraction of human neutrophils by zonal differential sedimentation.

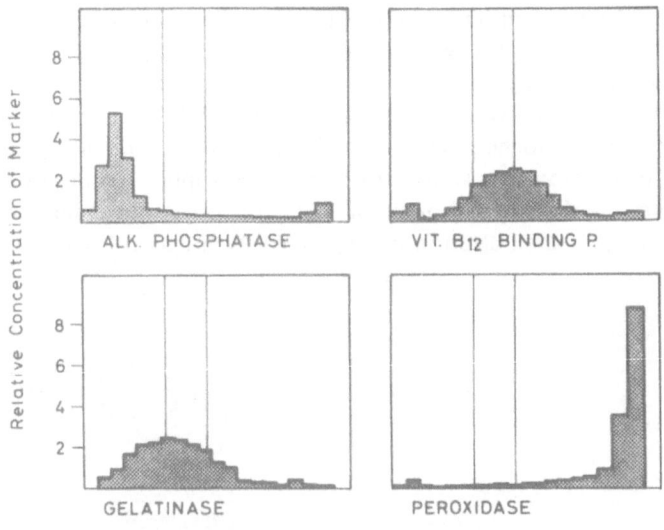

Figure 3. Resolution of four populations of subcellular particles from human blood neutrophils by zonal differential sedimentation. A novel population of storage organelles containing gelatinase is identified. The experimental conditions are identical to those presented in Figure 1, lower graphs. The azurophil granules (peroxidase) are found at the outer limit and the specific granules (vitamin B_{12}-binding protein) in the middle of the gradient. Alkaline phosphatase indicates the position of membrane fragments of various subcellular origin. The particles containing gelatinase distribute at an intermediate position between the membranes and the specific granules. They are smaller than the specific granules and are clearly larger, in terms of mass, than the membrane fragments. Vertical lines indicate the modal relative sedimentation velocities of the specific granules and the novel organelles. (From Dewald *et al.*, 1982.)

IV. RELEASE OF ENZYMES AND OTHER EXPORT PROTEINS

A. Granule Discharge into Phagocytic Vacuoles

The disappearance of the granules from neutrophils engaged in phagocytosis had already been observed by Metchnikoff and his contemporaries. A real-life account of this phagocytosis-dependent process was obtained many years later by phase-contrast microscopy and microcinematography (Robineaux and Frederick, 1955; Hirsch, 1962), and a detailed description of the discharge of the granules into phagocytic vacuoles (which actually proved that Metchnikoff's understanding of degranulation was correct) was then provided by Cohn and Hirsch (1960 a, b) and by Zucker-Franklin and Hirsch (1964) using both biochemical and electron microscopic techniques.

Once the granules were characterized, the question arose as to whether both

types would be released into vacuoles. In a cytochemical study of rabbit heterophil leukocytes, Bainton (1973) found evidence to suggest that the fusion of
specific and azurophil granules with phagocytic vacuoles is sequential. Unfortunately, this type of investigation is not feasible with human neutrophils because
of the lack of a cytochemical marker for the specific granules. On the other
hand, the high peroxidase activity of human neutrophils has been of invaluable
help in assessing the site and mode of discharge of the azurophil granules. This
point can be illustrated electron micrographically. Figures 4 and 5 show human

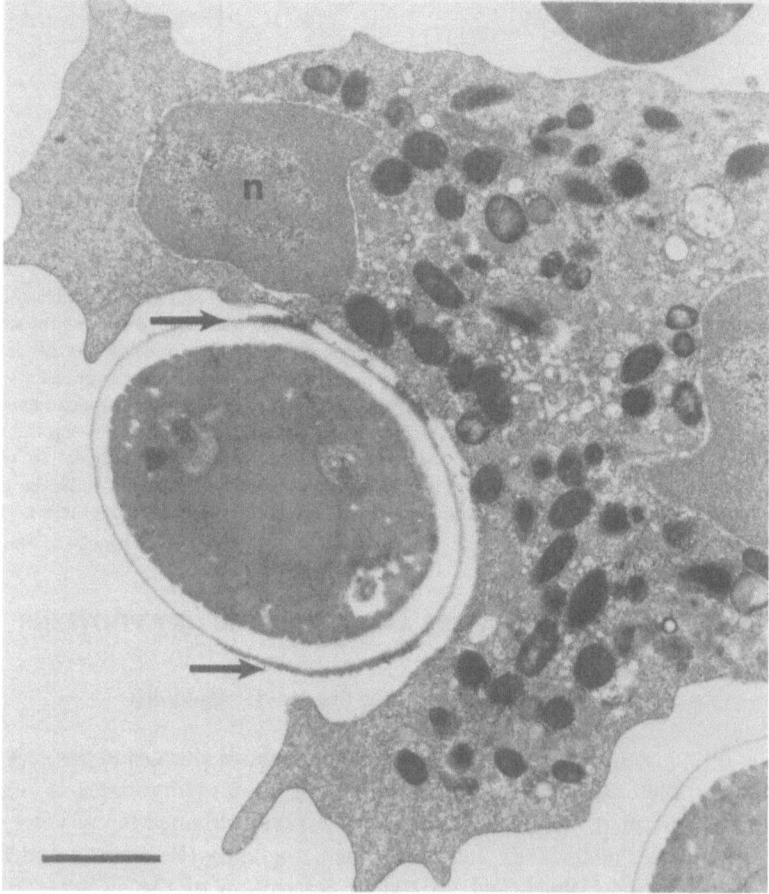

Figure 4. Partial electron microscopic view of a human peripheral blood neutrophil in
the process of phagocytosing a yeast cell. The forming vacuole is still wide open, but granular
discharge has already occurred. At three sites on the surface of the yeast cell, deposits of
peroxidase-positive azurophil granule content are clearly seen (arrows), (n) nucleus. Scale bar =
1 μm.

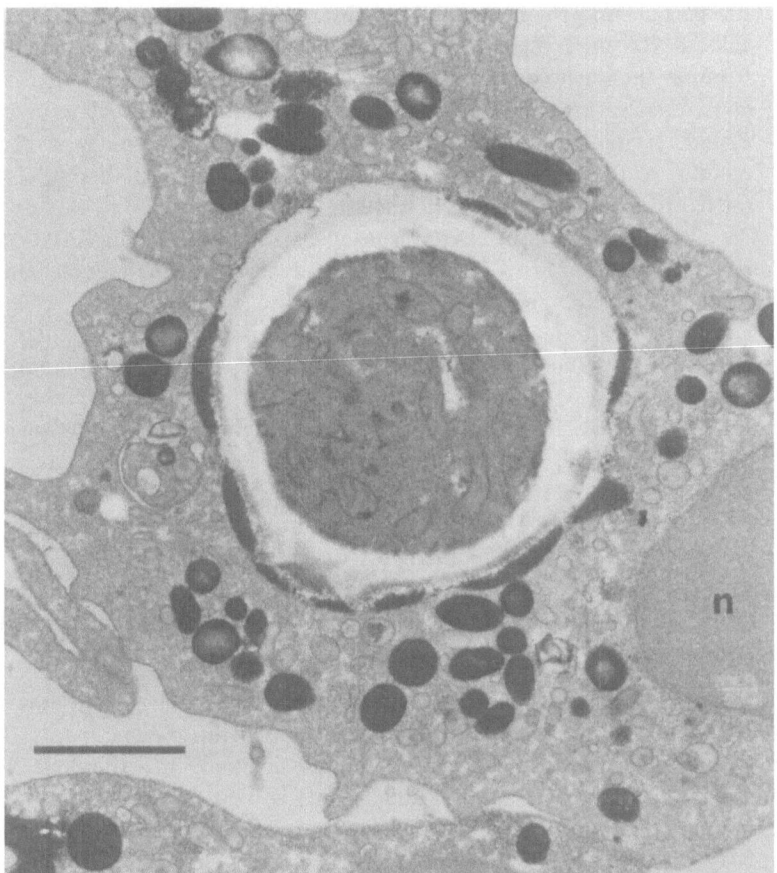

Figure 5. Partial electron microscopic view of a human peripheral blood neutrophil that has phagocytosed a yeast cell. Staining for peroxidase activity reveals the azurophil granules. Many of these granules have already fused with the phagocytic vacuole. Large amounts of peroxidase-positive granule content are seen in close apposition with the endocytosed yeast, (n) nucleus. Scale bar = 1 μm.

neutrophils in the process of phagocytosing opsonized yeast cells—our preferred particles for morphological studies, since they induce the formation of large phagocytic vacuoles and are not degraded intracellularly. Two situations are shown: an early contact between a neutrophil and a particle (Fig. 4) and a complete phagocytic vacuole (Fig. 5). These and similar electron micrographs from many laboratories provide essential information about the fate of the azurophil granules:

1. The discharge of azurophil granules is initiated by the contact between

the particle and the neutrophil membrane. The granules which, in resting cells, never enter the ectoplasm are seen in contact with the membrane forming the vacuole. Fusion and release of the granule contents is the consequence. This early event occurs long before the vacuole is completed. It remains restricted to that portion of the neutrophil plasma membrane that is stimulated by particle contact and is therefore committed to forming a phagocytic vacuole.

2. Granule discharge is massive, resulting in a very high concentration of enzymes in the thin space between the membrane of the vacuole and the particulate target.

3. The loss of significant amounts of granule enzymes into the phagocyte environment from still incomplete vacuoles is a common consequence of phagocytosis.

4. Since granule discharge already occurs into incomplete vacuoles, neutrophils have the capacity to attack and degrade in a directed way extracellular substrates that are too large to be engulfed. An even more telling view of the extent of granule discharge into phagocytic vacuoles is provided by electron microscopic study of freeze-fractured neutrophils. The surfaces of phagocytic vacuoles exposed by this technique reveal by their bumpy appearance the sites of fusion of innumerable granules (Amherdt et al., 1978).

Although qualitative in nature, these electron microscopic observations help rationalize the more complete data provided by biochemical experiments. That phagocytosing neutrophils release granule-bound enzymes into the pericellular environment was first observed by Ohta (1964) and by Burke et al., (1964). These findings were confirmed and expanded in many laboratories (see Henson, 1971a; May et al., 1970; Weissmann et al., 1971 for early references). It was then found that the extent of release increased with the phagocytic load and the size of the particles used (Henson, 1971a; Wright and Malawista, 1972; Henson et al., 1972; Leffell and Spitznagel, 1975), in agreement with the notion of enzymes escaping from incomplete vacuoles. Related experiments by Henson (1971b), who used immune complexes attached to membrane filters as the stimulus, showed—as one would expect from the morphological observation—that surface stimulation even by particles that cannot be internalized is sufficient to induce granule discharge. An important observation was that the release of specific granule contents, i.e., lysozyme and lactoferrin, was more rapid and more abundant than that of azurophil granule enzymes, such as acid glycosidases, myeloperoxidase, and neutral proteinase (Taichman et al., 1972; Leffell and Spitznagel, 1974, 1975; Bentwood and Henson, 1980). This finding suggested that the discharge of specific granules (which cannot be monitored microscopically) may be regulated in a different manner from that of the azurophils.

Of particular interest, in this respect, is the investigation by Leffell and Spitznagel (1974, 1975). These investigators exposed human neutrophils to Latex beads covered with immune complexes or different immunoglobulins and determined the proportions of lactoferrin and myeloperoxidase released into the phagosomes and to the exterior. They recovered lactoferrin mainly in the medium and myeloperoxidase mainly in the phagosome fraction, suggesting a difference in the mechanisms of release of specific and azurophil granules.

It is possible that lactoferrin escapes more easily to the exterior if one assumes, as suggested by the data of Bainton (1973) with rabbit heterophils, that specific granules fuse rapidly at early stages of vacuole formation. The simplest interpretation of these findings, however, is that specific granules, in contrast to the azurophils, are discharged both into phagocytic vacuoles and at plasma membrane sites not engaged in particle uptake.

B. Phagocytosis-Independent Release of Granule Contents

The interaction with a particulate target (and the ensuing phagocytosis) is the ultimate and most potent stimulus for neutrophils. Before engaging in phagocytosis, however, neutrophils respond to chemotactic signals. Chemotactic factors and other soluble molecules that interact with binding or affinity sites on the neutrophil membrane were found to induce exocytosis. Stimulus-dependent enzyme release by neutrophils is often studied after pretreatment of the cells with cytochalasin B, a compound that markedly enhances their responsiveness. In this section we describe the responses of untreated (i.e., normal) neutrophils and deal with cytochalasin B-treated cells separately.

Woodin (1962) and Woodin and Wieneke (1964) were the first to show convincingly that neutrophils selectively secrete granule enzymes. In rabbit heterophil leukocytes treated with leukocidin, vitamin A, or streptolysin O (Woodin and Wieneke, 1964, 1966), these workers observed the release of β-glucuronidase, myeloperoxidase, and some other enzymes later found to be stored in the azurophil granules (Baggiolini et al., 1969), but did not observe an apparent release of aldolase, a cytosol marker. This work emphasized the importance of calcium ions for release and suggested that both calcium and adenosine triphosphate (ATP) are necessary for the coalescence between granules and plasma membrane.

Unfortunately, the thorough and systematic studies of Woodin and Wieneke have not been followed up in other laboratories. Leukocidin and streptolysin-O were shown to induce abundant exocytosis of azurophil granule contents, in strong contrast with all other soluble stimuli, considered in this section. It would appear important to test such bacterial products on human neutrophils with today's knowledge of the distinct subcellular storage compartments of these cells. Release of granule contents independent of phagocytosis was subsequently reported by Estensen et al. (1974). These investigators showed that phorbol myristate acetate (PMA) induces the rapid release of lysozyme in a concentration-dependent fashion, but little or no release of β-glucuronidase and myeloperoxidase, and concluded that selective discharge of specific granules was taking place. The effect of PMA was confirmed by Goldstein *et al.* 1974, 1975*a*); further information was provided by Wright *et al.* (1977), who showed that the selective release of lysozyme induced by PMA resulted in a marked reduction of the size of the specific granule fraction recovered upon subcellular fractionation. No release of enzymes from the azurophil granules and no change in their subcellular fractionation profiles was observed.

In connection with this demonstration of the selective effect of PMA on exocytosis from specific granules, an inconsistency of the original studies should be pointed out. Estensen *et al.* (1974) reported that alkaline phosphatase was released together with lysozyme, apparently in keeping with a gradual loss of histochemical alkaline phosphatase reactivity (White and Estensen, 1974). Alkaline phosphatase, however, is not a specific granule enzyme in human neutrophils (Bretz and Baggiolini, 1974; Spitznagel *et al.*, 1974). It was recognized as a marker of the specific granules of rabbit heterophils (Baggiolini *et al.*, 1969) but was subsequently shown to be associated with the granule membrane and not to be part of the granule content (Bretz and Baggiolini, 1973). This explains why, even in the case of the rabbit, little alkaline phosphatase activity is liberated upon phagocytosis (Henson, 1971*a*). A similar pattern and extent of enzyme release was found to be induced by the ionophore A23187 in the presence of calcium (Goldstein *et al.*, 1974; Koza *et al.*, 1975). Again, lysozyme release was paralleled by a loss of specific granules, as evidenced by subcellular fractionation (Wright *et al.*, 1977). Concanavalin A, another agent known to bind to the neutrophil membrane (Ryan *et al.*, 1974), also induced the selective discharge of specific granules (Hoffstein *et al.*, 1976). Its effect resulted from the interaction with mannosyl residues of membrane glycoproteins, as suggested by the inhibition of release with α-methyl-mannoside.

Enzyme release induced by peptides and other factors formed during infection and inflammation is of particular interest because of its possible implications in neutrophil physiology. The effect of $C5a_{des\ Arg}$, or zymosan-activated serum, was studied in a number of laboratories, in most cases, however, on cytochalasin B-treated neutrophils only. In normal neutrophils, C5a was found to induce some exocytosis from specific but not from azurophil granules (Henson *et al.*, 1978; Bentwood and Henson, 1980). These results are in accord with those of Goldstein *et al.* (1975*b*), who showed that C5a stimulates human neutrophils to produce superoxide, but not to release β-glucuronidase, and those of Wright and Gallin (1979), who observed lysozyme but no β-glucuronidase release by adherent human neutrophils exposed to partially purified C5a. Chemotactic factors extracted from bacterial culture filtrates (Becker *et al.*, 1974) and the synthetic chemotactic peptides, formylmethionyl-leucyl-phenylalanine, (fMet-Leu-Phe) and analogues, originally described by Schiffmann *et al.* (1975) also induce the release of granule enzymes. Lysozyme was regularly released to a greater extent than β-glucuronidase; this process was accentuated by pretreatment of the neutrophils with cytochalasin B (Becker and Showell, 1974; Showell et al., 1976). The release of specific granule contents by human neutrophils stimulated with fMet-Leu-Phe or pepstatin was reported in subsequent work (Fehr and Dahinden, 1979; Dahinden and Fehr, 1980). Pepstatin is a pentapeptide of microbial origin that binds to the fMet-Leu-Phe receptor of neutrophils (Nelson et al., 1979). In our study on gelatinase secretion (Dewald et al., 1982) we found that fMet-Leu-Phe, PMA, and A23187 induce significant release of the specific granule constituent vitamin B_{12}-binding protein, but no release of β-glucuronidase from normal human neutrophils. Selective exocytosis of specific granule contents was also found with leukocytic pyrogen, another peptide of biological interest (Klempner et al., 1978).

Two kinds of cellular lipids were recently shown to activate neutrophils: leukotriene B_4 (LTB_4) and platelet-activating factor (PAF). It should be noted that both agents are produced by activated neutrophils and are acting as stimuli on the same cells. LTB_4 and its unstable precursor LTA_4 were identified as products of human neutrophils supplied with arachidonic acid and stimulated with the ionophore A23187 by Borgeat and Samuelsson (1979) and Radmark et al. (1980). LTB_4 was subsequently found to be released by neutrophils exposed to opsonized zymosan (Claessen et al., 1981) or fMet-Leu-Phe (Jubiz et al., 1982). Under the latter conditions, the 20-hydroxy and the 1,20-dioic acid derivatives of LTB_4, formed by ω-oxidation, were also identified as products (Jubiz et al., 1982).

A possible role of LTB_4 in inflammation was suggested by the work of Ford-Hutchinson et al. (1980), who showed that LTB_4 induces chemokinesis and aggregation of human neutrophils with a potency comparable to that of C5a and fMet-Leu-Phe and far superior to that of monohydroxy-eicosanoids. LTB_4 is also equipotent with C5a as a chemotactic agent (Goetzl and Pickett, 1981; Showell et al., 1982) and is proinflammatory (Bray et al., 1981). Several investigators have reported that LTB_4 induces exocytosis by cytochalasin-B-treated neutrophils (Goetzl and Pickett, 1980; Rae and Smith, 1981). In rabbit neutrophils, exocytosis was reported to depend fully on the presence of cytochalasin B. However, a study by Hafstrom et al. (1981) documents a significant selective release of lysozyme from normal human neutrophils. A number of papers concur in showing that fMet-Leu-Phe is both more potent and more effective than LTB_4 in inducing exocytosis (Goetzl and Pickett, 1980; Rae and Smith, 1981; Hafstrom et al., 1981; Feinmark et al., 1981; Showell et al., 1982). The secretory effects described appear to be specific for LTB_4. 5-Hydroxy-eicosatetraenoic acid (5-HETE), LTC_4, and two LTB_4 isomers produced concomitantly with LTB_4 were found to be inactive (Hafstrom et al., 1981). PAF or AGEPC, a plasmalogen with the structure 1-O-alkyl-2-acetyl-sn-glyceryl-3-phosphocholine (Benveniste et al., 1979; Demopoulos et al., 1979), is produced by neutrophils undergoing phagocytosis or challenged with soluble stimuli (Sanchez-Crespo et al., 1980; Camussi et al., 1981) by a process that appears to be independent of the respiratory burst and granule discharge (Betz and Henson, 1980). The effect of PAF on neutrophil secretion is still unclear. Shaw et al. (1981), Smith and Bowman (1982), and Ingraham et al. (1982) reported that PAF induces exocytosis by neutrophils only upon treatment with cytochalasin B. Jouvin-Marche et al. (1982), however, who compared synthetic PAF with its 2-lyso derivative and lysophosphatidylcholine, showed a concentration-dependent release of sizable amounts of lysozyme and small but significant amounts of β-glucuronidase and acid phosphatase from normal human neutrophils incubated for 1 hr with 0.01 and 0.1 μM PAF. At even lower concentrations, synthetic PAF enhanced the release of specific and azurophil granule enzymes induced by phagocytosis of opsonized zymosan.

Release of specific granule contents was also observed in the absence of added stimuli. Corcino et al. (1970) reported the liberation of relatively large amounts of vitamin B_{12}-binding protein by human neutrophils incubated at 37°C in Hank's balanced salt solution. This finding can be interpreted today as discharge of specific granules, the subcellular store of vitamin B_{12}-binding proteins. Similarly, Goldstein et al. (1974) observed the release of some lysozyme in the presence of calcium and phosphate ions, in the absence of an added stimulus.

C. Exocytosis from Smaller Storage Organelles

We have already pointed out that one or more populations of small storage organelles, distinct from the granules, are revealed by subcellular fractionation of neutrophil homogenates. The recent discovery of gelatinase as an exclusive constituent (Murphy et al., 1980) made it possible to study some of the properties of this storage compartment in living neutrophils (Dewald et al., 1982). Gelatinase is released after challenge of the neutrophils with soluble or particulate stimuli. Exocytosis from this compartment is more rapid and much more extensive than from specific and azurophil granules, as illustrated in Figures 6 and 7. Figure 6 shows the time course of release induced by PMA at moderate concentration and during phagocytosis of opsonized zymosan. Within 30 min, 50–70% of the gelatinase is liberated; most of this activity is already detectable in the incubation medium within 10 min of stimulation. In both cases, there is significant release of vitamin B_{12}-binding protein from the specific granules, whereas release of β-glucuronidase, a constituent of the azurophil granules, is observed only during phagocytosis. The latter finding illustrates the differential discharge of the two types of granules and is in accord with the data obtained in several other laboratories, as discussed above. The left-hand graphs of Fig. 6 show that a considerable proportion of the gelatinase is released even in the absence of added stimuli, provided that the blood samples or the buffy coats from which the neutrophils are prepared are aged in the cold for some time (24 hr in our case).

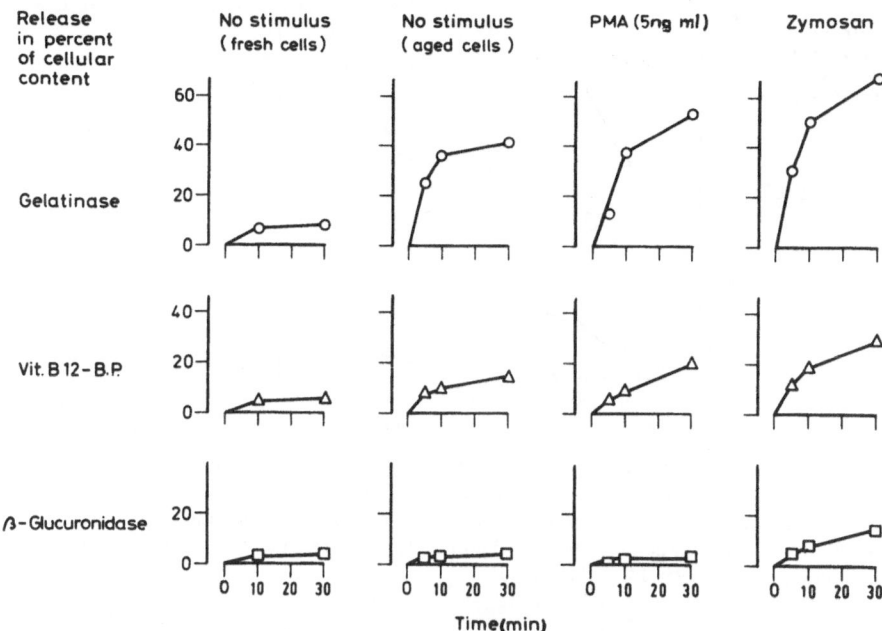

Figure 6. Time course of the release of gelatinase (small secretory organelles), vitamin B_{12}-binding protein (specific granules) and β-glucuronidase (azurophil granules) from human neutrophils. Freshly prepared cells were exposed to phorbol myristate acetate (PMA) or opsonized zymosan, and the percentage of markers released into the incubation medium was determined. Fresh cells and cells prepared from buffy coats of donor blood aged at 4°C for 24 hr were incubated as above without the addition of stimuli. (From Dewald *et al.*, 1982.)

Under these conditions, small but significant amounts of vitamin B_{12}-binding protein are also released from the specific granules, which agrees with the observations of Corcino *et al.* (1970) and Goldstein *et al.* (1974) mentioned in Section IV. B. Figure 7 illustrates the dependence of secretion on the concentration of the stimuli. Increasing levels of PMA and A23187 induce a progressive release of gelatinase up to 80% of the cellular content within 10 min. The response to fMet-Leu-Phe is different: gelatinase release reaches a plateau corresponding to about 25% of the initial cellular content, already at very low stimulus concentrations. The secretion of vitamin B_{12}-binding protein follows a similar pattern, but at a much lower level. Exocytosis from the specific granules is marked after PMA or A23187 stimulation, but only minimal after fMet-Leu-Phe stimulation. A similar situation is encountered with activated serum as a source of $C5a_{des\ Arg}$. Whereas release of gelatinase reaches 30–40%, release of vitamin B_{12}-binding protein does not exceed 10% (Table II). The discrete effects of chemotactic peptides on normal neutrophils have often been overlooked. Most

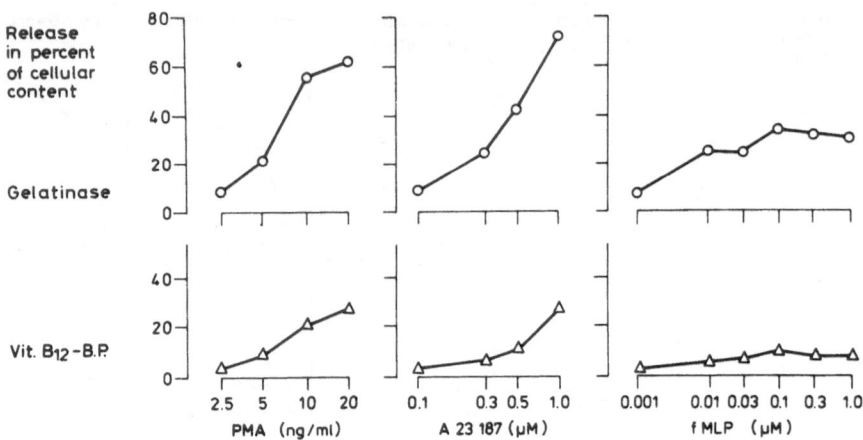

Figure 7. Secretion of gelatinase and vitamin B_{12}-binding protein from freshly prepared human neutrophils stimulated with phorbol myristate acetate (PMA), A23187, and fMet-Leu-Phe (fMLP), with dependence on stimulus concentration. The amount of markers released into the incubation medium in 10 min is expressed as a percentage of the initial cellular content. (From Dewald *et al.*, 1982.)

investigators reported that pretreatment with cytochalasin B was required for the induction of enzyme release with chemotactic peptides.

D. Exocytosis After Treatment with Cytochalasin B

Several investigators have reported that cytochalasin B enhances the extracellular release of granule enzymes by neutrophils exposed to phagocytosable

Table II. Release of Gelatinase and Vitamin B_{12}-Binding Protein from Freshly Prepared Normal Human Neutrophils Incubated with Activated Serum

Stimulus[a]	Dilution	N	Release (%) of cellular content (mean ± SD)		
			Gelatinase	Vitamin B_{12}-binding protein	β-Glucuronidase
None (control)	—	5	7.0 ± 1.9	3.2 ± 0.8	2.6 ± 0.9
Zymosan-treated serum	1:3	3	37.3 ± 14.6[b]	10.0 ± 3.5[b]	2.3 ± 1.5 (NS)
Zymosan-treated serum + EACA	1:30 or 1:60	5	31.2 ± 8.4[b]	8.6 ± 2.0[b]	2.8 ± 0.8 (NS)

[a]Fresh human serum was activated by incubation with 5 mg zymosan per milliliter at 37°C for 30 min. 1 M ε-aminocaproic acid (EACA) was added to prevent the conversion of C5a into C5a$_{\text{des Arg}}$ (Fernandez and Hugli, 1976).
[b]Statistical difference with respect to control, $P < 0.01$; NS, not significantly different from control.

particles (Davies *et al.*, 1973; Henson and Oades, 1973; Skosey *et al.*, 1973; Zurier *et al.*, 1973). Cytochalasin B-treated neutrophils recognize particles normally, but are unable to ingest them, due to impaired microfilament function. As in phagocytosis, discharge of granules occurs at the sites of interaction between cell and particle but, since phagosomes are not formed, the enzymes liberated are largely recovered in the extracellular milieu (Weissmann *et al.*, 1975). For this reason, cytochalasin B was used widely in studies of phagocytic enzyme release. It was subsequently found that this compound actually modifies the responsiveness of neutrophils to different types of stimuli. Cytochalasin B was found to (1) facilitate the aggregation induced by bacterial chemotactic peptides (O'Flaherty *et al.*, 1977) and C5a (Craddock *et al.*, 1978); (2) enhance the respiratory burst induced by C5a, concanavalin A, fMet-Leu-Phe, or A23187 (Goldstein *et al.*, 1975b; Zabucchi *et al.*, 1978; Becker *et al.*, 1979; Bennett *et al.*, 1980); and (3) enhance enzyme release in response to these and other soluble stimuli. Cytochalasin B, however, changes the quality of the release response and its uncritical use has introduced some confusion about the secretory properties of neutrophils.

Figure 8 shows the secretory pattern of human neutrophils exposed to fMet-

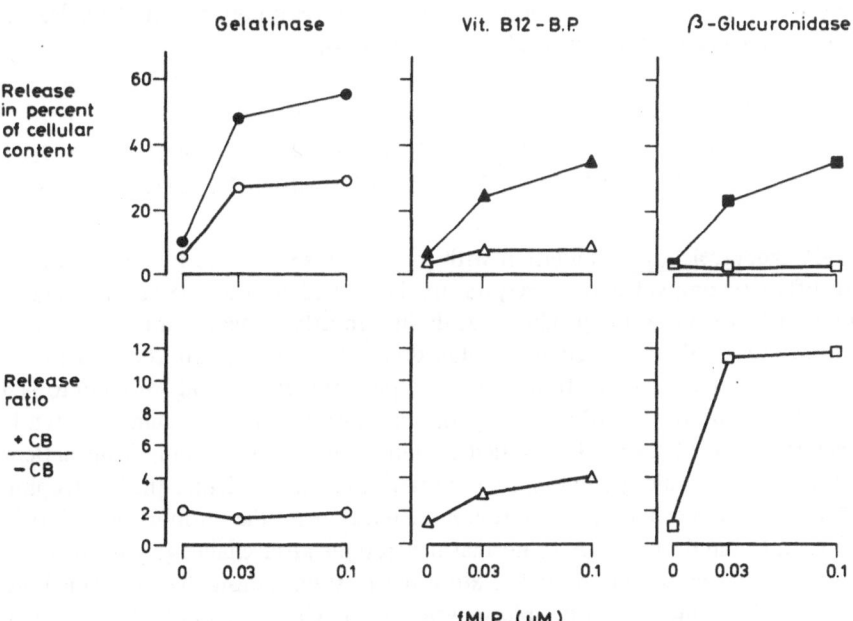

Figure 8. Release of gelatinase, vitamin B_{12}-binding protein and β-glucuronidase in response to increasing concentrations of fMet-Leu-Phe (fMLP) by normal (open symbols) and cytochalasin B-treated (filled symbols) human neutrophils. The upper row of graphs shows the percentage of markers released in 10 min. The lower row of graphs shows the ratios of the percentage release obtained with (+CB) and without (–CB) cytochalasin B pretreatment.

Leu-Phe and the modifications caused by cytochalasin B. As pointed out in Figure 7, under these experimental conditions, normal cells release about one-third of their gelatinase, as well as some vitamin B_{12}-binding protein, but no β-glucuronidase. Pretreatment with cytochalasin B enhances exocytosis from the gelatinase-containing organelles and the specific granules to different extents and modifies the cell so as to permit exocytosis from the azurophil granules, which are retained by normal neutrophils. With the knowledge of these properties, one can take advantage of the stimulus-enhancing effect of cytochalasin B for the study of conditions and agents that induce or modulate exocytosis and other neutrophil responses (see, e.g., Weissmann et al., 1975). In fact, many of the agents now established as stimuli for neutrophils were originally investigated in experiments with cytochalasin B-treated cells. This applies to the studies of fMet-Leu-Phe and congeners (Showell et al., 1976), anaphylatoxins (Goldstein et al., 1975a; Chenoweth and Hugli, 1978, 1980), leukotrienes (Goetzl and Pickett, 1980; Feinmark et al., 1981), and PAF (Shaw et al., 1981).

The mechanism of action of cytochalasin B is still a matter of speculation. Enhanced exocytosis could result from the breakdown or paralysis of the ectoplasmic microfilament network, which prevents granule contact with the plasma membrane (Henson et al., 1979). Such an effect on microfilaments could also relieve restrictions on the motility of membrane components and thus lead to general enhancement of neutrophil responsiveness.

V. RESPIRATORY BURST AND RELEASE OF ARACHIDONIC ACID OXYGENATION PRODUCTS IN RELATIONSHIP TO EXOCYTOSIS

Phagocytosis and stimulation with most agents shown to induce exocytosis are often accompanied by a respiratory burst and by the liberation of arachidonic acid oxygenation products. Although mostly concomitant, these important responses of stimulated neutrophils do not appear to be interdependent.

That enzyme release from the azurophil granules during phagocytosis is not dependent on or influenced by the respiratory burst was demonstrated by Baehner et al. (1969), who studied degranulation of neutrophils from patients affected by chronic granulomatous disease. In these patients, the neutrophils, which lack a respiratory burst response, released similar proportions of three azurophil granule enzymes as normal neutrophils after challenge with different types of phagocytosable particles. More recent studies show that the same holds true for release induced by nonphagocytic stimuli. Goldstein et al. (1975b) found that C5a induces superoxide production but no release of β-glucuronidase by human neutrophils. When the same cells are pretreated with cytochalasin B, a rapid secretion of β-glucuronidase is observed without a comparable increase in superoxide production. Using anion channel blockers, Korchak et al. (1980) obtained a strong inhibition of the release of lysozyme and β-glucuronidase induced in human neutrophils by immune complexes or A23187 but no decrease in the production of superoxide. A dissociation of degranulation and superoxide production was also obtained by Cotter et al. (1981) by means of a monoclonal antibody raised against human neutrophils, which markedly decreased the release of myeloperoxidase and lysozyme induced in cytochalasin B-treated cells by different stimuli without affecting superoxide formation. Finally, in our recent study on the release of gelatinase from human neutrophils (Dewald et al., 1982), we found a number of conditions leading to abundant enzyme secretion without enhanced production of superoxide.

In neutrophils, as in many other cells, stimulation induces the release of arachidonic acid from membrane phospholipids. Free arachidonate is transformed via two oxygenation pathways. Cyclooxygenase yields the endoperoxide, prostaglandin G_2 (PGG_2), from which prostaglandins (Higgs et al., 1975; Zurier and Sayadoff, 1975) and thromboxanes (Higgs et al., 1976; Goldstein et al., 1978) are formed. 5-Lipoxygenase yields 5-hydroperoxy-eicosatetraenoic acid (5-HPETE), which is then reduced to its 5-hydroxy derivative (Borgeat et al., 1976; Stenson and Parker, 1979) or converted into leukotrienes (Borgeat and Samuelsson, 1979; Radmark et al., 1980; Hansson and Radmark, 1980).

Cyclooxygenase products such as PGD_2, PGE_2, and PGI_2 were found to inhibit stimulus-dependent enzyme release by cytochalasin B-treated neutrophils (Weissmann et al., 1975; Smith and Iden, 1980). In view of this action, which is believed to result from a rise in intracellular cyclic adenosine monophosphate (cAMP) (Weissmann et al., 1975), one would expect cyclooxygenase inhibitors to enhance enzyme release. The effects of the common nonsteroidal anti-inflammatory drugs, all of which inhibit cyclooxygenase, were studied in many laboratories (cf. Northover, 1977; Smith, 1978, 1979; Smith and Iden, 1980; Smolen and Weissmann, 1980). These drugs were generally found to lower enzyme release induced by soluble or particulate stimuli. Their effects were mostly moderate, and the concentrations required were at the upper limit of the plasma levels obtained clinically. Most investigators agree that the observed decrease in enzyme release does not depend on the inhibition of cyclooxygenase, as suggested by Smolen and Weissmann (1980). The latter workers suggested that products of the lipoxygenase pathway may mediate enzyme release and superoxide formation in neutrophils. In similar experiments, Smith et al. (1981) came to the opposite conclusion. Most recently, however, the same laboratory (Smith et al., 1982) reported that U-60,257, an inhibitor of leukotriene synthesis (Bach et al., 1982), blocked LTB_4 formation by human neutrophils challenged with A23187 and inhibited, in cyclochalasin B-treated cells, the formation of superoxide and the release of β-glucuronidase and lysozyme induced by A23187 or fMet-Leu-Phe. It is thus conceivable that lipoxygenase products may favor enzyme release. More powerful and more selective lipoxygenase inhibitors, however, are needed to properly test this possibility.

VI. A NEW LOOK AT SECRETION BY NEUTROPHILS

In this review of exocytosis by neutrophils, we have given a detailed description of the characteristics of the secretory responses of these cells to a variety of stimuli. Exocytosis of the contents of the two types of granules follows different rules. Azurophil granules are discharged only when neutrophils interact with phagocytosable particles, while specific granules are discharged upon interaction of the cells with both particulate and soluble stimuli. In the latter case, specific granule constituents are released directly into the pericellular environment, indicating that these granules can function as secretory organelles.

In recent studies, we identified a novel storage compartment in human neutrophils, consisting of small, vesicle-like secretory organelles containing gelatinase (Dewald *et al.*, 1982). Gelatinase release after stimulation is both rapid and extensive. As judged from the results obtained so far, it is always paralleled, albeit at a low level, by the release of the specific granule marker vitamin B_{12}-binding protein.

Studies of the biochemical properties of the novel secretory organelles and of their discharge on stimulation will provide much needed information on the role of secretory events in the early stages of neutrophil mobilization, adherence, diapedesis, and directed movement in the tissues.

VII. REFERENCES

Amherdt, M., Baggiolini, M., Perrelet, A., and Orci, L., 1978, Freeze-fracture of membrane fusions in phagocytosing polymorphonuclear leukocytes, *Lab. Invest.* **39**:398.

Avila, J. L., and Convit, J., 1973, Human polymorphonuclear leukocyte enzymes. I. Assay of acid hydrolases and other enzymes, *Biochim. Biophys. Acta* **293**:397.

Bach, M. K., Brashler, J. R., Smith, H. W., Fitzpatrick, F. A., Sun, F. F., and McGuire, J. C., 1982, 6,9-Deepoxy-6,9-(phenylimino)-6,8-prostaglandin I_1, (U-60,257), a new inhibitor of leukotriene C and D synthesis: in vitro studies, *Prostaglandins* **23**:759.

Baehner, R. L., Karnovsky, M. J., and Karnovsky, M. L., 1969, Degranulation of leukocytes in chronic granulomatous disease, *J. Clin. Invest.* **48**:187.

Baggiolini, M., 1972, The enzymes of the granules of polymophonuclear leukocytes and their functions, *Enzyme* **13**:132.

Baggiolini, M., Hirsch, J. G., and de Duve, C., 1969, Resolution of granules from rabbit heterophil leukocytes into distinct populations by zonal sedimentation, *J. Cell Biol.* **40**: 529.

Baggiolini, M., de Duve, C., Masson, P. L., and Heremans, J. F., 1970a, Association of lactoferrin with specific granules in rabbit heterophil leukocytes, *J. Exp. Med.* **131**:559.

Baggiolini, M., Hirsch, J. G., and de Duve, C., 1970b, Further biochemical and morphological studies of granule fractions from rabbit heterophil leukocytes, *J. Cell Biol.* **45**:586.

Baggiolini, M., Bretz, U., and Dewald, B., 1978, Subcellular localization of granule enzymes, in: *Neutral Proteases of Human Polymorphonuclear Leukocytes* (K. Havemann, and A. Janoff, eds.), pp. 3–17, Urban & Schwarzenberg, Baltimore and Munich.

Bainton, D. F., 1973, Sequential degranulation of the two types of polymorphonuclear leukocyte granules during phagocytosis of microorganisms, *J. Cell Biol.* **58**:249.

Bainton, D. F., and Farquhar, M. G., 1966, Origin of granules in polymorphonuclear leukocytes: Two types derived from opposite faces of the Golgi complex in developing granulocytes, *J. Cell Biol.* **28**:277.

Bainton, D. F., and Farquhar, M. G., 1968, Differences in enzyme content of azurophil and specific granules of polymorphonuclear leukocytes. II. Cytochemistry and electron microscopy of bone marrow cells, *J. Cell Biol.* **39**:299.

Bainton, D. F., Ullyot, J. L., and Farquhar, M. G., 1971, The development of neutrophilic polymorphonuclear leukocytes in human bone marrow. Origin and content of azurophil and specific granules, *J. Exp. Med.* **134**:907.

Becker, E. L., and Showell, H. J., 1974, The ability of chemotactic factors to induce lysosomal enzyme release. II. The mechanism of release, *J. Immunol.* **112**:2055.

Becker, E. L., Showell, H. J., Henson, P. M., and Hsu, L. S., 1974, The ability of chemotactic factors to induce lysosomal enzyme release. I. The characteristics of the release, the importance of surfaces and the relation of enzyme release to chemotactic responsiveness, *J. Immunol.* **112**:2047.

Becker, E. L., Sigman, M., and Oliver, J. M., 1979, Superoxide production induced in rabbit polymorphonuclear leukocytes by synthetic chemotactic peptides and A23187: the nature of the receptor and the requirement for Ca^{2+}, *Am. J. Pathol.* **95**:81.

Bennett, J. P., Cockcroft, S., and Gomperts, B. D., 1980, Use of cytochalasin B to distinguish between early and late events in neutrophil activation, *Biochim. Biophys. Acta* **601**:584.

Bentwood, B. J., and Henson, P. M., 1980, The sequential release of granule constituents from human neutrophils, *J. Immunol.* **124**:855.

Benveniste, J., Tencé, M., Varenne, P., Bidault, J., Boullet, C., and Polonsky, J., 1979, Semisynthesis and proposed structure of platelet-activating factor (PAF): PAF-acether, an alkyl ether analog of lysophosphatidylcholine, *C. R. Acad. Sci. [D] (Paris)* **289**:1037.

Betz, S. J., and Henson, P. M., 1980, Production and release of platelet-activating factor (PAF); dissociation from degranulation and superoxide production in the human neutrophil, *J. Immunol.* **125**:2756.

Borgeat, P., and Samuelsson, B., 1979, Arachidonic acid metabolism in polymorphonuclear leukocytes: Effects of ionophore A23187, *Proc. Natl. Acad. Sci. (USA)* **76**:2148.

Borgeat, P., Hamberg, M., and Samuelsson, B., 1976, Transformation of arachidonic acid and homo-γ-linolenic acid by rabbit polymorphonuclear leukocytes, *J. Biol. Chem.* **251**:7816.

Bray, M. A., Ford-Hutchinson, A. W., and Smith, M. J. H., 1981, Leukotriene B_4: An inflammatory mediator in vivo, *Prostaglandins* **22**:213.

Bretz, U., and Baggiolini, M., 1973, Association of the alkaline phosphatase of rabbit polymorphonuclear leukocytes with the membrane of the specific granules, *J. Cell Biol.* **59**:696.

Bretz, U., and Baggiolini, M., 1974, Biochemical and morphological characterization of azurophil and specific granules of human neutrophilic polymorphonuclear leukocytes, *J. Cell Biol.* **63**:251.

Burke, J. S., Uriuhara, T., Macmorine, D. R. L., and Movat, H. Z., 1964, A permeability factor released from phagocytosing PMN-leukocytes and its inhibition by protease inhibitors, *Life Sci.* **3**:1505.

Camussi, G., Aglietta, M., Coda, R., Bussolino, F., Piacibello, W., and Tetta, C., 1981, Release of platelet-activating factor (PAF) and histamine. II. The cellular origin of human PAF: Monocytes, polymorphonuclear neutrophils and basophils, *Immunology* **42**:191.

Chenoweth, D. E., and Hugli, T. E., 1978, Demonstration of specific C5a receptor on intact human polymorphonuclear leukocytes, *Proc. Natl. Acad. Sci. (USA)* **75**:3943.

Chenoweth, D. E., and Hugli, T. E., 1980, Human C5a and C5a analogs as probes of the neutrophil C5a receptor, *Mol. Immunol.* **17**:151.

Claessen, H.-E., Lundberg, U., and Malmsten, C., 1981, Serum-coated zymosan stimulates the synthesis of leukotriene B_4 in human polymorphonuclear leukocytes. Inhibition by cyclic AMP, *Biochem. Biophys. Res. Commun.* 99:1230.

Cohn, Z. A., and Hirsch, J. G., 1960a, The isolation and properties of the specific cytoplasmic granules of rabbit polymorphonuclear leukocytes, *J. Exp. Med.* 112:983.

Cohn, Z. A., and Hirsch, J. G., 1960b, The influence of phagocytosis on the intracellular distribution of granule associated components of polymorphonuclear leukocytes, *J. Exp. Med.* 112:1015.

Corcino, J., Krauss, S., Waxman, S., and Herbert, V., 1970, Release of vitamin B_{12}-binding protein by human leukocytes in vitro, *J. Clin. Invest.* 49:2250.

Cotter, T. G., Spears, P., and Henson, P. M., 1981, A monoclonal antibody inhibiting human neutrophil chemotaxis and degranulation, *J. Immunol.* 127:1355.

Craddock, P. R., White, J. G., and Jacob, H. S., 1978, Potentiation of complement (C5a)-induced granulocyte aggregation by cytochalasin B, *J. Lab. Clin. Med.* 91:490.

Dahinden, C., and Fehr, J., 1980, Receptor-directed inhibition of chemotactic factor-induced neutrophil hyperactivity by pyrazolon derivatives. Definition of a chemotactic peptide antagonist, *J. Clin. Invest.* 66:884.

Davies, P., Fox, R. I., Polyzonis, M., Allison, A. C., and Haswell, A. D., 1973, The inhibition of phagocytosis and facilitation of exocytosis in rabbit polymorphonuclear leukocytes by cytochalasin B, *Lab. Invest.* 28:16.

Demopoulos, C. A., Pinckard, R. N., and Hanahan, D. J., 1979, Platelet-activating factor. Evidence for 1-*O*-alkyl-2-acetyl-*sn*-glyceryl-3-phosphorylcholine as the active component (a new class of lipid chemical mediators), *J. Biol. Chem.* 254:9355.

Dewald, B., Rindler-Ludwig, R., Bretz, U., and Baggiolini, M., 1975, Subcellular localization and heterogeneity of neutral proteases in neutrophilic polymorphonuclear leukocytes, *J. Exp. Med.* 141:709.

Dewald, B., Bretz, U., and Baggiolini, M., 1982, Release of gelatinase from a novel secretory compartment of human neutrophils, *J. Clin. Invest.* 70:518.

de Duve, C., and Wattiaux, R., 1966, Functions of lysosomes, *Annu. Rev. Physiol.* 28:435.

de Duve, C., de Barsy, T., Poole, B., Trouet, A., Tulkens, P., and Van Hoof, F., 1974, Commentary. Lysosomotropic agents, *Biochem. Pharmacol.* 23:2495.

Estensen, R. D., White, J. G., and Holmes, B., 1974, Specific degranulation of human polymorphonuclear leukocytes, *Nature* 248:347.

Fehr, J., and Dahinden, C., 1979, Modulating influence of chemotactic factor-induced cell adhesiveness on granulocyte function, *J. Clin. Invest.* 64:8.

Feinmark, S. J., Lindgren, J. A., Claessen, H.-E., Malmsten, C., and Samuelsson, B., 1981, Stimulation of human leukocyte degranulation by leukotriene B_4 and its ω-oxidized metabolites, *FEBS Lett.* 136:141.

Fernandez, H. N., and Hugli, T. E., 1976, Partial characterization of human C5a anaphylatoxin. I. Chemical description of the carbohydrate and polypeptide portions of human C5a, *J. Immunol.* 117:1688.

Ford-Hutchinson, A. W., Bray, M. A., Doig, M. V., Shipley, M. E., and Smith, M. J. H., 1980, Leukotriene B, a potent chemokinetic and aggregating substance released from polymorphonuclear leukocytes, *Nature* 286:264.

Goetzl, E. J., and Pickett, W. C., 1980, The human PMN leukocyte chemotactic activity of complex hydroxy-eicosatetraenoic acids (HETEs), *J. Immunol.* 125:1789.

Goetzl, E. J., and Pickett, W. C., 1981, Novel structural determinants of the human neutrophil chemotactic activity of leukotriene B, *J. Exp. Med.* 153:482.

Goldstein, I. M., Horn, J. K., Kaplan, H. B., and Weissmann, G., 1974, Calcium-induced lysozyme secretion from human polymorphonuclear leukocytes, *Biochem. Biophys. Res. Commun.* 60:807.

Goldstein, I. M., Hoffstein, S. T., and Weissmann, G., 1975a, Mechanisms of lysosomal enzyme release from human polymorphonuclear leukocytes. Effects of phorbol myristate acetate, *J. Cell. Biol.* **66**:647.

Goldstein, I. M., Roos, D., Kaplan, H. B., and Weissmann, G., 1975b, Complement and immunoglobulins stimulate superoxide production by human leukocytes independently of phagocytosis, *J. Clin. Invest.* **56**:1155.

Goldstein, I. M., Malmsten, C. L., Kindahl, H., Kaplan, H. B., Radmark, O., Samuelsson, B., and Weissmann, G., 1978, Thromboxane generation by human peripheral blood polymorphonuclear leukocytes, *J. Exp. Med.* **148**:787.

Hafstrom, I., Palmblad, J., Malmsten, C. L., Radmark, O., and Samuelsson, B., 1981, Leukotriene B_4—a stereospecific stimulator for release of lysosomal enzymes from neutrophils, *FEBS Lett.* **130**:146.

Hansson, G., and Radmark, O., 1980, Leukotriene C_4: Isolation from human polymorphonuclear leukocytes, *FEBS Lett.* **122**:87.

Henson, P. M., 1971a, The immunologic release of constituents from neutrophil leukocytes. II. Mechanisms of release during phagocytosis and adherence to nonphagocytosable surfaces, *J. Immunol.* **107**:1547.

Henson, P. M., 1971b, Interaction of cells with immune complexes: Adherence, release of constitutents, and tissue injury, *J. Exp. Med.* **134**:114.

Henson, P. M., and Oades, Z. G., 1973, Enhancement of immunologically induced granule exocytosis from neutrophils by cytochalasin B, *J. Immunol.* **110**:290.

Henson, P. M., Johnson, H. B., and Spiegelberg, H. L., 1972, The release of granule enzymes from human neutrophils stimulated by aggregated immunoglobulins of different classes and subclasses, *J. Immunol.* **109**:1182.

Henson, P. M., Zanolari, B., Schwartzman, N. A., and Hong, S. R., 1978, Intracellular control of human neutrophil secretion. I. C5a-induced stimulus-specific desensitization and the effects of cytochalasin B, *J. Immunol.* **121**:851.

Henson, P. M., Hollister, J. R., Musson, R. A., Webster, R. O., Spears, P., Henson, J. E., and McCarthy, K. M., 1979, Inflammation as a surface phenomenon: Initiation of inflammatory processes by surface-bound immunologic components, in: *Advances in Inflammation Research* (G. Weissmann, B. Samuelsson, and R. Paoletti, eds.), pp. 341–352, Raven Press, New York.

Higgs, G. A., McCall, E., and Youlten, L. J. F., 1975, A chemotactic role for prostaglandins released from polymorphonuclear leucocytes during phagocytosis, *Br. J. Pharmacol.* **53**:539.

Higgs, G. A., Bunting, S., Moncada, S., and Vane, J. R., 1976, Polymorphonuclear leukocytes produce thromboxane A_2-like activity during phagocytosis, *Prostaglandins* **12**:749.

Hirsch, J. G., 1962, Cinemicrophotographic observations on granule lysis in polymorphonuclear leukocytes during phagocytosis, *J. Exp. Med.* **116**:827.

Hoffstein, S., Soberman, R., Goldstein, I., and Weissmann, G., 1976, Concanavalin A induces microtubule assembly and specific granule discharge in human polymorphonuclear leukocytes, *J. Cell. Biol.* **68**:781.

Ingraham, L. M., Coates, T. D., Allen, J. M., Higgins, C. P., Baehner, R. L., and Boxer, L. A., 1982, Metabolic, membrane, and functional responses of human polymorphonuclear leukocytes to platelet-activating factor, *Blood* **59**:1259.

Jouvin-Marche, E., Poitevin, B., and Benveniste, J., 1982, Platelet-activating factor (PAF-acether), an activator of neutrophil functions, *Agents Actions* **12**:716.

Jubiz, W., Radmark, O., Malmsten, C., Hansson, G., Lindgren, J. A., Palmblad, J., Udén, A.-M., and Samuelsson, B., 1982, A novel leukotriene produced by stimulation of leukocytes with formylmethionylleucylphenylalanine, *J. Biol. Chem.* **257**:6106.

Kane, S. P., and Peters, T. J., 1975, Analytical subcellular fractionation of human granulocytes with reference to the localization of vitamin B_{12}-binding proteins, *Clin. Sci. Mol. Med.* **49**:171.

Klempner, M. S., Dinarello, C. A., and Gallin, J. I., 1978, Human leukocytic pyrogen induces release of specific granule contents from human neutrophils, *J. Clin. Invest.* **61**: 1330.

Korchak, H. M., Eisenstat, B. A., Hoffstein, S. T., Dunham, P. B., and Weissmann, G., 1980, Anion channel blockers inhibit lysosomal enzyme secretion from human neutrophils without affecting generation of superoxide anion, *Proc. Natl. Acad. Sci. (USA)* **77**:2721.

Koza, E. P., Wright, T. E., and Becker, E. L., 1975, Lysosomal enzyme secretion and volume contraction induced in neutrophils by cytochalasin B, chemotactic factor and A23187, *Proc. Soc. Exp. Biol. Med.* **149**:476.

Leffell, M. S., and Spitznagel, J. K., 1972, Association of lactoferrin with lysozyme in granules of human polymorphonuclear leukocytes, *Infect. Immun.* **6**:761.

Leffell, M. S., and Spitznagel, J. K., 1974, Intracellular and extracellular degranulation of human polymorphonuclear azurophil and specific granules induced by immune complexes, *Infect. Immun.* **10**:1241.

Leffell, M. S., and Spitznagel, J. K., 1975, Fate of human lactoferrin and myeloperoxidase in phagocytizing human neutrophils: Effects of immunoglobulin G subclasses and immune complexes coated on latex beads, *Infect. Immun.* **12**:813.

May, C. D., Levine, B. B., and Weissmann, G., 1970, Effects of compounds which inhibit antigenic release of histamine and phagocytic release of lysosomal enzyme on glucose utilization by leukocytes in human, *Proc. Soc. Exp. Biol. Med.* **133**:758.

Murphy, G., Reynolds, J. J., Bretz, U., and Baggiolini, M., 1977, Collagenase is a component of the specific granules of human neutrophil leukocytes, *Biochem. J.* **162**:195.

Murphy, G., Bretz, U., Baggiolini, M., and Reynolds, J. J., 1980, The latent collagenase and gelatinase of human polymorphonuclear neutrophil leucocytes, *Biochem. J.* **192**:517.

Nelson, R. D., Ackerman, S. K., Fiegel, V. D., Bauman, M. P., and Douglas, S. D., 1979, Cytotaxin receptors of neutrophils: evidence that F-methionyl peptides and pepstatin share a common receptor, *Infect. Immun.* **26**:996.

Northover, B. J., 1977, Effect of indomethacin and related drugs on the calcium ion-dependent secretion of lysosomal and other enzymes by neutrophil polymorphonuclear leucocytes in vitro, *Br. J. Pharmacol.* **59**:253.

O'Flaherty, J. T., Kreutzer, D. L., Showell, H. J., and Ward, P. A., 1977, Influence of inhibitors of cellular function on chemotactic factor-induced neutrophil aggregation, *J. Immunol.* **119**:1751.

Ohta, H., 1964, A biochemical study on the neutrophilic granules isolated in a pure state from leukocyte homogenate, *Acta Haematol. Jpn.* **27**:555.

Radmark, O., Malmsten, C., Samuelsson, B., Goto, G., Marfat, A., and Corey, E. J., 1980, Leukotriene A. Isolation from human polymorphonuclear leukocytes, *J. Biol. Chem.* **255**:11828.

Rae, S. A., and Smith, M. J. H., 1981, The stimulation of lysosomal enzyme secretion from human polymorphonuclear leucocytes by leukotriene B_4, *J. Pharm. Pharmacol.* **33**:616.

Robineaux, J., and Frederick, J., 1955, Contribution à l'étude des granulations neutrophiles des polynucléaires par la microcinematographie en contraste de phase, *C.R. Soc. Biol. (Paris)* **149**:486.

Ryan, G. B., Borysenko, J. Z., and Karnovsky, M. J., 1974, Factors affecting the redistribution of surface-bound concanavalin A on human polymorphonuclear leukocytes, *J. Cell Biol.* **62**:351.

Sanchez-Crespo, M., Alonso, F., and Egido, J., 1980, Platelet-activating factor in anaphylaxis and phagocytosis. I. Release from human peripheral polymorphonuclears and monocytes during the stimulation by ionophore A23187 and phagocytosis but not from degranulating basophils, *Immunology* **40**:645.

Schiffmann, E., Corcoran, B. A., and Wahl, S. M., 1975, N-Formylmethionyl peptides as chemoattractants for leucocytes, *Proc. Natl. Acad. Sci. (USA)* **72**:1059.

Shaw, J. O., Pinckard, R. N., Ferrigni, K. S., McManus, L. M., and Hanahan, D. J., 1981, Activation of human neutrophils with 1-*O*-hexadecyl/octadecyl-2-acetyl-*sn*-glyceryl-3-phosphorylcholine (platelet activating factor), *J. Immunol.* **127**:1250.

Showell, H. J., Freer, R. J., Zigmond, S. H., Schiffmann, E., Aswanikumar, S., Corcoran, B., and Becker, E. L., 1976, The structure–activity relations of synthetic peptides as chemotactic factors and inducers of lysosomal enzyme secretion for neutrophils, *J. Exp. Med.* **143**:1154.

Showell, H. J., Naccache, P. H., Borgeat, P., Picard, S., Vallerand, P., Becker, E. L., and Sha'afi, R. I., 1982, Characterization of the secretory activity of leukotriene B$_4$ toward rabbit neutrophils, *J. Immunol.* **128**:811.

Skosey, J. L., Chow, D., Damgaard, E., and Sorensen, L. B., 1973, Effect of cytochalasin B on response of human polymorphonuclear leukocytes to zymosan, *J. Cell Biol.* **57**:237.

Smith, R. J., 1978, Nonsteroid anti-inflammatory agents: Regulators of the phagocytic secretion of lysosomal enzymes from guinea-pig neutrophils, *J. Pharmacol. Exp. Ther.* **207**:618.

Smith, R. J., 1979, The guinea pig neutrophil calcium-dependent lysosomal enzyme secretory process. Inhibition by nonsteroid anti-inflammatory agents, *Biochem. Pharmacol.* **28**: 2739.

Smith, R. J., and Bowman, B. J., 1982, Stimulation of human neutrophil degranulation with 1-*O*-octadecyl-2-*O*-acetyl-*sn*-glyceryl-3-phosphorylcholine: Modulation by inhibitors of arachidonic acid metabolism, *Biochem. Biophys., Res. Commun.* **104**:1495.

Smith, R. J., and Iden, S. S., 1980, Pharmacological modulation of chemotactic factor-elicited release of granule-associated enzymes from human neutrophils. Effects of prostaglandins, nonsteroid anti-inflammatory agents and corticosteroids, *Biochem. Pharmacol.* **29**:2389.

Smith, R. J., Sun, F. F., Iden, S. S., Bowman, B. J., Sprecher, H., and McGuire, J. C., 1981, An evaluation of the relationship between arachidonic acid lipoxygenation and human neutrophil degranulation, *Clin. Immunol. Immunopathol.* **20**:157.

Smith, R. J., Sun, F. F., Bowman, B. J., Iden, S. S., Smith H. W., and McGuire, J. C., 1982, Effect of 6,9-Deepoxy-6,9-(phenylimino)-6,8-prostaglandin 1$_1$ (U-60,257), and inhibitor of leukotriene synthesis, on human neutrophil function, *Biochem. Biophys. Res. Commun.* **109**:943.

Smolen, J. E., and Weissmann, G., 1980, Effects of indomethacin, 5,8,11,14-eicosatetraynoic acid, and p-bromophenacyl bromide on lysosomal enzyme release and superoxide anion generation by human polymorphonuclear leukocytes, *Biochem. Pharmacol.* **29**:533.

Sopata, I., and Dancewicz, A. M., 1974, Presence of a gelatin-specific proteinase and its latent form in human leucocytes, *Biochem. Biophys. Acta* **370**:510.

Spitznagel, J. K., Dalldorf, F. G., Leffell, M. S., Folds, J. D., Welsh, I. R. H., Cooney, M. H., and Martin, L. E., 1974, Character of azurophil and specific granules purified from human polymorphonuclear leukocytes, *Lab. Invest.* **30**:774.

Stenson, W. F., and Parker, C. W., 1979, Metabolism of arachidonic acid in ionophore-stimulated neutrophils. Esterification of a hydroxylated metabolite into phospholipids, *J. Clin. Invest.* **64**:1457.

Taichman, N. S., Pruzanski, W., and Ranadive, N. S., 1972, Release of intracellular constituents from rabbit polymorphonuclear leukocytes exposed to soluble and insoluble immune complexes, *Int. Arch. Allergy* **43**:182.

Weissmann, G., 1971, The molecular basis of acute gout, *Hosp Pract* **6**:43.

Weissmann, G., Dukor, P., and Zurier, R. B., 1971, Effect of cyclic AMP on release of lysosomal enzymes from phagocytes, *Nature (New Biol.)* **231**:131.

Weissman, G., Goldstein, I., Hoffstein, S., Chauvet, G., and Robineaux, R., 1975, Yin/Yang modulation of lysosomal enzyme release from polymorphonuclear leukocytes by cyclic nucleotides, *Ann. NY Acad. Sci.* **256**:222.

West, B. C., Rosenthal, A. S., Gelb, N. A., and Kimball, H. R., 1974, Separation and characterization of human neutrophil granules, *Am. J. Pathol.* **77**:41.

Wetzel, B. K., Horn, R. G., and Spicer, S. S., 1967, Fine structural studies on the development of heterophil, eosinophil and basophil granulocytes in rabbits, *Lab. Invest.* **16**:349.

White, J. G., and Estensen, R. D., 1974, Selective labilization of specific granules in polymorphonuclear leukocytes by phorbol myristate acetate, *Am. J. Pathol.* **75**:45.

Woodin, A. M., 1962, The extrusion of protein from the rabbit polymorphonuclear leucocyte treated with staphylococcal leucocidin, *Biochem. J.* **82**:9.

Woodin, A. M., and Wieneke, A. A., 1964, The participation of calcium, adenosine triphosphate and adenosine triphosphatase in the extrusion of the granule proteins from the polymorphonuclear leucocytes, *Biochem. J.* **90**:498.

Woodin, A. M., and Wieneke, A. A., 1966, The secretion of protein by the polymorphonuclear leucocyte treated with streptolysin 0, *Exp. Cell Res.* **43**:319.

Wright, D. G., and Gallin, J. I., 1979, Secretory responses of human neutrophils: Exocytosis of specific (secondary) granules by human neutrophils during adherence *in vitro* and during exudation *in vivo*, *J. Immunol.* **123**:285.

Wright, D. G., and Malawista, S. E., 1972, The mobilization and extracellular release of granular enzymes from human leukocytes during phagocytosis, *J. Cell Biol.* **53**:788.

Wright, D. G., Bralove, D. A., and Gallin, J. I., 1977, The differential mobilization of human neutrophil granules. Effects of phorbol myristate acetate and ionophore A23187, *Am. J. Pathol.* **87**:273.

Zabucchi, G., Soranzo, M. R., Berton, G., Romeo, D., and Rossi, F., 1978, The stimulation of the oxidative metabolism of polymorphonuclear leukocytes: Effect of colchicine and cytochalasin B, *J. Reticuloendothel. Soc.* **24**:451.

Zucker-Franklin, D., and Hirsch, J. G., 1964, Electron microscope studies on the degranulation of rabbit peritoneal leukocytes during phagocytosis, *J. Exp. Med.* **120**:569.

Zurier, R. B., and Sayadoff, D. M., 1975, Release of prostaglandins from human polymorphonuclear leukocytes, *Inflammation* **1**:93.

Zurier, R. B., Hoffstein, S., and Weissmann, G., 1973, Cytochalasin, B: Effect on lysosomal enzyme release from human leukocytes, *Proc. Natl. Acad. Sci. (USA)* **70**:844.

Chapter 9

Mechanisms of Regulating the Respiratory Burst in Leukocytes

Linda C. McPhail and Ralph Snyderman

Laboratory of Immune Effector Function
Howard Hughes Medical Institute and Division of Rheumatic and
Genetic Diseases
Department of Medicine
Duke University Medical Center
Durham, North Carolina 27710

I. THE RESPIRATORY BURST

When leukocytes encounter opsonized microorganisms or a variety of inflammatory stimuli, their utilization of oxygen is substantially enhanced. This phenomenon was first observed as increased oxygen uptake by the stimulated cells (Baldridge and Gerard, 1933; Sbarra and Karnovsky, 1959) and was correlated with the production of hydrogen peroxide (Iyer *et al.*, 1961). Concomitant with the alterations in respiration, enhanced glucose oxidation via the hexose monophosphate shunt occurs as well (Sbarra and Karnovsky, 1959). In recent years, it has become clear that oxygen utilization in activated phagocytic cells can proceed by one electron reduction steps, and that the initial product is probably superoxide anion (O_2^-) (Babior *et al.*, 1973). Two molecules of O_2^- can then interact in a dismutation reaction, resulting in the formation of hydrogen peroxide (H_2O_2). These reactions are outlined in Eqs. (1) and (2):

$$O_2 + e^- \rightarrow O_2^- \tag{1}$$

$$2O_2^- + 2H^+ \rightarrow O_2^- + H_2O_2 \tag{2}$$

Several other reactive oxygen species may also be generated during the respiratory burst. The three-electron reduction product of oxygen, hydroxyl radical ($OH\cdot$), can be formed by the interaction of O_2^- and H_2O_2 when trace amounts of metal ions are present (Haber and Weiss, 1934)[Eqs. (3)–(5)], and evidence that leukocytes produce OH· or similar oxidizing radicals has been reported (Johnston et al., 1975; Weiss et al., 1977; Tauber and Babior, 1977; Rosen and Klebanoff, 1979b). Equations (3) and (4) show the reactions proposed by Haber and Weiss for the formation of OH· using iron as the metal catalyst:

$$O_2^- + Fe^{3+} \rightarrow O_2 + Fe^{2+} \tag{3}$$

$$Fe^{2+} + H_2O_2 \rightarrow Fe^{3+} + OH^- + OH \cdot \tag{4}$$

The sum of the two individual reactions can be written as follows:

$$O_2^- + H_2O_2 \rightarrow O_2 + OH^- + OH \cdot \tag{5}$$

During the respiratory burst, leukocytes also emit light. This phenomenon, called chemiluminescence, was originally ascribed to the decay of an excited form of oxygen termed singlet oxygen (Allen et al., 1972). There is however, no direct evidence that leukocytes produce singlet oxygen, and the actual source of chemiluminescence is currently unknown (McPhail et al., 1979; Foote et al., 1980).

Phagocytic cells, then, are capable of converting oxygen into potentially toxic species. The role of oxygen radicals in the antimicrobial and inflammatory activities of phagocytes and the mechanisms of stimulating these cells to produce oxygen radicals are the subjects of this review.

II. ROLE OF OXIDATIVE METABOLISM IN MICROBIAL KILLING

A. Studies Using Normal Cells or Oxygen Radical-Generating Systems

Several lines of evidence suggest that oxygen-dependent mechanisms are important in the microbicidal activity of leukocytes. Bactericidal activity, but not phagocytosis, is considerably depressed in vitro under hypoxic or anaerobic conditions (Selvaraj and Sbarra, 1966; Mandell, 1974). Furthermore, the removal of oxygen radicals by chemical scavengers or specific enzymes inhibits the killing capacity of phagocytes (Johnston et al., 1975). Oxygen radicals produced by chemical or enzymatic generating systems are destructive to microorganisms (Babior et al., 1975; Klebanoff, 1974; DeChatelet et al., 1975b; Drath and Karnovsky, 1974; Rosen and Klebanoff, 1979a). These studies have shown that either H_2O_2 or O_2^- have lethal effects. However, these two oxygen metabolites are much more effective in combination (Rosen and Klebanoff, 1979a), which supports a role for a product of their interactions, presumably hydroxyl radical [see Eq. (5)]. The bactericidal activity of H_2O_2 is also dramatically augmented in the presence of the enzyme myeloperoxidase (MPO) and a halide (Klebanoff, 1967). In most instances, circulating phagocytes secrete MPO (see Chapter 8, this volume) concomitantly with the triggering of H_2O_2 generation, and this system may also be an important microbicidal mechanism (Klebanoff, 1975). Here, the actual toxic species is probably hypochlorous acid, which can be formed by the $MPO-H_2O_2$ catalyzed oxidation of chloride ion [see Eq. (6)] (Agner, 1972; Harrison and Schultz, 1976; Weiss et al., 1982; Foote et al., 1983):

$$H_2O_2 + Cl^- \xrightarrow{MPO} OCl^- + H_2O \qquad (6)$$

Thus, leukocytes possess several oxygen-dependent mechanisms that are potentially bactericidal. The individual contribution of any particular mechanism has been difficult to determine and may vary with the target organism.

B. Phagocyte Oxidative Defects

Some insight into the relative contribution of different microbicidal mechanisms has been gained by the study of several experiments of nature, i.e., genetic defects that result in microbicidal abnormalities. Three important defects have been extensively investigated: (1) chronic granulomatous disease (CGD), in which the enzyme system responsible for converting oxygen into superoxide anion is defective; (2) hereditary myeloperoxidase deficiency; and (3) specific granule deficiency.

1. Chronic Granulomatous Disease

First described in 1957 (Berendes et al., 1957; Landing and Shirkey, 1957), CGD is characterized by increased susceptibility to recurrent bacterial infections. Leukocytes from these patients undergo normal phagocytosis and degranulation (Kaplan et al., 1968; Stossel et al., 1972; Baehner et al., 1969) but have a pronounced defect in their ability to kill most bacteria, particularly staphylococci and gram-negative enterics (Holmes et al., 1966; Quie et al., 1967). Leukocytes from patients with CGD do not respond with an increase in oxidative metabolism during phagocytosis (Holmes et al., 1967), supporting the dependence of cellular bactericidal activity on the respiratory burst.

The nature of the basic molecular defect in CGD has been controversial, and several enzyme deficiencies have been reported (reviewed by DeChatelet, 1978; Johnston and Newman, 1977; and Babior, 1978). The major controversy has centered around whether NADH or NADPH is the substrate providing reducing equivalents for O_2 (Baehner and Karnovsky, 1968; Segal and Peters, 1976; Hohn and Lehrer, 1975; McPhail et al., 1977; Curnutte et al., 1975). Most studies support NADPH as the physiological substrate, although purification of the enzyme will be necessary before the true substrate specificity can be determined.

Recent evidence has suggested that this NADPH oxidase activity is actually a multicomponent electron transport system consisting of a flavoprotein, a b-type cytochrome, and possibly ubiquinone. These studies are discussed in more detail in Section III. Conceivably a defect in any component required for activation of the enzyme system could result in CGD, and recent reports suggest that several different genetic forms of the disease exist. The classic X-linked form of CGD appears to be caused by the absence of the cytochrome b component of the NADPH oxidase system (Segal et al., 1983). An X-linked variant has also been described, in which the oxidase system has a decreased affinity for NADPH (Lew et al., 1981). A third defect was reported in which the patient's cells contained a normal cytochrome b component but had no detectable levels of the flavoprotein (Gabig, 1983). Identification of a specific defect in the autosomal recessive form of the disease has not been made, but it is likely that several different genetic deficiencies can exist. Possibilities include defects in a part of the mechanism of activation of the oxidase system, an alteration in a component of the oxidase itself, or complete absence of one or more of the components.

2. Myeloperoxidase Deficiency

Another disease characterized by an oxidative bactericidal defect is hereditary myeloperoxidase deficiency. In contrast to CGD, these patients have few recurrent infections, suggesting either that the $MPO-H_2O_2$-halide bactericidal system is of minor importance in vivo or that leukocytes from these patients have developed alternative bactericidal mechanisms (Lehrer and Cline, 1969; Klebanoff, 1970). Kinetic studies of the respiratory burst in leukocytes have shown that while the duration of the burst is brief in normal cells, it is much more prolonged in leukocytes from MPO-deficient patients (Rosen and Klebanoff, 1976; Nauseef et al., 1983). Other evidence has suggested that MPO may be a component of a normal control mechanism for inactivating the NADPH oxidase system (Jandl et al., 1978). Conceivably, then, in MPO-deficient cells, the increased persistence of oxygen radicals is sufficient for normal killing of most microorganisms (Klebanoff and Pincus, 1971; Rosen and Klebanoff, 1976). The isolated $MPO-H_2O_2$-halide system has been shown to have potent microbicidal, tumoricidal, and inflammatory activities (reviewed in Klebanoff, 1980) and the ability of normal leukocytes to mediate cytotoxic effects can be reduced by inhibitors which block MPO activity (Klebanoff, 1970). It is likely, then, that normal oxygen-dependent microbicidal activity depends on the joint action of MPO and the oxygen radical-generating system.

3. Specific Granule Deficiency

Leukocytes from several patients with increased susceptibility to bacterial infection were found to lack contents of specific granules (Strauss et al., 1974; Komiyama et al., 1979; Breton-Gorius et al., 1980; Gallin et al., 1982; Boxer et al., 1982). One of the components of specific granules is the iron-containing protein, lactoferrin. Lactoferrin has been shown to enhance production of hydroxyl radical by leukocyte particulate fractions containing the activated NADPH oxidase system (Ambruso and Johnston, 1981). The enhancement was dependent on the presence of iron bound to the protein, suggesting the involvement of the Haber-Weiss reactions [see Eqs. (3)-(5)]. The microbicidal defect in these cells may therefore reflect a deficiency of OH· production (Johnston, 1982). Indeed, leukocytes from two of these patients did have abnormally low levels of OH· production but had normal O_2^- generation (Ambruso et al., 1982b; Boxer et al., 1982). However, differentiated HL-60 promyelocytic leukemic cells completely deficient in lactoferrin can generate OH·, or similar oxidizing radicals (Newburger and Tauber, 1982). Studies on additional patients and cell lines will be necessary to resolve the role of lactoferrin in OH· production.

Further support for the possibility that OH· is important for optimal bactericidal activity is provided by studies of leukocytes from newborns. Their cells have a mild bactericidal defect (Wright et al., 1975; Shigeoka et al., 1979; Mills et al., 1979) and it has been shown that leukocytes from newborns are depressed in their ability to generate OH· but show normal or elevated levels of O_2^- production (Ambruso et al., 1979). This observation can be further correlated with decreased levels of lactoferrin in these cells (Ambruso et al., 1982a). Thus, the available evidence is strongly suggestive of an important role for OH· or similar oxidizing radicals in leukocyte microbicidal activity.

III. ENZYMATIC BASIS OF THE RESPIRATORY BURST

Identification of the enzyme responsible for converting oxygen to toxic products has been the subject of great interest and controversy for more than a decade. A number of enzymes have been proposed, including a soluble NADH oxidase (Baehner and Karnovsky, 1968; Badwey and Karnovsky, 1979), a particulate NADH oxidase (Briggs et al., 1977; Segal and Peters, 1976), glutathione peroxidase (Holmes et al., 1970), and a particulate NADPH oxidase (Patriarca et al., 1971; Hohn and Lehrer, 1975; DeChatelet et al., 1975a; Curnutte et al., 1975; Babior et al., 1976; McPhail et al., 1976). Other laboratories have been unable to confirm the earlier findings that glutathione peroxidase or a soluble NADH oxidase is deficient in chronic granulomatous disease (Holmes and Good, 1972; DeChatelet et al., 1976a). Most of the recent studies have supported a particulate NADPH oxidase activity as the respiratory burst enzyme in human neutrophils. This enzyme activity is almost undetectable in unstimulated, or resting, cells and increases dramatically when the cells are stimulated by phagocytosis (Hohn and Lehrer, 1975; DeChatelet et al., 1975a; Babior et al., 1976; McPhail et al., 1976). Moreover, the normal phagocytosis-associated increase in NADPH oxidase activity does not occur in cells from patients with CGD (Hohn and Lehrer, 1975; DeChatelet et al., 1975a; Curnutte et al., 1975; McPhail et al., 1977).

The activated enzyme is membrane bound and has been extensively studied using a postnuclear particulate fraction from broken cell preparations. The activity has a neutral pH optimum (Babior et al., 1976; Suzuki and Lehrer, 1980) and can use either NADPH or NADH as substrate (Babior et al., 1976; Iverson et al., 1977). The apparent Michaelis Constant (K_m) for NADPH ($\sim 50\ \mu M$) is about 10-fold lower than the K_m obtained for NADH (Babior et al., 1976; Iverson et al., 1977; Tauber and Goetzl, 1979; Cohen et al., 1980a,c; Suzuki and Lehrer, 1980; Light et al., 1981; McPhail and Snyderman, 1983), supporting NADPH as the physiological substrate. The stoichiometry of the reaction carried out by the enzyme is not yet clear (Light et al., 1981; Babior et al., 1976; Suzuki and Lehrer, 1980), probably because the enzyme preparations studied so far have been quite crude. However, a general reaction can be written as follows:

$$\left.\begin{array}{c} \text{NADPH} \\ \text{NADP}^+ \end{array}\right) \left(\begin{array}{c} \text{O}_2 \\ \text{O}_2^- \end{array}\right. \tag{7}$$

The enzyme activity can be partially solubilized from the membrane by means of detergents, and the properties of the solubilized enzyme are quite similar to those of the particulate enzyme (Gabig et al., 1978; Gabig and Babior, 1979; Tauber and Goetzl, 1979; Babior and Peters, 1981). Further purification has been difficult because solubilization yields are low and the solubilized activity is extremely unstable. However, ongoing efforts in several laboratories hold promise that purification will be accomplished in the near future.

The subcellular location of the enzyme activity has been controversial. Sucrose density gradient separation techniques have suggested a location either in the granule population (Patriarca et al., 1973; Iverson et al., 1978) or in the plasma membrane (Dewald et al., 1979; Yamaguchi et al., 1982). Other membrane isolation techniques have also supported a plasma membrane location (Cohen et al., 1980a,c). These results were obtained in stimulated cells, since the enzyme is measurable only when activated, and it is conceivable that the enzyme location is different in unstimulated cells. Final resolution of subcellular location will likely depend on the development of an antibody to the oxidase or its components.

Recent evidence has suggested that the respiratory burst "enzyme" is actually a multicomponent system similar to known electron transport chains. The concept was initially proposed by Segal et al. (1978), who described a cytochrome b present in normal human neutrophils that was absent in several patients with CGD. Through the efforts of several laboratories this concept has evolved into a model system consisting of a flavoprotein moiety (Babior and Kipnes, 1977; Gabig and Babior, 1979; Light et al., 1981), the b-type cytochrome (Millard et al., 1979; Borregaard et al., 1979, 1982; Segal and Jones, 1980; Sloan et al., 1981; Cross et al., 1982; Gabig et al., 1982; Segal et al., 1983) and possibly a ubiquinone component (Sloan et al., 1981; Crawford and Schneider, 1982;

Cunningham *et al.*, 1982). The possible pathway of electron transport can be outlined as follows:

$$
\begin{pmatrix} \text{NADPH} \\ \text{NADP}^+ \end{pmatrix} \begin{pmatrix} \text{FAD}^+ \\ \text{FADH}_2 \end{pmatrix} \begin{pmatrix} \text{quinone}_{(\text{red})} \\ \text{quinone}_{(\text{ox})} \end{pmatrix} \begin{pmatrix} \text{cyt. b}_{(\text{ox})} \\ \text{cyt. b}_{(\text{red})} \end{pmatrix} \begin{pmatrix} \text{O}_2^- \\ \text{O}_2 \end{pmatrix} \quad (8)
$$

Initially, two electrons are transferred from NADPH to the flavoprotein. They are then transported one at a time, to the b cytochrome, possibly through the participation of ubiquinone 50. The final step is transfer of an electron to O_2, resulting in formation of O_2^-. It should be emphasized that this model is hypothetical. Recently, it has been reported that the flavoprotein and cytochrome b moities of the activated oxidase system can be resolved into separate fractions (Gabig, 1983). This technique should permit reconstitution experiments to be undertaken, which will be necessary to determine the pathway of electron transport.

Recent evidence has also suggested that components of the oxidase system may be located in separate sites in the cell and are assembled during activation of the respiratory burst (Rossi *et al.*, 1980; Sloan *et al.*, 1981; DeChatelet *et al.*, 1982; Borregaard *et al.*, 1983). This concept is appealing, since assembly of components as a step in the activation process could be a powerful regulatory mechanism (see Section V).

Most of the studies described above were carried out using human or guinea pig neutrophils. A particulate NADPH oxidase activity also exists in monocytes and macrophages (McPhail *et al.*, 1981b; Chaudhry *et al.*, 1982; Sasada *et al.*, 1983; Hoffman and Autor, 1980; Lew and Stossel, 1981). The K_m for NADPH in these reports is similar to that for the neutrophil activity. However, one study reported about a 2-fold increase in the K_m for the human monocyte compared with the neutrophil enzyme in paired experiments (Chaudhry *et al.*, 1982). It seems unlikely, however, that the enzyme is different in monocytes, since monocytes share with neutrophils the respiratory burst defect observed in CGD (Musson *et al.*, 1982; Mandell and Hook, 1969; Chaudhry *et al.*, 1982). A decrease in K_m for NADPH has also been reported for the oxidase activity from lipopolysaccharide-elicited mouse macrophages in comparison with the activity from resident macrophages (Sasada *et al.*, 1983). Undoubtedly, the crudeness of the preparations used for K_m determinations could introduce artifacts, and comparison of purified enzymes will be necessary to determine whether differences truly exist.

IV. ACTIVATION OF THE RESPIRATORY BURST

Although the nature of the respiratory burst enzyme has been extensively studied, less effort has been directed toward understanding the mechanism of activation of the enzyme system. Activation is initiated at the plasma membrane of the cell either by stimulus-receptor coupling or by one of several nonreceptor-mediated mechanisms. A heterogeneous array of particulate and soluble stimuli can trigger the respiratory burst, raising the possibility that more than one mechanism exists for activation of the oxidase system. The stimuli that do not act through known or postulated receptors, i.e., ionophores, are of interest, since their mechanisms of action, if understood, may suggest possible transductional events. However, it is important to consider that an intermediate step proposed by studies using only one stimulus may not hold for all stimuli.

The following major approaches have been used to study activation mechanisms: (1) correlating changes in the levels of potential intermediates with activation of the respiratory burst; (2) examining the effect of agents which inhibit or augment potential intermediates on respiratory burst activity; and (3) comparing normal cells with cells from patients with CGD for the presence or absence of changes or for any differences in characteristics of the changes. Although the evidence obtained from these studies is indirect and does not prove participation of any particular intermediate, candidates may be suggested that can be examined more extensively. On the basis of stimulus–response mechanisms in other cell types, a number of second messengers are candidates for participation in activation of the respiratory burst. These include cyclic nucleotides, arachidonate or its metabolites, and calcium and/or other ion fluxes. Several criteria should be met by any intermediate: (1) the onset of a change in its level should precede the onset of the respiratory burst; (2) inhibition or enhancement of its level should appropriately affect respiratory burst activity; and (3) reconstitution of the intermediate with the remainder of the transductional machinery should activate the oxidase system. None of the possible intermediates has yet been shown to fulfill all these criteria.

A. Cyclic Nucleotides

Several stimuli that induce a respiratory burst, e.g., chemoattractants, the calcium ionophore A23187, immune complexes, also induce a transient rise in the level of cAMP in human neutrophils (Herlin *et al.,* 1978; Simchowitz *et al.,* 1980*b;* Smolen *et al.,* 1980). After stimulation with chemoattractants, levels of cAMP were shown to increase 2- to 3-fold, peak at 5–15 sec, and return to basal levels by 2–5 min. Levels of cGMP remained unchanged during stimulation, although earlier reports stated that cGMP did accumulate in response to chemoattractants, phorbol myristate acetate (PMA), or A23187 (Hatch *et al.,* 1977; Smith and Ignarro, 1975). The reported increase in cAMP preceded onset of O_2^- generation, implying that cAMP may be an intermediate. However, these investigators found that treatment of cells with cAMP agonists causing a sustained increase in cAMP levels did not provoke O_2^- release and actually inhibited stimulus-induced O_2^- generation, in agreement with the inhibition of the respiratory burst by cAMP agonists previously observed at other laboratories (May et al., 1970; Qualliotine et al., 1972; Cox and Karnovsky, 1973; Nakagawara and Minakami, 1975; Goldstein et al., 1976; Lehmeyer and Johnston, 1978). Several of these prior studies also found that treatment with agents that increase cGMP levels had no effect on respiratory burst activity (Nakagawara and Minakami, 1975; Lehmeyer and Johnston, 1978; Simchowitz et al., 1980b).

Further evidence supporting a role for cAMP and not cGMP in affecting stimulus-induced responses is given by a report, using immunocytochemistry, of the appearance of cAMP on the granulocyte cell surface early during phagocytosis coincident with the appearance of granule products (Pryzwansky et al., 1981). No changes were observed in the distribution of cGMP at this time point (30 sec of phagocytosis). These investigators also found that the regulatory subunit of type 1 cAMP-dependent protein kinase appeared with cAMP on the cell surface at the site of newly forming phagosomes. This observation is consistent with the possibility that the rise in cAMP levels after stimulation of the cell could activate a protein kinase involved in the regulation of the respiratory burst enzyme. On the basis of the evidence described above, this cAMP-mediated regulation is more likely to control an inactivation mechanism, rather than an activation process.

B. Arachidonic Acid and Its Metabolites

Addition of various stimuli to neutrophils results in the release of arachidonic acid from membrane phospholipids and conversion of arachidonate to several hydroxylated and prostanoid metabolites (Higgs et al., 1976; Zurier and Sayadoff, 1975; Goldstein et al., 1978; Wentzell and Epand, 1979; Borgeat and Samuelsson, 1979; Hirata et al., 1979; Stenson and Parker, 1979; Goetzel and Sun, 1979; Walsh et al., 1981). The release of arachidonate is probably achieved by activation of a phospholipase, either a phospholipase C followed by the action of diacylglycerol lipase (Pike and Snyderman, 1981) or a phospholipase A_2 (Hirata et al., 1979; Walsh et al., 1981) or both (Takenawa et al., 1983), and the release requires a transmethylation reaction when triggered by N-formyl peptides (Pike and Snyderman, 1981; Hirata et al., 1979). Certain products of the lipoxygenase pathway of arachidonate metabolism, particularly leukotriene B_4 and 12-L-hydroxy-eicosatetraenoic acid, have been reported to trigger activation of the respiratory burst (Goetzl et al., 1977; Serhan et al., 1982b), but several other metabolites appear to be inactive (Goetzl et al., 1980). Moreover, inhibitors of arachidonate metabolism (indomethacin, nordihydroguaiaretic acid, 5, 8,11,14-eicosatetraynoic acid, and p-bromophenacyl bromide) decrease the magnitude of the respiratory burst induced by fMet-Leu-Phe, PMA, and opsonized zymosan (Simchowitz et al., 1979; Smolen and Weissmann, 1980; Rossi et al.,

1981; Stocker and Richter, 1982). However, other investigators have found that indomethacin and 5,8,11,14-eicosatetraynoic acid had no effect on O_2^- generation triggered by PMA or immunoglobulin-coated filters (Badwey et al., 1981; Lehmeyer and Johnston, 1978). The basis for the differences using PMA as stimulus may be that different inhibitors were used by the different investigators and may also relate to the specificity problems associated with the use of inhibitors in general. Interestingly, PMA, a potent inducer of the respiratory burst (Repine et al., 1974; DeChatelet et al., 1976a), does not appear to trigger the release of arachidonate (Walsh et al., 1981). This implies that arachidonate or its metabolites may be intermediates in activating the respiratory burst for some, but not all stimuli.

Arachidonic acid itself has been shown to trigger oxidative metabolism in human neutrophils (Badwey et al., 1981; Ochs and Reed, 1981). Inhibitor studies suggested that the response to arachidonate is not mediated by a metabolite (Badwey et al., 1981), and other fatty acids can also stimulate the respiratory burst (Kakinuma and Minakami, 1978; Heyneman and Bauwens-Monbaliu, 1981; Badwey et al., 1981), implying that the arachidonate released by some stimuli could directly mediate activation of the respiratory burst. It is possible that other products of phospholipase C-mediated phosphatidylinositol turnover may influence activation of oxidative metabolism. Phosphatidic acid has been shown to act as a calcium ionophore in liposomes, and it is generated before the onset of O_2^- release in human neutrophils (Cockcroft et al., 1980; Serhan et al., 1981; Serhan et al., 1982a; Serhan et al., 1983). Diacylglycerol can activate the calcium and phospholipid-dependent protein kinase (protein kinase C) from rat brain (Kishimoto et al., 1980). Phosphorylation is a common activation mechanism for enzymes, and it is tempting to speculate that such a mechanism may be operating in neutrophils for triggering the respiratory burst. This will be discussed in Section IV. C. Presently, however, the precise role that arachidonate release and phosphatidylinositol turnover may have in the activation of the burst is unclear.

C. Calcium and Calcium-Dependent Protein Kinases

Considerable evidence has accumulated that calcium is an important second messenger in many cell types, including leukocytes. Several stimuli of leukocytes have been shown to induce an increase in permeability of the cell membrane to calcium (Gallin and Rosenthal, 1974; Naccache et al., 1977; Molski et al., 1981). In the presence of the ionophores A23187 and X537, which increase membrane permeability to calcium, calcium alone can activate the respiratory burst (Schell-Frederick, 1974; Romeo et al., 1975). Finally, the ability of a variety of stimuli to trigger oxidative metabolism is dependent on calcium. Removal of extracellular calcium inhibits activation mediated by fMet-Leu-Phe, concanavalin A, fluoride ion, or digitonin (Cohen and Chovaniec, 1978; Lehmeyer et al., 1979; Simchowitz and Spilberg, 1979a; Curnutte et al., 1979; Smolen et al., 1981). This suggests the possibility that a calcium influx is involved in the activation mechanisms used by these stimuli. In support of this, it has been shown that inhibition of calcium fluxes with lanthanum ion or verapamil depress activation by fMet-Leu-Phe or cytochalasin D (Simchowitz and Spilberg, 1979a; Matsumoto et al., 1979).

Several lines of evidence have suggested that intracellular calcium changes may be more important for signal transduction than an influx of extracellular calcium. Generation of O_2^- triggered by either PMA or immune complexes is not affected by the absence of extracellular calcium (Lehmeyer et al., 1979; Smolen et al., 1981), and the response to several other stimuli is reduced, but not completely blocked by the presence of EGTA (Smolen et al., 1981). However, an inhibitor of intracellular calcium translocation, 8-(N,N-diethylamino)-octyl 3,4, 5-trimethoxybenzoate hydrochloride (TMB-8), could block activation by PMA and immune complexes and was more effective than EGTA with fMet-Leu-Phe or A23187 as stimuli (Matsumoto et al., 1979; Smith and Iden, 1981; Smolen et al., 1981).

In further support of a role for intracellular calcium changes, several investigators have shown that calcium is rapidly released from intracellular stores during stimulation. This was initially suggested by the observation that in the absence of extracellular calcium, several stimuli induce a calcium efflux (Gallin and Rosenthal, 1974; Barthelemy et al., 1977; Naccache et al., 1977). These results were extended by the ultrastructural demonstration of changes in the intracellular location of calcium during stimulation (Cramer and Gallin, 1979; Hoffstein, 1979). Further evidence has been obtained using the fluorescent probe, chlorotetracycline, which incorporates into the cell membrane and responds to changes in calcium concentration. Results suggest that calcium is rapidly lost from the membrane during stimulation and that the release precedes the onset of O_2^- generation (Naccache et al., 1979; Takeshige et al., 1980; Smolen and Weissmann, 1982).

The mechanism by which free intracellular calcium could mediate activation of the respiratory burst is still a matter of speculation. One possibility is through the action of calmodulin, a protein of widespread distribution in mammalian cells (Cheung, 1980). Calmodulin has been demonstrated in phagocytic cells (Chafouleas et al., 1979; Lew and Stossel, 1981; Takeshige and Minakami, 1981; Jones et al., 1982). A number of investigators have shown that calmodulin antagonists of varying specificities can inhibit O_2^- generation triggered by several stimuli (Cohen et al., 1980b; Alobaidi et al., 1981; Lew and Stossel, 1981; Smolen et al., 1981; Takeshige and Minakami, 1981; Ochs and Reed, 1981; Stocker and Richter, 1982). The influence of calcium, EGTA, purified calmodulin, or calmodulin antagonists on the activated NADPH oxidase system has been examined by several investigators (Cohen et al., 1980b; Lew and

Stossel, 1981; Takeshige and Minakami, 1981; Jones *et al.,* 1982). However, the results are not consistent, possibly because of differences in cell source or enzyme preparation and assay techniques. Therefore, no firm conclusions can be made as yet as to the role of calmodulin in regulating NADPH oxidase activity or in activating the respiratory burst.

A second possible enzyme for mediation of calcium effects is the calcium- and phospholipid-dependent protein kinase C (Takai *et al.,* 1979; Kuo *et al.,* 1980; Minakuchi *et al.,* 1981). Phosphorylation and dephosphorylation of proteins occur rapidly after stimulation of leukocytes (Schneider *et al.,* 1981; Andrews and Babior, 1983), suggesting that protein kinases and phosphatases are activated. Although cells from two patients with CGD had identical phosphorylation patterns (Andrews and Babior, 1983), this does not rule out a role for phosphorylation, since the defect in these patients' cells could be at some step after the phosphorylation event. The primary basis for proposing protein kinase C as a possible effector for calcium in leukoyctes is the observation made recently that phorbol diesters can directly bind to and activate protein kinase C in rat brain extracts (Castagna *et al.,* 1982; Niedel *et al.,* 1983) and in the granulocytic cell line, HL-60 (J. Niedel, personal communication). Since PMA is a potent activator of the respiratory burst in leukoyctes, protein kinase C could be the mechanism by which phorbol diesters induce this response. It has recently been reported that protein kinase C is the predominant kinase present in human neutrophils (Minakuchi *et al.,* 1981; Helfman *et al.,* 1983) and that it is also present in rabbit neutrophils (Huang *et al.,* 1983). Another interesting property of the phospholipid-dependent protein kinase C is that it also can be activated by diacylglycerol and calcium (Kishimoto *et al.,* 1980; Kuo *et al.,* 1980). As described in Section IV.B, several stimuli of leukocyte function trigger the breakdown of phosphatidylinositol, resulting in the formation of diacylglycerol. Thus, a second mechanism for activation of protein kinase C, that is independent of phorbol diesters, could exist in leukocytes.

We recently examined the role of various lipids in the activation of protein kinase C in human neutrophil extracts; some of our results are given in Table I. Similar to the observations in other cell types, human neutrophil protein kinase C can be efficiently activated by diacylglycerol and phosphatidylserine in a calcium-dependent fashion. No activation is observed in the absence of added lipid or with the addition of diolein alone. Phosphatidylserine alone could activate; however, the presence of diolein increased the affinity of protein kinase C for calcium (not shown). An unexpected finding was that arachidonic acid itself could activate protein kinase C. Activation by arachidonate was potentiated by diolein, but without an affinity shift for calcium (not shown). The presence of arachidonate did not further enhance the level of activity obtained with the combination of phosphatidylserine and diolein. We also demonstrated that PMA was a potent activator of human neutrophil protein kinase activity in the absence of calcium. These results clearly show that three mechanisms for

Table I. Effect of Various Lipids on Activation of Human Neutrophil
Protein Kinase C

Lipid added[a]	^{32}P Incorporated into histone[b,c] (cpm/40 μg extract protein)[d]	
	$-Ca^{2+}$	$+Ca^{2+}$
None	5,202 ± 27 (2)	4,841 ± 183 (3)
Diolein (2 μg/ml)	5,167 ± 950 (2)	5,046 ± 313 (3)
Phosphatidylserine (20 μg/ml)	6,791 ± 1,591 (2)	36,523 ± 3,317 (2)
Phosphatidylserine + diolein	6,716 ± 1,571 (3)	68,732 ± 5,040 (5)
Arachidonate (35 μg/ml)	4,855 ± 527 (3)	20,373 ± 790 (4)
Arachidonate + diolein	5,596 ± 204 (3)	35,217 ± 1,492 (4)
Arachidonate + diolein + phosphatidylserine	4,530 ± 516 (3)	64,399 ± 7,304 (5)
Phorbol myristate acetate (300 ng/ml) (+ phosphatidylserine, + diolein)	61,588 ± 2,413 (2)	58,473 (1)

[a]Lipids were added from freshly made stock. Aliquots of diolein and phosphatidylserine in chloroform were evaporated and resuspended in H_2O by sonication. Arachidonate was dissolved in 100% ethanol and diluted with H_2O to 25% ethanol, and pH was adjusted to neutrality just before use. Phorbol myristate acetate was in dimethyl sulfoxide.
[b]Protein kinase C assay was performed as described by Helfman et al. (1983) in the presence of 0.4 mM EGTA and in the presence or absence of 2.0 mM added calcium.
[c]Total number of experiments performed with each stimulus is given in parentheses.
[d]Triton X-100 extracts of unstimulated human neutrophils were prepared as described by Helfman et al. (1983).

activation of protein kinase C potentially exist in human neutrophils. In the presence of phosphatidylserine, receptor-mediated release of diacylglycerol could activate protein kinase C, possibly without a local change in calcium concentration. Release of arachidonate, either alone or with diacylglycerol, is a second possible mechanism of activation. An increase in calcium concentration would likely be required as well, possibly induced by products of arachidonate, itself, i.e., LTB$_4$ (Serhan et al., 1982a). The third mechanism is the direct activation of protein kinase C by phorbol diesters, such as PMA, in the absence of calcium or changes in calcium concentration. Indeed, our preliminary data suggest that PMA causes a marked increase in the affinity of the kinase for calcium. Taken together, these results support a model proposing the participation of protein kinase C in activation of the respiratory burst.

D. Transmembrane Potential and Ion Fluxes

One of the earliest responses to a stimulus in leukocytes is a change in membrane potential, as measured either indirectly, using lipophilic probes, in neutrophils (Utsumi et al., 1977; Korchak and Weissmann, 1978; Seligmann et al., 1980; Simchowitz et al., 1980a; Whitin et al., 1980) or directly, using microelectrodes, in macrophages (Gallin and Gallin, 1977). The initial change appears to be a depolarization (Seligmann and Gallin, 1980; Kuroki *et al.*, 1982), which is likely caused by movement of specific ions, as yet unidentified. Fluxes of calcium, sodium, and potassium occur after stimulation of the cell (Naccache *et al.*, 1977; Gallin and Gallin, 1977; Simchowitz and Spilberg, 1979*b*), any or all of which could influence membrane potential.

These membrane potential changes appear to be linked to activation of the respiratory burst. The normal membrane depolarization observed in response to fMet-Leu-Phe or PMA is absent in cells from some patients with CGD (Whitin *et al.*, 1980; Seligmann and Gallin, 1980). However, cells from at least one CGD patient had a normal depolarization response (Lew *et al.*, 1981), suggesting that depolarization is not sufficient for triggering of the respiratory burst and also that depolarization is not itself a consequence of oxygen radical production. Although several conditions that inhibit membrane depolarization also depress the stimulation of oxidative metabolism (Whitin *et al.*, 1980; Korchak and Weissmann, 1980; Simchowitz and Spilberg, 1979*b*), membrane depolarization induced by high extracellular potassium levels, gramicidin or ouabain does not trigger the respiratory burst or influence the normal oxidative response to fMet-Leu-Phe (Kuroki *et al.*, 1982; Della Bianca *et al.*, 1983). Thus, the precise relationship of membrane potential changes to activation of the respiratory burst is still unclear.

V. MULTIPLE MECHANISMS OF ACTIVATION

Evidence has accumulated suggesting that not all stimuli share the same transductional pathway for activation of the respiratory burst. Some stimuli (fMet-Leu-Phe, Con A) demonstrate a marked dependence on extracellular calcium, while others (immune complexes, PMA) do not (Lehmeyer *et al.*, 1979; Simchowitz and Spilberg, 1979*a*; Smolen *et al.*, 1981; Smith and Ignarro, 1980). Activation of oxidative metabolism by some stimuli (fMet-Leu-Phe, C5a) is enhanced by the presence of cytochalasin B, while activation by others (PMA) is unaffected (Lehmeyer *et al.*, 1979; Webster *et al.*, 1980; Boxer *et al.*, 1979). Generation of O_2^- triggered by fMet-Leu-Phe can be inhibited by low concentrations of aliphatic alcohols, while O_2^- release by PMA is unaffected (Yuli *et al.*, 1982). Also, two patients have been described whose cells did not respond to some stimuli with increased oxidative metabolism, similar to CGD, but their cells responded normally to other stimuli (Weening *et al.*, 1976; Harvath and Andersen, 1979).

Further evidence was provided by McPhail *et al.* (1981*a*) who showed that neutrophils exposed to the nonpenetrating protein-reactive agent, *p*-diazobenzenesulfonic acid (DASA), were able to produce O_2^- at normal levels in response to some stimuli, such as PMA, A23187, and sodium fluoride, but not to others, such as fMet-Leu-Phe, Con A. In contrast, lysosomal enzyme release induced by all stimuli was normal, suggesting that the inhibition of O_2^- release was not due to inhibition of binding. The inhibitory effect of DASA on the ability of Con A to stimulate O_2^- release and the inability of DASA to inhibit PMA-induced O_2^- generation had been described previously (Goldstein *et al.*, 1977; Badwey *et al.*, 1980). These results implied that a DASA-susceptible surface protein was involved in a transduction mechanism used only by certain stimuli and suggested the existence of more than one mechanism of activation.

Measurements in the aforementioned experiments were of O_2 consumption and O_2^- release by intact cells. This left open the possibility that the differences between stimuli were actually due to activation of separate respiratory burst enzymes. We have recently compared the Michaelis constants of the NADPH and NADH oxidase activities found in particulate fractions isolated from cells stimulated by chemoattractants, A23187, or PMA (McPhail and Snyderman, 1983). The results are given in Table II. No significant difference (F test) in the apparent K_m for NADPH was found using different stimuli. The K_m for NADH of the enzyme activated by fMet-Leu-Phe was 10-fold higher (450 μM). These values are in agreement with those previously reported for oxidase activity (see Section III). The variation in V_{max} shown in Table II indicates that the total amount of enzyme activated was stimulus dependent. These results suggested that the same enzyme was activated by dissimilar stimuli.

Table II. K_m and V_{max} Values for NADPH Oxidase Activity Triggered by Various Stimuli

Stimulus[a]	K_m[b,c] (M)	V_{max}[b,c] (nmol O_2^-/min per mg)
fMet-Leu-Phe	59 ± 4 (4)	3.3 ± 0.8 (4)
A23187	60 ± 6 (3)	2.2 ± 0.7 (3)
PMA, 1 min	54 ± 4 (3)	4.6 ± 0.7 (3)
PMA, 15 min	44 ± 6 (3)	22.7 ± 4.8 (3)

[a]Neutrophils were treated with the indicated stimulus for various times in the presence of cytochalasin B, and particulate fractions were isolated as described previously (McPhail and Snyderman, 1983). Conditions of stimulation were 10^{-6} M fMet-Leu-Phe for 1 min; 5×10^{-6} M A23187 for 5 min; 1.6×10^{-6} M phorbol myristate acetate (PMA) for 1 min; or 1.6×10^{-6} M PMA for 15 min.

[b]K_m and V_{max} were determined in each individual experiment by Lineweaver-Burk analysis of data obtained at 9 to 10 substrate concentrations using the assay for NADPH oxidase activity described by McPhail and Snyderman (1983). These values were combined for the mean ± SEM shown.

[c]Total number of experiments performed with each stimulus is given in parentheses.

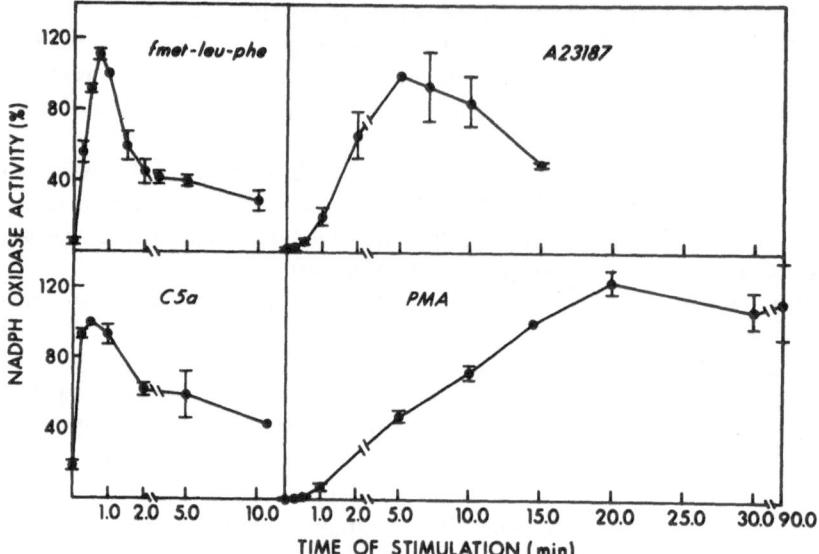

Figure 1. Kinetics of activation of NADPH oxidase by various stimuli. Neutrophils were exposed for the indicated times to either 10^{-6} M fMet-Leu-Phe, 10^{-7} M C5a, 5×10^{-6} M A23187, or 1.6×10^{-6} M phorbol myristate acetate (PMA) in the presence of cytochalasin B. Particulate fractions were then isolated and assayed as described by McPhail and Snyderman (1983). Data are expressed as the mean ±SEM of two to eight experiments at each time point, except for only one experiment at 10 min with C5a. Reproduced from *J. Clin. Invest.*, 1983, **72**:196, by copyright permission of the American Society for Clinical Investigation.

Examination of the temporal pattern of activation by different stimuli provided the first direct evidence that the mechanism of activation of NADPH oxidase varies with the stimulus. As shown in Figure 1, oxidase activation by chemoattractants began rapidly (no detectable lag in particulate fractions), peaked by 45 sec, and then declined. In contrast, activation by A23187 or PMA began after a lag of 15–30 sec and proceeded more slowly. A23187-mediated activation peaked at 5 min and then declined gradually. Activation by PMA plateaued at 20 min and did not decline for as long as 90 min. These data also suggest the existence of different stimulus-dependent regulatory mechanisms. Oxidase activation by chemoattractants is rapidly suppressed, while levels of enzyme activated by PMA remain constant for long periods of time. Thus, chemoattractants, but not PMA, appear to trigger directly an inactivation mechanism as well as an activation process.

These results did not distinguish whether the pathways used by different stimuli were totally independent or whether they converged at some step before activation of the oxidase itself. If exposure of cells to one stimulus could influence activation by a second stimulus, we reasoned that the two stimuli might share a common intermediate. This possibility had been suggested by studies in intact cells, showing that initial exposure of human neutrophils or monocytes either to chemoattractants (Van Epps and Garcia, 1980; English *et al.*, 1981; Kitagawa and Takaku, 1981) or to several nonchemotactic soluble stimuli (Fletcher and Gallin, 1982; Badwey *et al.*, 1982; Kitagawa *et al.*, 1980) potentiated the oxidative response to another stimulus. This was extended by Bender *et al.* (1983) to show that the level of NADPH oxidase activated by PMA was increased, but the K_m for NADPH was unchanged, by pre-exposure of neutrophils to chemoattractants. We undertook to examine systematically the effect of initial treatment of cells with one stimulus on both the kinetics of activation of NADPH oxidase and the level of oxidase activity achieved by stimulation with a second agent.

Cells were sequentially exposed to a series of heterologous or homologous stimuli, and levels of oxidase activity in particulate fractions were examined. As shown in Figure 2, cells were stimulated with 10^{-6} *M* fMet-Leu-Phe for 5 min, during which time NADPH oxidase levels peaked and declined. Cells given a second dose of fMet-Leu-Phe (10^{-6} *M*) showed no restimulation of oxidase

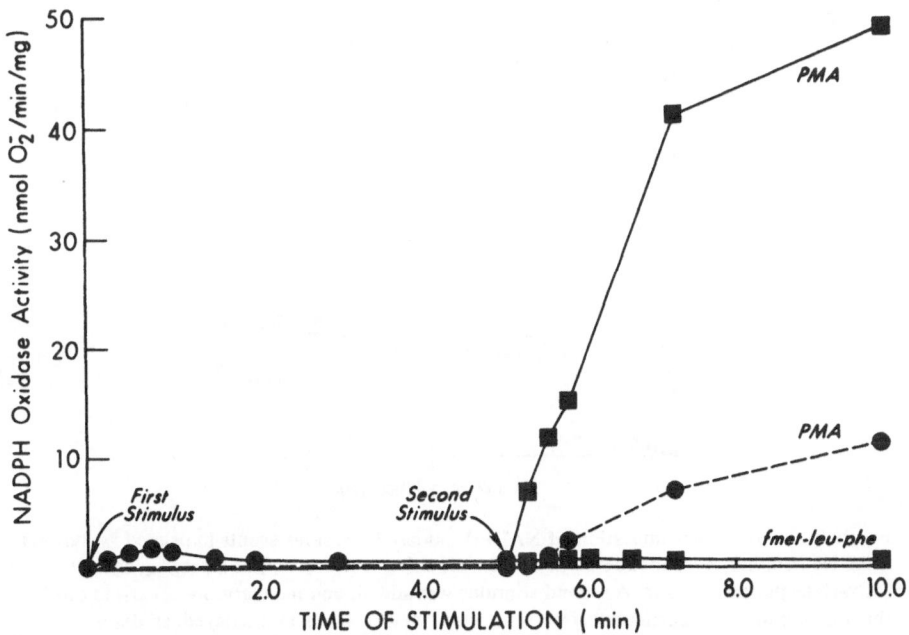

Figure 2. Temporal pattern of NADPH oxidase activity from cells stimulated sequentially with the same or a different agent. Neutrophils at 5×10^7/ml were incubated for various times at $37°C$ with either buffer as the first stimulus (- - - -) or with 10^{-6} *M* fMet-Leu-Phe as the first stimulus (———). At 5 min either 10^{-6} *M* fMet-Leu-Phe or 1.6×10^{-6} *M* phorbol myristate acetate (PMA) was added, and incubation was carried out for the additional times indicated. Particulate fractions were then isolated and assayed as described by McPhail and Snyderman (1983).

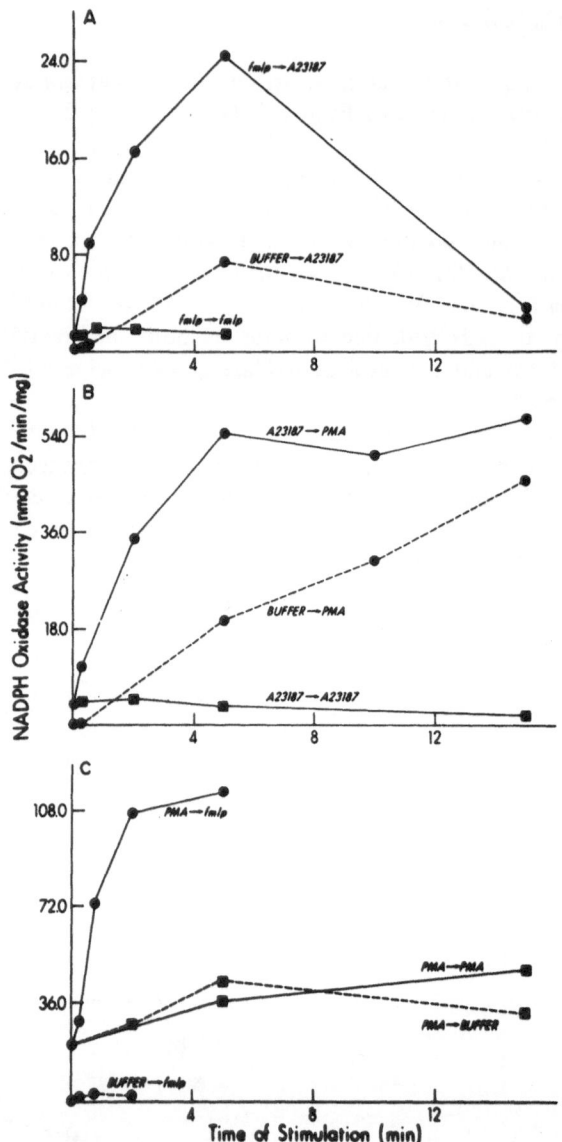

Figure 3. Kinetics of stimulation of NADPH oxidase by various agents in primed *vs.* normal cells. Neutrophils were incubated at 37°C with either buffer (----) or a priming agent (——) for various periods of time. A second stimulus was added, and incubation was carried out for the times indicated. Particulate fractions were then isolated and assayed as described by McPhail and Snyderman (1983). (A) Cells were exposed to buffer or 10^{-6} M fMet-Leu-Phe (fMLP) for 5 min, followed by either 10^{-6} M fMet-Leu-Phe or 10^{-5} M A23187. (B) Cells were exposed to buffer or 10^{-5} M A23187 for 15 min, followed by either 10^{-5} M A23187 or 1.6×10^{-6} M phorbol myristate acetate (PMA). (C) Cells were exposed to buffer or 1.6×10^{-7} M PMA for 20 min, followed by either 1.6×10^{-6} M PMA or 10^{-6} M fMet-Leu-Phe.

activity. However, in cells given PMA ($1.6 \times 10^{-6}\ M$) at 5 min, a marked enhancement of NADPH oxidase activation was apparent, as compared with control cells exposed initially to buffer alone. The enhancement was characterized by elimination of the normal lag period, a faster rate of activation, and achievement of activity levels 2- to 3-fold higher than normal. We have termed this enhancing effect "priming," which is similar in some respects to the potentiation of oxidative responses by bacterial products observed in macrophages (Pabst and Johnston, 1980). Priming for NADPH oxidase activation is also observed with other combinations of heterologous stimuli. As shown in Figure 3, fMet-Leu-Phe can prime for A23187, PMA can prime for fMet-Leu-Phe, and A23187 can prime for PMA. In contrast, cells exposed to any given stimulus are unresponsive to a second addition of the same stimulus. However, this unresponsiveness (homologous desensitization) depended on the concentration of stimulus used for the priming exposure. Figure 4 demonstrates that fMet-Leu-Phe at doses of $\leqslant 10^{-7}\ M$ could prime for itself. The ability of each stimulus to influence oxidase activation by other stimuli suggests that, although stimulus-dependent differences in the patterns of activation exist, a common intermediate is shared by all.

We were able to differentiate this shared priming step from the final activation of the oxidase in several ways. First, the ED_{50} for priming by a given stimulus

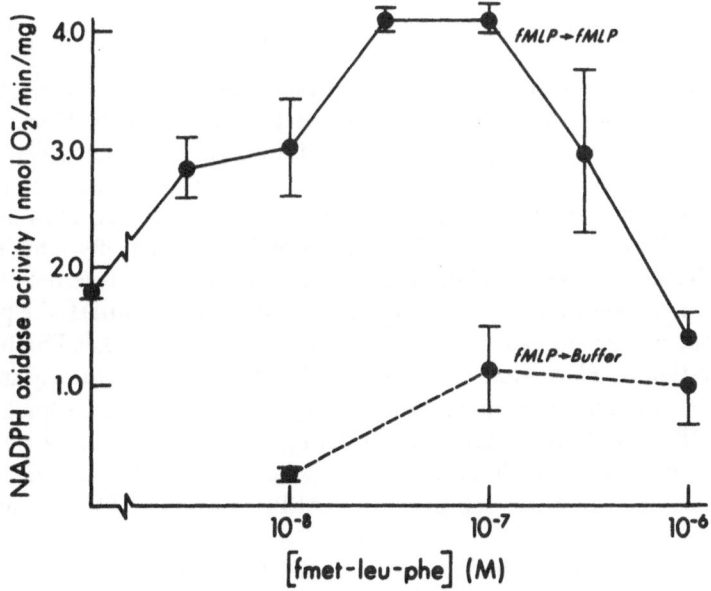

Figure 4. Effect of varying the concentration of fMet-Leu-Phe (fMLP) for priming on activation of NADPH oxidase by a second exposure to fMet-Leu-Phe. Neutrophils at 37°C were treated with various doses of fMet-Leu-Phe for 5 min and were then given either $10^{-6}\ M$ fMet-Leu-Phe (——) or buffer (- - - -) for 45 sec. Particulate fractions were then isolated and assayed as described by McPhail and Snyderman (1983).

Table III. ED_{50} Values for Priming versus Activation of
NADPH Oxidase by Different Stimuli

Stimulus[b]	ED_{50}[a]	
	Priming[c]	Activation[d]
f Met-Leu-Phe	$3.4 \times 10^{-8}\,M$	$2.9 \times 10^{-7}\,M$
Phorbol myristate acetate (PMA)	$5.0 \times 10^{-8}\,M$	$5.7 \times 10^{-7}\,M$
A23187	$1.6 \times 10^{-7}\,M$	$2.9 \times 10^{-6}\,M$

[a]ED_{50} values were calculated from curves obtained using 7–10 concentrations of each agent. Results are given as the mean of two experiments with each stimulus for priming and three to four experiments with each stimulus for activation.
[b]Neutrophils were stimulated in the presence of cytochalasin B, and particulate fractions were isolated and assayed as described by McPhail and Snyderman (1983).
[c]Priming conditions were as follows: f Met-Leu-Phe, 5 min, followed by $1.6 \times 10^{-6}\,M$ phorbol myristate acetate (PMA), 5 min; PMA, 20 min, followed by $10^{-6}\,M$ f Met-Leu-Phe, 45 sec; A23187, 15 min, followed by $1.6 \times 10^{-6}\,M$ PMA, 5 min. Values were corrected for any activity obtained with the priming stimulus alone.
[d]Activation conditions were as follows: f Met-Leu-Phe, 1 min; PMA, 15 min; A23187, 5 min.

was 10-fold lower than the ED_{50} for activation by that stimulus (Table III). Second, activation of NADPH oxidase by fMet-Leu-Phe could be blocked under conditions in which priming was still evident. In these experiments, we took advantage of several pharmacological manipulations that inhibit activation of the respiratory burst by fMet-Leu-Phe but that have no effect on PMA-mediated activation. Removal of extracellular calcium by EGTA markedly inhibited oxidase activation by fMet-Leu-Phe, and the inhibition could be reversed in a dose-dependent fashion by the addition of calcium (Fig. 5). In contrast, the presence or absence of calcium had little effect on the ability of fMet-Leu-Phe to prime for activation by PMA. Activation by fMet-Leu-Phe was also strongly inhibited by addition of 0.25% butanol or removal of cytochalasin B during stimulation of the cells (Fig. 6). However, priming by fMet-Leu-Phe for PMA was unaffected by butanol and was observed in the absence of cytochalasin B. None of these manipulations had any effect on activation of NADPH oxidase by PMA in unprimed cells.

These results suggest that activation of NADPH oxidase by different stimuli is the result of at least two distinct shared processes. The priming step can be pharmacologically separated from the actual activation step, and our evidence suggests that each step is triggered by a separate signal. Our previous data (McPhail and Snyderman, 1983, Fig. 1) implies that separate transductional

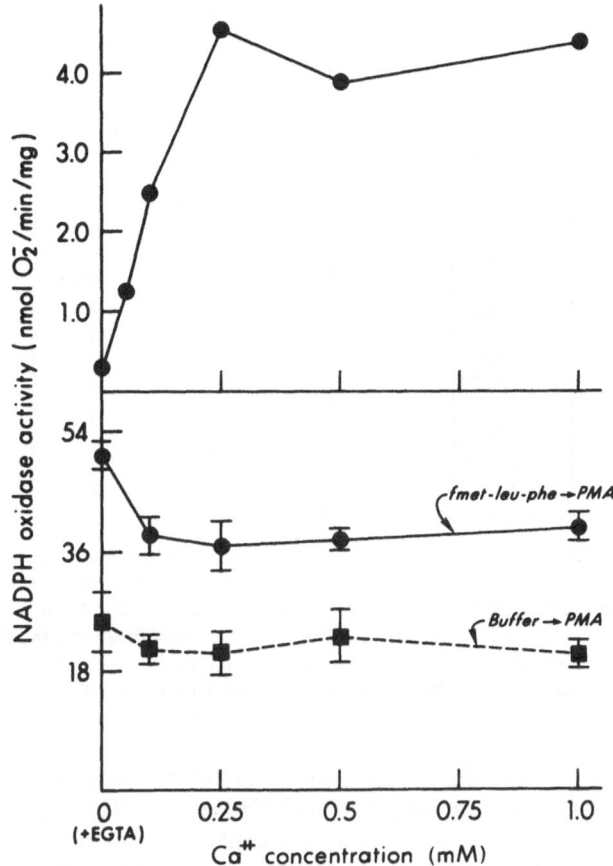

Figure 5. Effect of varying the concentration of calcium on activation *vs.* priming of NADPH oxidase by fMet-Leu-Phe. Neutrophils were suspended in saline, containing 5.0 m*M* Hepes at pH 7.4 and were incubated at 37°C in the presence of 3.0 m*M* EGTA or with the concentrations of CaCl$_2$ indicated. For activation, cells were stimulated with 10^{-6} *M* fMet-Leu-Phe for 45 sec. For priming, cells were exposed to buffer (----) or to 10^{-6} *M* fMet-Leu-Phe (——) for 5 min, followed by addition of 1.6×10^{-6} *M* phorbol myristate acetate (PMA) for an additional 15 min. Particulate fractions were then isolated and assayed.

pathways exist for different stimuli and, presumably, these occur before the final activation step. Also, other stimulus-specific regulatory mechanisms play a role, as evidenced by the homologous desensitization observed at high doses of each stimulus. The concentration of stimulus is critical for determining the signals that are transduced. Low doses of stimulus can trigger priming, but higher doses are required for signaling the final activation and for the homologous desensitization process. An intriguing hypothesis for a two-signal mechanism of NADPH

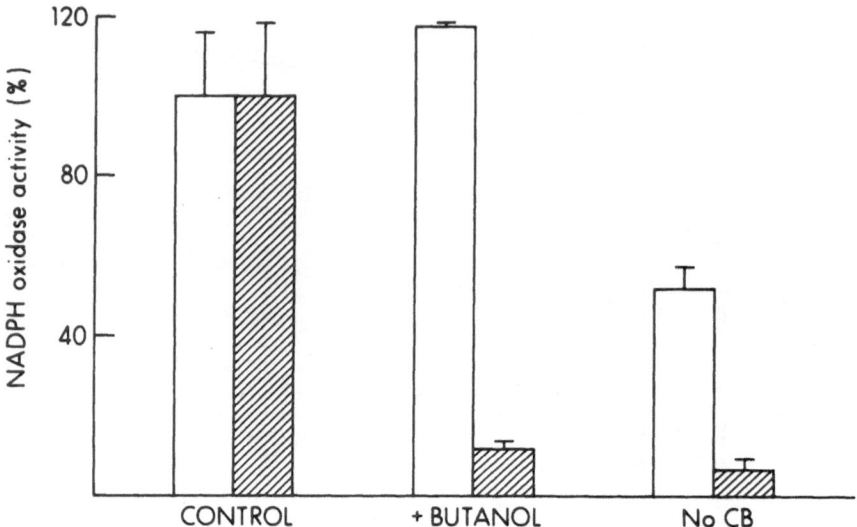

Figure 6. Effect of butanol and cytochalasin B (CB) on activation versus priming of NADPH oxidase by fMet-Leu-Phe. Neutrophils were incubated at 37°C in the presence or absence of 0.25% butanol (+CB) or in the presence or absence of 10^{-5} M CB for 5 min. (□) Activation conditions, exposure of cells to 10^{-6} M fMet-Leu-Phe for 45 sec. (■) Priming conditions, exposure of cells to 10^{-6} M fMet-Leu-Phe for 5 min, followed by 1.6 X 10^{-6} M phorbol myristate acetate for 5 min. Particulate fractions were then isolated and assayed.

oxidase activation incorporates our own and other recent observations that phorbol diesters activate protein kinase C (Castagna *et al.*, 1982; Niedel *et al.*, 1983) and that all or part of the oxidase complex may be translocated from an intracellular organelle to the plasma membrane during stimulation (Borregaard *et al.*, 1983). Thus, translocation of the oxidase system may be triggered by one signal, while phosphorylation of the enzyme complex may require a separate signal. Both signals would be necessary for activation to occur. If priming accomplished one of the signals, then a decrease in the lag time for activation might be expected. This has actually been observed in the case of PMA and A23187. We have also postulated the existence of one or more inactivation mechanisms for the oxidase and have proposed that oxidase activity is regulated by the balance between the rates of activation and inactivation (McPhail and Snyderman, 1983). A decrease in activation lag time caused by priming could change this balance and result in the enhanced levels of activity observed. Alternatively, it is possible that priming has inhibited the rate at which NADPH oxidase is inactivated. If inactivation of the oxidase is slowed or prevented by priming, a decrease in lag time for activation and potentiation of activity levels might be expected. We are currently exploring these possibilities for the nature of the priming step.

VI. MODEL FOR REGULATION OF NADPH OXIDASE

On the basis of our own studies, as well as the many others described herein, we have formulated a working model for the regulation of NADPH oxidase activity. We hypothesize that activation of NADPH oxidase is mediated by protein kinase C with the possible involvement of assembly and/or translocation of the oxidase complex. Activation of protein kinase C can be accomplished by several mechanisms, which can account for the different transductional mechanisms seen with different stimuli. First, PMA can activate the kinase directly. Second, stimuli such as chemoattractants and calcium ionophores could mediate activation by triggering phosphatidylinositol turnover and/or phospholipase A_2 activation. The resulting products, arachidonate and diacylglycerol, can activate protein kinase C directly in the presence of calcium. The increase in calcium concentration could be mediated by arachidonate metabolites, such as leukotriene B_4 and/or phosphatidic acid, which act as endogenous ionophores.

The inactivation pathway could be mediated by cAMP-dependent protein kinase. Increasing the levels of cAMP by pharmacological means results in inhibition of the respiratory burst (see Section IV.A). Both chemoattractants and the calcium ionophore A23187 trigger a rapid increase in levels of cAMP, while PMA does not (Smolen and Weissmann, 1981; Section IV.A). The patterns of the cAMP responses parallel to some degree the inactivation patterns observed for the oxidase triggered by chemoattractants and A23187 (McPhail and Snyderman, 1983) (see Fig. 1). The onset of the inactivation of the oxidase and the increase in cAMP occurs earlier and at a faster rate with chemoattractants, as compared with A23187. Although PMA does not trigger an early increase in cAMP levels, later time points (15–20 min) have not been analyzed. The plateau observed for oxidase activation by PMA (Fig. 1) could be caused by a delayed activation of cAMP-dependent protein kinase, or it could reflect saturation of either the available activation mechanism, i.e., protein kinase C, or the available oxidase. Thus, we are postulating that the level of NADPH oxidase activity in phagocytic cells is ultimately regulated by the rates of phosphorylation and dephosphorylation triggered by each stimulus. Evidence for direct phosphorylation and dephosphorylation of the oxidase complex does not yet exist, nor is it known whether a kinase activates and a phosphatase inactivates, or *vice versa*. These areas will undoubtedly be the focus of future research efforts.

VII. REFERENCES

Agner, K., 1972, Biological effects of hypochlorous acid formed by "MPO" peroxidation in the presence of chloride ions, in: *Structure and Function of Oxidation-Reduction Enzymes* (A. Akeson and A. Ehrenberg, eds.), Vol. 18, pp. 329–335, Pergamon Press, New York.

Allen, R. C., Sternholm, R. L., and Steele, R. J., 1972, Evidence for the generation of an electronic excitation state(s) in human polymorphonuclear leukocytes and its participation in bactericidal activity, *Biochem. Biophys. Res. Commun.* 47:679.

Alobaidi, T., Naccache, P. H., and Sha'afi, R. I., 1981, Calmodulin antagonists modulate rabbit neutrophil degranulation, aggregation and stimulated oxygen consumption, *Biochim. Biophys. Acta* 675:316.

Ambruso, D. R., and Johnston, R. B., Jr., 1981, Lactoferrin enhances hydroxyl radical production by human neutrophils, neutrophil particulate fractions and an enzymatic generating system, *J. Clin. Invest.* 67:352.

Ambruso, D. R., Altenburger, K. M., and Johnston, R. B., Jr., 1979, Defective oxidative metabolism in newborn neutrophils: Discrepancy between superoxide anion and hydroxyl radical generation, *Pediatrics* 64:722.

Ambruso, D. R., Bentwood, B., Henson, P. M., and Johnston, R. B., Jr., 1982a, Decreased hydroxyl radical generation and lactoferrin content in cord blood neutrophils, *Pediatr. Res.* 16:198A. (Abstr.)

Ambruso, D. R., Sasada, M., Nishiyama, H., Kubo, A., Komiyama, A., and Allen, R. H., 1982b, Studies of neutrophil function in a patient with specific granule deficiency, *Clin. Res.* 30:309A. (Abstr.)

Andrews, P. C., and Babior, B. M., 1983, Endogenous protein phosphorylation by resting and activated human neutrophils, *Blood* 61:333.

Babior, B. M., 1978, Oxygen-dependent microbial killing by phagocytes, *N. Engl. J. Med.* 298:659, 721.

Babior, B. M., and Kipnes, R. S., 1977, Superoxide-forming enzyme from human neutrophils: Evidence for a flavin requirement, *Blood* 50:517.

Babior, B. M., and Peters, W. A., 1981, The O_2^--producing enzyme of human neutrophil. Further properties, *J. Biol. Chem.* 256:2321.

Babior, B. M., Kipnes, R. S., and Curnutte, J. T., 1973, Biological defense mechanisms. The production by leukocytes of superoxide, a potential bactericidal agent, *J. Clin. Invest.* 52:741.

Babior, B. M., Curnutte, J. T., and Kipnes, R. S., 1975, Biological defense mechanisms. Evidence for the participation of superoxide in bacterial killing by xanthine oxidase, *J. Lab. Clin. Med.* 85:235.

Babior, B. M., Curnutte, J. T., and McMurrich, B. J., 1976, The particulate superoxide-forming system from human neutrophils. Properties of the system and further evidence supporting its participation in the respiratory burst, *J. Clin. Invest.* 58:989.

Badwey, J. A., and Karnovsky, M. L., 1979, Production of superoxide and hydrogen peroxide by an NADH oxidase in guinea pig polymorphonuclear leukocytes. Modulation by nucleotides and divalent cations, *J. Biol. Chem.* 254:11530.

Badwey, J. A., Curnutte, J. T., Robinson, J. M., Lazdins, J. K., Briggs, R. T., Karnovsky, M. J., and Karnovsky, M. L., 1980, Comparative aspects of oxidative metabolism of neutrophils from human blood and guinea pig peritonea: Magnitude of the respiratory burst, dependence upon stimulating agents, and localization of the oxidases, *J. Cell. Physiol.* 105:541.

Badwey, J. A., Curnutte, J. T., Karnovsky, M. L., 1981, cis-Polyunsaturated fatty acids induce high levels of superoxide production by human neutrophils, *J. Biol. Chem.* 256:12640.

Badwey, J. A., Curnutte, J. T., Berde, C. B., and Karnovsky, M. L., 1982, Cytochalasin E diminishes the lag phase in the release of superoxide by human neutrophils, *Biochem. Biophys. Res. Commun.* 106:170.

Baehner, R. L., and Karnovsky, M. L., 1968, Deficiency of reduced nicotinamide adenine dinucleotide oxidase in chronic granulomatous disease, *Science* 162:1277.

Baehner, R. L., Karnovsky, M. J., and Karnovsky, M. L., 1969, Degranulation of leukocytes in chronic granulomatous disease, *J. Clin. Invest.* **48**:187.

Baldridge, C. W., and Gerard, R. W., 1933, The extra respiration of phagocytosis, *Am. J. Physiol.* **103**:235.

Barthelemy, A., Paridaens, R., and Schell-Frederick, E., 1977, Phagocytosis-induced [45] calcium efflux in polymorphonuclear leukocytes, *FEBS Lett.* **82**:283.

Bender, J. G., McPhail, L. C., and Van Epps, D. E., 1983, Exposure of human neutrophils to chemotactic factors potentiates activation of the respiratory burst enzyme, *J. Immunol.* **130**:2316.

Berendes, H., Bridges, R. A., and Good, R. A., 1957, A fatal granulomatosus of childhood, *Minn. Med.* **40**:309.

Borgeat, P., and Samuelsson, B., 1979, Arachidonic acid metabolism in polymorphonuclear leukocytes: Effects of ionophore A23187, *Proc. Natl. Acad. Sci. (USA)* **76**:2148.

Borregaard, N., Staehr-Johansen, K., Taudorff, E., and Wandall, J. H., 1979, Cytochrome b is present in neutrophils from patients with chronic granulomatous disease, *Lancet* **1**:949.

Borregaard, N., Simons, E. R., and Clark, R. A., 1982, Involvement of cytochrome b_{-245} in the respiratory burst of human neutrophils, *Infect. Immun.* **38**:1301.

Borregaard, N., Heiple, J. M., Simons, E. R., and Clark, R. A., 1983, Subcellular localization of the b-cytochrome component of the microbicidal oxidase: Translocation during activation, *J. Cell. Biol.* **97**:52.

Boxer, L. A., Yoder, M., Bonsib, S., Schmidt, M., Ho, P., Jersild, R., and Baehner, R. L., 1979, Effects of a chemotactic factor, N-formyl-methionyl peptide on adherence, superoxide anion generation, phagocytosis, and microtubule assembly of human polymorphonuclear leukocytes, *J. Lab. Clin. Med.* **93**:583.

Boxer, L. A., Coates, T. D., Haak, R. A., Wolach, J., Hoffstein, S., and Baehner, R. L., 1982, Lactoferrin deficiency associated with altered granulocyte function, *N. Engl. J. Med.* **307**:404.

Breton-Gorius, J., Mason, D. Y., Buriot, D., Vilde, J. L., and Griscelli, C., 1980, Lactoferrin deficiency as a consequence of a lack of specific granules in neutrophils from a patient with recurrent infections: Detection by immunoperoxidase staining for lactoferrin and cytochemical electron microscopy, *Am. J. Pathol.* **99**:413.

Briggs, R. T., Karnovsky, M. L., and Karnovsky, M. J., 1977, Hydrogen peroxide production in chronic granulomatous disease. A cytochemical study of reduced pyridine nucleotide oxidases, *J. Clin. Invest.* **59**:1088.

Castagna, M., Takai, Y., Kaibuchi, K., Sano, K., Kikkawa, U., and Nishizuka, Y., 1982, Direct activation of calcium-activated, phospholipid-dependent protein kinase by tumor-promoting phorbol esters, *J. Biol. Chem.* **257**:7847.

Chafouleas, J. G., Dedman, J. R., Munjaal, R. P., and Means, A. R., 1979, Calmodulin. Development and application of a sensitive radioimmunoassay, *J. Biol. Chem.* **254**:10262.

Chaudhry, A. N., Santinga, J. T., and Gabig, T. G., 1982, The subcellular particulate NADPH-dependent O_2^--generating oxidase from human blood monocytes: Comparison to the neutrophil system, *Blood* **60**:979.

Cheung, W. Y., 1980, Calmodulin plays a pivotal role in cellular regulation, *Science* **207**:19.

Cockcroft, S., Bennett, J. P., and Gomperts, B. D., 1980, Stimulus–secretion coupling in rabbit neutrophils is not mediated by phosphatidyl inositol breakdown, *Nature* **288**:275.

Cohen, H. J., and Chovaniec, M. E., 1978, Superoxide production by digitonin-stimulated guinea pig granulocytes. The effects of N-ethyl maleimide, divalent cations, and glycolytic and mitochondrial inhibitors on the activation of the superoxide-generating system, *J. Clin. Invest.* **61**:1088.

Cohen, H. J., Chovaniec, M. E., and Davies, W. A., 1980a, Activation of the guinea pig granulocyte NAD(P)H-dependent superoxide generating enzyme: Localization in a plasma membrane enriched particle and kinetics of activation, *Blood* 55:355.

Cohen, H. J., Chovaniec, M. E., and Ellis, S. E., 1980*b*, Chlorpromazine inhibition of granulocyte superoxide production, *Blood* 56:23.

Cohen, H. J., Newburger, P. E., and Chovaniac, M. E., 1980*c*, NAD(P)H-dependent superoxide production by phagocytic vesicles from guinea pig and human granulocytes, *J. Biol. Chem.* 255:6584.

Cox, J. P., and Karnovsky, M. L., 1973, The depression of phagocytosis by exogenous cyclic nucleotides, prostaglandins, and theophylline, *J. Cell. Biol.* 59:480.

Cramer, E. B., and Gallin, J. I., 1979, Localization of submembranous cations to the leading end of human neutrophils during chemotaxis, *J. Cell. Biol.* 82:369.

Crawford, D. R., and Schneider, D. L., 1982, Identification of ubiquinone-50 in human neutrophils and its role in microbicidal events, *J. Biol. Chem.* 257:6662.

Cross, A. R., Higson, F. K., Jones, O. T. G., Harper, A. M., and Segal, A. W., 1982, The enzymic reduction and kinetics of oxidation of cytochrome b_{-245} of neutrophils, *Biochem. J.* 204:479.

Cunningham, C. C., DeChatelet, L. R., Spach, P. I., Parce, W., Thomas, M. J., Lees, C. J., and Shirley, P. S., 1982, Identification and quantitation of electron-transport components in human polymorphonuclear neutrophils, *Biochim. Biophys. Acta* 682:430.

Curnutte, J. T., Kipnes, R. A., and Babior, B. M., 1975, Defect in pyridine nucleotide dependent superoxide production by a particulate fraction from the granulocytes of patients with chronic granulomatous disease, *N. Engl. J. Med.* 293:628.

Curnutte, J. T., Babior, B. M., and Karnovsky, M. L., 1979, Fluoride-mediated activation of the respiratory burst in human neutrophils. A reversible process, *J. Clin. Invest.* 63:637.

DeChatelet, L. R., 1978, Initiation of the respiratory burst in human polymorphonuclear neutrophils: A critical review, *J. Reticuloendothel. Soc.* 24:73.

DeChatelet, L. R., McPhail, L. C., Mullikin, D., and McCall, C. E., 1975*a*, An isotopic assay for NADPH oxidase activity and some characteristics of the enzyme from human polymorphonuclear leukocytes, *J. Clin. Invest.* 55:714.

DeChatelet, L. R., Shirley, P. S., Goodson, P. R., and McCall, C. E., 1975*b*, Bactericidal activity of superoxide anion and of hydrogen peroxide: Investigations employing dialuric acid, a superoxide generating drug, *Antimicrob. Agents Chemother.* 8:146.

DeChatelet, L. R., Shirley, P. S., and Johnston, R. B., Jr., 1976*a*, Effect of phorbol myristate acetate on the oxidative metabolism of human polymorphonuclear leukocytes, *Blood* 47:545.

DeChatelet, L. R., Shirley, P. S., and McPhail, L. C., 1976*b*, Normal leukocyte glutathione peroxidase activity in patients with chronic granulomatous disease, *J. Pediatr.* 89:598.

DeChatelet, L. R., Lees, C. J., and Shirley, P. S., 1982, Separation of superoxide generation from NADP formation in subcellular fractions from human neutrophils, *Clin. Res.* 30: 363A. (Abstr.)

Della Bianca, V., Bellavite, P., De Togni, P., Fumarulo, K., and Rossi, F., 1983, Studies on stimulus-response coupling in human neutrophils. I. Role of monovalent cations in the respiratory and secretory response to *N*-formylmethionylleucylphenylalanine, *Biochem. Biophys. Acta* 755:497.

Dewald, B., Baggiolini, M., Curnutte, J. T., and Babior, B. M., 1979, Subcellular localization of the superoxide-forming enzyme in human neutrophils, *J. Clin. Invest.* 63:21.

Drath, D. B., and Karnovsky, M. L., 1974, Bactericidal activity of metal-mediated peroxide-ascorbate systems, *Infect. Immun.* 10:1077.

English, D., Roloff, J. S., and Lukens, J. N., 1981, Chemotactic factor enhancement of superoxide release from fluoride and phorbol myristate acetate stimulated neutrophils, *Blood* 58:129.

Fletcher, M. P., Seligmann, B. E., and Gallin, J. I., 1982, Correlation of human neutrophil secretion, chemoattractant receptor mobilization, and enhanced functional capacity, *J. Immunol.* **128**:941.

Foote, C. S., Abakerli, R. B., Clough, R. L., and Shook, F. C., 1980, On the question of singlet oxygen production in leukocytes, macrophages and the dismutation of superoxide anion, in: *Biological and Clinical Aspects of Superoxide and Superoxide Dismutase* (W. H. Bannister and J. V. Bannister, eds.), pp. 222–230, Elsevier–North Holland, New York.

Foote, C. S., Goyne, T. E., and Lehrer, R. I., 1983, Assessment of chlorination by human neutrophils, *Nature* **301**:715.

Gabig, T. G., 1983, The NADPH-dependent O_2^--generating oxidase from human neutrophils. Identification of a flavoprotein component that is deficient in a patient with chronic granulomatous disease, *J. Biol. Chem.* **258**:6352.

Gabig, T. G., and Babior, B. M., 1979, The O_2^--forming oxidase responsible for the respiratory burst in human neutrophils. Properties of the solubilized enzyme, *J. Biol. Chem.* **254**:9070.

Gabig, T. G., Kipnes, R. S., and Babior, B. M., 1978, Solubilization of the O_2^- forming activity responsible for the respiratory burst in human neutrophils, *J. Biol. Chem.* **253**:6663.

Gabig, T. G., Schervish, E. W., and Santinga, J. T., 1982, Functional relationship of the cytochrome b to the superoxide-generating oxidase of human neutrophils, *J. Biol. Chem.* **257**:4114.

Gallin, E. K., and Gallin, J. I., 1977, Interaction of chemotactic factors with human macrophages: Induction of transmembrane potential changes, *J. Cell. Biol.* **75**:277.

Gallin, J. I., and Rosenthal, A. S., 1974, The regulatory role of divalent cations in human granulocyte chemotaxis, *J. Cell. Biol.* **62**:594.

Gallin, J. I., Fletcher, M. P., Seligmann, B. E., Hoffstein, S., Cehrs, K., and Mounessa, N., 1982, Human neutrophil specific granule deficiency: A model to assess the role of neutrophil specific granules in the evolution of the inflammatory process response, *Blood* **59**:1317.

Goetzl, E. J., and Sun, F. F., 1979, Generation of unique monohydroxy-eiscosatetraenoic acids from arachidonic acid by human neutrophils, *J. Exp. Med.* **150**:406.

Goetzl, E. J., Woods, J. M., and Gorman, R. R., 1977, Stimulation of human eosinophil and neutrophil polymorphonuclear leukocyte chemotaxis and random migration by 12-L-hydroxy-5,8,10,14-eicosatetraenoic acid, *J. Clin. Invest.* **59**:179.

Goetzl, E. J., Brash, A. R., Tauber, A. I., Oates, J. A., and Hubbard, W. C., 1980, Modulation of human neutrophil function by monohydroxy-eicosatetraenoic acids, *Immunology* **39**:491.

Goldstein, I. M., Roos, D., Weissmann, G., and Kaplan, H. B., 1976, Influence of corticosteroids on human polymorphonuclear leukocyte function *in vitro*. Reduction of lysosomal enzyme release and superoxide production, *Inflammation* **1**:305.

Goldstein, I. M., Cerqueira, M., Lind, S., and Kaplan, H. B., 1977, Evidence that the superoxide-generating system of human leukocytes is associated with the cell surface, *J. Clin. Invest.* **59**:249.

Goldstein, I. M., Malmsten, C. L., Kindahl, H., Kaplan, H. B., Ridmark, O., Samuelsson, B., and Weissmann, G., 1978, Thromboxane generation by human peripheral blood polymorphonuclear leukocytes, *J. Exp. Med.* **148**:787.

Haber, F., and Weiss, J., 1934, The catalytic decomposition of hydrogen peroxide by iron salts, *Proc. R. Soc. Lond.(A)* **147**:332.

Harrison, J. E., and Schultz, J., 1976, Studies on the chlorinating activity of myeloperoxidase, *J. Biol. Chem.* **251**:1371.

Harvath, L., and Andersen, B. R., 1979, Defective initiation of oxidative metabolism in polymorphonuclear leukocytes, *N. Engl. J. Med.* **300**:1130.

Hatch, G. E., Nichols, W. K., and Hill, H. R., 1977, Cyclic nucleotide changes in human neutrophils induced by chemoattractants and chemoattractant modulators, *J. Immunol.* 119:450.

Helfman, D. M., Appelbaum, B. D., Vogler, W. R., and Kuo, J. F., 1983, Phospholipid-sensitive Ca^{2+}-dependent protein kinase and its substrates in human neutrophils, *Biochem. Biophys. Res. Commun.* 111:847.

Herlin, T., Petersen, C. S., and Esmann, V., 1978, The role of calcium and cyclic adenosine 3',5'-monophosphate in the regulation of glycogen metabolism in phagocytosing human polymorphonuclear leukocytes, *Biochim. Biophys. Acta* 542:63.

Heyneman, R. A., and Bauwens-Monbaliu, D., 1981, Kinetics of nicotinamide adenine dinucleotides in oleate-stimulated polymorphonuclear leukocytes, *FEBS Lett.* 127:87.

Higgs, G. A., Bunting, S., Moncada, S., and Vane, J. R., 1976, Polymorphonuclear leukocytes produce thromboxane A_2-like activity during phagocytosis, *Prostaglandins* 12:749.

Hirata, F., Corcoran, B. A., Venkatasubramanian, K., Schiffmann, E., and Axelrod, J., 1979, Chemoattractants stimulate degradation of methylated phospholipids and release of arachidonic acid in rabbit leukocytes, *Proc. Natl. Acad. Sci. (USA)* 76:2640.

Hoffman, M., and Autor, A. P., 1980, Production of superoxide anion by an NADPH-oxidase from rat pulmonary macrophages, *FEBS Lett.* 121:352.

Hoffstein, S. T., 1979, Ultrastructural demonstration of calcium loss from local regions of the plasma membrane of surface-stimulated human granulocytes, *J. Immunol.* 123:1395.

Hohn, D. C., and Lehrer, R. I., 1975, NADPH oxidase deficiency in X-linked chronic granulomatous disease, *J. Clin. Invest.* 55:707.

Holmes, B., and Good, R. A., 1972, Metabolic and functional abnormalities of human neutrophils, in: *Phagocytic Mechanisms in Health and Disease* (R. C. Williams, Jr., ed.), p. 51, Intercontinental Book Corp., New York.

Holmes, B., Quie, P. G., Windhorst, D. B., and Good, R. A., 1966, Fatal granulomatous disease of childhood: An inborn abnormality of phagocytic function, *Lancet* 1:1225.

Holmes, B., Page, A. R., and Good, R. A., 1967, Studies of the metabolic activity of leukocytes from patients with a genetic abnormality of phagocytic function, *J. Clin. Invest.* 46:1422.

Holmes, B., Park, B. H., Malawista, S. E., Quie, P. G., Nelson, D. L., and Good, R. A., 1970, Chronic granulomatous disease in females. A deficiency of leukocyte glutathione peroxidase, *N. Engl. J. Med.* 283:217.

Huang, C. K., Hill, J. H., Jr., Mackin, W. M., Bormann, B. J., and Becker, E. L., 1983, Effects of chemotactic factors on the protein phosphorylation of rabbit peritoneal neutrophils, *Fed. Proc.* 42:1080. (Abstr.)

Iverson, D., DeChatelet, L. R., Spitznagel, J. K., and Wang, P., 1977, Comparison of NADH and NADPH oxidase activities in granules isolated from human polymorphonuclear leukocytes with a fluorometric assay, *J. Clin. Invest.* 59:282.

Iverson, D. B., Wang-Iverson, P., Spitznagel, J. K., and DeChatelet, L. R., 1978, Subcellular localization of NAD(P)H oxidase(s) in human neutrophilic polymorphonuclear leukocytes, *Biochem. J.* 176:175.

Iyer, G. Y. N., Islam, M. F., and Quastel, J. H., 1961, Biochemical aspects of phagocytosis, *Nature* 192:535.

Jandl, R. C., Andre-Schwartz, J., Borges-DuBois, L., Kipnes, R. S., McMurrich, B. J., and Babior, B. M., 1978, Termination of the respiratory burst in human neutrophils, *J. Clin. Invest.* 61:1176.

Johnston, R. B., Jr., 1982, Defects of neutrophil function, *N. Engl. J. Med.* 307:434.

Johnston, R. B., Jr., and Newman, S. L., 1977, Chronic granulomatous disease, *Pediatr. Clin. North Am.* 24:365.

Johnston, R. B., Jr., Keele, B. B., Jr., Misra, H. P., Lehmeyer, J. E., Webb, L. S., Baehner, R. L., and Rajagopalan, K. V., 1975, The role of superoxide anion generation in phagocytic bactericidal activity. Studies with normal and chronic granulomatous disease leukocytes, *J. Clin. Invest.* **55**:1357.

Jones, H. P., Ghai, G., Petrone, W. F., and McCord, J. M., 1982, Calmodulin-dependent stimulation of the NADPH oxidase of human neutrophils, *Biochim. Biophys. Acta* **714**:152.

Kakinuma, K., and Minakami, S., 1978, Effects of fatty acids on superoxide radical generation in leukocytes, *Biochim. Biophys. Acta* **538**:50.

Kaplan, E. L., Laxdal, T., and Quie, P. G., 1968, Studies of polymorphonuclear leukocytes from patients with chronic granulomatous disease of childhood: Bactericidal capacity for streptococci, *Pediatrics* **41**:591.

Kishimoto, A., Takai, Y., Mori, T., Kikkawa, U., and Nishizuka, Y., 1980, Activation of calcium and phospholipid-dependent protein kinase by diacylglycerol, its possible relationship to phosphatidyl inositol turnover, *J. Biol. Chem.* **255**:2273.

Kitagawa, S., and Takaku, F., 1981, Effect of the chemotactic peptide on the subsequent superoxide releasing response in human polymorphonuclear leukocytes, *FEBS Lett.* **128**:5.

Kitagawa, S., Takaku, F., and Sakamoto, S., 1980, A comparison of the superoxide-releasing response in human polymorphonuclear leukocytes and monocytes, *J. Immunol.* **125**:359.

Klebanoff, S. J., 1967, A peroxidase-mediated antimicrobial system in leukocytes, *J. Clin. Invest.* **46**:1078.

Klebanoff, S. J., 1970, Myeloperoxidase: Contribution to the microbicidal activity of intact leukocytes, *Science* **169**:1095.

Klebanoff, S. J., 1974, Role of superoxide anion in the myeloperoxidase-mediated antimicrobial system, *J. Biol. Chem.* **249**:3724.

Klebanoff, S. J., 1975, Antimicrobial mechanisms in neutrophilic polymorphonuclear leukocytes, *Semin. Hematol.* **12**:117.

Klebanoff, S. J., 1980, Oxygen metabolism and the toxic properties of phagocytes, *Ann. Intern. Med.* **93**:480.

Klebanoff, S. J., and Pincus, S. H., 1971, Hydrogen peroxide utilization in myeloperoxidase-deficient leukocytes: A possible microbicidal control mechanism, *J. Clin. Invest.* **50**:2226.

Komiyama, A., Morosawa, H., Nakahata, T., Miyagawa, Y., and Akabane, T., 1979, Abnormal neutrophil maturation in a neutrophil defect with morphologic abnormality and impaired function, *J. Pediatr.* **94**:19.

Korchak, H. M., and Weissmann, G., 1978, Changes in membrane potential of human granulocytes antecede the metabolic responses to surface stimulation, *Proc. Natl. Acad. Sci. (USA)* **75**:3818.

Korchak, H. M., and Weissmann, G., 1980, Stimulus–response coupling in the human neutrophil. Transmembrane potential and the role of extracellular Na^+, *Biochim. Biophys. Acta* **601**:180.

Kuo, J. F., Anderson, R. G. G., Wise, B. C., Mackerlova, L., Salomonsson, I., Brackett, N. L., Katoh, N., Shoji, M., and Wrenn, R. W., 1980, Calcium-dependent protein kinase: Widespread occurrence in various tissues and phyla of the animal kingdom and comparison of effects of phospholipid, calmodulin, and trifluoperazine, *Proc. Natl. Acad. Sci. (USA)* **77**:7039.

Kuroki, M., Kamo, N., Kobatake, Y., Okimasu, E., Utsumi, K., 1982, Measurement of membrane potential in polymorphonuclear leukocytes and its changes during surface stimulation, *Biochim. Biophys. Acta* **693**:326.

Landing, B. H., and Shirkey, H. S., 1957, A syndrome of recurrent infections and infiltration of viscera by pigmented lipid histiocytes, *Pediatrics* **20**:431.

Lehmeyer, J. E., and Johnston, R. B., Jr., 1978, Effect of anti-inflammatory drugs and agents that elevate intracellular cyclic AMP on the release of toxic oxygen metabolites: Studies in a model of tissue-bound IgG, *Clin. Immunol. Immunopathol.* 9:482.

Lehmeyer, J. E., Snyderman, R., and Johnston, R. B., Jr., 1979, Stimulation of neutrophil oxidative metabolism by chemotactic peptides: Influence of calcium ion concentration and cytochalasin B and comparison with stimulation by phorbol myristate acetate, *Blood* 54:35.

Lehrer, R. I., and Cline, M. J., 1969, Leukocyte myeloperoxidase deficiency and disseminated candidiasis: The role of myeloperoxidase in resistance to *Candida* infection, *J. Clin. Invest.* 48:1478.

Lew, P. D., and Stossel, T. P., 1981, Effect of calcium on superoxide production by phagocytic vesicles from rabbit alveolar macrophages, *J. Clin. Invest.* 67:1.

Lew, P. D., Southwick, F. S., Stossel, T. P., Whitin, J. C., Simons, E., and Cohen, H. J., 1981, A variant of chronic granulomatous disease: Deficient oxidative metabolism due to a low-affinity NADPH oxidase, *N. Engl. J. Med.* 305:1329.

Light, D. R., Walsh, C., O'Callaghan, A. M., Goetzl, E. J., and Tauber, A. L., 1981, Characteristics of the cofactor requirements for the superoxide-generating NADPH oxidase of human polymorphonuclear leukocytes, *Biochemistry* 20:1468.

Mandell, G. L., 1974, Bactericidal activity of aerobic and anaerobic polymorphonuclear neutrophils, *Infect. Immun.* 9:337.

Mandell, G. L., and Hook, E. W., 1969, Leukocyte function in chronic granulomatous disease, *Am. J. Med.* 47:473.

Matsumoto, T., Takeshige, K., and Minakami, S., 1979, Inhibition of phagocytotic metabolic changes of leukocytes by an intracellular calcium-antagonist 8-(*N*, *N*-diethylamine)-octyl-3,4,5-trimethoxybenzoate, *Biochem. Biophys. Res. Commun.* 88:974.

May, C. D., Levine, B. B., and Weissmann, G., 1970, Effects of compounds which inhibit antigenic release of histamine and phagocytic release of lysosomal enzyme on glucose utilization by leukocytes in humans, *Proc. Soc. Exp. Biol. Med.* 133:758.

McPhail, L. C., and Snyderman, R., 1983, Activation of the respiratory burst enzyme in human polymorphonuclear leukocytes by chemoattractants and other soluble stimuli. Evidence that the same oxidase is activated by different transductional mechanisms, *J. Clin. Invest.* 72:192.

McPhail, L. C., DeChatelet, L. R., and Shirley, P. S., 1976, Further characterization of NADPH oxidase activity of human polymorphonuclear leukocytes, *J. Clin. Invest.* 58:774.

McPhail, L. C., DeChatelet, L. R., Shirley, P. S., Wilfert, C., Johnston, R. B., Jr., and McCall, C. E., 1977, Deficiency of NADPH oxidase activity in chronic granulomatous disease, *J. Pediatr.* 90:213.

McPhail, L. C., DeChatelet, L. R., and Johnston, Jr., R. B., 1979, Generation of chemiluminescence by a particulate fraction isolated from human neutrophils. Analysis of molecular events, *J. Clin. Invest.* 63:648.

McPhail, L. C., Henson, P. M., and Johnston, R. B., Jr., 1981a, Respiratory burst enzyme in human neutrophils. Evidence for multiple mechanisms of activation, *J. Clin. Invest.* 67:710.

McPhail, L. C., Musson, R. A., and Johnston, R. B., Jr., 1981b, Superoxide generation by human monocytes and monocyte-derived macrophages: Characterization of a monocyte subcellular NADPH oxidase, *Fed. Proc.* 40:4987. (Abstr.)

Millard, J. A., Gerard, K. W., and Schneider, D. L., 1979, The isolation from rat peritoneal leukocytes of plasma membrane enriched in alkaline phosphatase and a b-type cytochrome, *Biochem. Biophys. Res. Commun.* 90:321.

Mills, E. L., Thompson, T., Bjorksten, B., Filipovich, D., and Quie, P. G., 1979, The chemiluminescence response and bactericidal activity of polymorphonuclear neutrophils from newborns and their mothers, *Pediatrics* **63**:429.

Minakuchi, R., Takai, Y., Yu, B., and Nishizuka, Y., 1981, Widespread occurrence of calcium-activated, phospholipid-dependent protein kinase in mammalian tissues, *J. Biochem.* **89**:1651.

Molski, T. F. P., Naccache, P. H., Borgeat, P., and Sha'afi, R. I., 1981, Similarities in the mechanisms by which formyl-methionyl-leucyl-phenylalanine, arachidonic acid and leukotriene B_4 increase calcium and sodium influxes in rabbit neutrophils, *Biochem. Biophys. Res. Commun.* **103**:227.

Musson, R. A., McPhail, L. C., Shafran, H., and Johnston, R. B., Jr., 1982, Differences in the ability of human peripheral blood monocytes and *in vitro* monocyte-derived macrophages to produce superoxide anion, *J. Reticuloendothel Soc.* **31**:261.

Naccache, P. H., Showell, H. J., Becker, E. L., and Sha'afi, R. I., 1977, Transport of sodium, potassium, and calcium across rabbit polymorphonuclear leukocyte membranes. Effect of chemotactic factor, *J. Cell. Biol.* **73**:428.

Naccache, P. H., Volpi, M., Showell, H. J., Becker, E. L., Sha'afi, R. I., 1979, Chemotactic factor-induced release of membrane calcium in rabbit neutrophils, *Science* **203**:461.

Nakagawara, A., and Minakami, S., 1975, Generation of superoxide anions by leukocytes treated with cytochalasin E, *Biochem. Biophys. Res. Commun.* **64**:760.

Nauseef, W. M., Metcalf, J. A., and Root, R. K., 1983, Role of myeloperoxidase in the respiratory burst of human neutrophils, *Blood* **61**:483.

Newburger, P. E., and Tauber, A. I., 1982, Heterogeneous pathways of oxidizing radical production in human neutrophils and the HL-60 cell line, *Pediatr. Res.* **16**:856.

Niedel, J. E., Kuhn, L. J., and Vandenbark, G. R., 1983, Phorbol diester receptor copurifies with protein kinase C, *Proc. Natl. Acad. Sci. (USA)* **80**:36.

Ochs, D. L., and Reed, P. W., 1981, Inhibition of the neutrophil oxidative burst and degranulation by phenothiazines, *Biochem. Biophys. Res. Commun.* **102**:958.

Pabst, M. J., and Johnston, R. B., Jr., 1980, Increased production of superoxide anion by macrophages exposed *in vitro* to muramyl dipeptide or lipopolysaccharide, *J. Exp. Med.* **151**:101.

Patriarca, P., Cramer, R., Moncalvo, S., Rossi, F., and Romeo, D., 1971, Enzymatic basis of metabolic stimulation in leukocytes during phagocytosis: The role of activated NADPH oxidase, *Arch. Biochem. Biophys.* **145**:255.

Patriarca, P., Cramer, R., Dri, P., Fant, L., Basford, R. E., and Rossi, F., 1973, NADPH oxidizing activity in rabbit polymorphonuclear leukocytes: Localization in azurophilic granules, *Biochem. Biophys. Res. Commun.* **53**:830.

Pike, M. C., and Snyderman, R., 1981, Transmethylation reactions are required for initial morphologic and biochemical responses of human monocytes to chemoattractants, *J. Immunol.* **127**:1444.

Pryzwansky, K. B., Steiner, A. L., Spitznagel, J. K., and Kapoor, C. L., 1981, Compartmentalization of cyclic AMP during phagocytosis by human neutrophilic granulocytes, *Science* **211**:407.

Qualliotine, D., DeChatelet, L. R., McCall, C. E., and Cooper, M. R., 1972, Stimulation of oxidative metabolism in polymorphonuclear leukocytes by catecholamines, *J. Reticuloendothel. Soc.* **11**:263.

Quie, P. G., White, J. G., Holmes, B., and Good, R. A., 1967, *In vitro* bactericidal capacity of human polymorphonuclear leukocytes: Diminished activity in chronic granulomatous disease of childhood, *J. Clin. Invest.* **46**:668.

Repine, J. E., White, J. G., Clawson, C. C., Holmes, B. M., 1974, The influence of phorbol myristate acetate on oxygen consumption by polymorphonuclear leukocytes, *J. Lab. Clin. Med.* **83**:911.

Romeo, D., Zabucchi, G., Miani, M., and Rossi, F., 1975, Ion movement across leukocyte plasma membrane and excitation of their metabolism, *Nature* 253:542.

Rosen, H., and Klebanoff, S. J., 1976, Chemiluminescence and superoxide production by myeloperoxidase-deficient leukocytes, *J. Clin. Invest.* 58:50.

Rosen, H., and Klebanoff, S. J., 1979a, Bactericidal activity of a superoxide anion-generating system: A model for the polymorphonuclear leukocyte, *J. Exp. Med.* 149:27.

Rosen, H., and Klebanoff, S. J., 1979b, Hydroxyl radical generation by polymorphonuclear leukocytes measured by electron spin resonance spectroscopy, *J. Clin. Invest.* 64:1725.

Rossi, F., Patriarca, P., Berton, G., and De Nicola, G., 1980, Subcellular localization of the enzyme responsible for the respiratory burst in resting and phorbol myristate acetate activated leukocytes, in: *Biological and Clinical Aspects of Superoxide and Superoxide Dismutase* (W. H. Bannister and J. V. Bannister, eds.), pp. 193–200, Elsevier–North Holland, New York.

Rossi, F., Della Bianca, V., and Bellavite, P., 1981, Inhibition of the respiratory burst and of phagocytosis by nordihydroguaiaretic acid in neutrophils, *FEBS Lett.* 127:183.

Sasada, M., Pabst, M. J., and Johnston, R. B., Jr., 1983, Activation of mouse peritoneal macrophages by lipopolysaccharide alters the kinetic parameters of the superoxide producing NADPH oxidase, *J. Biol. Chem.* 258:9631.

Sbarra, A. J., and Karnovsky, M. L., 1959, The biochemical basis of phagocytosis. I. Metabolic changes during the ingestion of particles by polymorphonuclear leukocytes, *J. Biol. Chem.* 234:1355.

Schell-Frederick, E., 1974, Stimulation of the oxidative metabolism of polymorphonuclear leukocytes by the calcium ionophore A23187, *FEBS Lett.* 48:37.

Schneider, C., Zanetti, M., and Romeo, D., 1981, Surface-reactive stimuli selectively increase protein phosphorylation in human neutrophils, *FEBS Lett.* 127:4.

Segal, A. W., and Jones, O. T. G., 1980, Absence of cytochrome b reduction in stimulated neutrophils from both female and male patients with chronic granulomatous disease, *FEBS Lett.* 110:111.

Segal, A. W., and Peters, T. J., 1976, Characterization of the enzyme defect in chronic granulomatous disease, *Lancet* 1:1363.

Segel, A. W., Jones, O. T. G., Webster, D., and Allison, A. C., 1978, Absence of a newly described cytochrome b from patients with chronic granulomatous disease, *Lancet* 1:949.

Segal, A. W., Cross, A. R., Garcia, R. C., Borregaard, N., Valerius, N. H., Soothill, J. F., and Jones, O. T. G., 1983, Absence of cytochrome b_{-245} in chronic granulomatous disease. A multicenter European evaluation of its incidence and relevance, *N. Engl. J. Med.* 308:245.

Seligmann, B. E., and Gallin, J. I., 1980, Use of lipophilic probes of membrane potential to assess human neutrophil activation. Abnormality in chronic granulomatous disease, *J. Clin. Invest.* 66:493.

Seligmann, B. E., Gallin, E. K., Martin, D. L., Shain, W., and Gallin, J. I., 1980, Interaction of chemotactic factors with human polymorphonuclear leukocytes: Studies using a membrane potential sensitive cyanine dye, *J. Membr. Biol.* 52:257.

Selvaraj, R. J., and Sbarra, A. J., 1966, Relationship of glycolytic and oxidative metabolism to particle entry and destruction in phagocytosing cells, *Nature* 211:1272.

Serhan, C., Anderson, P., Goodman, E., Dunham, P., and Weissmann, G., 1981, Phosphatidate and oxidized fatty acids are calcium ionophores. Studies employing arsenazo III in liposomes, *J. Biol. Chem.* 256:2736.

Serhan, C. N., Fridovich, J., Goetzl, E. J., Dunham, P. B., and Weissmann, G., 1982a, Leukotriene B_4 and phosphatidic acid are calcium ionophores. Studies employing arsenazo III in liposomes, *J. Biol. Chem.* 257:4746.

Serhan, C. N., Radin, A., Smolen, J. E., Korchak, H., Samuelsson, B., and Weissmann, G., 1982b, Leukotriene B$_4$ is a complete secretagogue in human neutrophils: A kinetic analysis, *Biochem. Biophys. Res. Commun.* 107:1006.

Serhan, C. N., Broekman, M. J., Korchak, H. M., Smolen, J. E., Marcus, A. J., and Weissmann, G., 1983, Changes in phosphatidylinositol and phosphatidic acid in stimulated human neutrophils. Relationship to calcium mobilization, aggregation and superoxide radical generation, *Biochim. Biophys. Acta* 762:420.

Shigeoka, A. O., Santos, J. I., and Hill, H. R., 1979, Functional analysis of neutrophil granulocytes from healthy, infected, and stressed neonates, *J. Pediatr.* 95:454.

Simchowitz, L., and Spilberg, I., 1979a, Generation of superoxide radicals by human peripheral neutrophils activated by chemotactic factor. Evidence for the role of calcium, *J. Lab. Clin. Med.* 93:583.

Simchowitz, L., and Spilberg, I., 1979b, Chemotactic factor-induced generation of superoxide radicals by human neutrophils: Evidence for the role of sodium, *J. Immunol.* 123:2428.

Simchowitz, L., Mehta, J., and Spilberg, I., 1979, Chemotactic factor-induced generation of superoxide radicals by human neutrophils. Effect of metabolic inhibitors and antiinflammatory drugs, *Arthritis Rheum.* 22:755.

Simchowitz, L., Atkinson, J. P., and Spilberg, I., 1980a, Stimulus-specific deactivation of chemotactic factor-induced cyclic AMP response and superoxide generation by human neutrophils, *J. Clin. Invest.* 66:736.

Simchowitz, L., Fischbein, L. C., Spilberg, I., and Atkinson, J. P., 1980b, Induction of a transient elevation in intracellular levels of adenosine-3',5'-cyclic monophosphate by chemotactic factors: An early event in human neutrophil activation, *J. Immunol.* 124:1482.

Sloan, E. P., Crawford, D. R., and Schneider, D. L., 1981, Isolation of plasma membrane from human neutrophils and determination of cytochrome b and quinone content, *J. Exp. Med.* 153:1316.

Smith, R. J., and Iden, S. S., 1981, Modulation of human neutrophil superoxide anion generation by the calcium antagonist 8-(*N,N*-diethylamino)-octyl-(3,4,5-trimethoxy) benzoate hydrochloride, *J. Reticuloendothel. Soc.* 29:215.

Smith, R. J., and Ignarro, L. J., 1975, Bioregulation of lysosomal enzyme secretion from human neutrophils: Roles of guanosine 3':5'-monophosphate and calcium in stimulus–secretion coupling, *Proc. Natl. Acad. Sci. (USA)* 72:108.

Smolen, J. E., and Weissmann, G., 1980, Effects of indomethacin, 5,8,11,14-eicosatetraynoic acid, and *p*-bromophenacyl bromide on lysosomal enzyme release and superoxide anion generation by human polymorphonuclear leukocytes, *Biochem. Pharmacol.* 29:533.

Smolen, J. E., and Weissmann, G., 1981, Stimuli which provoke secretion of azurophil enzymes from human neutrophils induce increments in adenosine cyclic 3'-5'-monophosphate, *Biochim. Biophys. Acta* 672:197.

Smolen, J. E., and Weissmann, G., 1982, The effect of various stimuli and calcium antagonists on the fluorescence response of chlorotetracycline-loaded human neutrophils, *Biochim. Biophys. Acta* 720:172.

Smolen, J. E., Korchak, H. M., and Weissmann, G., 1980, Increased levels of cyclic adenosine-3',5'-monophosphate in human polymorphonuclear leukocytes after surface stimulation, *J. Clin. Invest.* 65:1077.

Smolen, J. E., Korchak, H. M., and Weissmann, G., 1981, The roles of extracellular and intracellular calcium in lysosomal enzyme release and superoxide anion generation by human neutrophils, *Biochim. Biophys. Acta* 677:512.

Stenson, W. F., and Parker, C. W., 1979, Metabolism of arachidonic acid in ionophore-stimulated neutrophils, *J. Clin. Invest.* 64:1457.

Stocker, R., and Richter, C., 1982, Involvement of calcium, calmodulin and phospholipase A in the alteration of membrane dynamics and superoxide production of human neutrophils stimulated by phorbol myristate acetate, *FEBS Lett.* 147:243.

Stossel, T. P., Root, R. K., and Vaughan, M., 1972, Phagocytosis in chronic granulomatous disease and the Chediak–Higashi syndrome, *N. Engl. J. Med.* 286:120.

Strauss, R. G., Bove, K. E., Jones, J. F., Mauer, A. M., and Fulginiti, V. A., 1974, An anomaly of neutrophil morphology with impaired function, *N. Engl. J. Med.* 290:478.

Suzuki, Y., and Lehrer, R. I., 1980, NAD(P)H oxidase activity in human neutrophils stimulated by phorbol myristate acetate, *J. Clin. Invest.* 66:1409.

Takai, Y., Kishimoto, A., Iwasa, Y., Kawahara, Y., Mori, T., and Nishizuka, Y., 1979, Calcium-dependent activation of a multifunctional protein kinase by membrane phospholipids, *J. Biol. Chem.* 254:3692.

Takenawa, T., Homma, Y., and Nagai, Y., 1983, Role of Ca^{2+} in phosphatidylinositol response and arachidonic acid release in formylated tripeptide or Ca^{2+} ionophore A23187-stimulated guinea pig neutrophils, *J. Immunol.* 130:2849.

Takeshige, K., and Minakami, S., 1981, Involvement of calmodulin in phagocytotic respiratory burst of leukocytes, *Biochem. Biophys. Res. Commun.* 99:484.

Takeshige, K., Nabi, Z. F., Tatscheck, B., and Minakami, S., 1980, Release of calcium from membranes and its relation to phagocytotic metabolic changes: A fluorescence study on leukocytes loaded with chlortetracycline, *Biochem. Biophys. Res. Commun.* 95:410.

Tauber, A. I., and Babior, B. M., 1977, Evidence for hydroxyl radical production by human neutrophils, *J. Clin. Invest.* 60:374.

Tauber, A. I., and Goetzl, E. J., 1979, Structural and catalytic properties of the solubilized superoxide-generating activity of human polymorphonuclear leukocytes. Solubilization, stabilization in solution, and partial characterization, *Biochemistry* 18:5576.

Utsumi, K., Sugiyama, K., Miyahara, M., Naito, M., Awai, M., and Inoue, M., 1977, Effect of concanavalin A on membrane potential of polymorphonuclear leukocyte monitored by fluorescent dye, *Cell Struct. Func.* 2:203.

Van Epps, D. E., and Garcia, M. L., 1980, Enhancement of neutrophil function as a result of prior exposure to chemotactic factor, *J. Clin. Invest.* 66:167.

Walsh, C. E., Waite, B. M., Thomas, M. J., and DeChatelet, L. R., 1981, Release and metabolism of arachidonic acid in human neutrophils, *J. Biol. Chem.* 256:7228.

Webster, R. O., Hong, S. R., Johnston, R. B., Jr., and Henson, P. M., 1980, Biological effects of the human complement fragments C5a and C5a$_{des Arg}$ on neutrophil function, *Immunopharmacology* 2:201.

Weening, R. S., Roos, D., Weemaes, C. M. R., Homan-Muller, J. W. T., and van Schaik, M. L. T., 1976, Defective initiation of the metabolic stimulation in phagocytizing granulocytes: A new congenital defect, *J. Lab. Clin. Med.* 88:757.

Weiss, S. J., King, G. W., and Lobuglio, A. F., 1977, Evidence for hydroxyl radical generation by human monocytes, *J. Clin. Invest.* 60:370.

Weiss, S. J., Klein, R., Slivka, A., and Wei, M., 1982, Chlorination of taurine by human neutrophils. Evidence for hypochlorous acid generation, *J. Clin. Invest.* 70:598.

Wentzell, B., and Epand, R. M., 1978, Stimulation of the release of prostaglandins from polymorphonuclear leukocytes by the calcium ionophore A23187, *FEBS Lett.* 86:255.

Whitin, J. C., Chapman, C. E., Simons, E. R., Chovaniec, M. E., and Cohen, H. J., 1980, Correlation between membrane potential changes and superoxide production in human granulocytes stimulated by phorbol myristate acetate. Evidence for defective activation in chronic granulomatous disease, *J. Biol. Chem.* 255:1874.

Wright, W. C., Jr., Ank, B. J., Herbert, J., and Stiehm, E. R., 1975, Decreased bactericidal activity of leukocytes of stressed newborn infants, *Pediatrics* 56:569.

Yamaguchi, T., Sato, K., Shimada, K., and Kakinuma, K., 1982, Subcellular localization of O_2^- generating enzyme in guinea pig polymorphonuclear leukocytes: Fractionation of subcellular particles by using a Percoll density gradient, *J. Biochem.* 91:31.

Yuli, I., Tomonaga, A., and Snyderman, R., 1982, Chemoattractant receptor functions in human polymorphonuclear leukocytes are divergently altered by membrane fluidizers, *Proc. Natl. Acad. Sci. (USA)* 79:5906.

Zurier, R. B., and Sayadoff, D. M., 1975, Release of prostaglandins from human polymorphonuclear leukocytes, *Inflammation* 1:93.

Chapter 10

Nonoxidative Antimicrobial Reactions of Leukocytes

John K. Spitznagel

Department Microbiology and Immunology
School of Medicine
Emory University
Atlanta, Georgia 30322

I. INTRODUCTION

Neutrophil polymorphonuclear granulocytes (PMNs) comprise the first line of cellular defense against a variety of common bacteria and fungi. Since Metchnikoff discovered the role of PMNs in defense against infection, much research has focused on the mediation of their antimicrobial activities (Metchnikoff, 1905). At first this work sought what may now be thought of as antibiotic-like components of PMNs with direct antimicrobial action. Research emphasis then began to shift as the capacity of PMNs to utilize O_2 during phagocytosis began to be recognized (Karnovsky, 1962). With the recognition by Holmes *et al.* (1968) of the oxidative defect in the PMNs of children with X-linked chronic granulomatous disease, many workers concentrated on oxygen dependent antimicrobial functions of PMNs. Klebanoff (1975) suggested that PMN antimicrobial mechanisms might be classified as either O_2 dependent or O_2 independent. Klebanoff and Clark (1978) also suggested that oxidative mechanisms, especially those dependent on myeloperoxidase, carry the principal burden of intraleukocytic killing in PMNs. Currently developing evidence suggests, however, that O_2-independent mechanisms may carry more of the burden of antimicrobial action than has been appreciated (Kossack *et al.*, 1981; Okamura and Spitznagel, 1982; Weiss *et al.*, 1982; Rest *et al.*, 1982).

PMNs migrate and phagocytize with energy derived through iodoacetate-sensitive glycolysis. They perform these functions independent of oxygen (Karnovsky, 1962). It is less well recognized that PMNs under stringent anaerobic conditions mobilize antimicrobial systems effective against various bacteria (Mandell, 1974; Okamura and Spitznagel, 1982; Weiss *et al.*, 1982), fungi (Lehrer, 1972), and even protozoans (Rein *et al.*, 1980). Further evidence for the importance of oxygen-independent mechanisms also derives from recent observations that PMNs of a chronic granulomatous disease patient were as effective as normal PMNs at killing *Neisseria gonorrhoeae* (Rest *et al.*, 1982), even though they were predictably incapable of reducing oxygen for antimicrobial effects (Quie *et al.*, 1967; Holmes *et al.*, 1968). A number of workers have attempted to abrogate PMN antimicrobial capacities with anaerobic conditions. They have only partially succeeded. In most instances even the most stringent anaerobic conditions only incompletely blocked killing. This suggested that O_2-independent mechanisms backed up those that are O_2 dependent (see, e.g., results in McRipley and Sbarra, 1967a; Holmes *et al.*, 1968; Klebanoff and Hamon, 1972; Lehrer and Cline, 1969).

It is the purpose of this chapter to review developments in knowledge of O_2-independent antimicrobial action of PMNs since the time of Metchnikoff (1905). A number of reviews have dealt with various aspects of these developments, including those by Skarnes and Watson (1957), Hirsch (1960a), Klebanoff (1975), Spitznagel (1980), and Root and Cohen (1981). We are all particularly indebted to Klebanoff and Clark (1978) for their superbly documented critical review.

Several subjects are relevant to O_2-independent microbicidal actions: antimicrobial cationic proteins, neutral proteinases, lysozyme, lactoferrin, small peptides, association of O_2-independent systems with PMN cytoplasmic granules, degranulation, intraphagosomal milieu (including hydrogen ion concentration and organic acids), evidence for role of O_2-independent mediators in intraleukocytic killing, cooperation of O_2-independent and O_2-dependent systems, ontogeny of the O_2-independent systems, and genetic or acquired defects and models of defects.

Many workers have contributed their identification and analysis of putatively antimicrobial substances to our understanding of the PMN, the mechanisms of their action, and the role they may play in resistance to infection. However, as Skarnes and Watson (1957) pointed out, the isolation from tissues and tissue fluids of substances with primary or secondary antimicrobial activity under *in vitro* conditions does not establish their role in host defense. It is essential to show that these substances exist as such in normal and infected tissues or that they are derived by physiological mechanisms from processes in normal tissues and body fluids. It is equally important to explore carefully the cell biology of systems that putatively deliver the substance to microbial forms that gain access to tissue or tissue fluids. It must be shown that they are antimicrobial in the phagolysosomal microenvironment. Not surprising is the finding that there are practically no instances in which all the necessary information is available. I have, however, tried in this chapter to examine existing information in these terms.

II. CATIONIC PROTEINS

From 1891 to 1912 a number of research papers appeared describing anti-microbial substances associated with pus or peripheral white blood cells (e.g., Hankin, 1891; Buchner, 1894; Denys and Havet, 1894; Schattenfroh, 1897; Korschun, 1908; Schneider, 1909; Kling, 1910; Zinsser, 1910; Weil, 1911; Manwaring, 1912). Several of these accounts suggested that these substances might be proteins. Two reports were especially noteworthy because they clearly suggested that the antimicrobial resembled protamine, the basic protein of salmon sperm (Kossell, 1896; Petterson, 1905).

All the above preparations were derived from pus or other cell mixtures. Generally the precise identity of the cell or cells of origin remained unknown, as did subcellular distribution. The primitive state of biochemistry precluded clear characterization of the antimicrobial proteins. There were exceptions. Ehrlich, for example, identified granules in the cytoplasm of certain leukocytes and, with the help of basic and acidic dyes, concluded that the granules of PMNs contained, among other things, basic substances (Ehrlich and Lazarus, 1900). Also exceptional was the work of Kanthack and Hardy (1894), who first described degranulation in phagocytizing granulocytes and showed that *Bacillus anthracis* that came in contact with granulocytes triggered degranulation and then ceased to grow. *B. anthracis* in the same preparations that were not in contact, and thus failed to trigger degranulation, continued to elongate and divide.

Soon basic proteins and cytoplasmic granules were essentially forgotten until research interest again focused on their role in antimicrobial mechanisms of tissue 40 years later. At that time Bloom and co-workers (Bloom and Blake, 1948; Bloom *et al.*, 1951) prepared from hog thymus a lysine-rich cationic protein active against *Micrococcus pyogenes* (*Staphylococcus aureus*), beta-hemolytic streptococci, *Escherichia coli*, and *Bacillus anthracis*. These investigators observed that the substance bound to bacterial cells—nucleic acids, DNA, or RNA—inhibited this binding. Subsequently Skarnes and Watson (1956) described an antimicrobial protein from lysates of whole rabbit PMNs. Skarnes and Watson (1957) revived the concept of leukins and applied the term to that protein.

A. Leukin

Skarnes and Watson (1956) and later Skarnes (1967) described the isolation, from lactic acid lysates of rabbit PMN, of an arginine-rich protein antimicrobial for gram-positive pathogens. Leukin was from bulk suspensions of peritoneal exudate and no histochemical or immunochemical studies were undertaken. It was impossible to ascertain the origin of the protein. However, leukin was positively charged due to a relatively high proportion of basic amino acids. Skarnes and Watson proposed it might in fact be a histone. And substantial numbers of publications have appeared (Miller *et al.*, 1942; Katchalski *et al.*, 1953; Burger and Stahmann, 1952; Hirsch, 1958; Spitznagel, 1961 *a, b;* Miller and Watson, 1969; Crawford, 1971; Pelletier and Delaunay, 1972) showing conclusively *in vitro* that histones and other proteins bearing a net positive charge have primary antimicrobial action. It has been awkward, however, to relate histones to antimicrobial defense for histones exist bound to DNA in the cell nucleus, a circumstance that suggests that they could only participate in antimicrobial defenses under conditions of cell death, necrosis, and deoxyribonuclease activity.

B. Phagocytin

This material was prepared from rabbit and from human PMNs by Hirsch (1956 *a*, 1960 *b*). It was at first believed antimicrobial only for gram-negative bacteria (Hirsch, 1956 *b*), but later both gram-negative and gram-positive organisms were found sensitive (Hirsch, 1960 *b*). The supposed resistance of gram-positive bacteria and the fact that phagocytin was extractable with weak citric acid buffer (histone was not) convinced Hirsch that phagocytin was different than histone. Later evidence (Cohn and Hirsch, 1960 *b*) showed that phagocytin was confined to cytoplasmic granules of PMNs and immensely strengthened the position that phagocytin was not histone. Cationic electrophoresis with phagocytin prepared in my laboratory and on samples kindly provided by Hirsch revealed that rabbit phagocytin was a heterogeneous substance having many cationic components, several of them more cationic than lysozyme, which was also present.

C. Antimicrobial Cationic Granule Proteins

It was clearly important to ask whether cationic proteins have in fact any role in response to infection. Using histochemical methods, Spitznagel and Chi (1963) showed that *E. coli* in experimentally induced cutaneous abscesses in rabbits and in guinea pigs appeared to have been coated with arginine-rich cationic proteins. The presence of PMNs with similarly reactive cytoplasmic granules in the lesions strongly suggested that these proteins had been brought to the lesions by emigrating PMNs, which then phagocytized the bacteria, exposing them to the granule proteins. Cytochemistry and *in vitro* phagocytic experiments soon showed that such granules were normal constituents of the cytoplasm of PMNs. The proteins were transferred from the granules to bacteria phagocytized by the PMNs. It was found that the bacteria coated with the proteins could no longer replicate (Spitznagel and Chi, 1963).

Zeya and colleagues then isolated a series of antimicrobial arginine-rich cationic proteins, first from guinea pig PMN granules (Zeya and Spitznagel, 1963; 1966 *a, b*) and then from rabbit PMN granules (Zeya and Spitznagel, 1966 *c;* Zeya *et al.*, 1966) (see Table I). The rabbit proteins demonstrated selective activity

Table I. Cationic Antimicrobial Granule Proteins from PMNs[a] and Macrophages: Amino Acids[b]

| | G. pig PMN[c] | Rabbit PMN | | | Rabbit AM[d] | | Human PMN | | | | BPI[i] | ACP[k] | |
	LP[e]	I[f]	II[f]	III[f]	MCP1[g]	MCP2[g]	CL[h] I	II	III	59 kd[j]	57 kd[j]	37 kd[j]
Aspartic acid	7.5	0.43	0.5	1.67	1.26	3.44	9.3	8.8	9.2	8.5	9.29	10.59
Glutamic acid	9.1	4.1	4.4	3.9	5.33	9.34	11.9	11.7	12.0	9.1	9.4	9.04
Glycine	6.1	5.7	5.7	6.16	9.30	12.30	9.7	9.2	9.6	5.9	6.3	10.81
Alanine	6.4	8.5	8.4	9.4	9.31	9.74	6.6	6.3	6.0	5.5	6.38	6.34
Valine	5.8	4.3	4.4	4.0	2.39	3.02	7.5	7.1	8.0	7.9	6.94	6.74
Leucine	9.4	10.3	12.4	9.8	8.01	8.02	8.4	8.0	7.6	10.6	10.4	7.21
Isoleucine	4.9	7.1	6.4	6.1	4.02	3.17	4.9	5.4	5.6	5.5	5.47	2.27
Serine	3.4	1.4	0.8	1.7	3.69	11.20	7.5	6.7	6.8	7.8	8.5	7.28
Threonine	5.6	0.8	0.4	0.77	0.66	2.01	5.7	5.4	4.8	4.2	4.5	5.44
Cystine	3.5	14.2	14.3	13.5	18.70	9.82	—	3.4	2.4	—	ND[l]	ND[l]
Methionine	1.1	0.2	0.1	0.39	0.2	0.95	—	1.7	1.6	3.3	2.6	1.10
Proline	6.2	6.7	5.8	7.0	6.05	4.72	5.3	5.3	4.4	7.9	6.1	12.48
Phenylalanine	4.2	2.3	2.5	2.9	2.63	2.48	2.6	2.9	2.8	5.8	5.68	4.21
Tyrosine	1.2	0.0	0.0	0.7	0.20	0.75	1.8	2.1	1.6	3.3	2.75	0.67
Histidine	0.7	3.5	2.7	2.7	2.57	2.93	2.2	2.1	2.4	3.6	4.36	5.19
Lysine	8.5	0.9	1.7	3.8	0.31	1.16	1.8	1.3	1.2	7.8	7.80	1.63
Arginine	15.5	31.3	30.0	25.3	25.50	14.90	14.1	13.4	13.6	3.3	3.04	9.00

[a]Polymorphonuclear leukocytes (neutrophils).
[b]Amino acids per 100 residues. Tryptophan not measured.
[c]Guinea pig PMNs.
[d]Alveolar macrophages.
[e]Lysosomal protein of guinea pig PMNs (Zeya and Spitznagel, 1966).
[f]Lysosomal protein of rabbit PMNs (Zeya and Spitznagel, 1968).
[g]Macrophage cationic protein (MCP) of rabbit alveolar macrophages (AM) (Patterson-Delafield et al., 1981).
[h]Chymotrypsin-like (CL) protein of human PMN lysosomes (Olsson and Venge, 1974).
[i]Bacterial permeability inducing (BPI) factor of human PMN lysosomes (Weiss et al., 1978).
[j]kd, kilodalton.
[k]Antibacterial cationic protein (ACP) of human PMN lysosomes (Shafer and Spitznagel, 1983).
[l]None detected.

against several gram-positive and gram-negative bacteria (Zeya and Spitznagel, 1966c). The cationic proteins of rabbit PMN granules were more numerous than those of guinea pig PMN but were similar in biochemical structure; the high content of arginine, the unusually prominent proportions of hydrophobic amino acids, the presence of significant half cystines, and the absence or low levels of tyrosine suggested relationships between proteins from the two species and the possibility of analogous biological actions (see Table I).

Recognition of these properties set a tentative standard for characterizing this category of antibacterial cationic granule protein and also defined some of the difficulties involved in studying them (Zeya and Spitznagel, 1968). Not taken into account at the time was the possible role of PMN granule proteases (Amrein and Stossel, 1980) in determining the character and recovery of the isolated proteins. Their role is considered in Section VI.

Extracts of granules from human PMNs included strongly cationic antimicrobial proteins (Welsh and Spitznagel, 1971). These proteins were more cationic than lysozyme which migrated to the cathode at pH 4.5 on cellulose acetate treated with cetyltrimethylammonium bromide. Their antimicrobial activity was primarily directed against gram-negative rods. One protein proved, with sodium dodecyl sulfate-reducing polyacrylamide gel (SDS-PAGE-mercaptoethanol electrophoresis) to have an apparent molecular weight of ~36 kilodaltons (kd) (Modrzakowski and Spitznagel, 1979).

Shafer and co-workers (Shafer et al., 1983; Shafer and Spitznagel, 1983) extended these findings identifying in extracts of diisopropyl fluorophosphate (DFP)-treated leukemic PMN granules an arginine-rich (see Table I), hydrophobic amino-acid rich protein (MW estimated 37 kd in SDS-PAGE-mercaptoethanol). Resolution depended on ion-exchange chromatography with CM Sephadex eluted with a salt gradient at pH 5.0 and exclusion chromatography with Sephadex G-75. The protein had primary antimicrobial effects on wild-type *Salmonella typhimurium* LT-2 and its outer membrane mutants as well as on *E. coli* and piliated opaque and piliated transparent *Neisseria gonorrhoeae*. An apparently identical protein can be isolated from PMNs not treated with DFP to inhibit proleolysis. With the same separation scheme both DFP-treated and -untreated PMNs also yielded a 57-kd protein estimated with SDS-PAGE-reducing gels. This material was rich in lysine and hydrophobic amino acids. Neither cationic protein was a protease, nor was either one contaminated with detectable protease. The amino acid composition of both is shown in Table I. Certain of properties of the 57-kd protein resembled those of bacterial permeability factor (BPI), as reported by Weiss et al. (1978) (see Table I).

In addition to the above, evidence has been garnered for the presence of antimicrobial cationic granular proteins in PMNs of other species, including the chicken (Brune and Spitznagel, 1973) and rat (Hodinka and Modrzakowski, 1983).

In addition to defining the antibacterial properties of certain cationic proteins of guinea pig PMN, Zeya and Spitznagel (1966a) found that the proteins killed *Candida albicans* as well. Lehrer *et al.* (1975) extended this work and found that PMNs of humans, rabbits, and guinea pigs have cationic proteins lethal for several species of *Candida.* Moreover, Patterson-Delafield *et al.* (1981) and Lehrer *et al.* (1980) have extended their work to alveolar macrophages of the rabbit, which they find have cationic anticandidal proteins (Table I). Evidently the cationic proteins of these alveolar macrophages are modulated by systemic injections of bacille de Calmette Guérin (BCG).

D. Cationic Granule Proteins of Eosinophil Granulocytes

The granules of eosinophils of humans (Gleich *et al.*, 1976; Ohlsson *et al.*, 1977) and of guinea pigs (Gleich *et al.*, 1973, 1974) are associated with several basic or cationic proteins that are rich in arginine. These cationic proteins are toxic for schistosomula of *Schistosoma mansoni* (Butterworth *et al.*, 1979), *Trichinella spiralis* larvae (Wassom and Gleich, 1979), and bloodstream forms of *Trypanosoma cruzi* (Kierszenbaum *et al.*, 1981). It is curious that these proteins, although toxic for higher parasites, are only weakly antibacterial (Gleich *et al.*, 1974). There is nothing about their amino acid composition that suggests they would differ so in their biological behavior from the cationic proteins of rabbit PMN granules. They are in addition to their importance in eosinophils incidental contaminants in purification procedures intended to recover PMN antimicrobial proteins (Ohlsson *et al.*, 1977). It is possible that knowledge of their amino acid sequences would lead to better understanding of their toxicity for higher parasites and would explain their failure to kill bacteria.

E. Cathepsin G as Cationic Antimicrobial Protein

This chymotrypsin-like proteolytic enzyme was described independently by Olsson and Venge (1974) and by Starkey and Barrett (1976). It had antimicrobial activity apparently independent of its enzymic activity and killed *Streptococcus faecalis, Staphylococcus aureus, Escherichia coli*, and *Pseudomonas aeruginosa* (Odeberg and Olsson, 1976) and *Acinetobacter* 199A (Thorne *et al.*, 1976). Neither heat inactivation nor DFP treatments that eliminated its chymotryptic-like activity diminished the antimicrobial action of cathepsin G. Although one of the cationic antibacterial proteins (Shafer *et al.*, 1983) from human PMN granules resembled to some extent cathepsin G, it differed with respect to molecular size and hydrophobic amino acids, had no chymotryptic or other demonstrated enzymic action, and its antimicrobial action (ID_{50} ~1 $\mu g/ml$ for *E. coli*) was much greater than that of cathepsin G.

F. Bacterial Permeability Increasing Factor

Changes in the permeability of actinomycin D with respect to outer membrane defective *Escherichia coli* have been used (Beckerdite *et al.*, 1974) to screen potentially antimicrobial fractions prepared from lysates of rabbit peritoneal exudate leukocytes. A protein complex isolated according to these criteria comprised bacterial permeability increasing factor (BPI) and a phospholipase A_2 (Beckerdite *et al.*, 1974; Weiss *et al.*, 1975). Antimicrobial action was attributed to the nonphospholipase protein, BPI. The phospholipase appeared to attack phospholipids in the bacterial membrane but not to kill the bacteria. The isolation procedure began with whole cell lysates, hence the significance of such a complex for *in vivo* antimicrobial action was uncertain. Cationic proteins are well known for their tendency to complex with other proteins. BPI, possibly associated with the cytoplasmic granules, might easily have become associated with phospholipase from sources other than the granules possibly the PMN cytosol or PMN nucleus during preparative procedures. More recently this same group of investigators has announced isolation of a BPI from human leukemic granulocytes. This BPI (Table I) is a 59-kd protein rich in lysine and hydrophobic amino acids. It has an isolectric point of 9.8. It is said to crossreact immunologically with rabbit BPI. It has no demonstrated enzymic activity (Weiss *et al.*, 1978). Shafer *et al.* (1983), as noted above, have obtained a protein with nearly identical amino acid compositions from PMN human, granule lysates. It remains to be determined what relationships exist between the proteins described by Weiss and those recovered by Shafer. The goat antibody reported by Weiss *et al.* (1978) and monoclonal antibodies we have raised (Spitznagel *et al.*, in preparation) should be useful for this purpose.

In summary, PMNs of all species thus far investigated have analogous families of cationic antimicrobial proteins. These proteins are best prepared from the cytoplasmic granules of the PMN. The granules are the source of much of the antimicrobial armamentarium of the PMN. Moreover, granules represent only a small fraction of the proteins in the whole PMN. Removal of the granules from other cell components simplifies isolation of granule proteins. In any event, the common pattern is that the proteins are rich in basic amino acid (usually arginine) and also rich in hydrophobic amino acids. In two (perhaps identical) instances, BPI and 57-kd protein (Table I), the principal basic amino acid is lysine. In the 38-kd antimicrobial protein (Shafer *et al.*, 1983), the principal basic amino acid is arginine. These proteins also have large proportions, greater than 50%, of hydrophobic amino acids. Their properties are consistent with those of proteins that might be expected to produce antibacterial effects.

G. Antimicrobial Action of Cationic Granule Proteins

Interest in the antimicrobial action of cationic proteins anticipated by many years the recognition that these potent agents are associated with granules of the

PMN cytoplasm. As noted in Section II, it was recognized very early that this class of antibacterial proteins carries net positive charges at or near physiological pH (Kossell, 1896; Petterson, 1905). This property of polypeptides and proteins has long been viewed as a necessary but insufficient determinant of antimicrobial capacity (Miller et al., 1942; Bloom and Blake, 1948; Bloom et al., 1951; Burger and Stahmann, 1952; Katchalski et al., 1953; Skarnes and Watson, 1956; Hirsch, 1958; Spitznagel, 1961a,b). The general inference has been that the cationic amino acids donate protons to form bonds with electronegative substituents accessible at microbial surfaces. These substituents are capable of forming poorly dissociated organic salt linkages. Early formal investigations of these relationships relied on the use of antibacterial polycations such as protamines and histones in model systems (Miller et al., 1942; Katchalski et al., 1953; Hirsch, 1958; Spitznagel, 1961a, b; Miller and Watson, 1969). However, the upsurge in cell biology made it clear that histones were probably not involved as actual mediators of antimicrobial mechanisms in phagocytosis. In 1963, Spitznagel and Chi (1963) demonstrated with rabbit PMNs that arginine-rich cationic proteins of PMN cytoplasmic granules are transported, and become bound during phagocytosis, bacteria lodged in normally aseptic tissues. They also submitted evidence that these cationic proteins were probably involved in the death of the bacteria. These findings were later confirmed at the ultrastructural level in rabbit and chicken PMNs (MacRae and Spitznagel, 1975).

Many studies have amply confirmed the tenacious binding of antibacterial proteins of the PMN granule to microbial cells (Cohn and Hirsch, 1960b; Spitznagel, 1961a; Zeya and Spitznagel, 1966a). In these reports a principal evidence submitted in support of electrostatic interaction at microbial surfaces was the inhibition of killing and cytochemical changes by polyanions such as RNA and DNA. This finding was exemplified by work with protamine and histone (Hirsch, 1958; Spitznagel, 1961a, b) and, more to the point, with cationic granule proteins (Zeya and Spitznagel, 1966b), in which it was shown that endotoxin could inhibit microbicidal action as well as did other anionic polymers. This work was subsequently extended by Modrzakowski and Spitznagel (1979) to human cationic granule proteins.

That microbicidal binding was not solely dependent on cationicity was clear from work that showed, for example, that the powerfully cationic granule proteins of eosinophils have only weak antibacterial capacities (Archer and Hirsch, 1963; Gleich et al., 1974). Moreover, with rabbit granule proteins, each had unique antimicrobial spectra that could not readily be related either to its relative cationicity or to principal catonic amino acids (Zeya and Spitznagel, 1968; Modrzakowski et al., 1979).

An interesting feature of the antimicrobial proteins, in addition to their cationicity and their tendency to bind to bacteria and endotoxin (Cohn and Hirsch, 1960b; Spitznagel and Chi, 1963; Zeya and Spitznagel, 1966b; Modrzakowski and Spitznagel, 1979; Weiss et al., 1980; Shafer and Spitznagel, 1983), was their strikingly high proportion of hydrophobic amino acids (Table I). These proteins tended to bind tenaciously to relatively hydrophobic chromatography media, including Biorex 70. They could only be dislodged from these media with high salt concentrations plus 8 M urea. Even with these harsh conditions yields were poor.

Evidence that the adsorption to bacterial cells involved hydrophobic bonds has heretofore been largely inferential. For example, a number of investigators have shown that enterobacteriaceae such as *Salmonella typhimurium* resist the antimicrobial actions of cationic granule proteins in proportion to the length of the polysaccharide core and O side chains of their outer membrane lipopolysaccharides (LPS) (Friedberg and Shilo, 1970; Tagesson and Stendahl, 1973; Rest *et al.*, 1977; Weiss *et al.*, 1980). Thus parent smooth bacterial forms with complete LPS resisted killing by the cationic proteins. Fifty percent of the fully smooth *Salmonella typhimurium* LT2 suspensions were killed only by >60 μg cationic granule protein/ml, while 50% of the very rough Re mutant were killed by ≤5 μg of cationic granule proteins/ml) (Rest *et al.*, 1978*a*). Similar results have been obtained with crude, mixed (specific plus azurophil) granule extracts (Rest *et al.*, 1977) (see Section VII for further information concerning granule types and their associations with various proteins) and with extracts of isolated human azurophil granules (Rest *et al.*, 1978*a*) and BPI (Weiss *et al.*, 1980).

Evidence for direct adsorption of the proteins to the bacteria has been published (Modrzakowski and Spitznagel, 1979; Weiss *et al.*, 1980). The results of Modrzakowski and Spitznagel (1979) suggested that overall the fully smooth, more resistant, *Salmonella* bound antibacterial components more efficiently than did the more sensitive deep rough mutants, and the LPS isolated from them did likewise. Weiss *et al.* (1980) apparently found the opposite with BPI. The reason for the discrepancy could be that Modrzakowski and Spitznagel used a mixture of granule proteins, while Weiss *et al.* used a more homogeneous protein. However, greater binding by rough strains would be consistent with a role for binding due to hydrophobic effects, since rough bacterial surfaces are hydrophobic relative to smooth ones. In any event, the relative size of the amphipathic LPS molecules in the outer membrane of *Salmonella typhimurium* mutants changes with transitions from rough to smooth (Smit *et al.*, 1975). The polysaccharide head group becomes shorter, while the hydrophobic tail group (lipid A), although it is unchanged in size, is larger relative to the head group in the rough organisms as compared with the smooth organisms.

H. Mechanisms of Antimicrobial Action

Cationic proteins bind to, and in all likelihood permeate, many microbial surfaces. The most important result from the point of view of the host is the early failure of microbial replication (see, e.g., Rest *et al.*, 1978*a*; and Weiss *et al.*, 1976). As far as the microbial cells are concerned, membrane permeability (Zeya and Spitznagel, 1966*b*) is altered and transport mechanisms fail (Odeberg and

Olsson, 1976). These changes have been observed in relationship to microbial contact with a variety of products, including fractions of lysates from whole PMNs (Beckerdite *et al.*, 1974), cationic proteins purified from extracts of cytoplasmic granules of guinea pig or rabbit PMN (Zeya and Spitznagel, 1966b), highly purified but still heterogeneous fractions from rabbit PMN lysates (Weiss *et al.*, 1977), a chymotrypsin-like cationic protein from human PMNs (Odeberg and Olsson, 1976), and a permeability increasing protein from human PMN granules (BPI) (Weiss *et al.*, 1978).

It has been recognized that polyanions (Zeya and Spitznagel, 1966b; Modrza-kowski and Spitznagel, 1979) block the antibacterial action of cationic granule proteins. Divalent cations, especially magnesium, also have the capacity to block the antimicrobial action of histone (Hirsch, 1958), phagocytin (Hirsch, 1956b), chymotrypsin-like cationic protein (Odeberg and Olsson, 1976), and highly purified rabbit PMN factor subsequently compared with BPI (Weiss *et al.*, 1976; Elsbach *et al.*, 1979). Weiss *et al.* (1976) found they could reverse the membrane permeability affects of BPI with Mg^{2+} and Ca^{2+}. Moreover, with Mg^{2+} they succeeded in reversing phospholipase A_2-mediated (Weiss and Elsbach, 1977) hydrolysis of the bacterial phospholipids. It is noteworthy that Mg^{2+} was reported to reverse microbial membrane damage due to complement-mediated damage (Muschel and Jackson, 1963). These effects of divalent cations suggest that they may have the capacity to displace the antimicrobial polycations from the electronegative substituents at the bacterial surface.

In any event, gram-negative bacteria are generally less resistant than gram-positive bacteria to the cationic granule proteins. This finding has concentrated investigative efforts on the mediation of gram-negative bacterial death. With respect to gram-negative bacteria, it is necessary to consider how cationic proteins adsorb to their outer membranes and damage the bacterial cells. It was early suspected (see Section II) that ionic forces were involved. Thus the cationic proteins have been supposed to provide protons that interact with negatively charged groups in bacterial cell walls (Hirsch, 1958; Zeya and Spitznagel, 1966a, b; Weiss *et al.*, 1980). The evidence for this has been largely indirect, and the nature of the binding anions in the microbial cell walls has been essentially unknown. Spitznagel (1961b) suggested that the action of cationic granule proteins might be analogous to that of polymyxin B. Shafer and Spitznagel (1983) took advantage of the newer knowledge of the antimicrobial action of polymyxin B and showed that the 37-kd and 57-kd cationic antimicrobial proteins purified from PMN granule extracts to high degrees of homogeneity bind, as does polymyxin B, to negatively charged pyrophosphate groups associated with the lipid A hydrophobic tail of LPS. Shafer's results also indicated that the hydrophobic components of the protein reacted with the long chain acyl substituents of the lipid A. These are the first results involving lipid A in the action of the antimicrobial cationic proteins of PMN granules. Early work (Friedberg and Shilo, 1970; Tagesson and Stendahl, 1973; Rest *et al.*, 1977, 1978a; and Weiss *et al.*, 1980) can be interpreted to suggest that the hydrophilic polysaccharides of the core and O antigens provide smooth gram-negative cell walls with outer membranes thermodynamically unfavorable to solution of the highly hydrophobic cationic proteins, from PMN granules. This suggestion arises from the greater resistance of smooth as compared with rough *Salmonella* and *Escherichia coli.*

There is thus substantial evidence that the outer membrane of the microbial cell is the site of action of the cationic granule proteins. It seems reasonable to conclude that the cationic and hydrophobic properties of the antibacterial proteins mediate this. How these substances damage or gain access to the cytoplasmic membrane is another question. Current concepts of the gram-negative cell wall suggest that damage may be mediated at the adhesion sites, the junctions between outer and inner membranes (Konisky, 1979), something in the way that colicins enter *Escherichia coli.* The roles of outer membrane proteins of the bacteria have not yet been explored. They deserve to be considered because they have a role in the action of colicins on gram-negative bacteria. Colicins are rather large proteins. The thermodynamic barriers they face in reaching the cytoplasmic bacterial membrane may be similar to those of the PMN granule proteins. The nature of the membrane damage mediated by the granule proteins remains a mystery. Ultrastructural studies with gram-negative rods treated with antibacterial leukocyte proteins have failed to reveal morphologically identifiable lesions (Van Houte *et al.*, 1977).

The effect of pH on antimicrobial action of cationic granule proteins is complex (Rest *et al.*, 1977) but a broad pH optimum for killing exists between pH values of 5 to 8. The effect of pH evidently depends on the character of the bacterial surface. With the chymotrypsin-like protein, Odeberg and Olsson found antimicrobial effects to be enhanced at pH 6.8 and higher. Weiss *et al.* (1978) found optimum killing with BPI to occur between pH 6 and pH 8 with *E. coli.*

Other investigators have shown that the effects of cationic proteins on bacteria include suppression of oxygen uptake by aerobes. The question of respiration, energy production, and the action of cationic granule proteins has been addressed in gram-positive bacteria. Gladstone and Walton, for example, showed that iron and haematin blocked the staphylocidal action of rabbit cationic granule proteins (Gladstone, 1973; Gladstone *et al.*, 1974; Gladstone and Walton, 1970, 1971). Walton and Gladstone (1976) have extended this work to show that anaerobiasis, various inhibitors of respiration, and agents that alter cellular energetics of the bacteria (e.g., dinitrophenol and valinomycin) inhibit profoundly the staphylocidal action of cationic rabbit granule proteins. Further investigation suggested the cytoplasmic membrane was the site of antimicrobial action of the cationic proteins (Walton and Gladstone, 1975). Walton (1978) showed that membrane damage was attributable to the action of $3500\text{-}M_r$ and $14{,}500\text{-}M_r$ cationic rabbit granule proteins. This action was considered comparable, although not identical, to that of protamine.

In other kinds of studies, Ginsburg *et al.* (1973) found that lytic action due to enzymes in leukocyte lysates acting on gram-positive cocci was blocked by both cationic and anionic electrolytes. Hallgren and Venge (1976) found that human cationic granule proteins enhanced ingestion of complexes formed between *Staphylococcus* protein A and IgG. Pelletier and Delauney (1972) describe hanced bactericidal action by PMN and macrophages to a kind of opsonic action mediated by histones.

Investigation of resistance to PMN granule proteins in pathogenic bacteria other than *Salmonella* promises to yield additional information concerning mechanisms of interaction between bacteria and host. Daly *et al.* (1982) showed that *N. gonorrhoeae* were about as resistant to human PMN azurophil granule proteins as were *E. coli* and *S. typhimurium.* Curiously, decreased resistance to human antimicrobial cationic proteins accompanied chromosomal mutation to low-level penicillin resistance in two strains of gonococci. Increased crosslinking known to exist in the peptidoglycan of certain of these mutant gonococci appeared related to or linked to the reduced resistance to the antimicrobial proteins. Isogenic opaque and transparent variants of gonococci were equally resistant to granule proteins, as were piliated and nonpiliated variants. The genetic and biochemical relationships remain to be precisely characterized. Rest (1979) found that piliation made no difference in sensitivity of *N. gonorrhoeae* to human granule proteins. Buck and Rest (1981) found evidence that the bactericidal components of granule extract rapidly inhibited capacity of *N. gonorrhoeae* to form colonies and that permeability to actinomycin D was slightly increased. Macromolecular synthesis, however, did not fail for about 45 min. Addition of Mg^{2+} blocked killing. Buck and Rest (1981) concluded the action of the granule proteins on *N. gonorrhoeae* resembled that of BPI on *E. coli*, as reported by Weiss *et al.* (1980).

Antimicrobial action of PMN granule proteins of human and other species is not solely directed at bacteria. Human, rabbit, and guinea pig PMNs all have cationic granule proteins that kill *Candida* species (Lehrer *et al.*, 1975). Moreover, Lehrer and colleagues have shown that rabbit alveolar macrophages have at least two cationic arginine-rich proteins that are increased by BCG injection. It remains to be seen whether the macrophages produce these themselves or whether they scavenge them from effete PMNs. These proteins described by Lehrer's group were active against *Candida* species and gram-positive bacteria, such as *Bacillus subtilis*, *Listeria monocytogenes*, and *Streptococcus faecalis.* Gram-negative bacteria were least sensitive (Patterson-Delafield *et al.*, 1980). Further experimentation showed rapid (within 2 min) suppression of O_2 uptake and rapid loss of intracellular rubidium (Patterson-Delafield *et al.*, 1981). These observations suggested that these proteins damaged microbial membranes and interfered with respiration and were consistent with those of Walton (1978) discussed in Section II. They also were consistent with evidence that rabbit PMN cationic protein inhibited mitochondrial respiration (Penniall *et al.*, 1972).

I. Summary

The existing evidence suggests that PMN granules of all species studied have cationic proteins relatively rich in basic amino acids and rich in hydrophobic amino acids. They have antimicrobial capacities independent of molecular oxygen availability. These proteins vary substantially in number and structure between species. Their antimicrobial action involves a temperature-independent very rapid binding step, as well as a temperature- and time-dependent killing step. Binding may be inhibited by hydrophilic polyanions, including polysaccharide chains of smooth enterobacteriaceae, or it may be inhibited by Mg^{2+}. The binding sites for the 37-kd and 57-kd proteins are probably similar to those of polymyxin B, pyrophosphate substituents of lipid A, and the long-chain acyl substituents of lipid A in the outer membranes of gram-negative bacteria. The resulting damage involves the cytoplasmic membrane of gram-negative bacteria by undefined mechanisms. Cytoplasmic membranes of gram-positive bacteria and *Candida* species are also damaged, but the role of the gram-positive cell envelope constituents other than this has not been investigated.

III. NEUTRAL PROTEASES AND ANTIMICROBIAL ACTIVITY

Neutral proteases are associated with human PMNs (Mounter and Atiyeh, 1960; Frankel-Conrat *et al.*, 1966) as well as with PMNs of rat (Anderson and Irwin, 1973; Calamai and Spitznagel, 1982), rabbit (Davies *et al.*, 1970), dog (Ohlsson, 1971), pig (Kopitar and Lebez, 1975), and horse (Koj *et al.*, 1976). The name neutral protease simply signifies proteolytic enzymes optimally active at or slightly above pH 7.0. The antimicrobial effects of these enzymes has principally been studied with human PMN proteases. Prominent among the neutral proteases of human PMNs are elastase (Janoff and Scherer, 1968; Ohlsson and Olsson, 1974) and chymotryptic-like enzyme (Rindler-Ludwig *et al.*, 1974; Schmidt and Havemann, 1977; Odeberg *et al.*, 1975). The chymotryptic-like enzyme has also been isolated from spleen and is called cathepsin G (Starkey and Barrett, 1976). In addition, PMNs of several species, including human PMNs, have collagenolytic activity (Lazarus *et al.*, 1968a,b; Murphy *et al.*, 1977, 1982).

All these proteases possess intrinsic interest, but only the chymotryptic-like enzyme and elastase have been implicated in antimicrobial activity. The evidence for the antimicrobial action of chymotrypsin-like enzyme has been discussed in Section II. It is only necessary to repeat here that its antimicrobial activity appears to be related to its action as cationic protein and has little to do with its enzymtic activity. These findings have been extended to show that it is active against *Candida parapsilosis* (Drazin and Lehrer, 1977).

The antibacterial action of PMN elastases seems to depend on their capacity to degrade proteins of gram-negative rods (Blondin and Janoff, 1976). More precise studies with *Acinetobacter* 199A have revealed that this action involved the cleavage of outer membrane protein to smaller subunits (Thorne *et al.*, 1976). This action removed certain proteins, making the other outer membrane proteins susceptible to cleavage by cathepsin G and cathepsin B. Cathepsin G, cathepsin B, cathepsin D, and elastase were (compared with lysozyme) only 5–10% lytic for *Micrococcus lysodiekticus* and even more slowly lytic for *S. aureus*. Only elastase could enhance lysozyme activity. Cathepsin G, elastase, and cathepsin D were bactericidal for *Acinetobacter* (Thorne *et al.*, 1976).

The outer membrane proteins of the *Gonococcus* are sensitive to cleavage by human PMN elastase. Nonpiliated gonococci (colony types 3 and 4) were used for these experiments (Rest and Pretzer, 1981). A PMN fraction that had both elastase and cathepsin G activity hydrolyzed protein I (the principal outer membrane protein) and protein II species (the opacity associated proteins). More recent studies by R. F. Rest (personal communication, 1983) have shown that highly purified PMN elastase not only cleaves these proteins, but is bactericidal for the *Gonococcus*.

It appears that both the neutral proteolytic enzymes and some of the enzymes functioning at pH optima greater or less than 7.4 can both digest microbial structures and kill selected bacteria. The range of antimicrobial activity for granule proteases should be investigated with a wide variety of clinically important microbes.

IV. LYSOZYME

Among the cationic antimicrobial proteins of PMNs, monocytes, and macrophages, lysozyme is unique. It is bacteriolytic, cleaving and degrading the peptidoglycan of many bacterial cell walls through its action as an endoacetyl muramidase (Strominger and Ghuysen, 1967). This enzyme converts the bacteria to virtual or actual spheroplasts (Muschel and Jackson, 1963). The bacterial cytoplasmic membranes then rupture because of the steep, negative gradient between intramicrobial and extramicrobial osmotic pressures. The resulting expulsion of cytoplasm from the bacteria (Wilson and Spitznagel, 1968) contributes to their ultimate dissolution, but indigestible debris may remain (Wang-Iverson *et al.*, 1978). The debris act as local tissue irritants, sometimes for long periods, although the bacteria are unable to replicate (Cromartie *et al.*, 1977; Spitznagel *et al.*, 1983). Other bacteriolytic enzymes have been described in animal tissue extracts—some highly purified (Thorne *et al.*, 1976) and some quite crude (Nieman *et al.*, 1954)—but none is as effectively bacteriolytic as lysozyme.

A. Character and Distribution

Lysozyme was first defined (Fleming, 1922; Fleming and Allison, 1922) as an enzyme widely distributed in tissues and body fluids of many animals. Early interest in the possible role of lysozyme in immunity to infection or as a possible therapeutic agent was rapidly dampened by the realization that relatively few bacteria were directly sensitive to its action and the realization that none of these sensitive bacteria was a high-grade pathogen (Salton, 1957; Chipman and Sharon, 1969). Despite this disappointment, the work of Fleming showing lysozyme to be a constituent of blood serum, of leukocytes, and of most bodily secretions emphasized the unusual nature of the enzyme. When the nature of the enzymic products of lysozyme digestion were demonstrated (Salton, 1957), it appeared especially interesting that animal cells would produce a powerful enzyme with its principal substrates in bacterial cell walls and not in animal tissues.

Subsequently lysozyme was crystallized from the whites of hens eggs, becoming available for, and a focus of, biochemical and X-ray crystallographic research. Its primary structure was ascertained independently by Jolles *et al.* (1963) and by Canfield (1963). Lysozyme was found to be a relatively cationic 14.5-kd protein with a single peptide chain. The protein was shown to be widely distributed in the tissues of various animal species, including the eggs of all birds. Most animal lysozymes are closely related to hen's egg lysozyme, with the primary structure of the loop region being highly conserved. For reasons not entirely clear, mammalian lysozymes tend to be more active enzymatically than the lysozyme of bird eggs.

Birds have a second lysozyme of 18 kd, which is coded by a completely different gene. Its enzymic behavior and specificities differ from those of hen's egg lysozyme. This lysozyme is only expressed in the eggs of a few birds, but it is expressed in the PMNs of chicken and duck and may be expressed in the PMNs of all birds (Hindenberg *et al.*, 1974). It is noteworthy that bird PMNs lack myeloperoxidase (MPO) (Brune *et al.*, 1972; Brune and Spitznagel, 1973). Possession of two PMN lysozymes may be compensatory for the absence of MPO and therefore uniquely advantageous to birds.

It is important to realize that certain other animal species, including goats, sheep, certain monkeys, cats, and hamsters, have virtually no lysozyme in their PMNs (Rausch *et al.*, 1974; Rausch and Moore, 1975); also, the cow has no lysozyme in its tears as well as none in its PMNs (Padgett and Hirsch, 1967). There is no clearly apparent correlation, inverse or direct, between lysozyme content and other enzymic activity among the PMNs of various mammals (Rausch and Moore, 1975). There is also no clear correlation between lysozyme in different species and resistance or susceptibility to various infections. Thus, available information fails to provide any obvious basis upon which to extend existing hypotheses concerning the biological role of lysozyme.

It might be useful, however, to measure and compare levels of lysozyme, cationic antimicrobial proteins, and myeloperixodase in the PMNs of many species in order to discover whether any patterns suggestive of compensatory roles could be discerned. For example, Gennaro *et al.* (1983) have described in the lysozyme-deficient bovine PMN a novel granule having several antimicrobial cationic proteins that distinctly differ from those described heretofore in other species. As with the presence of two different lysozymes in PMNs of birds, the presence of this granule and its proteins in PMNs of cattle tempts speculation.

B. Antimicrobial Action

Lysozyme is one of the best understood of the enzymes. It cleaves the bacterial cell walls at the β 1–4 linkages between N-acetylmuramic acid and N-acetylglucosamine in the glycan backbone of the bacterial cell wall peptidoglycan. The cleavage products have been identified (Salton, 1957; Heymann *et al.*, 1964; Strominger and Tipper, 1974), and the relationship of lysozyme structure to its action has been demonstrated with X-ray crystallography (discussed by Chipman and Sharon, 1969; Strominger and Ghuysen, 1967). Substrate requirements of lysozyme have been defined (Ghuysen, 1974). Conditions for the optimum activity of lysozyme are, within limits, likely to be present in phagolysomes.

Considerable research has focused on the microbial factors inhibiting lysozyme cleavage of cell walls. Gram-positive bacteria have thick cell walls replete with various polysaccharides, proteins, and lipids. In general, walls of gram-positive organisms resist cleavage owing to O-acetyl groups ester-linked to the peptidoglycans (Brumfitt *et al.*, 1958; Strominger and Ghuysen, 1967; Glick *et al.*, 1972; Gallis *et al.*, 1976). The presence of free amino substituents on the glucosamines of cell walls also may interfere with lysozyme activity (Hayashi *et al.*, 1973), as may the degree of substitution of peptide subunits on the N-acetylmuramic acid units of the glycan backbone (Strominger and Ghuysen, 1967). With gram-negative organisms, however, lysozyme is unable to permeate the outer membrane. When the outer membrane is disrupted by treatment with alkali (Zinder and Arndt, 1956), with heat (Warren *et al.*, 1955; Becker and Hartsell, 1954; Noller and Hartsell, 1961), with chelating agents (Repaske, 1956; Repaske, 1958; Bryan, 1974; Witholt *et al.*, 1976), or with cationic amphipathic molecules such as polymyxin (Warren, 1957), sensitivity to lysozyme increases. Other manipulations that enhance lysozyme action on gram-negative rods include various enzyme treatments (Thorne *et al.*, 1976; Neiman, 1954) and antibody and complement (Amano *et al.*, 1954; Inouye *et al.*, 1959; Muschel and Jackson, 1963; Wardlaw, 1962; Gemsa *et al.*, 1966; Davis *et al.*, 1966; Glynn and Milne, 1967; Davis *et al.*, 1968; Wilson and Spitznagel, 1968; Glynn, 1969). The common factor in enhancement of lysozyme activity against gram-negative bacteria is the disruption of the outer membrane to allow lysozyme access to the peptidoglycan. This action leads to the lysis of the organism (e.g., Wilson and Spitznagel, 1968). The virtual spheroplasts formed by the lysozymal degradation of the cell wall readily lyse in the relatively low osmotic pressure of the tissue the microenvironment.

The extent to which and the way in which lysozyme affects microbes other than bacteria is not well known. It is reported, however, that lysozyme can inhibit growth of *Coccidioides immitis* in the spherule phase (Collins and Pappagianis, 1974). Lysozyme has been implicated in host resistance to *Cryptococcus neoformans* (Gadebusch and Johnson, 1966). Lysozyme is also known to have candidacidal properties, possibly mediated by a lytic action (Kamaya, 1970). It has been invoked in host resistance to *Candida albicans* (Lehrer *et al.*, 1975; Diamond and Krzeskcki, 1978).

C. Role in Serum and in Phagocytes

The literature contains numerous excellent studies that have dealt with the role of lysozyme in serum mediated bacteriolysis of gram-negative bacteria (Inoue *et al.*, 1959; Muschel and Jackson, 1963; Wardlaw, 1962; Gemsa *et al.*, 1966; Davis *et al.*, 1966, 1968; Glynn and Milne, 1967; Wilson and Spitznagel, 1968; Glynn, 1969). Serum from normal persons has a low but constant content of lysozyme. (Some degree of bacteriolysis occurs with the bactericidal action of serum.) On the basis of these studies, it can be concluded that the complement components of serum are bactericidal for serum-sensitive strains, but bacteriolysis does not occur unless lysozyme is present.

Serum lysozyme is only active against a few gram-positive bacteria owing to various biochemical structures of the gram-positive cell walls (see Section IV). Moreover, serum lysozyme concentrations are such that the attack on some gram-positive bacteria might be too slow to be bactericidal. What have these considerations to do with the lysozyme in PMNs? With gram-negative organisms, the encounter with serum complement might enhance their vulnerability to lysozyme insufficiently for them to be killed in serum. But the effects of complement might suffice to render them vulnerable to the much higher concentrations of lysozyme available in PMNs or macrophages. These considerations would probably not have any bearing on the fate of gram-positive bacteria. However, Leijh *et al.* (1979) found complement components necessary in the system in order for human monocytes to be maximally bactericidal for *Staphylococcus aureus* and *Staphylococcus epidermidis* as well as *Escherichia coli*. Thus it is conceivable that opsonization with serum enhances intracellular lysozyme action on both gram-positive and gram-negative bacteria, although a mechanism cannot be proposed for such action on gram-positive bacteria. The role of complement and its relationship to a role for intracellular lysozyme remain to be investigated.

The actual participation of lysozyme in the death of bacteria during phago-cytosis has not been rigorously demonstrated. What has been demonstrated is that the dissolution of bacterial cells phagocytized by PMNs is related to the relative resistance of their cell walls to lysozyme digestion *in vitro*. Thus Brumfitt *et al.* (1958) and Brumfitt and Glynn (1961) were able to show that wild-type *Micrococcus lysodiekticus* were readily lysed in the phagolysosomes of PMNs and macrophages. In contrast to the wild-type bacteria, *M. lysodiekticus* selected for ability to grow on lysozyme were resistant to lysis and survived phagocytosis. Similarly, inhibitors of lysozyme interfered with lysis of *M. lysodiekticus* by phagocytes. The cell walls of group A streptococci are naturally highly resistant to lysozyme (see Section IV.B). Even though group A streptococci die rapidly after being phagocytized by PMNs, their walls resist digestion and persist inside the PMNs that have phagocytized them (Glick *et al.*, 1972).

D. Lysozyme Deficiency

Finally, it should be re-emphasized that animals normally deficient in lyso-zyme (Padgett and Hirsch, 1967; Rausch and Moore, 1975) fail to show any disability clearly associated with this deficiency. Moreover, rabbits found to bear a mutation leading to absence of lysozyme did not show responses to infection markedly different from normal animals (Prieur *et al.*, 1974). A 40-year-old man presenting with a myeloproliferative disorder and partial lysozyme deficiency suffered decreased resistance and inability to eliminate infections due to low-grade bacterial pathogens, but no evidence was available that the lysozyme deficiency was responsible. Absence of specific granules, demonstrated total deficiency of lactoferrin, or both, seemed more likely than partial lysozyme deficiency to be responsible for the compromised state of this patient (Spitznagel *et al.*, 1972). It is thus difficult to define the biological role of lysozyme in PMN granules. Clearly lysozyme degrades microbial cells under favorable circumstances, and this will facilitate bacterial killing. However, study of a large number of lysozyme-deficient families, if such can be identified, and their response to infection will probably be necessary in order to advance understanding in this area.

V. LACTOFERRIN

Lactoferrin was first described by Sorensen and Sorensen (1939). Subse-quently purified and characterized as having an MW of ~76,000 (Masson, 1970; Bullen *et al.*, 1978), this iron-binding protein resembles transferrin in certain amino acid sequences among its cysteic peptides, suggesting a common ancestral protein (Bluard-Deconinck *et al.*, 1974). However, lactoferrin is primarily found in various secretions, milk, tears, saliva, nasal and bronchial secretions, bile, urine, seminal fluid, cervical mucus, and polymorphonuclear leukocytes (Masson, 1970; Masson and Heremans, 1966; Baggiolini *et al.*, 1970; Bullen *et al.*, 1978). In the peripheral blood of humans and in their bone marrow lactoferrin is confined to the secondary (specific) granules of neutrophilic granulocytes just as it is confined in blood and marrow of rabbits. Lactoferrin concentration in serum is 0.01 μM compared with transferrin at 30 μM (Bullen *et al.*, 1978). The actual physiological role of lactoferrin is still unknown. However, its capacity to bind metals, especially iron and copper with high binding constants at both physiological and very low pH (Masson, 1970; Bullen *et al.*, 1978), suggests it has a role in iron or copper metabolism. Lactoferrin binds iron even at pH 2, while transferrin cannot bind iron below pH 4.5. Perhaps, as Van Snick *et al.* (1974) suggested, it participates in return of iron to reticuloendothelial pools and is involved in the hypoferremia of inflammation. This explanation is not easily reconciled with the distribution of lactoferrin except during active inflammatory reaction. This distribution, taken together with the capacity of lactoferrin for binding iron, suggests, for example, that it might have a role in defense against infection. For example, lactoferrin is not just packaged in the specific granules; it is secreted by them during phagocytosis into the phagolysosome onto the surface of the PMN and into the surrounding medium (Leffell and Spitznagel, 1975; Pryzwansky *et al.*, 1979 *b*). Thus the substance is present throughout the scene of antimicrobial events. Its presence in secretions positions it in the fluids that bathe most epithelial surfaces as, for example, in the gut lumen, bronchial mucosa, and mammary ducts (see above).

A. Antimicrobial Action

Lactoferrin has primary antimicrobial capacities (Masson and Heremans, 1966; Masson, 1970; Oram and Reiter, 1968; Reiter *et al.*, 1975; Bullen, 1975; Bullen *et al.*, 1972, 1978; Kirkpatrick *et al.*, 1971; Arnold *et al.*, 1977; Bishop *et al.*, 1976). In growth medium lactoferrin is bacteriostatic (Arnold *et al.*, 1982; Bishop *et al.*, 1976; Bullen, 1975; Bullen *et al.*, 1972; Bullen and Wallis, 1977). The effect is due to iron-unsaturated lactoferrin (apolactoferrin) and it is antagonized by iron or haematin (Arnold *et al.*, 1982; Bullen, 1975; Bullen *et al.*, 1972, 1978; Bullen and Wallis, 1977; Weinberg, 1971, 1974). Bullen *et al.* (1978) placed *E. coli* 0111/134 into the intestines of newborn guinea pigs. Infant guinea pigs so inoculated and then fed haematin (50 μg by mouth) turned out to have intestinal populations of *E. coli* 0111/134 100,000 times greater than those of controls not given haematin. Guinea pig milk normally has lactoferrin unsaturated with iron. This apolactoferrin may have inhibited *E. coli* by complexing iron normally available to the *E. coli* in the gut. The inference was drawn that the *E. coli* proliferated more extensively in the haematin-fed guinea pigs due to experimentally increased iron in the gut, exceeding the binding capacity of the available lacto-ferrin. The bacteria were no longer deprived of iron. Bacteriostasis failed to occur. Antibody was said to participate with lactoferrin in this bacteriostatic reaction in the gut. Cow milk contains both lactoferrin and transferrin. Milk strongly inhibits *E. coli*, but the system is complex, being inhibited by citrate. Citrate is supposed to complex the iron. The iron of the iron–citrate complex is then more available to the bacteria than iron complexed by lactoferrin. Addition of bicar-bonate also reverses the antimicrobial effects due to lactoferrin in milk (Reiter *et al.*, 1975; Bishop *et al.*, 1976).

Bullen *et al.* (1978) state that the following outcomes are possible when different species of bacteria are incubated in serum. Some may grow, some are killed rapidly, and others show bacteriostasis. Presumably bacteria able to grow in the presence of iron-chelating proteins possess specific mechanisms for acquiring iron from transferrin (or lactoferrin) either through binding of iron to a cell-surface receptor or through secretion by the bacterial cells of a low-molecular-weight iron chelator that can capture iron from the iron–protein complex. The resulting chelate is then taken up by the bacteria (Weinberg, 1971, 1974). Both bactericidal and bacteriostatic effects can be reversed by saturation of the protein with Fe^{3+} or by heme compounds (Bullen *et al.*, 1978). The precise function of antibody and complement in these systems is unclear, but Bullen *et al.* (1978) claim they cannot function in the absence of unsaturated iron-binding proteins. Lactoferrin in PMNs is iron unsaturated and exists in a low-iron environment in the PMN phagolysosome (Bullen *et al.*, 1978). Studies with a variety of bacteria (*Clostridium welchi, Proteus aeruginosa, Escherichia coli, Listeria monocyto-genes, Candida albicans* and other "fungi," *Mycobacterium, Vibrio cholerae, Neisseria meningitidis*, and *Neisseria gonorrhoeae*) have led to the conclusion that their iron requirements could be limiting to their capacity to replicate in a host. The iron-binding capacity of lactoferrin and transferrin was the important limit-ing factor on iron supplies, and additions of iron in growth media inhibited the bacteriostasis achieved due to iron-unsaturated lactoferrin.

Recently Arnold, in contrast to Bullen, described a strictly bactericidal lacto-ferrin system (Arnold *et al.*, 1977, 1980, 1981, 1982). This system depended on incubation of bacteria in non-growth-sustaining media with unsaturated lactoferrin followed by subcultures of the suspended bacteria. Several organisms were reported sensitive: *Streptococcus mutans, Streptococcus salivarius, Streptococcus mitis, Streptococcus pneumoniae, Escherichia coli, Vibrio cholerae, Proteus aer-uginosa*, and *Candida albicans*. Various organisms were resistant, such as *Strepto-coccus pyogenes, Streptococcus lactis, Staphylococcus aureus, Staphylococcus epidermidis*, various *Escherichia coli* strains, *Enterobacteria cloaca, Salmonella newport*, and *Shigella sonnei*. The *Streptococcus pneumonia* was rough and be-came resistant to lactoferrin when its capsule production was enhanced by mouse passage. In this system simple addition of iron did not inhibit antimicrobial action due to lactoferrin. Nevertheless, iron unsaturation of the lactoferrin was a strict necessity. Saturation of the lactoferrin with Fe^{3+} before use in the antimicrobial system eliminated its antimicrobial action. Careful experiments showed that these effects of lactoferrin were different from those due to iron starvation (Arnold *et al.*, 1982). Removal of adhered lactoferrin from bacteria failed to rescue them from death.

B. Role of Lactoferrin in PMNs

Cited above were several publications that strongly suggest that O_2-independent killing mechanisms were functional under conditions of stringent anaerobiasis and in PMNs of patients with CGD that were unable to reduce molecular O_2 to O_2^- and related products. In species other than man, especially in the rabbit, ample evidence exists that iron and haematin can reverse the antimicrobial powers of polymorphs (Gladstone, 1973; Galdstone and Walton, 1970, 1971; Galdstone *et al.*, 1974; Walton, 1978; Walton and Gladstone, 1975, 1976). However, Bullen and Wallis (1977) found that reversal of microbicidal action with additions of iron was much more dramatic when the iron was introduced into PMN phagolysosome, as a complex of antiferritin–ferritin. This enhanced effect was attributed to the greater access of iron to the lactoferrin compared with the poor access achieved with iron salts, ferritin, or haematin alone. Unfortunately, these experiments are intrinsically complex, difficult to control, and difficult to interpret.

Other approaches to studies on the role of lactoferrin were attempted by Wang-Iverson *et al.* (1978). These workers purged human PMNs of their specific granules and lactoferrin with the action of phorbol myristate acetate (PMA). The PMNs thus depleted retained substantial capacity for phagocytosis and intraleuko-cytic killing. There was, however, a definite reduction in killing capacity as compared with control PMNs even though the PMA-treated cells retained brisk hexose monophosphate shunt responses to phagocytic challenge. The antimicrobial effects may have been reduced due to absence of specific granules and lacto-ferrin, but the complexity of the experimental system leaves much for further investigation.

C. Lactoferrin Deficiency

A more promising approach to the possible antimicrobial action of lacto-ferrin in PMNs is to identify and study patients with PMN lactoferrin deficiency, specific granule deficiency, or both deficiencies. A few such patients have been identified. Their specific granule and lactoferrin deficiencies have been established with various combinations of immunocytochemistry, electron microsopy, and cell fractionation.

In each instance other cell parameters such as chemotaxis, phagocytosis, intraleukocytic killing of various bacteria, O_2 metabolism, enzyme activities, and ultrastructure have been studied. The first such case was presented by Spitznagel *et al.* (1972) (Table II). This 42-year-old patient was diagnosed as having a myeloproliferative syndrome (Philadelpha chromosome positive). During his 14-month course, the patient suffered repeated infections due to opportunistic pathogens that resisted antimicrobial therapy. The essential fact was that his PMNs showed greatly impaired intraleukocytic killing for the organisms that caused his infections. His PMNs were completely devoid of specific granules or lactoferrin. They showed 50% of normal lysozyme levels. However, PMN azurophil granules and myeloperoxidase (MPO) were at normal levels. Azurophil granules degranulated in response to phagocytic challenge. It was concluded that the lactoferrin-specific granule deficiency accounted for much of this compromised host's susceptibility to infection.

Since that time several other cases have been reported, including those by Strauss *et al.* (1974), Parmley *et al.* (1975), Komiyama *et al.* (1979), Breton-Gorius *et al.* (1980), and Gallin *et al.* (1982). One of these cases was the subject of two of the reports, i.e., those by Breton-Gorius *et al.* (1980) and by Gallin *et al.* (1982). The common defect in these patients has been their unusual susceptibility to various infections and their lack of specific granules. In only two patients has absence of lactoferrin been documented. It can only be assumed that it was absent from the PMNs of the other patients (Table II).

One patient (Spitznagel *et al.*, 1972) almost certainly had an acquired deficiency. The other patients had genetically determined disease. The genetically determined disease appeared compatible with life, although the quality of the life was impaired. In all patients examined intraleukocytic killing of bacteria was reduced, but the specific organisms differed from patient to patient. Defects have been described for PMNs and adhesion (Oseas *et al.*, 1981), although these have not been observed in all patients. The patient of Breton-Gorius was shown by Gallin to have impaired chemotaxis, reduced binding of chemoattractants, and normal adhesion. This patient had abnormal phagocytic parameters, including oxidative metabolism and reduced introleukocytic killing. Thus, even genetically determined specific granule and lactoferrin deficiency appear unlikely to provide clear-cut or uniform answers. Still, the cases studied indicate that for normal antimicrobial phagocytosis due to PMNs, specific granules and lactoferrin are essential. The precise relationships of the various defects remain to be defined.

VI. SMALL PEPTIDES

Small peptides as a potentially promising source of materials with antimicrobial activity have been largely overlooked. An exception is the work of Modrzakowski and Paranavitana (1981), which has shown antimicrobial activity in peak D isolated from crude granule extracts of human granulocytes with chromatography

Table II. Summary of Five Cases of Specific Granule Deficiency[a]

| Age/Sex | Infections | Neutrophils | | Intraleukocytic antimicrobial action | Chemotaxis | Specific granules | Lactoferrin | Neutrophil alkaline phosphatase |
		Peripheral count	Morphology					
14/M[b]	Staphylococcal skin and respiratory	Normal	Bilobed nuclei	Candida normal, staphylococci impaired	Impaired	Absent	ND[i]	Absent
7/F[c]	Abscesses, otitis mastoiditis, eczema due to Staphylococcus aureus, Pseudomonas aeruginosa	Normal	Bilobed nuclei, nuclear blebs clefts, pockets	Staphylococci impaired	Impaired	Absent or rare	ND[i]	Present in <3% of PMNs
43/M[d]	Recurrent lung, skin, blood; Hemophilus parainfluenza, Staphyloccus aureus, Proteus rettgeri, Klebsiella pneumonia Pseudomonas aeruginosa, Enterobacter cloacae, Enterococcus, Actinetobacter	Elevated during infections	Philadelphia 1 chromosome, 63% of cells otherwise normal; frequently bilobed	Impaired for E. coli, P. rettgeri, Streptococcus; normal for S. aureus	Normal	Absent	Absent	Normal

Patient	Clinical infections						
5½/F[e]	Ear, throat, diarrhea; oral lesions due to *Pseudomonas*, *Klebsiella*, and *Escherichia coli*	Severe neutropenia	Multiple small lobes, notched nuclei	ND[i]	Decreased	Absent	ND[i]	Markedly decrease
6/M[f]	Staphylococcal skin infection; infections by *Pneumococcus*, *Candida albicans*	Normal	Bilobed nuclei	Normal activity against *Staphylococcus aureus* and *Serratia marcescens*	Normal	Absent	Absent	Decreased
9/M[g]	Severe scalp infections, *Proteus mirabilis*, *Staphylococcus*	Normal	Normal	Slightly decreased, *S. aureus*	Impaired[h] decreased fMet-Leu-Phe receptors	Absent	Absent	Not detected

[a] Adapted and augmented from (Breton-Gorius et al., 1982). The 6-year-old boy and the 9-year-old boy were actually the same patient observed at different stages of development.
[b] Patient described by Strauss et al. (1974).
[c] Patient described by Komiyama et al. (1979).
[d] Patient described by Spitznagel et al. (1972).
[e] Patient described by Parmley et al. (1975).
[f] Patient described by Breton-Gorius et al. (1980).
[g] Patient of Breton-Gorius (see footnote a) at age 9 by Gallin et al. (1982).
[h] Several abnormalities of membrane receptors, function, aggregation, and charge are described in detail in the original paper.
[i] ND, no data.

on Sephadex G-75. The activity was manifested against *Acinetobacter*. The peptides had manifest MW of ~9000 kd. Their antimicrobial action was time and temperature dependent. They were more active against stationary-phase than against logarithmic-phase bacteria. The proteolytic enzymes pronase and trypsin eliminated antimicrobial activity but heat failed to inactivate the antimicrobial action of these small peptides. Microbial resistance was increased proportionally as the carbon chain lengths of fatty acids in the growth substrate were increased.

These peptides rendered liposomes formed from lipid of *Acinetobacter* leaky for glucose. The peak D peptides were ineffectual against *Salmonella typhimurium* or *S. albus* and only slightly active against *Streptococcus faecalis* and *Staphylococcus aureus*. These peptides are of interest because they are cationic and of low molecular weight. Most are evidently products of proteolysis that occurs during degranulation under low pH conditions.

The D peak is a well-recognized portion of the effluent from granule proteins prepared without efforts to curb proteolysis and passed over Sephadex G-75. The influence of proteolysis for the end result of attempts to prepare proteins from PMNs has been stressed (Amrein and Stossel, 1980). It is important to recognize that these fragments may be derived from any of the granule or associated proteins. Whatever their origin, these or similar fragments are probably formed during the naturally occurring degranulation of phagocytosis, since pH and other conditions would favor proteolysis (Rouse, 1925*a,b;* Mandell, 1970; Kakinuma, 1970; Jensen and Bainton, 1973; Jacques and Bainton, 1978). There is a very real possibility that such fragments are available *in vivo* in phagolysosomes of PMNs in high concentration, where they may have antimicrobial capacity for some species of bacteria or other microbes. The possibility should be investigated that proteolytic cleavage is important in the activation of higher-molecular-weight antimicrobial components. From the granules of species such as the rabbit and the rat, isolation of antimicrobial arginine-rich, highly cationic peptides or proteins of ~10,000 MW have been reported (Zeya and Spitznagel, 1968; Walton, 1978; Hodinka and Modrzakowski, 1983). The experiments with rat and rabbit PMNs have not to my knowledge been repeated under conditions inhibitory for proteolysis. It cannot be assumed that such cationic proteins would fail to appear during preparation in the presence of DFP. Still the possibility has to be considered and remains to be investigated that these relatively small proteins in rodent PMNs are in fact products of proteolytic cleavage.

VII. ASSOCIATION OF O$_2$-INDEPENDENT SUBSTANCES WITH CYTOPLASMIC GRANULES OF PMNs

The first suggestion that antimicrobial activity might be associated with a granule fraction of leukocytes was made by Fishman and Silverman (1957) and Fishman *et al.* (1957). Phagocytin then turned out to be associated with the cytoplasmic granules of PMNs of rabbits and humans (Cohn and Hirsch, 1960*b*). Following these reports, substantial evidence for the association of O_2-independent antimicrobial substances with PMN granules has continued to appear.

A. Cationic Antimicrobial Proteins

The antimicrobial, cationic, arginine-rich, proteins of rabbit PMNs proved to be associated with the granules of rabbit PMNs (Zeya and Spitznagel, 1963, 1966*a,b,* 1968, 1971; Zeya *et al.,* 1966*a*).

Human PMNs carry their cationic O_2-independent antimicrobial components in their granules, as first shown by Welsh and Spitznagel (1971). These findings have been repeatedly verified with crude granule preparations from human PMNs (Buck and Rest, 1981; Daly *et al.,* 1982; Olsson and Venge, 1972; Rest, 1979; Rest *et al.,* 1977, 1978*a;* Shafer *et al.,* 1983; Thorne *et al.,* 1976; Weiss *et al.,* 1978). Moreover, the principal antimicrobial activity for *S. typhimurium, E. coli,* and *N. gonorrhoeae* has been shown to be most concentrated in the azurophil (primary) granules, especially those with buoyant density of ∼1.21 (Rest *et al.,* 1978*a*). The exact localization of BPI (Weiss *et al.,* 1978) and the 57-kd and 37-kd antimicrobial proteins (Shafer *et al.,* 1983) have yet to be established. However, the apparent concentration of antimicrobial activity in the primary granules (buoyant density 1.21) suggests that one or all of the above are located there.

B. Proteolytic Enzymes

Other substances demonstrating antimicrobial activity, such as the chymotryptic-like cationic protein (cathepsin G) (Olsson and Venge, 1972) and elastase (Thorne *et al.,* 1976), have been localized in the azurophil granules (DeWald *et al.,* 1975; Ohlsson *et al.,* 1977; Rausch *et al.,* 1978) of human PMNs.

The localizations described above were accomplished for the most part with granules resolved from leukocyte cytoplasm with isopycnic centrifugation in sucrose density gradients. However, immunocytocytochemical methods have verified these findings. In addition, MacRae and Spitznagel (1975) have shown with ultrastructural histochemistry that cationic proteins are concentrated in the azurophil granules of rabbit and chicken PMNs.

C. Lysozyme

Lysozyme, another antimicrobial protein of PMNs, has been shown to be associated with their cytoplasmic granules (Cohn and Hirsch, 1960*a;* Spitznagel *et al.,* 1974; Zeya and Spitznagel, 1963; Baggiolini *et al.,* 1969; Bretz and Baggiolini, 1974; Brune and Spitznagel, 1973) in rabbit, human, chicken, and guinea pig granules, as well as in the granules of several other species. Exceptions are the PMNs and PMN granules of cow, goat, sheep, cat, hamsters, and several species of monkeys, all of which lack lysozyme (Rausch and Moore, 1975). Lysozyme is now known to be distributed between the specific and the azurophil granules in human PMNs (Spitznagel *et al.*, 1974; Bretz and Baggiolini, 1974; Rest *et al.*, 1978*b*) as it is in rabbit and rat PMNs.

D. Lactoferrin

Lactoferrin is distributed in the specific (secondary) granules along with approximately one-half the lysozyme in rabbit (Baggiolini *et al.*, 1970). The same distribution obtains in the human polymorphonuclear leukocytes (Leffell and Spitznagel, 1972; Spitznagel *et al.*, 1974; Wang-Iverson *et al.*, 1978).

E. Influence of Species and Genetic Abnormalities

In addition to the above antimicrobial cationic proteins, lysozyme, and lactoferrin described in human and rabbit PMNs, antimicrobial cationic proteins have been described in a large granule type found in bovine PMNs. These granules are apparently neither azurophils or specifics. They are a third large granule type recently described by Gennaro *et al.* (1982, 1983). The granules have buoyant densities of 1.20, 1.21, and 1.23, respectively; one-half the lactoferrin is in the 1.21-granule, while the rest plus cationic antibacterial protein ($<$20 kd) are in the 1.23-density granules. These findings in addition to those of Brune and Spitznagel (1973) and Hindenburg *et al.* (1974), who showed that two molecularly distinct lysozymes are present in the cytoplasmic granules of chicken PMNs suggest that careful investigation of various species may well reveal additional O_2-independent antimicrobial substances.

Finally, it is noteworthy that the observation that lactoferrin and approximately one-half the lysozyme of human PMNs are associated with the specific granules is convincingly supported by studies on patients who lack specific granules. In their PMNs lactoferrin is completely absent. Their PMN lysozyme levels are about 50% of normal (Spitznagel *et al.*, 1972; Breton-Gorius *et al.*, 1980; Strauss *et al.*, 1974; Gallin *et al.*, 1982). Similar deficiencies have been induced in PMNs exposed to phorbol myristate acetate (Wang-Iverson *et al.*, 1978). In addition, lactoferrin synthesis coincides with formation of specific granule in human marrow myelocytes Pryzwansky *et al.* (1979*a*). Rausch *et al.* 1978) found that the giant granules of PMNs from humans with Chediak-Higashi syndrome had lactoferrin incorporated in them along with various azurophil granule proteins.

It is important to mention that the cytoplasmic granules of eosinophils are associated with highly cationic arginine-rich proteins (Archer and Hirsch, 1963; Gleich *et al.*, 1973, 1974; Ohlsson *et al.*, 1977). The Charcot–Leyden crystal found in eosinophil granules comprises the major cationic protein (Gleich *et al.*, 1976).

F. Summary

The various O_2-independent antimicrobial substances of PMNs and of eosinophils are associated with one or another class of cytoplasmic granule. In humans the cationic antimicrobial proteins are associated with the azurophil granules; cathepsin G, elastase, and lysozyme are also associated with them. Lactoferrin and lysozyme are associated with the specific granules. The same principles apply to granulocytes of other animals, but with variations in the proteins and in the characteristics of the granules peculiar to each species.

VIII. DEGRANULATION

First recognized 90 years ago, this event is a concomitant of phagocytosis and is crucial for delivery of O_2-independent antimicrobial systems to their targets. Guinea pig peritoneal granulocytes, upon coming in contact with viable *Bacillus anthracis*, rapidly lost their cytoplasmic granules, which seemed to vanish against the bacillary cell walls. The bacilli that came in contact with the granules stopped growing, while nearby bacilli not in contact with phagocytes continued to grow (Kanthack and Hardy, 1894). This phenomenon was independently rediscovered by Robineaux and Frederic (1955), Hirsch and Cohn (1960, 1964), and Cohn and Hirsch (1960*b*).

A. Membrane Fusion and Phagolysosome Formation

Ultrastuctural studies then showed that granule membrane fused with the membranes of the phagosomes. A communication opened from the granule to phagosome, forming a single structure. This structure, the phagolysosome (Zucker-Franklin and Hirsch, 1964), contained the phagocytized particle and the granule matrix. Histochemical experiments revealed cationic arginine-rich proteins in the matrices of granules in rabbit and guinea pig PMNs. These cationic proteins reacted with the surfaces of phagocytized bacteria, an event accompanied by death of the bacteria (Spitznagel and Chi, 1963). Ultrastructural histochemistry then confirmed that cationic proteins were present in the azurophil (primary) granules of rabbit PMNs and that these proteins interacted with phagocytized particles subsequent to membrane fusion and formation of the phagolysosome (Macrae and Spitznagel, 1975). Experiments with PMNs of chickens revealed similar findings.

B. Translocation of Granule Proteins

Pryzwansky *et al.* (1979*b*) further showed that as soon as 5–15 sec after contact between challenge particle and phagocytic cell, a protein marker for specific granules, lactoferrin, and markers for azurophil granules, MPO, cathepsin G, and elastase appeared about the challenge particle. They appeared near or on the cell surface evidently at the mouth of the nascent phagolysosome. Thus contact between phagocytic challenge particles and O_2-independent and O_2-dependent antimicrobial systems occurred very soon after phagocytosis was initiated. The particle, granule components, enzymes, and cationic proteins all became components of the phagolysosomes. The separate fusion, first of specific and then of azurophil granules with phagolysosome, was reported based on ultrastuctural studies (Bainton, 1973).

Stossel *et al.* (1971) documented the presence of lysosomal enzymes in phagolysosomes induced in PMNs with paraffin oil droplets. Leffell and Spitznagel (1974, 1975) found that both specific granule and azurophil granule contents appeared in phagolysosomes formed by human PMNs in response to polystyrene particles coated with antigen–antibody complexes or heat-aggregated human immunoglobulin. They found that lactoferrin for the most part actually left the PMNs and entered the extracellular fluid, while MPO remained associated with the phagolysosomes. Segal *et al.* (1980) have performed similar experiments and obtained essentially the same results. They found, however, that the kinetics of degranulation of acid hydrolases were slower than the kinetics for MPO and lactoferrin. They concluded the acid hydrolase came exclusively from a third granule compartment within the PMN.

C. Stimuli for Degranulation

The stimuli for and consequences of degranulation have been studied in considerable detail (see, e.g., review in Klebanoff and Clark, 1978). The detailed mechanisms of degranulation involve cell biology beyond the scope of this chapter. However, in summary it is clear that while degranulation is a central event in antimicrobial phagocytosis, it can and does occur independently (Goldstein *et al.*, 1975) of phagocytosis. Thus it is of interest in the broader aspects of the inflammatory response. Experimentally, in suspension, degranulation without phagocytosis occurred when PMNs were briefly pretreated with an inhibitor of microfilaments, such as cytochalasin B. Similar degranulation also occurred when the cells were attached to a large, solid substrate. Under these conditions the soluble mediators, such as the anaphylotoxin C5a or the chemotactic peptide formyl methionyl-leucyl-phenylalanine (fMet-Leu-Phe), induced receptor-mediated granule secretion (Henson and Oades, 1975).

However, degranulation probably happens most often in connection with phagocytosis. Degranulation during phagocytosis is probably a receptor-mediated function, but the necessary stimuli are not entirely understood. For example, Leffell and Spitznagel (1974, 1975) found that while uncoated polystyrene Latex beads were phagocytized by human PMNs, the beads hardly induced any degranulation into phagosomes (phagolysosome formation). Beads coated with antigen-antibody complexes or heat-aggregated immunoglobulin did induce degranulation and phagolysosome formation. Complement was not required in the system, and IgG$_3$ was most potent in inducing degranulation, while IgG$_4$ was practically inactive in inducing degranulation into phagolysosomes. Henson and Oades (1975) have shown that aggregated immunoglobulin alone stimulates degranulation when phagocytized or when encountered on unphagocytosable surfaces. Evidently either Fc or C3 fragments alone stimulate degranulation on appropriate surfaces (Henson and Oades, 1975).

Receptors for both Fc and C3b are well established as components of PMN plasma membrane. Other receptors that for example bind mannose are available. Further details concerning these receptors and their functions in endocytosis are to be found in a recent review by Steinman *et al.* (1983). In any event, the nature of the stimuli and the plasma membrane receptors will place major constraints on the degranulation of PMNs. Cyclic adenosine monophosphate (cAMP) is readily demonstrated with immunocytochemistry at the site of membrane perturbation. Cyclic guanosine monophosphate (cGMP) is seen with immunocytochemistry in the portion of the PMN most remote from the perturbation. That the cAMP is actively involved is reflected by the demonstration in the PMN cytoplasm of the receptor subunit of the cAMP phosphoprotein kinase (Pryzwansky *et al.*, 1981).

D. Membrane Function in Degranulation

According to Smolen *et al.* (1980), various stimuli, including complement and immune complexes, induced changes in membrane potential of PMNs in <10 sec. This change was followed quickly by release of lysosomal enzymes and superoxide generation. Smolen's stop-flow experiments revealed that secretion followed different stimuli by times dependent on the quality of the stimulant. The quantity of stimulant primarily influenced the magnitude of response. The various responses seemingly could be dissociated. Smolen has also implicated phospholipase and lipoxygenase mediators in degranulation events (Smolen and Weissmann, 1980). More recently this group (Smolen and Weissmann, 1981) presented evidence for two groups of PMN stimulants or secretagogues, i.e., complete secretagogues (inducing degranulation of both azurophil and specific granule) and incomplete ones (producing degranulation only by specific granules). The complete secretagogues induced transient elevation of cAMP. The incomplete secretagogues did not. This finding could be one of the first clues concerning molecular control of degranulation through second messengers. Evidently Fc and C3b receptors recognize complete secretagogues. No physiologically incomplete secretagogues were demonstrated, although chemoattractants were always tested, in the presence of cytochalasin B. Conconavalin A and phorbol myristate acetate were the only incomplete secretagogues tested. Demonstrations of physiological but incomplete secretagogues would be of great interest.

E. Ion Flux and Arachidonic Acid Metabolites

Ion fluxes are temporally related to degranulation induced with soluble mediators such as C5a and fMet-Leu-Phe. Thus substantial influxes of Na^+ and Ca^{2+} occur within 30 sec of stimulation. Substantial effluxes of K^+ occur (Naccache et al., 1977). This and other evidence suggests that calmodulin influences degranulation (Alobaidi et al., 1981). O'Flaherty et al. (1979) have found that two drugs that block arachidonic acid metabolism, i.e., 5,8,11,14-eicosatetraynoic acid and indomethacin, block degranulation induced by C5a and fMet-Leu-Phe. This finding suggests that metabolites of arachidonic acid may modulate degranulation.

F. Microtubules and Microfilaments

Substantial evidence suggests that microtubules are involved in degranulation and that microfilaments may be involved as well. Precisely what they do remains to be defined. Evidence for involvement is summarized in Chapter 5 of the recent book by Klebanoff and Clark (1978).

G. Mechanisms of Membrane Fusion

The mechanisms of membrane fusion between granule and phagosomal membranes and the establishment of communications between these two compartments have yet to be clarified. Electron microsopic examinations have revealed rather unusual granulations in the protein of granule membranes of PMNs. It is possible that these granulations are involved in membrane recognition and fusion during phagocytosis (Baggiolini et al., 1976). If so, they might be important in directing the orderly traffic among plasma membrane, phagosome, lysosomes, and phagolysosomes. Studies on the proteins of specific and azurophil granule membranes showed that they are unique and that some of them are indeed exposed on the cytoplasmic face of the granules. Comparison with cell-surface proteins showed substantial differences in proteins from the specific and azurophil granule membranes, although there were four polypeptides in common (Brown et al., 1983). These findings were also consistent with a role for these proteins in granule to granule and granule to plasma membrane recognition. The role of membrane in endocytosis, including phagocytosis, has been exhaustively reviewed in a recent article by Steinman *et al.* (1983). Although the model systems explored therein primarily involved macrophages, fibroblasts, and other cells, the principles in all likelihood are applicable to PMNs as well.

H. Disorders of Degranulation

Diseases in which disorders of degranulation are prominent so far appear to be infrequent and limited in number. Prominent and most studied among them is the Chediak–Higashi syndrome, a disorder characterized by partial albinism, recurrent pyogenic infections, and abnormally large granules in all lysosome-containing cells. These patients are eventually afflicted with lymphomatous disease. The Chediak–Higashi syndrome is transmitted in an autosomal recessive pattern. Premature fusion of azurophil and specific granules occurs as the PMNs differentiate (Rausch *et al.*, 1978). Premature fusion results in effective abrogation of granule function.

Dysfunction of actin in PMNs has been shown to cause ineffectual intraleukocytc killing and decreased resistance to infection. Ultrastructural studies revealed relatively few microfilaments in the cortical areas of the PMNs of such patients (Boxer *et al.*, 1974). Some suggestion of excessive degranulation was found in experiments with the PMNs of these patients. This would be consistent with observations showing that the antifilament drug cytochalasin B facilitates degranulation without phagocytosis.

I. Summary

That degranulation exists is indisputable. It is clearly a mechanism through which highly reactive proteins can be delivered in high concentrations to phagocytized particles such as microbial cells. Unphagocytosable surfaces, i.e., areas that exceed the limits that permit the PMN to enclose them completely in vesicles of membrane also cause degranulation. Degranulation is crucial in delivery and application of O_2-independent antimicrobial mechanisms. It will be of great value to the pharmacology of inflammation to understand in detail the mechanisms and modes of control for degranulation of PMN.

IX. INTRAPHAGOSOMAL MILIEU

The phagolysosome is a membrane-bound structure that varies in size, depending on the number and volume of particles ingested by the PMN. If one considers the phagolysosomal membrane of PMNs to be closely apposed to the particle (Steinman *et al.*, 1983), a minimum volume for a phagocytic vesicle fitted to one or two *E. coli* could be ~0.07 μm^3 or 0.14 μm^3. Since the organism itself would, at least at the outset, be impermeable to proteins from the host cell, the actual volume would have to be reduced by the volume of the particle itself and the space available for fluid and solutes might be very small indeed. The point is that any solutes placed into this space by degranulation granules would be very concentrated. For example, if assuming that one specific granule has 3.2×10^{-8} μg of lactoferrin (Leffell and Spitznagel, 1972) and that the entire vesicle of 0.14 μm^3 would be filled with solvent, the concentration of lactoferrin could achieve 3×10^{-3} M. Arnold *et al.* (1980) have shown that concentrations of 4.2×10^{-6} M lactoferrin may be bactericidal for *E. coli*. The cationic proteins of the azurophil granule are active in the range of 10^{-8}-10^{-9} M. It is likely that highly microbicidal concentrations of azurophil granule proteins are readily established in the phagolysosome.

A. Hydrogen Ion Concentration

The hydrogen ion concentration in PMN phagocytic vacuoles has long been a focus of research interest. This is appropriate, since each granule constitutent entering the phagolysome expresses its activity within a relatively narrow pH range. There is general agreement that the pH after some period of time is low (Rouse, 1925a,b; Sprick, 1956; Pavlov and Soloviev, 1967; Mandell, 1970; Kakinuma, 1970; Jensen and Bainton, 1973; Reijngoud and Tager, 1973, 1975; Jacques and Bainton, 1978). Estimates have ranged from as low as pH 3.0 (Rous, 1925a) to pH 6.5 (Mandell, 1970). The pH may be relatively high, e.g., 6.5 at 3 min, after initiation of phagocytosis with rabbit PMNs and fall to pH 4.0 after 7-15 min (Jensen and Bainton, 1973). Similar results were obtained with human PMNs (Jacques and Bainton, 1978). The methods of measurement have classically depended on color change in indicator dyes. In more recent times the dyes selected have been fluorescent. Color change has been measured not by visual comparison, but with a spectrofluorometer. Kakinuma (1970) used a different approach, in which 5,5-dimethyl-2,4-oxazolidinedione distribution across cell membranes was measured in guinea pig PMNs. An estimated intracellular pH of 6.85-7.05 was measured 10 min after phagocytosis of *E. coli*. Various problems beset this technique, as they do the indicator dye techniques. For example, it measures the intracellular pH for the whole cell. With certain assumptions, Kakinuma estimated the pH in the phagocytic vacuole to be 5.5-6.0.

Another way of estimating intravacuolar pH is to consider the pH requirements of enzymes shown to act there. Elastase of human PMNs, for example, has a pH optimum of ~8.0. Elastase activity decreases substantially at pH 7.2 and is inactive at pH 6.0. There is evidence that PMN elastase attacks and digests bacterial proteins during phagocytosis (Blondin and Janoff, 1976). On such grounds it is likely that the internal environment of the elastase is in the range of 7.0-8.0 for sufficient time for this digestion to occur. The general position is that the pH may be about 7.0 at 3 min after phagocytosis begins and will be anywhere from 4.5 to 6.0 after 10 to 15 min.

The fall in pH of the phagolysosome has been attributed to lactic acid production (Kakinuma, 1970) and to movement of protons and anions across the phagolysosomal membrane (Reijngoud and Tager, 1973, 1975; Goldman and Rottenberg, 1973). Recent studies by Segal et al. (1981) show that pH in normal human PMN phagolysosome first rises to 7.8 and then falls to 6.0–6.5. The PMNs of patients with chronic granulomatous disease fail to show this initial rise; instead, there is simply a rapid fall in intravascular pH. Since these cells either lack the cytochrome b_{245} found in normal cells (X-linked form of CGD) or fail to reduce it (autosomal form) (Segal et al., 1983). Segal suggests that the cytochrome b_{245} may serve as an electron-transport system that optimizes pH conditions for killing by other antimicrobial mechanisms. Segal and colleagues have further suggested that the impaired intraleukocytic action of PMNs displayed by patients with CGD could in part be due to defective control of intravacuolar pH.

B. Antimicrobial Action Due to pH and Fatty Acids

It has long been recognized that some microorganisms are intolerant of low pH (Avery and Cullen, 1919; Lord and Nye, 1919) and the organisms themselves may reduce the pH of the medium (Avery and Cullen, 1919). Fatty acids of various chain lengths have been shown to exert antimicrobial effects on various bacteria, as have other organic acids and ketone bodies (Dubos, 1950, 1953; Nieman, 1954; Kodicek, 1949) and long-chain fatty acids (Galbraith and Miller, 1973a-c, Galbraith et al., 1971). Thus intolerant microbes might die in the low pH existing in established phagolysosomes. They might even contribute to that low pH by producing acids themselves. Another concept of fatty acid toxicity suggests that auto-oxidation of unsaturated fatty acids provides additional antibacterial effects (Gutteridge et al., 1981). Since the potential for such oxidation is present in phagolysosome of PMNs, this possibility cannot be dismissed. Thus the presence of fatty acids in the phagolysosome could add to its antimicrobial activity either directly or through oxidation.

C. Influence of Exogenous Substances in the Phagolysosome

1. Viruses and Iron

Exogenous influences and substances may modify conditions within the phagolysosome. Influenza virus is said, for example, to inhibit degranulation (Abramson et al., 1982b) and intraleukocytic killing for S. aureus (Abramson et al., 1982a). Iron appears to inhibit intraleukocytic killing, but the mechanism is different from that due to influenza virus. Probably it interferes with action of lactoferrin or cationic proteins (see Section X) (Bullen and Wallis, 1977; Gladstone, 1973; Gladstone and Walton, 1970, 1971, 1974; Walton, 1978; Walton and Gladstone, 1975, 1976).

2. Bacteria

Interference with intraleukocytic killing may be mediated by products of bacteria. For example, the lipopolysaccharide in the outer membranes of *S. typhimurium* that inhibits the antimicrobial action of cationic azurophil granule proteins of human PMNs (Modrzakowski and Spitznagel, 1979). Also, *Brucella* may inhibit degranulation (Kreutzer *et al.*, 1979) and so may *Legionella pneumophilia* (Horwitz and Silverstein, 1981). Finally, the toxic sulfolipids of mycobacteria have been shown to prevent lysosome–phagosome fusion in macrophages (Goren, 1983). Thus a number of substances can interfere with phagolysosomal functions; some of these interfering substances are products of bacterial surfaces (Costerton *et al.*, 1979). In this connection, there may be differences in rates of fusion between phagosomes and lysosomes, depending on the kind of stimulus operating. Differences in these rates could substantially alter the outcome of interactions between bacteria and PMNs (Amano *et al.*, 1981).

3. Antibody and Complement

Serum antibody and complement components probably contribute to intraleukocytic antimicrobial action. Of course, antibody and complement are important for rapid phagocytosis and degranulation, but they may be important in another way especially with gram-negative bacteria. Ample evidence testifies that antibody plus complement damages the outer membranes of gram-negative bacteria and permits lysozyme to reach the peptidoglycan of the gram-negative cell wall (Amano *et al.*, 1954; Muschel and Jackson, 1963; Wilson and Spitznagel, 1968; Davis *et al.*, 1966; Gemsa *et al.*, 1966; Davis *et al.*, 1968). A number of reports (Menzel *et al.*, 1978; Bjornson *et al.*, 1980; Tedesco *et al.*, 1981; Melby and Midtvedt, 1981) have suggested that antibody and complement components of serum enhance intraleukocytic killing by effects other than opsonization. The organisms studied were *E. coli* and *Bacteroides*. The effect seemingly was not confined to action against gram-negative bacteria. Other investigators have presented evidence to support similar action with *S. aureus* in granulocytes (Solberg *et al.*, 1976) and in monocytes (Leijh *et al.*, 1979). Another exogenous influence invoked has been that due to antibiotics. Even with concentrations at only a fraction of the mean inhibitory concentration (MIC) for the antibiotic intraleukocytic killing was enhanced (Root *et al.*, 1981).

D. Influence of Granule Components

The milieu of phagolysosomes will be heavily influenced by the composition of the lysosomes with which they fuse (see Sections VII and VIII, which deal with association of O_2-independent systems with, respectively, granules and degranulation). Attention should be directed to the concept that substances may interact to provide an enhanced antimicrobial environment. For example, two enzymes may interact. Thorne *et al.* (1976) have shown that the granule proteases may enhance each other or lysozyme. Weiss has shown that a phospholiphase A may enhance antimicrobial action of an antibacterial fraction of rabbit PMNs (Weiss and Elsbach, 1977; Weiss *et al.*, 1979). Other evidence indicates that proteolytic enzyme and lysozyme may be synergistic (Becker and Hartsell, 1954, 1955; Berlin and Neujahr, 1968). Ginsburg's group has suggested that enzyme cocktails may have superior activity compared with single enzyme (Ginsburg *et al.*, 1973; Ne'eman *et al.*, 1976). Since the specific and azurophil granules contribute a rich mixture of enzymes including several glyosidases (Rest *et al.*, 1978b) the effects in phagolysosomes may be exalted well beyond those effects that have been achieved *in vitro*.

E. Species Differences

Phagolysosomal environments probably differ between species. There are substantial differences between the azurophil granules, specific granules, and other granules in man as well as in cow (Gennaro *et al.*, 1983), rabbit (Britz and Lowther, 1981), rat (Calamai and Spitznagel, 1982), chicken (Brune and Spitznagel, 1973; Hindenburg *et al.*, 1974), and various other animals (Rausch and Moore, 1975). Each system is so complex that it is difficult to find microbial probes that will permit appropriate comparative studies of intraleukocytic killing between different species. It is hoped that microbial genetics will prove helpful in developing target bacteria suitable for such work.

F. Role in Antimicrobial Action

Is the phagolysosome absolutely necessary for antimicrobial action of PMNs? Densen and Mandell (1978) have presented evidence that at least with the gonococcus the phagolysosome is necessary. In fact, the only paper I have been able to find that asserts otherwise is one by Okamura *et al.* (1979), in which cytochalasin B-treated PMNs killed *E. coli*, although they were unable to ingest them. Whether killing was due to O_2-dependent or O_2-independent mechanisms was not ascertained. If the attempted phagocytosis that characterizes interaction between very large organisms and PMNs provides a contact equivalent to that of a phagolysosome (Diamond and Krzeskcki, 1978), degranulation will occur between the attached PMNs and the microbial surface. In that case indeed there are probably no instances where killing occurs without a phagolysosome.

G. Abnormalities in Disease

Do genetic defects in phagolysosome formation occur? This is not clear. However, it is likely that in Chediak–Higashi syndrome and in actin disorders there are abnormalities involving phagolysosomes. Moreover, the work of Segal

et al. (1981) (Section IX.A) suggests that pH control may be abnormal in phagolysosomes of patients with chronic granulomatous disease. In any of these situations the phagolysosomal defect or defects are most likely secondary and not
primary.

H. Summary

The phagolysosome may be seen as the crucible in which the final events of
microbial killing take place and microbial degradation begins. Crucial elements
of the phagolysosome are the membrane surrounding it, the antimicrobial and
hydrolytic enzymic proteins degranulating into it, the pH control, ionic composition, and exclusion or neutralization of inhibitory substances. It is also likely
that the serum antibodies and the complement cascade encountered by bacteria
before phagocytosis enhance the antimicrobial action in the phagolysosome. One
of the research challenges of the coming years is to elucidate the complex actions of this organelle.

X. EVIDENCE OF A ROLE FOR O_2-INDEPENDENT MEDIATORS IN INTRALEUKOCYTIC KILLING DUE TO PMNs

It has been relatively easy to demonstrate *in vitro* that the granule proteins
of PMNs have antimicrobial activity and that molecular oxygen is unnecessary.
It has been more difficult to demonstrate *in vivo* the reality of their participation in intraleukocytic killing. This is primarily because it is difficult to create
rigorously anaerobic environments and to conduct in them experiments with
complete phagocytic systems. Such experiments are on record—some of them
even approach the ideal of stringent anaerobiasis. These studies testify that
anaerobic PMNs phagocytize and kill various bacteria. Curiously, some of the
earliest experiments of this kind were designed to show that exclusion of O_2
diminished the antimicrobial capacities of PMNs. Exclusion of O_2 did diminish
these capacities to some extent, but to a surprising degree they also demonstrated the capacity of PMNs even in nitrogen atmospheres to kill several species
of bacteria (McRipley and Sbarra, 1967*a,b;* Selvaraj and Sharra, 1966; Klebanoff
and Hamon, 1972). In these experiments the investigators may have assumed
that residual killing could be attributed to residual oxygen however no controls
for this possibility were included.

A. Antimicrobial Action in Chronic Granulomatous Disease

Other evidence that has favored a role for O_2-independent mechanisms in the
mediation of antimicrobial action has been reported for the antimicrobial defect
in chronic granulomatous disease. Chronic granulomatous disease of childhood
has, since its elucidation (Holmes *et al.,* 1968), served as a paradigm for demon-

strating the importance of O_2 for antimicrobial systems of PMNs. Yet, examination of most reports of this disease show that PMNs of patients with CGD have usually retained a measurable capacity to kill bacteria (Holmes *et al.*, 1968; Repine *et al.*, 1977, 1981a,b). The organisms most often tested have been *Staph. aureus* or *Serratia marcescens*, catalase producers that are notoriously frequent pathogens in CGD. Because they have catalase they are considered to release no H_2O_2 and to in fact be able to eliminate H_2O_2 in their vicinity. *S. viridans* is frequently used to challenge CGD PMN as well. These PMNs kill them readily. Catalase-negative streptococci produce H_2O_2 and may commit suicide in CGD PMNs because such PMNs have normal amounts of MPO (Kaplan, 1968). Delworth and Mandel (1977) studied four adult CGD patients. The data showed that these patients' PMNs killed appreciable numbers of *S. aureus* under aerobic conditions, but neither normal nor CGD cells killed *S. aureus* to any extent under anaerobic conditions. This seems to suggest that the CGD cells retained enough O_2-reducing capacity to mediate decreased but measurable killing under aerobic conditions. It remains to be seen whether some unsuspected factor contributed to killing under aerobic conditions or interfered with killing under anaerobic conditions. Since no assay of O_2-independent granule components was made, it could be postulated that O_2-independent components were actually lacking. There is no evidence for this speculation, but there is also not very much that opposes it.

Other experiments with the PMNs of CGD patients have contributed to the concept of O_2-independent killing mechanisms. Rest *et al.* (1982) have shown that *N. gonorrhoeae* are killed as efficiently in CGD PMNs as they are in PMNs of normal persons. Rest did not include experiments with anaerobic cells in his work. Thus his experiment is different from that of Delworth and Mandell.

Recently published work suggests with even more dramatic experimental data that CGD leukocytes are actively antimicrobial and that this activity is perhaps 70% diminished compared with control PMNs (Segal *et al.*, 1981). This work also presents evidence that the pH in phagolysosomes of PMNs from CGD patients falls rapidly and directly to pH 6.0. Normal PMNs show a rise initially and then a fall, but the vacuolar pH never drops much below 7.0. These findings, if verified, will support the concept that O_2-independent mechanisms function and will suggest that they function to better advantage if the pH of the phagolysosome is in the optimum range for antibacterial activity due to the phagolysosomal contents. In other words, the efficiency of the O_2-independent mechanisms would, according to this concept, appear to depend on pH control mediated by cytochrome c_{-245} and molecular oxygen.

B. O_2-Independent Mechanisms in PMNs of Birds

Still other material suggesting the existence of O_2-independent mechanisms exists in the literature. For example, chicken PMNs are devoid of MPO (Brune and Spitznagel, 1973), yet they have various cationic proteins (Brune and Spitznagel, 1973) and two rather than one molecularly distinct lysozyme (Hindenburg *et al.*, 1974). Chicken PMNs have active antimicrobial capacity (Brune *et al.*, 1972). Curiously, they failed to produce extracellularly detectable reduction products of O_2 during phagocytosis (Pennial and Spitznagel, 1975). The inference could be drawn that for antimicrobial action, chicken PMNs rely heavily on nonoxidative mechanisms.

C. Inhibitory Effects of Iron and Other Substances

Other experiments that favor O_2-independent mechanisms include studies with staphylococci loaded with iron salts (Repine *et al.*, 1981*b*) or with the substance dimethyl sulfoxide (DMSO) used as a scavenger for free hydroxyl ion (Repine *et al.*, 1981*a*). In experiments with iron, it was found that iron loading enhanced killing of *S. aureus* by H_2O_2. However, iron-loaded staphylococci were not more sensitive to killing by either normal or CGD PMNs. In experiments with DMSO, the drug reduced killing of *S. aureus* due to normal PMNs only slightly and had no effect on killing of *S. aureus* due to CGD PMNs. Unfortunately this kind of experiment is so complex that it cannot be adequately controlled, and the results are difficult to interpret.

D. Phagocytosis in Anaerobic Conditions

Somewhat more critical experiments have been reported by workers specifically interested in the putative O_2-independent antimicrobial mechanisms of human PMNs (Lehrer, 1972; Mandell, 1974; Bjornson *et al.*, 1980; Okamura and Spitznagel, 1982; Weiss *et al.*, 1982). The principal advantages in these experiments were the use of greater rigor not just in obtaining anaerobiosis, but in ensuring maintenance of anaerobiosis with appropriate controls. In addition, other techniques proved useful, such as monitoring the production of superoxide anion in a heavily challenged phagocytic system. In one set of experiments (Bjornson *et al.*, 1980), the phagocytic challenge bacteria were *Bacteroides*. These organisms themselves are so sensitive to oxygen toxicity that the continued viability of control suspensions of bacteria throughout the experiment served to monitor exclusion of O_2. In all these systems, anaerobic PMNs demonstrated antimicrobial capacity of anaerobic PMNs. For example, Mandell (1974) tested human PMNs against *S. epidermidis, Enterococcus, S. viridans, P. aeruginosa, Peptostreptococcus anaerobius, Bacteroides fragilis, C. perfringens*, and *Peptococcus magnus* and found that all were killed as well by PMNs under nitrogen as by PMNs under air. *Staphylococcus aureus* (two strains), *E. coli, S. marcescens, Klebsiella pneumoniae, P. vulgaris*, and *S. typhimurium* managed to survive to a greater extent in anaerobic PMNs than they did in aerobic PMNs.

Nevertheless, even these organisms were killed, although in lesser numbers. Mandell pointed out that the latter organisms were implicated in infections among nearly 72% of Baehner's series of CGD patients (quoted by Mandell, 1974). *Staphylococcus aureus* was the most resistant organism to anaerobic killing in Mandell's experiments. It has also resisted most granule proteins except the chymotryptic-like cationic protein (Odeberg and Ollson, 1976). It would have been more useful if the characteristics, e.g., roughness and smoothness of the gram-negative strains, had been stated. In experiments with rabbit PMNs Weiss *et al.* (1982) found no difference in aerobic and anaerobic killing of *S. epidermidis* and *S. typhimurium* MR10 (rough strain). They also compared ingestion and killing of smooth *S. typhimurium* under aerobic conditions with PMNs of normal and CGD patients. The CGD patients' PMNs had the capacity to kill *Salmonella*.

These experiments were all mutually confirmatory. They did not, however, give any specific indication concerning the source of antibacterial action in PMNs. Okamura and Spitznagel (1982) took advantage of Rest's demonstration (Rest *et al.*, 1977, 1978) that antimicrobial cationic proteins from azurophil granules kill *S. typhimurium* LT2 and that outer membrane mutants of LT-2 show ordered resistance to these antimicrobial preparations in proportion to the length (completeness) of the polysaccharide chains of their outer membrane lipopolysaccharides. Okamura compared the *in vitro* resistance of these mutants to the granule proteins of human PMNs with the resistance of these mutants to antimicrobial action due to anaerobic PMNs. The results showed that the resistance of these strains to anaerobic PMNs was ordered in the same way as killing due to granule proteins. Aerobic killing was similarly ordered. Phagocytosis by anaerobic and aerobic PMNs was similar. It therefore appeared highly likely that the antimicrobial proteins of the granules were responsible for the intraleukocytic killing. The results were especially interesting in light of the results of others (Kossack *et al.*, 1981), which showed that killing of *S. typhimurium* by PMNs appeared independent of the degree to which they stimulate oxidative metabolism in PMNs under aerobic conditions. Okamura's findings along with those of Weiss *et al.* (1982) and Kossack *et al.* (1981) suggest that O_2-independent mechanisms may be mainly responsible for the killing of *Salmonella* in human and rabbit PMNs. Finally, it should be mentioned that O_2-independent mechanisms of granulocytes evidently can kill *Candida albicans* (Lehrer *et al.*, 1975, 1980). Thus the action of O_2-independent antimicrobial mechanisms is not confined to bacteria.

E. Summary

In summary, convincing evidence exists that PMNs can kill a variety of microbes in atmospheres nearly devoid of oxygen. Moreover, PMNs of patients with CGD, although incapable of reducing molecular oxygen, are nonetheless able to kill *Salmonella, Neisseria,* staphylococci, and other organisms. The available data suggest that this killing in both kinds of experiment is due to O_2-independent mechanisms. In experiments with a series of *Salmonella* outer membrane mutants, evidence suggests that the granule proteins are responsible.

XI. COOPERATION BETWEEN O_2-INDEPENDENT AND O_2-DEPENDENT ANTIMICROBIAL SYSTEMS

Cooperation of this kind has not been extensively documented. There are some experiments that support the possibility. For example, it has been shown that killing and lysis of gram-negative bacteria may be synergistic in mixtures of hydrogen peroxide, ascorbic acid, and lysozyme (Miller and Watson, 1969). Since all these components might be present in PMN phagolysosome, they might contribute to antibacterial action there. Another demonstration, in this instance of synergisms between PMN elastase or chymotryptic-like cationic proteins and myeloperoxidase, has been described (Odeberg and Olsson, 1976). Again all the necessary components presumably will be present in the human PMN phagolysosome, so that the components of the system will definitely be present. Whether they will in fact function in this fashion in the PMN remains to be tested. Ambruso and Johnston (1981) have recently described a system in which they show that iron bound to lactoferrin was 5000 times more effective than free iron in enhancing formation of the cytoxic free hydroxy radical from superoxide anion and H_2O_2. This is an especially exciting revelation, since it suggests a regulatory role of lactoferrin in PMN production of free hydroxy radical.

XII. ONTOGENY OF THE O_2-INDEPENDENT ANTIMICROBIAL SYSTEMS

The development of this system is closely related to the development of the PMN in the bone marrow. The elegant work of Bainton *et al.* (1971) has shown how, in the bone marrow, the myeloblast transits to become a promyelocyte with the initiation of two events: synthesis of myeloperoxidase in the Golgi apparatus and formation of azurophil granules containing the myeloperoxidase on the concave inner face of the Golgi apparatus. The differentiation of promyelocytes to myelocytes is signaled by the formation of specific granules on the convex outer face of the Golgi apparatus. The ultrastructure of these early granulocytes continues to change as the PMNs continue to mature. Formation of azurophil granules stops. The nucleus condenses and assumes its characteristic polylobar morphology. Ribosomes, rough endoplasmic reticulum, mitochondria, and Golgi complex all are reduced in number, size, or both. Characteristic morphology has been described with light microscopy for all these stages (reviewed in Klebanoff and Clark, 1978).

The history of the appearances of cathepsin G (chymotrypsin-like cationic antimicrobial protein), elastase, lysozyme, and lactoferrin (see O_2-independent mechanisms, discussed in Sections II–VII) and MPO, a component of the O_2-dependent antimicrobial system, was traced in relationship to the events described by Bainton. With immunofluorescence histocytochemistry, Pryzwansky et al. (1979a) showed that cathepsin G, elastase, and MPO were all synthesized in promyelocytes and placed in the azurophil granules. In contrast, lactoferrin only began to be synthesized in myelocytes. Lysozyme was synthesized in both promyelocytes and myelocytes. It appeared in both azurophil and specific granules. Further confirmation of the above analysis of the development of PMN granules was reported by Rausch et al. (1978), who demonstrated the origin and composition of the giant granules of PMNs from children with Chediak–Higashi disease.

From the stage of the promyelocyte, granules in PMNs of children with Chediak–Higashi syndrome fuse. Azurophils fuse first with azurophils. The specifics fuse with specifics and then azurophils fuse with specifics. Premature granule fusion in the absence of phagocytosis and phagosome formation is the central fault. The biochemical basis for this fault remains to be ascertained.

In summary, the development of the proteins of the O_2-independent antimicrobial systems appears to coincide with the differentiation of azurophil and specific granules of PMNs in the marrow. This process requires about 7.5 days (Bainton et al., 1971). Studies to date do not identify the developmental pattern of accessory systems such as actin fibers, microtubules, and surface receptors. These are beyond the scope of this chapter. However, it is clear that without suitable differentiation of the entire cell, the antimicrobial systems cannot be efficiently delivered.

XIII. GENETIC DEFECTS RELEVANT TO O_2-INDEPENDENT ANTIMICROBIAL MECHANISMS

A. Specific Granule and Lactoferrin

Genetically determined or acquired deficiencies of one or more of these putative antimicrobial mechansims would provide opportunities to evaluate their role in antimicrobial phagocytosis. The only deficiency documented to date has been total absence of lactoferrin. This has been reported in only two patients (Spitznagel et al., 1972; Breton-Gorius et al., 1980). Both patients were also deficient in specific granules and had a partial lysozymal deficiency (Spitznagel et al., 1972) or vitamin B_{12}-binding protein deficiency. The latter deficiency was reported by Gallin et al. (1982), who studied in further detail the patient originally reported by Breton-Gorius (Breton-Gorius *et al.*, 1980). Other patients with specific granule deficiency has been reported, but those reports lacked measurements of lactoferrin (Straus *et al.*, 1974; Komiyama *et al.*, 1979; Parmley *et al.*, 1975). All these patients suffered recurrent infections. From their lesions were isolated *S. aureus, P. rettgeri, P. aeruginosa,* and *C. albicans.*

Owing to the additional complexities introduced by total specific granule deficiency, caution is appropriate in interpreting the problems in these patients. Gallin *et al.* (1982) made it clear that multiple functional abnormalities may be demonstrated, including decrease in PMN and monocyte accumulation in rebuck windows and premature disaggregation of PMNs after aggregation induced with fMet-Leu-Phe. Chemotaxis was decreased, as were binding of fMet-Leu-Phe and responses to fMet-Leu-Phe. Bactericidal activity, stimulated superoxide production, chemiluminescence, nitro-blue tetrazolium (NBT) reduction, and elicited changes in PMN membrane potential were all said to be abnormal. Thus specific granules were missing, and their absence was probably important. However, precisely which defects were attributable to lactoferrin deficiency and which attributable to other specific granule constituents could not be ascertained. Functions such as chemotaxis, hexosemonophosphate shunt activity, NBT reduction, and O_2 uptake were all normal in the PMNs of the patient reported by Spitznagel *et al.* (1972). Intraleukocytic killing of various opportunistic pathogens was depressed, however, compared with killing due to normal controls. Critical data concerning all the patients are summarized in Table II. In these cases lactoferrin and specific granule deficiency probably represent a defect in differentiation that occurs between the promyelocyte and myelocyte stages of PMN maturation in the marrow (Bainton *et al.*, 1971, Pryzwanski *et al.*, 1979a). This raises a number of questions concerning the molecular biology of the control of lactoferrin synthesis and specific granule formation that we cannot answer. Nevertheless, these issues may be open to investigation in the near future. Except for these patients, no documented cases of deficiency in other O_2-independent components are currently available.

As monoclonal or other immunospecific antibodies that recognize BPI, 57-kd, and 37-kd cationic antimicrobial proteins become available, they should be used to screen persons with histories of recurrent infections with *Proteus* sp., *Pseudomonas* sp., *Staphylococcus* sp., *Candida* sp., or other opportunistic pathogens. Immunocytochemical studies, enzyme-linked immunosorbent assay (ELISA), or both should be included in diagnostic studies on such patients in order to assess the status of their PMNs with respect to those proteins and with respect to lactoferrin. These appear to be the least cumbersome methods applicable to the problem. Transmission electron microscopy and sucrose-density centrifugal analysis of PMN subcellular organelles are expensive. Furthermore, these methods consume much time and blood. A high level of suspicion for such abnormalities should be raised in patients with recurrent infections and abnormalities in the antimicrobial capacities of their peripheral PMNs. Nuclear abnormalities in the PMNs along with apparent absence or reduction of neutrophil granules should quickly raise the question of specific granule deficiency, lactoferrin deficiency, or both.

B. Lysozyme Deficiency

Rabbits provide an example of lysozyme deficiency in animals normally having lysozyme in their PMN granules (Prieur et al., 1974). These isolated deficiencies appear not to have influenced the health of the rabbits adversely. Many animal species lack lysozyme in their PMNs without any apparent adverse effects on their health or leukocyte functions (Padgett and Hirsch, 1967; Rausch et al., 1974; Rausch and Moore, 1975). Evidence has recently been adduced that cattle that lack lysozyme (Padgett and Hirsch, 1967) carry a unique granule with antimicrobial proteins in their matrices (Gennaro et al., 1983). It is conceivable that this represents a compensatory mechanism. In the reverse sense, the presence of two catalytically and molecularly distinct lysozyme in chicken PMNs may somehow compensate for their complete lack of MPO (Brune and Spitznagel, 1973; Hindenburg et al., 1974).

C. Experimental Specific Granule Deficiency

An experimental model of specific granule deficiency that depends on the deprivation of normal PMNs of their specific granules and lactoferrin with phorbol myristate acetate has been examined (Wang-Iverson et al., 1978). The results showed that when specific granules had been removed, a measurable decrease in the intraleukocytic killing capacity of these cells was regularly observed. This defect did not appear attributable to impaired phagocytosis, to impaired hexose monophosphate shunt activity, or to diminished numbers of azurophil granules or depletion of MPO. As with genetically determined or acquired granule deficiency, the molecular basis for defective intraleukocytic killing could not be established.

Finally, it should be relatively easy to evaluate elastase and cathepsin G content of human PMNs. This should be possible either with enzymic analysis with highly specific substrates now available or with the use of immunocytochemical or enzyme-linked immunoassays. Only if this is done will we gain further insights into the realities of antimicrobial functions putatively due to these substances.

In summary, only lactoferrin deficiency in humans has been identified and studied. It has been detected only in patients with recurrent infections and has been complicated in each case by concomitant specific granule deficiency. Lysozyme deficiency has been observed in animals as a genetic defect. It also occurs naturally in many animal species. No compromise in host resistance has as yet been associated with either normal or mutational lysozyme deficiency. No documented deficiencies have been reported for BPI, 57-kd cationic antimicrobial protein, 37-kd cationic antimicrobial protein, elastase, or cathepsin G. Means for clinical identifications of abnormalities in these substances have been suggested.

XIV. SUMMARY

Increasingly abundant evidence supports the hypothesis that PMNs and perhaps alveolar macrophages have antimicrobial mechanisms independent of the presences of molecular oxygen for effective action against an array of bacteria and against some fungi. Eosinophils have mechanisms toxic for schistosomula and *Trichinella* larvae. In all instances the antimicrobial substances isolated have been cationic proteins and, in PMNs, associated with the azurophil cytoplasmic granules of the PMNs. Several of these substances have thus far demonstrated no enzymic function. Two of these substances are serine proteases but in one, chymotrypsin-like protein, the antimicrobial action depends on the cationic properties of the protein and is independent of the proteolytic action of the substance. In most instances, these proteins are cationic due to relatively large proportions of arginine. In two instances, a large proportion of lysine is present. All have high proportions (about 50%) of hydrophobic amino acid. Such proteins occur in the PMNs of man, rabbit, guinea pig, rat, cow, and chicken. The present view is that they are most active against gram-negative bacteria. At least two of them— 37-kd and 57-kd proteins (Shafer and Spitznagel, 1983)—act on *S. typhimurium* in a manner analogous to that of polymyxin B through binding to lipid A. Currently available results shows that anaerobic PMNs have substantial antimicrobial capacity. Whether this capacity is due to the O_2-independent mechanisms discussed in this chapter remains to be established with greater certainty.

XV. REFERENCES

Abramson, J. S., Mills, E. L., Giebink, G. S., and Quie, P., 1982*a*, Depression of monocyte and polymorphonuclear leukocyte oxidative metabolism and bactericidal capacity by influenza a virus, *Infect. Immun.* **35**:350.

Abramson, J. S., Lewis, J. C., Lyles, D. S., Heller, K. A., Mills, E. L., and Bass, D. A., 1982*b*, Inhibition of neutrophil lysosome–phagosome fusion associated with influenza virus infection *in vitro*, *J. Clin. Invest.* **June**:1393.

Alobaidi, T., Naccache, P. H., and Sha'afi, R. I., 1981, Calmodulin antagonists modulate rabbit neutrophil degranulation, aggregation and stimulated oxygen consumption, *Biochim. Biophys. Acta* **17**:675:316.

Amano, T., Inai, S., Seki, Y., Kashiba, S., Fujikawa, K., and Nishimura, S., 1954, Studies on the immune bacteriolysis. I. Accelerating effect on the immune bacteriolysis by lysozyme-like substance of leucocytes and egg-white lysozyme, *Med. J. Osaka Univ.* **4**:401.

Amano, F., Hashida, R., and Mizuno, D., 1981, Differences in the rates and extents of fusion between lysosomes and phagocytic vesicles containing different particles, *J. Biochem.* **89**:1847.

Ambruso, D. R., and Johnston, R. B., 1981, Lactoferrin enhances hydroxyl radical production by human neutrophils, neutrophil particulate fractions, and an enzymatic generating system, *J. Clin. Invest.* **67**:352.

Amrein, P. C., and Stossel, T. P., 1980, Prevention of degradation of human polymorphonuclear leukocyte proteins by disopropylfluorophosphate, *Blood* **56**:442.

Andersen, A. J., and Irwin, C., 1973, Some properties of neutral-acting proteases and actin degradative enzymes in rat leucocytes, *Life Sci.* **13**:601.

Archer, G. T., and Hirsch, J. G., 1963, Isolation of granules from eosinophil leukocytes and study of their enzyme contents, *J. Exp. Med.* **118**:277.

Arnold, R. R., Cole, M. F., and McGhee, J. R., 1977, A bactericidal effect for human lactoferrin, *Science* **197**:263.

Arnold, R. R., Brewer, M., and Gauthier, J. J., 1980, Bactericidal activity of human lactoferrin: Sensitivity of a variety of microorganisms, *Infect. Immun.* **28**:893.

Arnold, R. R., Russell, J. E., Champion, W. J., and Gauthier, J. J., 1981, Bactericidal activity of human lactoferrin: Influence of physical conditions and metabolic state of the target microorganism, *Infect. Immun.* **32**:655.

Arnold, R. R., Russell, J. E., Champion, W. J., Brewer, M., and Gauthier, J. J., 1982, Bactericidal activity of human lactoferrin. Differentiation from the stasis of iron deprivation, *Infect. Immun.* **35**:792.

Avery, O. T., and Cullen, G. E., 1919, Hydrogen ion concentration of cultures of pneumococci of the different types of carbohydrate media, *J. Exp. Med.* **30**:359.

Baggiolini, M., Hirsch, J. G., and de Duve, C., 1969, Resolution of granules from rabbit heterophil leukocytes into distinct populations by zonal sedimentation, *J. Cell. Biol.* **40**:529.

Baggiolini, M., de Duve, C., Masson, P. L., and Heremans, J. K., 1970, Association of lactoferrin with specific granules in rabbit heterophil leukocytes, *J. Exp. Med.* **131**:559.

Baggiolini, M., Amherdt, M., and Orci, L., 1976, Unusual membrane fracture faces in polymorphonuclear leukocyte granules, *Experientia* **32**:1400.

Bainton, D. F., 1973, Sequential degranulation of the two types of polymorphonuclear leukocyte granules during phagocytosis of microorganisms, *J. Cell. Biol.* **58**:249.

Bainton, D. F., Ullyot, J. L., and Farquhar, M. G., 1971, The development of neutrophilic, polymorphonuclear leucocytes in human bone marrow. Origin and content of azurophil and specific granules. *J. Exp. Med.* **134**:907.

Becker, M. E., and Hartsell, S. E., 1954, Factors affecting bacteriolysis using lysozyme in dual enzyme systems, *Arch. Biochem.* **53**:402.

Becker, M. E., and Hartsell, S. E., 1955, The synergistic action of lysozyme and trypsin in bacteriolysis, *Arch. Biochem.* **55**:257.

Beckerdite, S., Mooney, C., Weiss, J., Franson, R., and Elsbach, P., 1974, Early and discrete changes in permeability of *Escherichia coli* and certain other gram-negative bacteria during killing by granulocytes, *J. Exp. Med.* **140**:396.

Berlin, I., and Neujahr, H. Y., 1968, Studies of controlled lysis of washed cell suspensions of *Lactobacillus fermenti* and preparation of membrane-like fragments by a combined trypsin lysozyme treatment, *Acta Chem. Scand.* [B] **22**:2972.

Bishop, J. G., Schanbacher, F. L., Ferguson, L. C., and Smith, K. L., 1976, *In vitro* growth inhibition of mastitis-causing coliform bacteria by bovine apo-lactoferrin and reversal of inhibition by citrate and high concentrations of apo-lactoferrin, *Infect. Immun.* **14**:911.

Bjornson, A. B., Bjornson, H. S., and Kilko, B. P., 1980, Specificity of immunoglobulin in antibodies in normal human serum that participate in opsonophagocytosis and intracellular killing of *Bacteroides fragilis* and *Bacteroides thetaiotamicron* by human polymorphonuclear leukocytes, *Infect. Immun.* **30**:263.

Blondin, J., and Janoff, A., 1976, The role of lysosomal elastase in the digestion of *Escherichia coli* proteins by human polymorphonuclear leukocytes, *J. Clin. Invest.* **58**:971.

Bloom, W. L., and Blake, F. G., 1948, Studies on an anti-bacterial polypeptide extracted from normal tissues, *J. Infect. Dis.* **83**:116.

Bloom, W. L., Winters, M. G., and Watson, D. W., 1951, The inhibition of two anti-bacterial basic proteins by nucleic acids, *J. Bacteriol.* **62**:7.

Bluard-Deconinck, J., Masson, P. L., Osinski, P. A., and Heremanns, J. F., 1974, Amino acid sequence of cystic peptides of lactoferrin and demonstration of similarities between lactoferrin and transferrin, *Biochim. Biophys. Acta* **365**:311.

Boxer, L. A., Hedley-Whyte, E. T., and Stossel, T. P., 1974, Neutrophil actin dysfunction and abnormal neutrophil behavior, *N. Engl. J. Med.* **291**:1093.

Breton-Gorius, J., Mason, D. Y., Buriot, D., Vilde, J. L., and Griscelli, C., 1980, Lactoferrin deficiency as a consequence of a lack of specific granules in neutrophils from a patient with recurrent infections. Detection by immunoperoxidase staining for lactoferrin and cytochemical electron microscopy, *Am. J. Pathol.* **99**:413.

Bretz, U., and Baggiolini, M., 1974, Biochemical and morphological characterization of azurophil and specific granules of human neutrophilic polymorphonuclear leukocytes, *J. Cell. Biol.* **63**:251.

Britz, M. L., and Lowther, D. A., 1981, Some properties of neutral proteinases from lysosomes of rabbit polymorphonuclear leucocytes, *Aust. J. Exp. Biol. Med. Sci.* **59**:63.

Brown, W. J., Shannon, W. A., and Snell, W. J., 1983, Specific and azurophilic granules from rabbit polymorphonuclear leukocytes. II. Cell surface localization of granule membrane and content proteins before and after degranulation, *J. Cell. Biol.* **96**:1040.

Brumfitt, W., and Glynn, A. A., 1961, Intracellular killing of *Micrococcus lysodeikticus* by macrophages and polymorphonuclear leucocytes: A comparative study, *Br. J. Exp. Pathol.* **42**:408.

Brumfitt, W., Wardlaw, A. C., and Park, J. T., 1958, Development of lysozyme-resistance in *Micrococcus lysodiekticus* and its association with an increased O-acetyl content of the cell wall, *Nature* **181**:1783.

Brune, K., and Spitznagel, J. K., 1973, Peroxidaseless chicken leukocytes. Isolation and characterization of anti-bacterial granules, *J. Infect. Dis.* **127**:84.

Brune, K., Leffell, M. S., and Spitznagel, J. K., 1972, Microbicidal activity of peroxidaseless chicken heterophile leukocytes, *Infect. Immun.* **5**:283.

Bryan, C. S., 1974, Sensitization of *E. coli* to the serum bactericidal system and to lysozyme by ethleneglycoltetraacetic acid, *Proc. Soc. Exp. Biol. Med.* **145**:1431.

Buchner, H., 1894, Neuere Fortschritte in der Immunitatsfrage, *MMW* **41**:497.

Buck, P., and Rest, R. F., 1981, Effects of human neutrophil granule extracts on macromolecular synthesis in *Neisseria gonorrhoeae*, *Infect. Immun.* **33**:426.

Bullen, J. J., 1975, Iron-binding proteins in milk and resistance to *Escherichia coli* infection in infants, *Postgrad. Med. J.* **51**:67.

Bullen, J. J., and Wallis, S. N., 1977, Reversal of the bactericidal effect of polymorphs by a ferritin–antibody complex, *FEMS Lett.* **1**:117.

Bullen, J. J., Rogers, H. J., and Leigh, L., 1972, Iron-binding proteins in milk and resistance to *Escherichia coli* infection in infants, *Br. Med. J.* **1**:69.

Bullen, J. J., Rogers, H. J., and Griffiths, E., 1978, Role of iron in bacterial infection, *Curr. Top. Microbiol. Immunol.* **80**:1.

Burger, W. C., and Stahmann, M. A., 1952, The agglutination and inhibition of growth of bacteria by lysine polypeptides, *Arch. Biochem.* **39**:27.

Butterworth, A. E., Wassom, D. L., Gleich, G. J., Loegering, D. A., and David, J. R., 1979, Damage to schistosomula of *Schistosoma mansoni* induced directly by eosinophil major basic protein, *J. Immunol.* **122**:221.

Calamai, E. G., and Spitznagel, J. K., 1982, Characterization of rat polymorphonuclear leukocyte subcellular granules, *Lab. Invest.* **46**:597.

Canfield, R. E., 1963, The amino acid sequence of egg white lysozyme, *J. Biol. Chem.* **238**:2698.

Chipman, D. M., and Sharon, N., 1969, Mechanism of lysozyme action. Lysozyme is the first enzyme for which the relation between structure and function has become clear, *Science* **165**:454.

Cohn, Z. A., and Hirsch, J. G., 1960a, The isolation and properties of the specific cytoplasmic granules of rabbit polymorphonuclear leucocytes, *J. Exp. Med.* **112**:983.

Cohn, Z. A., and Hirsch, J. G., 1960b, The influence of phagocytosis on the intracellular distribution of granule-associated components of polymorphonuclear leucocytes, *J. Exp. Med.* **112**:1015.

Collins, M. S., and Pappagianis, D., 1974, Inhibition by lysozyme of growth of the spherule phase of *Coccidioides immitis in vitro*, *Infect. Immun.* **10**:616.

Costerton, J. W., Brown, M. R. W., and Sturgess, J. M., 1979, The cell envelope: Its role in infection, in: *Pseudomonas aeruginosa: Clinical Manifestations of Infection and Current Therapy* (R. G. Dogett, ed.), pp. 41–62, Academic Press, New York.

Crawford, J. J., 1971, Interaction of *Actinomyces* organisms with cationic polypeptides, I. Histochemical studies of infected human and animal tissues, *Infect. Immun.* **4**:632.

Cromartie, W. J., Craddock, J. H., Schwab, H. J., Anderle, S. K., and Yang, C., 1977, Arthritis in rats after systemic injection of streptococcal cells or cell walls, *J. Exp. Med.* **146**:1585.

Daly, J. A., Lee, T. J., Spitznagel, J. K., and Sparling, P. F., 1982, Gonococci with mutations to low-level penicillin resistance exhibit increased sensitivity to the oxygen-independent bactericidal activity of human polymorphonuclear leukocyte granule extracts, *Infect. Immun.* **35**:826.

Davies, P., Krakauer, K., and Weissmann, G., 1970, Subcellular distribution of neutral proteases and peptidases in rabbit polymorphonuclear leucocytes, *Nature* **228**:761.

Davis, S. D., Gemsa, D., and Wedgwood, R. J., 1966, Kinetics of the transformation of gram-negative rods to spheroplasts and ghosts by serum, *J. Immunol.* **96**:570.

Davis, S. D., Gemsa, D., Ianetta, A., and Wedgwood, R. J., 1968, Potentiation of serum bactericidal activity by lysozyme, *J. Immunol.* **101**:277.

Delworth, J. A., and Mandell, G. L., 1977, Adults with chronic granulomatous disease of childhood, *Am. J. Med.* **63**:233.

Densen, P., and Mandell, G. L., 1978, Gonococcal interactions with polymorphonuclear neutrophils: Importance of the phagosome for bactericidal activity, *J. Clin. Invest.* **62**:1161.

Denys, J., and Havet, J., 1894, Sur la part des leucocytes dans le pouvoir bactericide du sang de chien, *Cellule* **10**:7.

DeWald, B., Rindler-Ludwig, R., Bretz, U., and Baggiolini, M., 1975, Subcellular localization and heterogeneity of neutral proteases in neutrophilic polymorphonuclear leukocytes, *J. Exp. Med.* **141**:709.

Diamond, R. D., and Krzeskcki, R., 1978, Mechanisms of attachment of neutrophils to *Candida albicans* pseudohyphae in the absence of serum, and of subsequent damage to pseudophyphae by micorbicidal processes of neutrophils *in vitro*, *J. Clin. Invest.* **61**:360.

Drazin, R. E., and Lehrer, R. I., 1977, Fungicidal properties of a chymotrypsin-like cationic protein from human neutrophils: Adsorption to *Candida parapsilosis*, *Infect. Immun.* **17**:382.

Dubos, R. J., 1950, The effect of organic acids on mammalian tubercle bacilli, *J. Exp. Med.* **42**:319.

Dubos, R. J., 1953, Effect of ketone bodies and other metabolites on the survival and multiplication of staphylococci and tubercle bacilli, *J. Exp. Med.* **98**:145.

Ehrlich, P., and Lazarus, A., 1900, Histology of the blood. Reprinted from, *Histology of the Blood: Normal and Pathological,* Cambridge University Press, in: *The Collected Works of Paul E. Ehrlich,* Vol. I: *Histology, Biochemistry and Pathology* (F. Himmelweit, ed.), p. 215, Pergamon Press, London and New York, 1956.

Elsbach, P., Weiss, J., Franson, R. C., Beckerdite-Quagliata, S., Schneider, A., and Harris, L., 1979, Separation and purification of a potent bactericidal/permeability-increasing protein and a closely associated phospholipase A2 from rabbit polymorphonuclear leukocytes: Observations on their relationship, *J. Biol. Chem.* **254**:1100.

Fishman, M., and Silverman, M. S., 1957, Bactericidal activity of rat leucocytic extracts. I. Anti-bacterial spectrum and the subcellular localization of the bactericidal activity, *J. Exp. Med.* **105**:521.

Fishman, M., Cole, L. J., and Silverman, M. S., 1957, Bactericidal activity of rat leucocyte extracts. II. Characterization of the bactericidal substance in leucocyte mitochondrial extracts, *J. Exp. Med.* **105**:529.

Fleming, A., 1922, On a remarkable bacteriolytic element found in tissues and secretions, *Proc. R. Soc. Lond.* [*Biol.*] **93**:306.

Fleming, A., and Allison, V. D., 1922, Observations on a bacteriolytic substance ("lysozyme") found in secretions and tissues, *Br. J. Exp. Pathol.* **3**:252.

Frankel-Conrat, J., Chew, W. B., Pitlick, F., and Barber, S., 1966, Certain properties of leukocytic cathepsins in health and disease, *Cancer* **19**:1393.

Friedberg, D., and Shilo, M., 1970, Interaction of gram-negative bacteria with the lysosomal fraction of polymorphonuclear leukocytes, *Infect. Immun.* **1**:305.

Gadebusch, H. H., and Johnson, A. G., 1966, Natural host resistance to infection with Cryptococcus neoformans. IV. The effect of some cationic proteins on the experimental disease, *J. Infect. Dis.* **116**:551.

Galbraith, H., and Miller, T. B., 1973a, Effect of metal cations and PH on the anti-bacterial activity and uptake of long chain fatty acids, *J. Appl. Bacteriol.* **36**:635.

Galbraith, H., and Miller, T. B., 1973b, Effect of long chain fatty acids on bacterial respiration and amino acid uptake, *J. Appl. Bacteriol.* **36**:659.

Galbraith, H., and Miller, T. B., 1973c, Physicochemical effects of long chain fatty acids on bacterial cells and their protoplasts, *J. Appl. Bacteriol.* **36**:647.

Galbraith, H., Miller, T. B., Paton, A. M., and Thompson, J. K., 1971, Anti-bacterial activity of long chain fatty acids and the reversal with calcium, magnesium, ergocalciferol and cholesterol, *J. Appl. Bacteriol.* **34**:803.

Gallin, J. I., Fletcher, M. P., Seligmann, B. E., Hoffstein, S., Cehrs, K., and Mounessa, N., 1982, Human neutrophil-specific granule deficiency: A model to assess the role of neutrophil-specific granules in the evolution of the inflammatory response, *Blood* **59**:1317.

Gallis, H. A., Miller, S. E., and Wheat, R. W., 1976, Degradation of ^{14}C-labeled streptococcal cell walls by egg white lysozyme and lysosomal enzymes, *Infect. Immun.* **13**:1459.

Gemsa, D., Davis, S. D., and Wedgwood, R. J., 1966, Lysozyme and serum bactericidal action, *Nature* **210**:950.

Genarro, R., Romeo, D., DeWald, B., and Baggiolini, M., 1982, The bovine neutrophil: Separation and partial characterization of plasma membrane and cytoplasmic granules, in: *Biochemistry and Function of Phagocytes* (F. Rossi and P. Patriarca, eds.), pp. 277–281, Plenum Press, New York.

Gennaro, R., Dolzani, L., and Romeo, D., 1983, Potency of bactericidal proteins purified from the large granules of bovine neutrophils, *Infect. Immun.* 40:684.

Ghuysen, J., 1974, Substrate requirements of glycosidases for lytic activity on bacterial walls, in: *Lysozyme* (E. F. Osserman, R. E. Canfield, and S. Beychok, eds.), pp. 185–193, Academic Press, New York.

Ginsburg, I., Ne'eman, N., and Lahav, M., 1973, Effect of cationic and anionic polyelectrolytes and antibodies on the lysis of micrococci and streptococci by leukocyte lysates and lysozyme, *Isr. J. Med. Sci.* 9:663.

Gladstone, G. P., 1973, The effect of iron and haematin on the killing of staphylococci by rabbit polymorphonuclear leucocytes. With notes on the inhibition of iron of serum b-lysins and staphylocidal cationic proteins from polymorphonuclear leucocytes, in: *Contributions to Microbiology and Immunology*, Vol. 1: *Staphylococci and Staphylococcal Infections*, pp. 222–243, Karger, Basel.

Gladstone, G. P., and Walton, E., 1970, Effect of iron on the bactericidal proteins from rabbit polymorphonuclear leucocytes, *Nature* 227:849.

Gladstone, G. P., and Walton, E., 1971, The effect of iron and haematin on the killing of staphylococci by rabbit polymorphs, *Br. J. Exp. Pathol.* 52:452.

Gladstone, G. P., Walton, E., and Kay, U., 1974, The effect of cultural conditions on susceptibility of staphylococci to killing by the cationic proteins from rabbit polymorphonuclear leucocytes, *Br. J. Exp. Pathol.* 55:427.

Gleich, G. J., Loegering, D. A., and Maldonado, J. E., 1973, Identification of a major basic protein in guinea pig eosinophil granules, *J. Exp. Med.* 137:1459.

Gleich, G. J., Loegering, D. A., Kueppers, F., Bojoj, S. P., and Mann, K. G., 1974, Physicochemical and biological properties of the major basic protein from guinea pig eosinophil granules, *J. Exp. Med.* 140:313.

Gleich, G. J., Loegering, D. A., Mann, K. G., and Maldonado, J. E., 1976, Comparative properties of the Charcot-Leyden crystal protein and the major basic protein from human eosinophils, *J. Clin. Invest.* 57:633.

Glick, A. D., Ranhand, J. M., and Cole, R. M., 1972, Degradation of group A streptococcal cell walls by egg-white lysozyme and human lysosomal enzymes, *Infect. Immun.* 6:403.

Glynn, A. A., 1969, The complement lysozyme sequence in immune bacteriolysis, *Immunology* 16:463.

Glynn, A. A., and Milne, C. M., 1967, A kinetic study of the bacteriolytic and bactericidal action of human serum, *Immunology* 12:639.

Goldman, R., and Rottenberg, H., 1973, Ion distribution in lysosomal suspensions, *FEBS Lett.* 33:233.

Goldstein, I. M., Hoffstein, S. T., and Weissmann, G., 1975, Mechanisms of lysosomal enzyme release from human polymorphonuclear leucocytes, effect of phorbol myristate acetate, *J. Cell. Biol.* 66:647.

Goren, M. B., 1983, Some paradoxes of macrophage function in host defenses to intracellular pathogens, *Adv. Exp. Med. Biol.* 162:31.

Gutteridge, J. M. C., Paterson, S. K., Segal, A. W., and Halliwell, B., 1981, Inhibition of lipid peroxidation by the iron-binding protein lactoferrin, *Biochem. J.* 199:259.

Hallgren, R., and Venge, P., 1976, Cationic proteins of human granulocytes: Enhancement of phagocytosis of staphylococcus protein A–IgG complexes, *Inflammation* 3:237.

Hankin, E. H., 1891, A bacteria-killing globulin, *Proc. R. Soc. Lond.* [*Biol.*] 48:93.

Hayashi, H., Ariki, Y., and Ito, E., 1973, Occurrence of glucosamine residues with free amino groups in cell wall peptidoglycan from bacilli as a factor responsible for resistance to lysozyme, *J. Bacteriol.* 113:592.

Henson, P. M., and Oades, Z. G., 1975, Stimulation of human neutrophils by soluble and insoluble immunoglobulin aggregates. Secretion of granule constituents and increased oxidation of glucose, *J. Clin. Invest.* **56**:1053.

Heymann, H., Manniello, J. M., and Barkulis, S. S., 1964, Structure of streptococcal cell walls. III. Characterization of an alanine-containing glucosaminylmuramic acid derivative liberated by lysozyme from streptococcal glycopeptide, *J. Biol. Chem.* **239**:2981.

Hindenburg, A., Spitznagel, J. K., and Amrein, N., 1974, Isozymes of lysozyme in leukocytes and egg-white. Evidence for the species specific control of egg-white lysozyme synthesis, *Proc. Natl. Acad. Sci. (USA)* **71**:1653.

Hirsch, J. G., 1956a, Phagocytin: A bactericidal substance from polymorphonuclear leucocytes, *J. Exp. Med.* **103**:589.

Hirsch, J. G., 1956b, Studies of the bactericidal action of phagocytin, *J. Exp. Med.* **103**:613.

Hirsch, J. G., 1958, Bactericidal action of histone, *J. Exp. Med.* **108**:925.

Hirsch, J. G., 1960a, Anti-microbial factors in tissues and phagocytic cells, *Bacteriol. Rev.* **24**:133.

Hirsch, J. G., 1960b, Further studies on preparation and properties of phagocytin, *J. Exp. Med.* **111**:323.

Hirsch, J. G., and Cohn, Z. A., 1960, Degranulation of polymorphonuclear leucocytes following phagocytosis of microorganisms, *J. Exp. Med.* **112**:1005.

Hirsch, J. G., and Cohn, Z. A., 1964, Digestive and autolytic functions of lysosomes in phagocytic cells, *Fed. Proc.* **23**:1023.

Hodinka, R. L., and Modrzakowski, M. C., 1983, Bactericidal activity of granule contents from rat polymorphonuclear leukocytes, *American Society for Microbiology, Abstract Annual Meeting*, p. 91, p. 74.

Holmes, B., Page, A. R., Windhorst, D. B., Quie, P. G., White, J. G., and Good, R. A., 1968, The metabolic pattern and phagocytic function of leukocytes with children with chronic granulomatous disease, *Ann. NY Acad. Sci.* **155**:888.

Horwitz, M. A., and Silverstein, S. C., 1981, Interaction of the legionnaires' disease bacterium (*Legionella pneumophila*) with human phagocytes. I. *L. pneumophila* resists killing by polymorphonuclear leukocytes, antibody and complement, *J. Exp. Med.* **153**:386.

Inoue, K., Tanigawa, Y., Takubo, M., Satini, M., and Amano, T., 1959, Quantitative studies on immune bacteriolysis. II. The role of lysozyme in immune bacteriolysis, *Biken's J.* **2**:1.

Jacques, Y. V., and Bainton, D. F., 1978, Changes in pH within the phagocyte vacuoles of human neutrophils and monocytes, *Lab. Invest.* **39**:179.

Janoff, A., and Scherer, J., 1968, Mediators of inflammation in leukocyte lysosomes. IX. Elastinolytic activity in granules of human polymorphonuclear leukocytes, *J. Exp. Med.* **128**:1137.

Jensen, M. S., and Bainton, D. F., 1973, Temporal changes in pH within the phagocytic vacoule of the polymorphonuclear neutrophilic leukocyte, *J. Cell. Biol.* **56**:379.

Jolles, J., Jaurague-Adell, J., Bernier, I., and Jolles, P., 1963, La structure chimique du lysozyme de blanc d'oeuf de poule: Etude detaillée, *Biochem. Biophys. Acta* **78**:668.

Kakinuma, K., 1970, Metabolic control and intracellular pH during phagocytosis by polymorphonuclear leucocytes, *J. Biochem.* **68**:177.

Kamaya, T., 1970, Lytic action of lysozyme on *Candida albicans*, Mycopathologia (Den Haag), **42**:197.

Kamizuma, A., Morosanna, H., Hahaha, T., Niyagawa, Y., and Akabane, T., 1979, Abnormal neutrophil maturation in a neutrophil defect with morphologic abnormality and impaired function, *J. Pediatr.* **94**:19.

Kanthack, A. A., and Hardy, W. B., 1894, The morphology and distribution of wandering cells of mammaliae, *J. Physiol. (Lond.)* **17**:81.

Kaplan, E. L., Laxdal, T., and Quie, P. G., 1968, Studies of polymorphonuclear leukocytes from patients with chronic granulomatous disease of childhood: Bactericidal capacity for streptococci, *Pediatrics* **41**:591.

Karnovsky, M. L., 1962, Metabolic basis of phagocytic activity, *Physiol. Rev.* **42**:143.

Katchalski, E., Bichowski-Slomnitzki, L., and Volcani, B. E., 1953, The action of some water soluble poly-α-amino acids on bacteria, *Biochem. J.* **55**:671.

Kierszenbaum, F., Ackerman, S. J., and Gleich, G. J., 1981, Destruction of bloodstream forms of *Trypanosoma cruzi* by eosinophil granule major basic protein, *Am. J. Trop. Med. Hyg.* **30**:775.

Kirkpatrick, C. H., Green, I., Rich, R. R., and Schade, A. L., 1971, Inhibition of growth of *Candida albicans* by iron-unsaturated lactoferrin: Relation to host-defense mechanisms in chronic mucocutaneous candidiasis, *J. Infect. Dis.* **124**:539.

Klebanoff, S. J., 1975, Antimicrobial mechanisms in neutrophilic polymorphonuclear leukocytes, *Semin. Hematol.* **12**:117.

Klebanoff, S. J., and Clark, R. A., 1978, *The Neutrophil–Function and Clinical Disorders*, Elsevier–North-Holland, New York.

Klebanoff, S. J., and Hamon, C. B., 1972, Role of myeloperoxidase-mediated anti-microbial systems in intact leukocytes, *J. Reticuloendothel. Soc.* **12**:170.

Kling, C. A., 1910, Untersuchungen uber die bakterientotenden Eigenschatten der weisten Blutkorperchen, *Z. Immunitaetsforsch. Immunobiol.* **7**:1.

Kodicek, E., 1949, The effect of unsaturated fatty acids on gram-positive bacteria, *Symp. Soc. Exp. Biol.* **3**:217.

Koj, A., Chudzik, J., and Dubin, A., 1976, Substrate specificity and modification of the active center of elastase-like neutral proteinases from horse blood leukocytes, *Biochem. J.* **153**:397.

Komiyama, A., Morosama, H., Nahaha, T., Miyagawa, Y., and Akabane, T., 1979, Abnormal neutrophil maturation in a neutrophil defect with morphologic abnormality and impaired function, *J. Pediatr.* **94**:19.

Konisky, J., 1979, Specific transport systems and receptors for colicins and phages, in *Bacterial Outer Membranes, Isogeneic and Functions* (M. Inoue, ed.), pp. 336–337, Wiley, New York.

Kopitar, M., and Lebez, D., 1975, Intracellular distribution of neutral proteinases and inhibitors in pig leucocytes. Isolation of two inhibitors of neutral proteinases, *Eur. J. Biochem.* **56**:571.

Korschun, C. V., 1908, Sur l'action bactericide de l'extrait leucocytaire des lapins et des cobayes, *Ann. Inst. Pasteur* **22**:586.

Kossack, R. E., Guerrant, R. L., Densen, P., Schadelin, J., and Mandell, G. L., 1981, Diminished neutrophil oxidative metabolism after phagocytosis of virulent *Salmonella typhi*, *Infect. Immun.* 674.

Kossell, H., 1896, Uber die basichen stoffe des zellkerns, *Hoppe-Seylers Z. Physiol. Chem.* **22**:176.

Kreutzer, D. L., Dreyfus, L. A., and Robertson, D. C., 1979, Interaction of polymorpho-nuclear leukocytes with smooth and rough strains of *Brucella abortus*, *Infect. Immun.* **23**:737.

Lazarus, G. S., Brown, R. S., Daniels, J. R., and Fullmer, H. M., 1968a, Human granulocyte collagenase, *Science* **159**:1483.

Lazarus, G. S., Daniels, J. R., Brown, R. S., Bladen, H. A., and Fullmer, H. M., 1968b, Degradation of collagen by a human granulocyte collagenolytic system, *J. Clin. Invest.* **47**:2622.

Laffrell, M. S., and Spitznagel, J. K., 1972, Association of lactoferrin with lysozyme in granules of human polymorphonuclear leukocytes, *Infect. Immun.* **6**:761.

Laffrell, M. S., and, Spitznagel, J. K., 1974, Intracellular and extracellular degranulation of human polymorphonuclear azurophil and specific granules induced by immune complexes, *Infect. Immun.* **10**:1241.

Laffrell, M. S., and Spitznagel, J. K., 1975, Fate of human lactoferrin and myeloperoxidase in phagocytizing human neutrophils: Effects of immunoglobulin G subclasses and immune complexes coated on latex beads, *Infect. Immun.* **12**:813.

Lehrer, R. I., 1972, Functional aspects of a second mechanism of candidacidal activity by human neutrophils, *J. Clin. Invest.* **51**:2566.

Lehrer, R. I., and Cline, M. J., 1969, Interaction of *Candida albicans* with human leukocytes and serum, *J. Bacteriol.* **98**:996.

Lehrer, R. I., Ladra, K. M., and Hake, R. B., 1975, Nonoxidative fungicidal mechanisms of mammalian granulocytes: Demonstration of components with candidacidal activity in human, rabbit and guinea pig leukocytes, *Infect. Immun.* **11**:1226.

Lehrer, R. I., Ferrari, L. G., Patterson-Delafield, J., and Sorrell, T., 1980, Fungicidal activity of rabbit alveolar and peritoneal macrophages against *Candida albicans, Infect. Immun.* **28**:1001.

Leijh, P. C., Van den Barselaar, M. T., Van Zwet, T. L., Daha, M. R., and Van Furth, R., 1979, Requirement of extracellular complement and immunoglobulin for intracellular killing of micro-organisms by human monocytes, *J. Clin. Invest.* **63**:772.

Lord, F. T., and Nye, R. N., 1919, The relation of the *Pneumococcus* to hydrogen ion concentration, acid death-point, and dissolution of the organisms, *J. Exp. Med.* **30**:389.

MacRae, E. K., and Spitznagel, J. K., 1975, Ultrastructural localization of cationic proteins in cytoplasmic granules of chicken and rabbit polymorphonuclear leukocytes, *J. Cell. Sci.* **17**:79.

Mandell, G. L., 1970, Intraphagosomal pH of human polymorphonuclear neutrophils, *Proc. Soc. Exp. Biol. Med.* **134**:447.

Mandell, G. L., 1974, Bactericidal activity of aerobic and anaerobic polymorphonuclear neutrophils, *Infect. Immun.* **9**:337.

Manwaring, W. H., 1912, The nature of the bactericidal substance in leucocytic extract, *J. Exp. Med.* **16**:249.

Masson, P., 1970, *La lactoferrin: Proteine les Secretions Externes et des Leukocytes Neutrophiles*, Librairie Malôine, Paris.

Masson, P. L., and Heremans, J. F., 1966, Studies on lactoferrin, the iron-binding protein of secretions, *Protides Biol. Fluids* **14**:115.

McRipley, R. J., and Sbarra, A. J., 1967a, Role of the phagocyte in host–parasite interactions. XI. Relationship between stimulated oxidative metabolism and hydrogen peroxide formation, and intracellular killing, *J. Bacteriol.* **94**:1417.

McRipley, R. J., and Sbarra, A. J., 1967b, Role of the phagocyte in host–parasite interactions. XII. Hydrogen peroxidase-myeloperoxidase bacterial system in the phagocyte, *J. Bacteriol.* **94**:1425.

Melby, K., and Midtvedt, T., 1981, A study of the elimination phase of phagocytosis of 32P-labeled *Escherichia coli* by human polymorphonuclear cell, *Acta Pathol. Microbiol. Scand. [B]* **89**:37.

Menzel, J., Jungfer, H., and Gemsa, D., 1978, Contribution of immunoglobulins, M. and G., complement, and properdin to the intracellular killing of *Escherichia coli* by polymorphonuclear leukocytes, *Infect. Immun.* **19**:659.

Metchnikoff, E., 1905, *Immunity in Infective Diseases*, Cambridge University Press, Cambridge.

Miller, T. E., and Watson, D. W., 1969, Biochemical characterization of the anti-microbial histone released by deoxyribonuclease and lactic acid, *Proc. Soc. Exp. Biol.* **131**:339.

Miller, B F., Abrams, R., Dorfman, A., and Klein, M., 1942, Antibacterial properties of protamine and histone, *Science* **96**:428.

Modrzakowski, M. C., and Paranavitana, C. M., 1981, Bactericidal activity of fractionated granule contents from human polymorphonuclear leukocytes: Role of bacterial membrane lipid, *Infect. Immun.* 32:668.

Modrzakowski, M. C., and Spitznagel, J. K., 1979, Bactericidal activity of fractionated granule contents from human polymorphonuclear leukocytes: Antagonism of granule cationic proteins by lipopolysaccharide, *Infect. Immun.* 25:597.

Modrzakowski, M. C., Cooney, M. H., Martin, L. E., and Spitznagel, J. K., 1979, Bactericidal activity of fractionated granule contents from human polymorphonuclear leukocytes, *Infect. Immun.* 23:587.

Mounter, L. A., and Atiyeh, W., 1960, Proteases of human leukocytes, *Blood* 15:52.

Murphy, G., Reynolds, J. J., Bretz, U., and Baggiolini, M., 1977, Collagenese is a component of the specific granules of human neutrophil leucocytes, *Biochem. J.* 162:195.

Murphy, G., Reynolds, J. J., Bretz, U., and Baggiolini, M., 1982, Partial purification of collagenase and gelatinase from human polymorphonuclear leucocytes, *Biochem. J.* 203:209.

Muschel, J. H., Carey, W. F., and Baron, L. S., 1959, Formalism of bacterial protoplasts by serum components, *J. Immunol.* 82:38.

Muschel, J. H., and Jackson, J. E., 1963, Activity of the antibody complement system and lysozyme against rough gram negative organisms, *Proc. Soc. Exp. Biol. Med.* 113:881.

Naccache, P. H., Showell, H. J., Becker, E. L., and Sha'afi, R. I., 1977, Changes in ionic movements across rabbit polymorphonuclear leukocyte membranes during lysosomal enzyme release. Possible ionic basis for lysosomal enzyme release, *J. Cell. Biol.* 75:635.

Ne'eman, N., Duchan, Z., Lehav, M., Sela, M. N., and Ginsburg, I., 1976, The effect of leukocyte hydrolases on bacteria. VII. Bactericidal and bacteriolytic reactions mediated by leukocyte and tissue extracts and their modifications by polyelectrolytes, *Inflammation* 1:261.

Nieman, C., 1954, Influence of trace amounts of fatty acids on the growth of microorganisms, *Bacteriol. Rev.* 18:147.

Noller, E. C., and Hartsell, S. E., 1961, Bacteriolysis of Enterobacteriaceae. II. Pre- and colytic treatments potentiating the action of lysozyme, *J. Bact.* 81:492.

Odeberg, H., and Olsson, I., 1975, Antibacterial activity of cationic proteins from human granulocytes, *J. Clin. Invest.* 56:1118.

Odeberg, H., and Olsson, I., 1976, Mechanisms for the microbicidal activity of cationic proteins of human granulocytes, *Infect. Immun.* 14:1269.

Odeberg, H., Olsson, I., and Venge, P., 1975, Cationic proteins of human granulocytes. IV. Esterase activity. *Lab. Invest.* 32:86.

O'Flaherty, J. T., Showell, H. J., Ward, P. A., and Becker, E. L., 1979, A possible role of arachidonic acid in human neutrophil aggregation and degranulation, *Am. J. Pathol.* 96:799.

Ohlsson, K., 1971, Interaction between human or dog leucocyte proteases and plasma protease inhibitors, *Scand. J. Clin. Lab. Invest.* 28:225.

Ohlsson, K., and Olsson, I., 1974, The neutral proteases of human granulocytes. II. Isolation and partial characterization of granulcoyte elastases. *Eur. J. Biochem.* 42:519.

Ohlsson, K., Olsson, I., and Spitznagel, J. K., 1977, Localization of chymotrypsin-like cationic protein, collagenase and elastase in azurophil granules of human neutrophilic polymorphonuclear leukocytes, *Hoppe Seylers Z. Physiol. Chem.* 358:361.

Okamura, N., and Spitznagel, J., 1982, Outer membrane mutants of *Salmonella typhimurium* LT2 have lipopolysaccharide-dependent resistance to the bactericidal activity of anaerobic human neutrophils, *Infect. Immun.* 36:1086.

Okamura, N., Ishibashi, S., and Takano, T., 1979, Evidence for bactericidal activity of polymorphonuclear leukocytes without phagocytosis, *J. Cell. Biol.* 86:469.

Olsson, I., and Venge, P., 1972, Cationic proteins of human granulocytes. I. Isolation of the cationic proteins from the granules of leukaemic myeloid cells, *Scand. J. Haematol.* 9:204.

Olsson, I., and Venge, P., 1974, Cationic proteins of human granulocytes. II. Separation of the cationic proteins of leukemic myeloid cells, *Blood* 44:235.

Oram, J. D., and Reiter, B., 1968, Inhibition of bacteria by lactoferrin and other iron-chelating agents, *Biochim. Biophys. Acta* 170:351.

Oseas, R., Yang, H. H., Baehner, R. L., and Boxer, L. A., 1981, Lactoferrin: A promoter of polymorphonuclear leukocyte adhesiveness, *Blood* 57:939.

Padgett, G. A., and Hirsch, J. G., 1967, Lysozyme: Its absence in tears and leukocytes of cattle, *Aust. J. Exp. Biol. Med. Sci.* 45:569.

Parmley, R. T., Ogawa, M., Darby, C. P., and Spicer, S. S., 1975, Congenital neutropenia: Neutrophil proliferation with abnormal maturation, *Blood* 46:723.

Patterson-Delafield, J., Martinez, R. J., and Lehrer, R. I., 1980, Microbicidal cationic proteins in rabbit alveolar macrophages: A potential host defense mechanism, *Infect. Immun.* 30:180.

Patterson-Delafield, J., Szklarek, D., Martinez, R. J., and Lehrer, R. I., 1981, Microbicidal cationic proteins of rabbit alveolar macrophages: Amino acid composition and functional attributes, *Infect. Immun.* 31:723.

Pavlov, E. P., and Soloviev, V. N., 1967, Changes in the hydrogen ion concentration of cytoplasma during the phagocytosis of microbes stained with indicator dyes, *Bull. Eksp. Biol. Med.* 63:78.

Pelletier, M., and Delaunay, A., 1972, Modifications par des histones (P II), du pouvoir bactericide des polynucléaires et des macrophages, *Ann. Inst. Pasteur* 123:85.

Penniall, R., and Spitznagel, J. K., 1975, Chicken neutrophils: Oxidative metabolism in phagocytic cells devoid of myeloperoxidase, *Proc. Natl. Acad. Sci. (USA)* 72:5012.

Penniall, R., Holbrook, J. P., and Zeya, H. I., 1972, The inhibition of cytochrome oxidase by lysosomal cationic proteins of rabbit polymorphonuclear leukocytes, *Biochem. Biophys. Res. Commun.* 47:1270.

Petterson, A., 1905, Ueber die bakterigiden leukocytenstaffe und ihse Begieburg zur Immunitat centr. *Bakteriol. Parasitenk Abt. I* 39:423.

Prieur, D. J., Olson, H. M., and Young, D. M., 1974, Lysozyme deficiency—an inherited disorder of rabbits, *Am. J. Pathol.* 77:283.

Pryzwansky, K. B., Rausch, P. G., Spitznagel, J. K., and Herion, J. C., 1979a, Immunocytochemical distinction between primary and secondary granule formation in developing human neutrophils: Correlations with Romanovsky stains, *Blood* 53:179.

Pryzwansky, K. B., Macrae, E. K., Spitznagel, J. K., and Cooney, M. H., 1979b, Early degranulation of human neutrophils: Immunocytochemical studies of surface and intracellular phagocytic events, *Cell* 18:1025.

Pryzwansky, K. B., Steiner, A. L., Spitznagel, J. K., and Kapoor, C. L., 1981, Compartmentalization of cyclic AMP during phagocytosis by human neutrophilic granulocytes, *Science* 211:407.

Quie, P. G., White, J. G., Holmes, B., and Good, R. A., 1967, *In vitro* bacterial capacity of human polymorphonuclear leukocytes: Diminished activity in chronic granulomatous disease of childhood, *J. Clin. Invest.* 46:668.

Rausch, P. G., and Moore, T. G., 1975, Granule enzymes of polymorphonuclear neutrophils. A phylogenetic comparison, *Blood* 46:913.

Rausch, P. G., Canonico, P. G., and Chapple, F. E. III, 1974, Lysosomal characterization of monkey peripheral granulocytes during infection, *Fed. Proc.* 33:257.

Rausch, P. G., Pryzwansky, K. B., and Spitznagel, J. K., 1978, Immunocytochemical identification of azurophilic and specific granule markers in the giant granules of Chediak–Higashi neutrophils, *N. Engl. J. Med.* **298**:693.

Reijngoud, D. J., and Tager, J. M., 1973, Measurement of intralysosomal pH, *Biochim. Biophys. Acta* **297**:174.

Reijngoud, D. J., and Tager, J. M., 1975, Effect of ionophores and temperature on intralysosomal pH, *FEBS Lett.* **54**:76.

Rein, M. F., Sullivan, J. A., and Mandell, G. L., 1980, Trichomonacidal activity of human polymorphonuclear neutrophils: Killing by destruction and fragmentation, *J. Infect. Dis.* **142**:575.

Reiter, B., Brock, J. H., and Steel, E. D., 1975, Inhibition of *Escherichia coli* by bovine colostrum and postcolostral milk. II. The bacteriostatic effect of lactoferrin on a serum susceptible serum resistant strain of *E. coli, Immunology* **28**:83.

Repaske, R., 1956, Lysis of gram-negative bacteria by lysozyme, *Biochim. Biophys. Acta* **22**:189.

Repaske, R., 1958, Lysis of gram-negative organisms and the role of versene, *Biochim. Biophys. Acta* **30**:225.

Repine, J. E., and Clawson, C. C., 1977, Quantitative measurement of the bactericidal capability of neutrophils from patients and carriers of chronic granulomatous disease, *J. Lab Clin. Med.* **90**:522.

Repine, J. E., Fox, R. B., and Berger, E. M., 1981*a*, Dimethyl sulfoxide inhibits killing of *Staphylococcus aureus* by polymorphonuclear leukocytes, *Infect. Immun.* **31**:510.

Repine, J. E., Fox, R. B., Berger, E. M., and Harada, R. N., 1981*b*, Effect of staphylococcal iron content on the killing of *Staphylococcus aureus* by polymorphonuclear leukocytes, *Infect. Immun.* **32**:407.

Rest, R. F., 1979, Killing of Neiserria gonorrhoeae by human polymorphonuclear neutrophil granule extracts, *Infect. Immun.* **25**:574.

Rest, R. F., and Pretzer, E., 1981, Degradation of gonococcal outer membrane proteins by human neutrophil lysosomal proteases, *Infect. Immun.* **34**:62.

Rest, R. F., Cooney, M. H., and Spitznagel, J. K., 1977, Susceptibility of lipopolysaccharide mutants to the bactericidal action of human neutrophil lysosomal fractions, *Infect. Immun.* **16**:145.

Rest, R. F., Cooney, M. H., and Spitznagel, J. K., 1978*a*, Bactericidal activity of specific and azurophil granules from human neutrophils: Studies with outer-membrane mutants of *Salmonella typhimurium* LT-2, *Infect. Immun.* **19**:131.

Rest, R. F., Cooney, M. H., and Spitznagel, J. K., 1978*b*, Subcellular distribution of glycosidases in human polymorphonuclear leucocytes, *Biochem. J.* **174**:53.

Rest, R. F., Fischer, S. H., Ingham, Z. Z., Jones, J. F., 1982, Interaction of Neisseria gonorrhoeae with human neutrophils: Effects of serum and goncoccal opacity on phagocyte killings and chemiluminescence, *Infect. Immun.* **203**:737.

Rindler-Ludwig, R., Schmalzl, F., and Braunsteiner, H., 1974, Isolierung und charakterisierung der chymotrypsinahnlichen protease aus neutiophiler Granulozyten des menschen. *Schweiz. Med. Wochenschr.* **104**:132.

Robineaux, J., and Frederic, J., 1955, Contribution a'l'étude des granulations neutrophiles des polynucléaires par la microcinématographie en contraste de phase, *C. R. Soc. Biol. (Paris)*, **149**:486.

Root, R. K., and Cohen, M. S., 1981, The microbicidal mechanisms of human neutrophils and eosinophils, *Rev. Infect. Dis.* **142**:565.

Root, R. K., Isturiz, R., Molavi, A., and Metcalf, J. A., 1981, Interactions between antibiotics and human neutrophils in the killing of staphylococci. Studies with normal and cytochalasin B-treated cells, *J. Clin. Invest.* **67**:247.

Rouse, P., 1925a, The relative reaction within living mammalian tissues. I. General features vital staining with litmus, *J. Exp. Med.* 41:379.

Rouse, P., 1925b, The relative reaction within living mammalian tissues II. On the mobilization of acid material within cells, and the reaction as influenced by the cell state, *J. Exp. Med.* 41:399.

Salton, M. R. J., 1957, The properties of lysozyme and its action on microorganisms, *Bacteriol. Rev.* 21:82.

Schattenfroh, A., 1897, Ueber die bacterien-feindlichen eigenschafter der leukocyten, *Arch. Hyg. (Berl.)* 31:1.

Schmidt, W., and Havemann, K., 1977, Chymotrypsin-like neutral protease from lysosome of human polymorphonuclear leukocytes, *Hoppe Seylers Z. Physiol. Chem.* 358:555.

Schneider, R., 1909, Die baklterizide und hamolytische wirking der tierischen gewebsflussigkeiten und ihre beziehungen zu dem leukozyten, *Arch. Hyg. (Berl.)* 70:40.

Segal, A. W., Dorling, J., and Coade, S., 1980, Kinetics of fusion of the cytoplasmic granules with phagocytic vacuoles in human polymorphonuclear leukocytes, *J. Cell Biol.* 85:42.

Segal, A. W., Geisow, M., Garcia, R., Harper, A., and Miller, R., 1981, The respiratory burst of phagocytic cells is associated with a rise in vaculolar pH, *Nature* 290:406.

Segal, A. W., Cross, A. R., Garcia, R. C., Borregaard, N., Valerius, N. H., Soothill, J. F., and Jones, O. T. G., 1983, Absence of cytochrome b-245 in chronic granulomatous disease: A multicenter European evaluation of its incidence and relevance, *N. Engl. J. Med.* 308: 245.

Selvaraj, R. J., and Sbarra, A. J., 1966, Relationship of glycolytic and oxidative metabolism and particle entry and destruction in phagocytosing cells, *Nature* 211:1272.

Shafer, W. M., and Spitznagel, J. K., 1983, Sensitivity of Salmonella typhimurium to polymorphonuclear granulocyte extracts: Role of lipid A. *Molecular Concepts of Lipid A, Washington, D.C., April 6-8, 1983.*

Shafer, W. M., Martin, L. E., Yakrus, M., and Spitznagel, J. K., 1983, Fractionation of bactericidal activity from human granulocytes under conditions of serine protease inhibition, Abst. B161, *Am. Soc. Microbiol. Proc.* 141.

Skarnes, R. C., 1967, Leukin, a bactericidal agent from rabbit polymorphonuclear leucocytes, *Nature* 216:806.

Skarnes, R. C., and Watson, D. W., 1956, Characterization of leukin: An antibacterial factor from leucocytes active against gram-positive pathogens, *J. Exp. Med.* 104:829.

Skarnes, R. C., and Watson, D. W., 1957, Antimicrobial factors of normal tissues and fluids, *Bacteriol. Rev.* 21:273.

Smit, J., Hanio, Y., and Nakaido, H., 1975, Outer membrane of *Salmonella typhimurium* chemical analysis and freeze fracture studies with lipopolysaccharide mutants, *J. Bacteriol.* 124:942.

Smolen, J. E., and Weissmann, G., 1980, Effects of indomethacin, 5,8,11,14-eicosatetraynoic acid, and P-bromophenacyl bromide on lysosomal enzyme release and superoxide anion generation by human polymorphonuclear leukocytes, *Biochem. Pharmacol.* 29:533.

Smolen, J. E., and Weissmann, G., 1981, Stimuli which provide secretion of azurophil enzymes from human neutrophils induce increments in adenosine cyclic 3' to 5' monophosphate, *Biochem. Biophys. Acta* 672:197.

Smolen, J. E., Korchak, H. M., and Weissmann, G., 1980, Initial kinetics of lysosomal enzyme secretion and superoxide anion generation by human polymorphonuclear leukocytes, *Inflammation* 4:145.

Solberg, C. O., Christie, K. E., Larsen, B., and Tonder, O., 1976, Influence of antibodies and thermolabile serum factors on the bactericidal activity of human neutrophil granulocytes, *Acta Pathol. Microbiol. Scand.* [C] 84:112.

Sorenson, M., and Sorenson, S. P. L., 1939, The proteins in whey, *C. R. Lab. Carlsberg* **23**:55.

Spitznagel, J. K., 1961*a*, The effects of mammalian and other cationic polypeptides on the cytochemical character of bacterial cells, *J. Exp. Med.* **114**:1063.

Spitznagel, J. K., 1961*b*, Anti-bacterial effects associated with changes in bacterial cytology produced by cationic polypeptides, *J. Exp. Med.* **114**:1079.

Spitznagel, J. K., 1980, Oxygen independent systems in polymorphonuclear leukocytes in the reticuloendothelial system: A comprehensive treatise, 2, in: *Biochemistry and Metabolism* (A. J. Sbarra and R. R. Strauss, eds.), pp. 355–368. Plenum, New York.

Spitznagel, J. K., and Chi, H.-Y., 1963, Cationic proteins and antibacterial properties of infected tissues and leukocytes, *Am. J. Pathol.* **43**:697.

Spitznagel, J. K., Cooper, M. R., McCall, A. F., DeChatelet, L. R., and Welsh, I. R. H., 1972, Selective deficiency of granules associated with lysozyme and lactoferrin in human polymorphs (PMN) with reduced microbicidal capacity, *J. Clin. Invest.* **51**:93a.

Spitznagel, J. K., Dalldorf, F. G., Leffell, M. S., Folds, J. D., Welsh, I. R. H., Cooney, M. H., and Martin, L. E., 1974, Character of azurophil and specific granules purified from human polymorphonuclear leukocytes, *Lab. Invest.* **30**:774.

Spitznagel, J. K., Goodrum, K. J., and Warejcka, D. J., 1983, Rat arthritis due to whole group B streptococci, *Am. J. Pathol.* **112**:37.

Sprick, M. G., 1956, Phagocytosis of *M. tuberculosis* and *M. smegmatis* stained with indicator dyes, *Am. Rev. Respir. Dis.* **74**:552.

Starkey, P. M., and Barrett, A. J., 1976, Human cathepsin G. catalytic and immunological properties, *Biochem. J.* **155**:273.

Steinman, R. M., Nellman, I. S., Muller, W. A., and Cohn, Z. A., 1983, Endocytosis and the recycling of plasma membrane, *J. Cell Biol.* **96**:1.

Stossel, T. P., Ballard, T. D., and Mason, R. J., 1971, Isolation and properties of phagocytic vesicles from polymorphonuclear leukocytes, *J. Clin. Invest.* **50**:1745.

Strauss, R. G., Bove, K. E., Jones, J. R., Mauer, A. M., and Fulginiti, V. A., 1974, An anomaly of neutrophil morphology with impaired function, *N. Engl. J. Med.* **290**:478.

Strominger, J. L., and Ghuysen, J.-M., 1967, Mechanisms of enzymatic bacteriolysis, *Science* **156**:213.

Strominger, J. L., and Tipper, D. J., 1974, Structure of bacterial cell walls: The lysozyme substrate, in *Lysozyme* (E. Osserman, R. E. Canfield, and S. Beychok, eds.), pp. 169–184. Academic Press, New York.

Tagesson, C., and Stendahl, O., 1973, Influence of the cell surface lipopolysaccharide structure of *Salmonella typhimurium* on resistance to intracellular bactericidal systems, *Acta Pathol. Microbiol. Scand.* [B] **81**:473.

Tedesco, R., Rottini, G., and Patriarca, P., 1981, Modulating effect of the late-acting components of the complement system on the bactericidal activity of human polymorphonuclear leukocytes on *E. coli* 0111:B4, *J. Immunol.* **127**:1910.

Thorne, K. J. I., Oliver, R. C., and Barrett, A. J., 1976, Lysis and killing of bacteria by lysosomal proteinases, *Infect. Immun.* **14**:555.

Van Houte, A. J., Elsbasch, P., Verkleij, A., and Weiss, J., 1977, Killing of *Escherichia coli* by a granulocyte fraction occurs without recognizable ultrastructural alterations in the bacterial envelope, as studies by freeze-fracture electron microscopy, *Infect. Immun.* **15**:556.

Van Snick, J. L., Masson, P. L., and Heremanns, J. F., 1974, The involvement of lactoferrin in the hyposideremia of acute inflammation, *J. Exp. Med.* **140**:1068.

Walton, E., 1978, The preparation, properties and action on *Staphylococcus aureus* of purified fractions from the cationic proteins of rabbit polymorphonuclear leucocytes, *Br. J. Exp. Pathol.* **59**:416.

Walton, E., and Gladstone, G. P., 1975, A study of the action of the cationic proteins from rabbit polymorphonuclear leucocytes on the staphylococcal cell membrane, *Br. J. Exp. Pathol.* 56:459.

Walton, E., and Gladstone, G. P., 1976, Factors affecting the susceptibility of staphylococci to killing by the cationic proteins from rabbit polymorphonuclear leucocytes: The effects of alteration of cellular energetics and of various iron compounds, *Br. J. Exp. Pathol.* 57:560.

Wang-Iverson, P., Pryzwansky, K. B., Spitznagel, J. K., and Cooney, M. H., 1978, Bactericidal capacity of phorbol myristate acetate-treated human polymorphonuclear leukocytes, *Infect. Immun.* 22:945.

Wardlaw, A. C., 1962, The complement-dependent bacteriolytic activity of normal human serum. I. The effect of pH and ionic strength and the role of lysozyme, *J. Exp. Med.* 115:1231.

Warren, G. H., Gray, J., and Bartell, P., 1955, The lysis of *Pseudomonas aeruginosa* by lysozyme, *J. Bacteriol.* 70:614.

Warren, G. H., Gray, J., and Yurchenco, J. A., 1957, Effect of polymyxin on the lysis of *Neisseria catarrhalis* by lysozyme, *J. Bacteriol.* 74:788.

Wassom, D. L., and Gleich, G. J., 1979, Damage to *Trichinella spiralis* newborn larvae by eosinophil major basic protein, *Am. J. Trop. Med. Hyg.* 28:860.

Weil, E., 1911, Untersuchungen uber die keimtotende Kraft der weissen Blutkorperchen. *Arch. Hyg. (Berl.)* 74:289.

Weinberg, E. D., 1971, Roles of iron in host-parasite interactions, *J. Infect. Dis.* 124:401.

Weinberg, E. D., 1974, Iron and susceptibility to infectious disease, *Science* 184:952.

Weinberg, E. D., 1974, Iron and susceptibility to infectious disease. *Science* 184:952.

Weiss, J., and Elsbach, P., 1977, The use of a phospholipase A-less Escherichia coli mutant to establish the action of granulocyte phospholipase A on bacterial phospholipids during killing by a highly purified granulocyte fraction, *Biochim. Biophys. Acta* 466:23.

Weiss, J., Franson, R. C., Beckerdite, S., Schmeidler, K., and Elsbach, P., 1975, Partial characterization and purification of a rabbit granulocyte factor that increases permeability of *Escherichia coli, J. Clin. Invest.* 55:33.

Weiss, J., Franson, R. C., Schmeidler, K., and Elsbach, P., 1976, Reversible envelope effects during and after killing of escherichia coli by a highly-purified rabbit polymorphonuclear leukocyte fraction, *Biochim. Biophys. Acta* 436:154.

Weiss, J., Victor, M., Cross, A. S., and Elsbach, P. E., 1977, Sensitivity of K-1 encapsulated *Escherichia coli* to killing by the bactericidal/permeability-increasing protein of rabbit and human neutrophils, *Infect. Immun.* 38:1149.

Weiss, J., Elsbach, P., Olsson, I., and Odeberg, H., 1978, Purification and characterization of a potent bactericidal and membrane active protein from the granules of human polymorphonuclear leukocytes, *J. Biol. Chem.* 253:2664.

Weiss, J., Beckerdite-Quagliata, S., and Elsbach, P., 1979, Determinants of the action of phospholipases A on the envelope phospholipids of *Escherichia coli, J. Biol. Chem.* 254:11010.

Weiss, J., Beckerdite-Quagliata, S., and Elsbach, P., 1980, Resistance of gram-negative bacteria to purified bactericidal leukocyte proteins: Relation to binding and bacterial lipopolysaccharide structure, *J. Clin. Invest.* 65:619.

Weiss, J., Victor, M., Stendhal, O., and Elsbach, P., 1982, Killing of gram-negative bacteria by polymorphonuclear leukocytes, *J. Clin. Invest.* 69:959.

Welsh, I. R. H., and Spitznagel, J. K., 1971, Distribution of lysosomal enzymes, cationic proteins, and bactericidal substances in subcellular fractions of human polymorphonuclear leukocytes, *Infect. Immun.* 4:97.

Wilson, L. A., and Spitznagel, J. K., 1968, Molecular and structural damage of *Escherichia coli* produced by antibody, complement and lysozyme systems, *J. Bacteriol.* 96:1339.

Witholt, B., van Heerikhuizen, H., and de Leij, L., 1976, How does lysozyme penetrate through the bacterial outer membrane? *Biochim. Biophys. Acta* 443:534.

Zeya, H. I., and Spitznagel, J. K., 1963, Anti-bacterial and enzymatic basic proteins from leukocyte lysosomes: Separation and identification, *Science* 142:1085.

Zeya, H. I., and Spitznagel, J. K., 1966a, Cationic proteins of polymorphonuclear leukocyte lysosomes. I. Resolution of antibacterial and enzymatic activities, *J. Bacteriol.* 91: 750.

Zeya, H. I., and Spitznagel, J. K., 1966b, Cationic proteins of polymorphonuclear leukocyte lysosomes. II. Composition, properties and mechanism of anti-bacterial action, *J. Bacteriol.* 91:755.

Zeya, H. I., and Spitznagel, J. K., 1966c, Anti-microbial specificity of leukocyte lysosomal cationic proteins, *Science* 154:1059.

Zeya, H. I., and Spitznagel, J. K., 1968, Arginine-rich proteins of polymorphonuclear leukocyte lysosomes. Anti-microbial specificity and biochemical heterogeneity, *J. Exp. Med.* 127:927.

Zeya, H. I., and Spitznagel, J. K., 1971, Characterization of cationic protein-bearing granules of polymorphonuclear leukocytes, *Lab. Invest.* 24:229.

Zeya, H. I., Spitznagel, J. K., and Schwab, J. H., 1966, Anti-bacterial action of PMN lysosomal cationic proteins resolved by density gradient electrophoresis, *Proc. Soc. Exp. Biol.* 121:250.

Zinder, N. D., and Arndt, W. F., 1956, Production of protoplasts of *Escherichia coli* by lysozyme treatment, *Proc. Natl. Acad. Sci. (USA)* 42:586.

Zinsser, H., 1910, On bactericidal substances extracted from normal leucocytes, *J. Med. Res.* 22:397.

Zucker-Franklin, D., and Hirsch, J. G., 1964, Electron microscope studies on the degranulation of rabbit peritoneal leukocytes during phagocytosis, *J. Exp. Med.* 120:569.

Chapter 11

Clinical Disorders of Leukocyte Functions

Harry R. Hill

Departments of Pathology and Pediatrics
University of Utah School of Medicine
Salt Lake City, Utah 84132

I. INTRODUCTION

A. Historical Perspective

After being questioned by a colleague about my current endeavors with a large number of reprints, reference printouts, and writing pads apparent, I informed him that I was writing another review on clinical abnormalities of phagocyte function. Why write another such review, I was asked, as there are a number of these in the current literature (Gallin, 1981; Lohr and Snyderman, 1981; Hill, 1981a; Gallin *et al.*, 1980; Hill, 1982; Charette and Hill, 1980; Mills and Quie, 1980; Johnston and Newman, 1977; Baehner, 1974; Stossel, 1974). That's a very good question, which momentarily dimmed my enthusiasm for the project. I believe, however, that the study of phagocyte disorders has turned the corner from that of a purely descriptive, and somewhat inexact, science to one that is applying the rapidly developing tools of cell biology to look into the mechanisms of these fascinating disorders. Thus, cell surface receptors, membrane potential changes, ion fluxes, cyclic nucleotide alterations, protein phosphorylation, microtubule and microfilament function, as well as the various critical metabolic pathways, are being carefully dissected in polymorphonuclear keukocytes (PMNs), monocytes (Mns), and macrophages (Macs). The knowledge gained from these critically important cells in the host-defense mechanism is now spilling over into the study of other cell types, such as those in muscle, liver, bone, and nervous tissue, which are much more difficult to obtain and study. Thus, in many aspects of cell physiology, we—the phagocyte people—are at the forefront of knowledge and scientific investigation.

Almost a century ago, Metchnikoff (translated in 1905) pointed out the critical role of phagocytic cells in protecting the body from invasion by pyogenic microorganisms. Theodore Leber (1888) a German ophthalmologist, subsequently suggested that tropic migration of phagocytic cells to sites of irritation or microbial invasion was critical to host defense. It was not until 1954 (Janeway *et al.*, 1954), however, that the first group of patients was described who would turn out to have a defect in phagocyte function. These patients had marked lymphadenopathy, hepatosplenomegaly, and severe recurrent infections, but no defect was initially detectable in their host-defense system. Similar additional patients were described (Berendes *et al.*, 1957; Bridges *et al.*, 1959), and the syndrome was named fatal granulomatous disease of childhood because of the marked granuloma formation that occurred and the almost universal fatal outcome of the original patients. It was not until a decade later that Quie and associates (1967) demonstrated that the phagocytic cells of these patients had a profound defect in intracellular microbicidal activity against a variety of common pathogens, such as *Staphylococcus aureus*. Holmes *et al.* (1967) found that the patient's cells had a defect in oxidative metabolism that could account for the observed functional abnormality. In spite of these pioneering studies carried out more than 15 years ago, we still do not know the precise biochemical mechanisms involved in the various forms of what is now known as chronic granulomatous disease (CGD). We have, however, discovered a great deal about oxidative and nonoxidative microbicidal mechanisms within PMNs, Mns, and Macs and have learned enough about the infections that these patients suffer to be able to manage them successfully, in most instances, hence the change in name from "fatal" to "chronic" granulomatous disease.

The precise sequence of reports on clinical defects in phagocyte chemotaxis is a little more difficult to decipher. In my admittedly somewhat biased opinion, the first report of such a disorder was made by S. D. Davis *et al.* (1966). These investigators described two female patients with fair skin, reddish hair, severe eczema, dystrophic fingernail changes, severe sinopulmonary infections, and recurrent staphylococcal abscesses. The abscesses did not have a great deal of surrounding erythema and were not particularly tender. For this reason, they were termed "cold abscesses." These investigators suggested the term "Job's syndrome" to designate the symptom complex suffered by these patients, quoting from the book of Job in the introduction to their article: "So went Satan forth from the presence of the Lord, and smote Job with sore boils from the sole of his foot unto his crown." No abnormality in the host defense mechanism was detected in these patients, although the number of functional and metabolic assays was limited at that time.

In 1971, Miller *et al.* (1971) first described two patients with what was described as the lazy leukocyte syndrome. These young children had suffered recurrent stomatitis, otitis, gingivitis, and febrile episodes. In addition to a rather marked neutropenia in the presence of normal marrow granulocyte stores, these patients had defective *in vitro* tests for directed (chemotactic) and random

PMN migration. That same year, there was an explosion of papers on chemotaxis in the literature, as at least semiquantitative methods for assessing PMN movement were developed. Thus, defective cell migration was described in neonates (Miller, 1971), adult diabetics (Mowat and Baum, 1971b), and patients with rheumatoid arthritis (Mowat and Baum, 1971a).

Buckley et al. (1972) described two male patients with a syndrome almost exactly like that described by S. D. Davis et al. (1966) in that they had peculiar facies, chronic eczema, dystrophic fingernail changes, recurrent sinopulmonary infections, and repeated staphylococcal abscesses. These patients also had extreme elevation of serum immunoglobulin E. (Subsequent studies indicated that the classic Job's syndrome patients also had marked hyperimmunoglobulinemia E.) Buckley's patients were found to have (1) immediate skin hypersensitivity to *Staphylococcus aureus* and *Candida albicans* antigens; (2) decreased anamnestic antibody responses to diphtheria and tetanus; (3) poor primary antibody responses to several antigens; (4) lack of a response to dinitrochlorobenzene (DNCB); and (5) a variable decrease in lymphocyte responses to *Candida* antigen. Phagocyte function was not studied in these patients. Abnormal PMN chemotaxis was described in an older patient with hyper-IgE by Clark et al. (1973) and in three young children by Hill and Quie (1974b). Subsequently, in association with Drs. Wedgwood, Ochs, Clark, Klebanoff and Quie, I (Hill et al., 1974d) studied the chemotactic responsiveness of the original Job's syndrome patients described by S. D. Davis et al. (1966) and found them to have a marked defect in cell migration. Thus, as in the case of CGD of childhood, a considerable period of time had elapsed between the clinical description of the syndrome and the detection of an underlying defect in phagocyte function.

The first clinical abnormality in monocyte function was probably a patient described by Snyderman et al. (1973). The patient, a 9-year-old girl, had suffered repeated mucocutaneous *Candida* infections since infancy and had monocyte chemotactic responses that ranged from 2% to 11% of normal. Subsequent reports of abnormal monocyte function have been limited to patients with Wiskott-Aldrich syndrome (Altman et al., 1974), viral infections, and various forms of malignancies (Snyderman and Pike, 1978).

Since these original patients were described, an expanding list of additional phagocyte disorders have been reported in the literature. The present chapter does not concentrate on each of these syndromes or disease states, but instead is selective in examining only those that have been well documented, and in which something is known about the underlying mechanisms involved.

B. Clinical Presentation of Phagocyte Disorders: General Comments

If one questions the clinical significance of phagocyte disorders, consider for a moment what happens to persons with no functioning PMNs, such as those with severe congenital neutropenia, leukemia, or drug-induced absence of granulocytes. These patients die, or they suffer severe recurrent bacterial infections. Without adequate numbers of functioning phagocytic cells, the body is simply incapable of preventing massive invasion by a variety of microorganisms.

Phagocytic cells, including PMNs, Mns, and Macs, have a particularly important role in protecting the skin, mucous membranes, and linings of the respiratory and gastrointestinal tracts. As such, they form the first line of defense against microbial invasion. Miles (1964) and Miles *et al.* (1957) showed some very nice animal experiments that a critical 2- to 4-hr period exists after invasion by pathogenic organisms during which phagocytic cells must arrive at the site of invasion if infection is to be suppressed or contained. If not, the resulting infection leads to a larger local lesion or disseminates throughout the body of the animal. The clinical presentation of phagocyte disorders suggests that this is true in the human also. In order to be effective, phagocytic cells must adhere or attach to the vascular endothelium near the site of invasion or inflammation, engage in diapedesis through the vessel wall, move in a unidirectional fashion toward the site, adhere to and ingest the offending organism, and activate biochemical pathways important in intracellular microbial killing.

Patients whose phagocytes have defects in adhesion or cell motility generally suffer cutaneous abscesses with common pathogens such as *Staphylococcus aureus* or have mucous membrane lesions due to agents like *C. albicans*. If the defect is a profound one, lesions may contain few if any phagocytes. In contrast, most patients end up with large abscesses filled with PMNs that have arrived after the critical 2- to 4-hr period during which such cells can be effective in eradicating or suppressing infection. Thus, patients with Job's syndrome often have massive lesions containing numerous PMNs (S. D. Davis *et al.*, 1966). Mucocutaneous candidiasis is frequently observed in this group (Clark *et al.*, 1973; Snyderman *et al.*, 1973; Van Scoy *et al.*, 1975), as are recurrent pneumonias, sinusitis, and otitis media. Sepsis and systemic infection is less common, however, suggesting that the reticuloendothelial cell system in these patients may be at least partially intact. Periodontal disease and dental caries are prominent in patients with chemotactic disorders (Clark *et al.*, 1977; Cianciola *et al.*, 1977). Allergic manifestations are also quite common in patients with disorders of granulocyte chemotaxis (Hill, 1982).

Disorders of phagocyte microbicidal activity are also associated with cutaneous abscesses, pulmonary infections, and gastrointestinal problems (Johnston and Newman, 1977; Mills and Quie, 1980). In general, these patients tend to suffer more deep-seated and chronic infections, such as liver, lung, and abdominal abscesses. Osteomyelitis due to staphylococci and other agents is also common (Cohen *et al.*, 1981; Mills and Quie, 1980). Granuloma formation with obstructive complications in the abdomen, gastrointestinal, and urinary systems often occur (Griscom *et al.*, 1974; Johansen *et al.*, 1982).

C. Laboratory Assessment of Phagocyte Function

There is considerable controversy over the need for routine laboratory testing of phagocyte function. Arguments for and against the clinical use of such tests in the evaluation of patients as well as an analysis of the information to be gained from such testing is contained in the proceedings of a round table discussion which was held at the Second European Conference on Phagocytic Leukocytes in Trieste, Italy in 1980 (Hill and Patriarca, 1982). It was clear from the discussion that the European centers were more likely to employ a variety of functional assays in evaluating patients with recurrent infections when compared to centers in the United States. Although most tests were carried out in rather specialized research laboratories, several centers made these available through regular clinical laboratories. A table listing the tests performed in a number of different laboratories can be found on page 679 of that article (Hill and Patriarca, 1982).

There are a number of different techniques for screening the various phagocytic functions important in host defense. A brief description of these is presented here, because the type of test employed can have a direct bearing on the significance of a described clinical abnormality.

1. Phagocyte Adhesion and Aggregation

Granulocyte adherence is usually measured using columns filled with nylon fiber (MacGregor et al., 1974). Anticoagulated whole blood or isolated phagocytes can be used in this system. Adherence is dependent on the amount of the fiber employed, the incubation period, the presence of divalent cations, and to some extent the type of anticoagulant used. A variety of drugs such as ethanol, salicylates, and prednisone may impair granulocyte adherence, whereas inflammation increases attachment (MacGregor et al., 1974; Lentner et al., 1976). Granulocyte adherence to nylon fiber has been shown to correlate well with attachment to endothelial cell monolayers (MacGregor et al., 1978).

2. Aggregation

Neutrophil aggregation is commonly measured in a platelet aggregometer (Craddock et al., 1978; Hammerschmidt et al., 1980) or using an automatic cell counter that is capable of counting the number of different-size particles (aggregated versus nonaggregated) in a suspension (O'Flaherty et al., 1977). Both assays work well to determine the effects of an aggregating substance such as C5a or human serum on granulocyte aggregation, but they function less well to assess the tendency of a patients cells to aggregate or the degree of aggregation that has occurred in vivo. In several clinical conditions, however, it is possible to detect circulating aggregating activity in the serum or plasma of patients (Craddock et al., 1979).

3. Migration

Phagocyte chemotaxis may be assessed *in vivo* employing the classical skin window techniques of Rebuck and Crowley (1955). Alternatively, chambers may be employed to quantitate the actual amount of cellular infiltrate into a local lesion (Brayton *et al.*, 1970). The major problem with both of these techniques is in creating a standard skin lesion. Scraping an area with a scapel seldom leads to a reproducible lesion, hence the considerable inherent variability in the assays (Dale *et al.*, 1974). Stripping the outer layer of skin with adhesive tape has also been suggested as one means of overcoming this problem (Mass *et al.*, 1975). In our experience, creating a lesion of sufficient depth with this technique is very difficult, so that few cells migrate into the area. The difficulty in creating a standard lesion along with the fact that a number of tissue proteases and other inflammatory mediators are released by such local trauma have led most investigators to abandon such assays or to use them only to back up the results of *in vitro* tests (Hill and Patriarca, 1982; Miller, 1973). In attempts to overcome these problems, Hellum and Solberg (1977) have devised a method to create skin blisters with a suction device that appears to result in uniform lesions. Migrating cells are then trapped in a special chamber for use in further functional and biochemical assays.

It is possible that such an assay system may eventually prove more reliable and relevant to the clinical situation, but the patient is certainly inconvenienced by such a procedure, and infection or tissue damage could possibly develop at the local skin site. For these reasons, most tests of phagocyte motility are carried out *in vitro*. Perhaps the most popular method employs various modifications of a chamber designed by Boyden (1962). Cells are permitted to settle, or they may be cytocentrifuged onto Micropore filters (Ward *et al.*, 1965; Baum *et al.*, 1971; Hill *et al.*, 1974a, 1975). The filters are then placed in the chemotactic chambers. Chemotactic factors are added to the bottom of the chamber and media is added alone to the top in assays designed to measure directed migration. Random motility is measured in the absence of chemotactic factors, while stimulated random migration, or chemokinesis, is determined in the presence of a chemoattractant, but without a gradient being present (Keller *et al.*, 1977). The Micropore filters are constructed of polycarbonate or cellulose and have pores with a diameter of 3-5 μM for PMNs and up to 8 μM for monocytes or macrophages. It should be pointed out that lot-to-lot and even filter-to-filter variation is considerable, making reproducibility using these techniques a significant problem. This necessitates testing a patient on a number of different occasions, using multiple replicates in each experiment. One may assess motility visually or through the use of radioactively labeled cells. In the visual assays, the distance to the leading front of two to three cells can be assessed with a micrometer—the leading front method. In addition, the number of cells reaching a given depth or the distal side of the filter can be determined. We really do not know which method of quantitating chemotaxis is more relevant to the clinical situation.

Several isotopes have been employed to label phagocytes for *in vivo* or *in vitro* studies of migration. These include chromium-51 (Gallin *et al.*, 1973); technetium-99m (English and McPherson, 1977) and indium-111 (Weiblen *et al.*, 1979). In general, these procedures require rather extensive handling of the cells, hypotonic lysis of contaminating erythrocytes (which may also take up the label), and several washes to remove unincorporated label. While excessive handling does not preclude *in vitro* studies of the effects of various agents or conditions on cell migration, we feel that it may alter baseline chemotactic responses in cells obtained from patients with suspected disorders (Hill *et al.*, 1975). Still, the radiolabeling techniques remove some of the subjectivity in interpreting chemotaxis assays visually and permit a larger number of samples to be assessed at one time. The radiolabeled assays require that two filters be employed: one for the cells to migrate through and the other for the cells to enter and subsequently be counted. These assays obviously do not permit a leading front method of quantitation.

Recently another method for assessing chemotaxis has become quite popular, probably because of its simplicity and the lack of a requirement for expensive chemotaxis chambers (Cutler, 1974; Nelson *et al.*, 1975; Orr and Ward, 1978). The method employs a thin layer of agarose under which cells migrate on a plastic surface. Wells are cut into the agar and filled with the cell suspension, a chemoattractant or media alone (Fig. 1). After 16-18 hr for monocytes or 2-4 hr for PMNs, the plates are fixed, the agar may or may not be removed, and the movement of the cells is quantitated. The distance to the leading front of two to

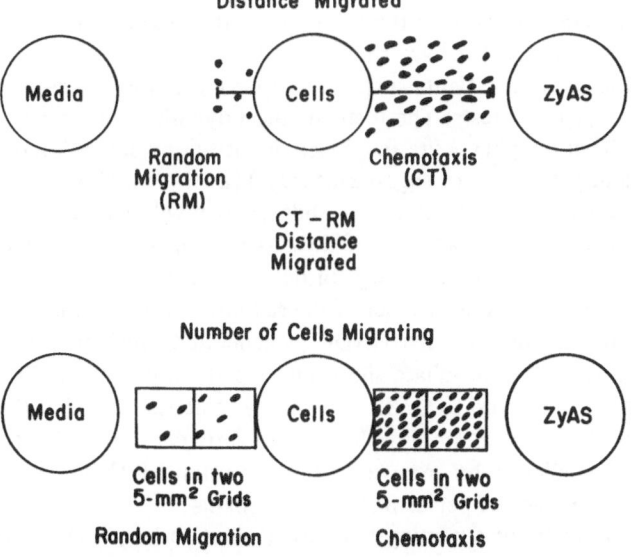

Figure 1. Evaluation of monocyte chemotaxis under agarose. ZyAS, zymosan-activated serum containing the chemoattractant, C5a. (From Hill *et al.*, 1983.)

three cells may be determined with a micrometer, or the number of cells moving into a reticule placed adjacent to the edge of the cell well may be counted (Fig. 1). Orr and Ward (1978) have shown that the technique is capable of measuring a dose–response effect and can differentiate random migration, chemokinesis, and chemotaxis. At least in our hands, the under-agarose system is less sensitive than the micropore filter method, so that a stronger chemoattractant is required in most instances. We believe that this can obscure the presence of defective chemotactic function in some patients. Nevertheless, the technique is a popular one and is readily adaptable for use in most laboratories.

4. Phagocytosis or Ingestion

Ingestion or particle uptake by phagocytes can be measured by several techniques, including the uptake of oil-red-O-coated particles (Stossel, 1973), radiolabeled bacterial uptake (Allred et al., 1979), or through the detection of metabolic activity of the cell following particle ingestion. The latter include assays dependent on nitroblue tetrazolium dye reduction (Johnston et al., 1969), chemiluminescence production (Hemming et al., 1976), or hexose monophosphate shunt activity (Holmes et al., 1967). In these assays, it is often quite difficult to distinguish between particle uptake and particle attachment to the surface of the cell. It is critical, therefore, to confirm by means of visual or electron microscopic techniques that ingestion has occurred.

5. Microbicidal Activity

The principle metabolic pathways important in oxygen-dependent microbicidal activity in phagocytes are shown in Figure 2. These pathways can be examined in the cells of patients suspected of having abnormalities in intracellular killing by a variety of tests. The histochemical dye nitroblue tetrazolium (NBT) is reduced within the phagocyte to a black deposit upon activation of the respiratory burst and generation of superoxide (O_2^-) (Baehner and Nathan, 1968). The test can be performed on PMA-coated slides, which will maximally stimulate the cells and result in more than 90% of the PMNs reducing the dye (Repine et al., 1979). As such, it is an excellent test for detecting chronic granulomatous disease and the heterozygous female carrier of the sex-linked form of the disorder.

During the respiratory burst $NADP^+$ is generated which subsequently stimulates the hexose monophosphate shunt and results in the metabolism of glucose to a five-carbon sugar and CO_2. If one employs glucose labeled at the 1-position with carbon-14, hexose monophosphate shunt activity can be estimated following a phagocytic challenge by measuring the evolution of $^{14}CO_2$ (Holmes et al., 1967). The test is easy to perform and quite reliable.

Additional tests for detecting respiratory burst activity include the detection of chemiluminescence (CL) production (Allen et al., 1974). Upon particle uptake or membrane perturbation, the microbicidal mechanism of the phagocyte is ac-

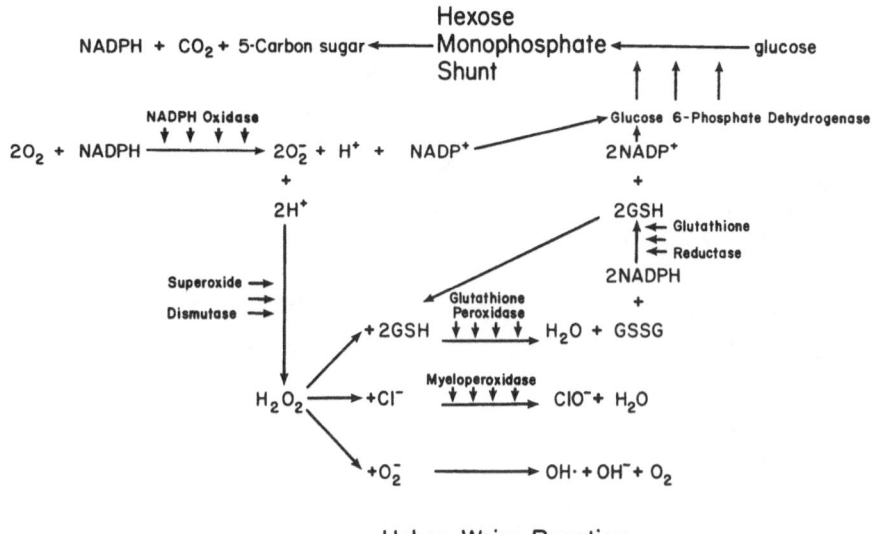

Haber-Weiss Reaction

Figure 2. Metabolic pathways important in oxygen-dependent phagocyte microbicidal activity. (From Hill, 1980.)

tivated and excited molecular oxygen species and carbonyl groups are generated. Upon decay back to the ground state, protons are released that can be quantitated in a liquid scintillation counter. While somewhat nonspecific because of the fact that a number of oxygen products lead to light generation (Cheson et al., 1976), the technique is quite sensitive in detecting respiratory burst activity and clearly differentiates between controls and patients with chronic granulomatous disease (Fig. 3). There is considerable variability in the assay from day to day, however, making it essential that daily controls be performed. This is especially true when luminol is employed to increase the amount of light generation. This compound, a cyclic hydrazide, is capable of reacting with an oxidizing agent to produce the electronically excited aminophthalate anion (Allen and Loose, 1976). This unstable intermediate relaxes to the ground state, emitting protons with such high-quantum efficiency that it amplifies the luminescence resulting from oxidative reactions occurring within stimulated leukocytes. In addition to increasing the variability of the CL response, luminol may either have some effect to initiate low-level respiratory burst activity or greatly enhance that occurring due to cell-to-cell contact (Allred et al., 1980). It also probably represents an added stress factor to the cell. Mills et al., (1980a, b) have suggested that this added stress can enable one to more readily detect the heterozygous carrier of chronic granulomatous disease.

The chemiluminescence assay is thus quite useful in screening for the metabolic defects of all forms of CGD (Stevens et al., 1978), myeloperoxidase defi-

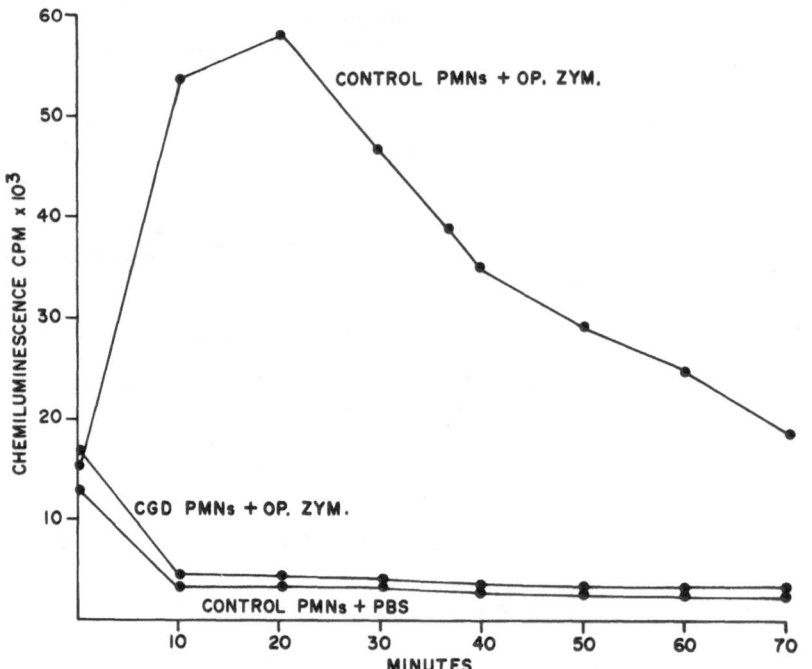

Figure 3. Chemiluminescence production by normal and chronic granulomatous disease (CGD) neutrophils exposed to opsonized zymosan. CPM, Counts per minute; PMNs, polymorphonuclear leukocytes.

ciency (Rosen and Klebanoff, 1976), and other congenital and acquired defects in phagocyte function (Shigeoka and Hill, 1978; Harvath and Andersen, 1979).

Actual assays of phagocytic uptake and microbial killing have been employed for a number of years and are still the "gold standard" in documenting an actual defect (Quie *et al.*, 1967). The various assays can be performed using differing bacteria to PMN ratios and with agents such as lysostaphin to destroy extracellular versus intracellular organisms. These assays are reasonably reliable and easily detect profound defects in microbicidal activity. They do not, however, have the sensitivity to screen for less prominent, partial defects in intracellular killing. An additional assay has been described in which the quantitation is dependent on the release of bacterial DNA (Friedlander, 1978).

More specific metabolic tests are available for detecting and quantitating superoxide (Bryant *et al.*, 1982), and H_2O_2 (Briggs *et al.*, 1977).

D. Abnormalities of Phagocyte Function: Real versus Artifactual

In general, most of the phagocyte functional assays are relatively simple to perform and do not require a great deal of expensive equipment. Unfortunately, however, there is always a certain degree of inherent variability in the assays as pointed out above. For this reason, it is important that patients suspected of having functional disorders be studied on several occasions and with multiple replicates per assay. It is also critical that artifacts in the methodology that result in apparent deficiencies be excluded. For instance, we once spent months examining a patient's serum that appeared to contain a cell-directed inhibitor of chemotaxis. After a number of different experiments, it became apparent that the abnormal result was secondary to an inhibitory effect on leukocyte settling rather than on actual cell movement. When suspended in the patient's serum or plasma, PMNs did not settle as rapidly onto the micropore filter in a Boyden chamber assay. When the cells were cytocentrifuged onto the filter, however, the inhibitory effect of the patient's serum disappeared completely. This is the major reason that we employ the cytocentrifuge in our chemotaxis assay system. One must always be aware that these *in vitro* assays involve extensive handling of the cells can induce artifacts. Only by critically examining reports of defective phagocyte function will we be able to rule out artifactual abnormalities or minor functional deficiencies that have no clinical significance.

II. ABNORMALITIES OF PHAGOCYTE ATTACHMENT, AGGREGATION, AND ADHESION

A. Enhanced Activity

Enhanced phagocyte attachment or aggregation has been reported in several clinical syndromes in which the PMN is thought to be a critical cell in inducing tissue damage. McCall *et al.* (1974) first indicated that intravascular activation of the complement cascade induced granulocytopenia and might act to aggregate leukocytes within the lung. Subsequently (Craddock *et al.*, 1977*a,b*) reported that in patients undergoing hemodialysis leukopenia often developed that was associated with a decrease in pulmonary function. These same investigators showed that infusion of sheep with autologous plasma that had been contacted with renal dialyzer cellophane resulted in the rapid development of leukopenia, doubling of the pulmonary artery pressure and a marked increase in pulmonary lymph effluent. Histologic studies revealed severe pulmonary vessel leukostasis and interstitial edema (Craddock *et al.*, 1977*a,b*). Contact between fresh plasma and the dialysis cellophane resulted in alternative pathway of complement activation, decreased factor B and C3, and consumption of hemolytic activity. MacGregor (1977) indicated that hemodialysis increases granulocyte adherence. Subsequently, the induction of PMN aggregation by serum was shown to be due to C5a (Hammerschmidt *et al.*, 1980). Circulating C5a may therefore cause the leukopenia and transient pulmonary dysfunction commonly observed during renal dialysis or cardiopulmonary bypass.

Other conditions associated with leukopenia and PMN accumulation in the lung include patients with gram-negative endotoxin shock, and those with what is termed the adult respiratory distress syndrome (ARDS). Pulmonary leukostasis, hypertension, and hypoxemia develop in this fulminant syndrome of respiratory failure (Jacob *et al.*, 1980), and circulating aggregatory activity toward PMNs can be detected in the plasma of patients (Hammerschmidt *et al.*, 1980). In all likelihood, PMNs aggregated and sequestered within the lung parenchyma contribute to the severe pulmonary damage observed in this syndrome (Hosea *et al.*, 1980). Recently, we have shown that the circulating PMNs of these patients are in a functionally and metabolically activated state and, thus, are probably primed to damage the endothelial and pulmonary tissue that they contact (Zimmerman *et al.*, 1983). Thus, under certain circumstances a variety of diffuse inflammatory processes may result in complement activation (Lentnek *et al.*, 1976). Circulating C5a, in turn, affects phagocytic cells—and perhaps the endothelial cells themselves—resulting in functional and biochemical alterations that favor tissue sequestration and the development of severe damage. Alternatively, other substances such as lactoferrin or arachidonic acid products, which increase in plasma during acute inflammatory processes, may be responsible for the leukostasis observed.

B. Decreased Activity

Decreased adhesion of granulocytes to nylon fiber columns can be induced by ethanol, prednisone, and aspirin (MacGregor *et al.*, 1974). In addition a heat-labile factor in the sera of homozygous β-thalassemia patients has been reported to depress adherence of PMNs (Bassaris *et al.*, 1982) to nylon fiber, but unfortunately the factor could not be well characterized.

An inherited abnormality of neutrophil adhesion was described by Crowley *et al.* (1980). The patient was a 5-year-old boy who suffered recurrent ear and skin infections and presented to the New Englnad Medical Center Hospital with a severe *Pseudomonas aeruginosa* infection of the larynx, trachea, and lungs. The patient's PMNs failed to attach to a plastic petri dish and did not spread on a surface as did normal PMNs. Chemotaxis as measured by a radiolabeled leukocyte technique was profoundly depressed as was ingestion as determined by uptake of paraffin oil droplets. Degranulation and intracellular bacterial killing were normal, however. Respiratory burst activity was decreased in the patient's PMNs after exposure to opsonized zymosan, but the soluble stimulant phorbol myristate acetate (PMA) evoked a normal response. Polyacrylamide gel electrophoresis (PAGE) of whole PMN homogenates from the patient revealed a striking absence of a high-molecular-weight protein of $\sim 110,000$. This protein was present in reduced levels both in patient's mother and in a female sibling, suggesting a congenital X-linked abnormality.

A patient with a similar clinical picture was recently described by Arnaout *et al.* (1982). This patient was an 8-year-old boy who suffered repeated skin and respiratory infections due to *Staphylococcus aureus* and *P. aeruginosa*. Functional PMN assays revealed decreased phagocytosis and degranulation in response to particulate stimuli, such as opsonized zymosan or IgG-coated sheep erythrocytes. In contrast to the previous patient, however, chemotaxis and random migration were entirely normal; adherence was not studied. Decreased respiratory burst activity occurred after exposure of the patient's PMNs to opsonized zymosan, but not to PMA. PAGE of PMN homogenates revealed the absence of a 150,000-dalton glycoprotein in the patient's cells as well as one-half the normal level of the protein in each of his parents. The precise role of this glycoprotein in receptor-mediated PMN function needs to be elucidated as well as its relationship to the protein that was missing in the patient described by Crowley *et al.* (1980).

Additional patients with decreased PMN adhesion or cell spreading have been described who suffered repeated infections and had delayed separation of the umbilical cord (Hayward *et al.*, 1979; Bowen *et al.*, 1980). The precise mechanism of the defect is unknown.

As indicated, most patients with decreased adhesion or attachment also have decreased chemotactic activity when tested *in vitro*. Thus, it is likely that cell attachment is essential to migration through a micropore filter or under an agarose layer. The one exception is the patient described by Arnaout *et al.* (1982), who certainly represents several paradoxes. Further elucidation of the abnormalities in this unusual case seems indicated.

III. CLINICAL SYNDROMES ASSOCIATED WITH ABNORMALITIES OF PHAGOCYTE MOTILITY

A. Newborn Infants

Newborn infants have a striking abnormality in PMN chemotaxis first suggested by Matoth (1952), who actually studied amoeboid movement rather than chemotaxis. Subsequently, Miller (1971) confirmed the profound nature of the defect in response to complement-generated chemotactic factors and speculated that the reason for the defect might be related to delayed maturation of critical enzymes in the neonatal cell. Defective monocyte and PMN chemotaxis was also found in neonatal cells by Klein *et al.* (1977), employing both a Boyden chamber assay and an under-agarose system. Chemotaxis of both types of cells remained extremely depressed up to 2 years of age and did not reach normal adult levels until 10 to 15 years of age. Pahwa *et al.* (1977) observed that Mn chemotaxis was normal in neonates, while PMN chemotaxis was depressed but not greatly when compared with adult PMNs (75%). The reason for the discrepancy between the two studies on Mn chemotaxis is unknown but may be related to the choice of assay systems.

Is the chemotactic defect in neonatal phagocytes a significant one? The answer to that question, I believe, is yes. The neonate is particularly susceptible to the development of cutaneous abscesses at sites of local trauma, such as from monitoring electrodes. Infants also commonly suffer from chronic mucocutaneous *Candida* infections associated with chemotactic defects. Respiratory infections such as those caused by group B streptococci are also extremely common during the neonatal period. (It is of interest that only neonates and other patients with suspected phagocyte abnormalities such as those with diabetes mellitus suffer from infections with group B streptococci.) These facts coupled with the known susceptibility of the neonate to overwhelming bacterial infection suggest strongly that the chemotactic abnormality is a clinically significant one.

What is the reason for abnormal PMN and perhaps Mn migration in the human neonate. Studies into the mechanisms involved have suggested that the ability of these cells to deform under negative pressure is greatly reduced (Miller, 1975). More recently, Kimura *et al.* (1981) have shown that the neonatal cell does not form concanavalin A (Con A) caps when incubated with colchicine, a microtubule-disrupting drug. This finding suggests that microtubules resist depolymerization and thus the cell remains rigid and relatively unmovable. This is in spite of the fact that the neonatal cell has been reported to have normal complement and Fc receptors as well as a normal number of receptors for the chemotactic peptide N-formyl-methionyl-leucyl-phenylalanine (Pross *et al.*, 1977; D. C. Anderson *et al.*, 1981). Recent studies suggest that a major functional abnormality of the neonatal PMN may result from its inability to redistribute adhesion sites from the leading edge to the tail, thus preventing forward movement. Additional studies on the mechanism of this defect are absolutely critical to a further understanding of the chemotactic process in general and of the neonatal PMN defect specifically.

B. Lazy Leukocyte Syndrome

Miller *et al.* (1971) reported two patients who suffered recurrent episodes of otitis media, stomatitis, gingivitis, and rhinitis. These patients also had a striking neutropenia but with normal marrow granulocyte stores and adequate myeloid precursors. Epinephrine and endotoxin had no effect on the peripheral PMN count, and Rebuck skin windows failed to show the appearance of PMNs. Chemotaxis of the patients' PMNs from peripheral blood and marrow aspirates was profoundly depressed in a filter-type assay. Random motility was also examined by observing the migration of leukocytes up into a vertically placed capillary tube and was also abnormal. In fact, an attempt was made to associate decreased random motility with release of granulocytes from marrow stores. To my knowledge, no additional patients with this exact syndrome have been reported and nothing is known of the mechanisms involved. Despite the described abnormalities, the patients apparently continued to grow well and suffer no life threatening infections.

C. Congenital Icthyosis

Miller *et al.* (1973) subsequently reported two additional kindreds in which affected children had congenital icthyosis and recurrent marked infections with *Trichophyton rubrum.* In contrast to the lazy leukocyte syndrome patients, these patients had normal peripheral PMN counts and no abnormal findings on bone marrow examinations. In addition to the *T. rubrum* infections, they also suffered from pneumonia, otitis media, and impetigo. One patient had a deep pelvic abscess, and both had a marked desquamative dermatitis. PMN function studies revealed depressed chemotactic function employing a filter assay, but normal random as measured by the capillary tube method described above. Decreased chemotactic activity was also detected in the fathers of both patients but not in other family members. These cases combined with the original lazy leukocyte syndrome patients led Miller to speculate that defective random migration as measured by the capillary tube method could be correlated with abnormal marrow release of PMNs, since the current patients had normal circulating PMNs and random migration. Unfortunately, groups of additional patients with neutropenia have not been studied by this technique, and no further conclusions can be drawn about the association between the test abnormality and marrow release of granulocytes. Nor have there been additional reports, to my knowledge, of similar patients with icthyosis and defective chemotaxis, although it is highly likely that an abnormality exists in these patients. One can only speculate about the mechanism(s) of abnormal chemotaxis in these patients. Severe skin disease may result in the generation of circulating inhibitors of PMN function. Prostaglandins are produced in the skin and would be a likely candidate for such a suppressive factor. IgE levels were also not reported in the patients. It is conceivable that these patients might be related to the hyperimmunoglobulinemia E patients who often have rather severe skin disease. Further delineation of this syndrome will have to await the detection of additional patients and more in-depth studies of the mechanisms involved.

D. Hyperimmunoglobulinemia E

The initial report of such patients was made by Davis *et al.* (1966), who described two young girls with peculiar facies, fair skin, reddish hair, recurrent staphylococcal abscesses, severe eczema, dystrophic fingernail changes, and recurrent sinopulmonary infections. The abscesses were somewhat unusual in that they were seldom accompanied by surrounding erythema or marked tenderness. For this reason they were termed cold abscesses. No specific abnormality was detected in the original two patients. Subsequently, Bannatyne *et al.* (1969) described a red-haired, female CGD patient and claimed to have found a microbicidal defect in Job's syndrome. Nevertheless, subsequent studies on the original two patients as well as numerous additional individuals with the syndrome have failed to detect any abnormality in microbicidal activity.

Buckley *et al.* (1972) later described two male patients with essentially the same syndrome of peculiar facies, chronic eczema, recurrent sinopulmonary infections, repeated staphylococcal abscesses, and dystrophic fingernail changes. Each was also found to have extreme hyperimmunoglobulinemia E and a variety of subtle immunological abnormalities. None of these, which were discussed in the introduction, would seem capable of causing the recurrent abscesses suffered by the patients (Hill, 1982) except for the immediate skin hypersensitivity reactions to *Staphylococcus aureus* and *C. albicans* antigens. Clark *et al.* (1973) then reported a female patient with recurrent abscesses and mucocutaneous candidiasis who had hyperimmunoglobulinemia E and defective chemotaxis. In 1974, Hill and Quie (1974*b*) described three unusual patients with extremely high serum immunoglobulin E (IgE) levels who had very early onset of severe eczema followed by multiple superficial and deep abscesses. The abscesses were almost always due to *Staphylococcus aureus*, although a few episodes of streptococcal skin infection also occurred. In contrast to the patients described by (Buckley *et al.*, 1972) and (Clark *et al.*, 1973), these patients had no problems with chronic *Candida* infection. Because most of their infections were abscesses caused by staphylococci, we concentrated on examining their PMN function. Phagocytosis and killing of *Staphylococcus aureus* and other pathogens by the patients cells were perfectly normal and their serum supported phagocytosis of these organisms. *In vitro* chemotactic assays employing a modified Boyden chamber technique (Hill *et al.*, 1974*a*, 1975) revealed a marked depression in chemotactic responsiveness which was present consistently in these three patients and was not related to the presence or absence of infection. Additional studies failed to reveal a circulating inhibitor of chemotactic activity in the serum or plasma of the patients. A striking feature of the three patients we studied was the marked pruritis and eczema that they suffered. The mothers often brought the children into the clinic with their hands wrapped or with long sleeve shirts pulled over their hands and tied, almost like a straitjacket. I soon found out the reason for this unusual habit when I freed the arms of one child to draw blood from an antecubital vein. The child immediately began to excoriate the anterior chest wall severely and was literally dripping blood down both sides within a few minutes. Even the slightest trauma on the skin of these children elicited a rather marked wheal and flare reaction, suggesting to us that increased release of histamine contributed to the clinical findings in these patients. Rivkin and

Becker (1972) had reported that histamine inhibited the chemotactic responses of rabbit PMNs. We (Hill and Quie, 1974b) found that it also inhibited human PMN chemotaxis, a finding that has subsequently been documented by R. Anderson et al. (1977). This effect is most likely through a H2 histamine receptor the stimulation of which results in elevated levels of cyclic $3'5'$-adenosine monophosphate (cAMP) in a number of tissues, such as the parietal cells of the stomach, the heart, and most of the cells of the immune system (Fig. 4).

A subsequent report by Van Scoy et al. (1975) indicated that the disease might be familial in nature with several generations of a kindred suffering from recurrent infection and hyperimmunoglobulinemia E and demonstrating decreased PMN chemotactic responsiveness.

Subsequently, we described (Hill et al., 1976a) three additional patients with hyperimmunoglobulinemia E and defective chemotaxis who had onset of diffuse urticaria before developing severe invasive staphylococcal disease, including sepsis and sepsis with pneumonia. Addition of burimamide to the cells of one of these patients partially reversed the apparent defect in chemotactic activity.

At that time we were not sure whether our patients were similar in nature to those described by S. D. Davis et al. (1966) or by Buckley et al. (1972). We had studied a red-haired girl with peculiar facies, severe eczema, recurrent abscesses, and hyperimmunoglobulinemia E who had defective chemotaxis. For this reason we believed that the Job syndrome patients most likely had a defect in PMN movement as the underlying reason for their recurrent abscesses.

Subsequently, Dr. Hans Ochs drew blood from the original Job's syndrome patients in Seattle and air expressed it to us in Minneapolis. Much to our dismay,

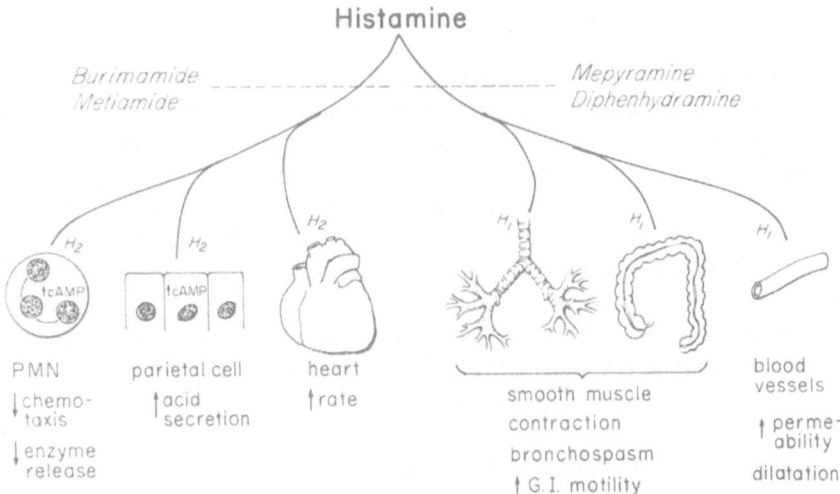

Figure 4. Effect of histamine on H1 and H2 receptors in various tissues. PMN, polymorphonuclear leukocyte. (From Hill et al., 1976a.)

the chemotactic function of these cells, which had been held *in vitro* for a total of 8–10 hr, was perfectly normal. Convinced that defective chemotaxis was a part of the syndrome, I traveled to Seattle where, in association with Drs. Hans Ochs, Robert Clark, Seymour Klebanoff, Paul Quie, and Ralph Wedgwood, we studied the original two Job's syndrome patients by both our chemotactic method (Hill *et al.*, 1974*b*, 1975) and the radiolabeled one employed by Dr. Clark's group (Gallin *et al.*, 1973). Both patients had a significant defect in PMN chemotactic responsiveness that at least partially corrected after *in vitro* incubation overnight (Hill *et al.*, 1974*d*). Subsequently a whole host of reports have appeared in the literature on similar patients with hyperimmunoglobulinemia E and recurrent infections (Chusid *et al.*, 1976; Dahl *et al.*, 1976; Jacobs and Norman, 1977; Weston *et al.*, 1977; Blum *et al.*, 1977; Issekutz *et al.*, 1978). Almost all have documented a chemotactic defect *in vitro* or *in vivo* in the patients, but the abnormality is a variable one necessitating serial testing (Hill *et al.*, 1976*b*; Issekutz *et al.*, 1978) in order to demonstrate the defect in some cases. Jacobs and Norman (1977) have also suggested a familial pattern of inheritance of the disease and linked transmission to HLA-B12 in one family. In addition to recurrent infections, at least one patient we studied went on to develop a histiocytic lymphoma of the brain (Bale *et al.*, 1977), an unusual tumor seen only in immunosuppressed transplant patients or in those with classic immunodeficiency syndromes such as the Wiskott–Aldrich syndrome. Thus, as in other immunodeficiencies, these patients may also be at increased risk for tumor cell development.

E. Allergic Disease and Recurrent Infections Without Hyperimmunoglobulinemia E

Additional patients have been described with milder allergic symptomatology, less severe infections, normal to slightly elevated IgE, and intermittent chemotactic defects that may or may not be related to the patients described above. These include infants with allergic gastrointestinal symptomatology, recurrent ear infections, and chronic diarrhea (Hill *et al.*, 1977) and adults with marked allergic rhinitis, recurrent abscesses, and bronchitis (Hill *et al.*, 1976*b*; Rubin *et al.*, 1978). *In vitro* exposure of the patients cells to an allergen to which they are sensitive results in a decrease in chemotactic function (Rubin *et al.*, 1978).

Schopfer *et al.* (1979) and later Berger *et al.* (1980) reported that the hyperimmunoglobulinemia E patients have elevated levels of specific IgE directed against *Staphylococcus aureus* and *C. albicans*, their most frequent pathogens. Still, the sera of these patients did not interfere with the interaction of these organisms with the patient's neutrophils, so a direct inhibitory or antiopsonic effect is unlikely. It may be that these patients actually have IgE-mediated allergic reactions to *Staphylococcus aureus* and *C. albicans*, resulting in mediator release, which could then depress the acute inflammatory response and permit infection to go unchecked. Further studies are needed to document or disprove such a possibility.

There are also other potential mechanisms that could explain at least some of the infections suffered by these patients. McGeady and Buckley (1975), Gallin et al. (1980), and Ogden et al. (1979) have observed depressed lymphocyte responses in severe eczema patients. Gallin et al. (1980) observed an inverse relationship between the concentration of IgE in a patient's plasma and the response of that patients lymphocytes to Con A. In addition, a lymphocyte derived inhibitor of PMN chemotaxis may be produced by the lymphocytes of these patients (Gallin et al., 1980). Further mechanistic studies are obviously needed to clarify the defects in the hyperimmunoglobulinemia E syndrome.

F. Hyperimmunoglobulinemia A

Four siblings with increased serum levels of IgA, neutropenia, eosinophilia, and defective PMN chemotaxis have been reported by Björksten and Lundmark (1976). Each sibling suffered recurrent pneumonia, otitis media, and abscesses. Eczema was present in three patients, but there was no elevation of IgE. Depressed antibody responses to immunization and depressed delayed hypersensitivity skin tests were noted. No serum inhibitors of chemotaxis were detected. Witemeyer and Van Epps (1976) described two similar patients who had depressed chemotactic activity. Both had normal IgA and IgE and all other immunologic function tests were normal.

G. Actin Dysfunction

Boxer et al. (1974) reported a 7-month-old child who presented with a history of recurrent vesicular skin lesions, abscesses, and blepharitis. Rebuck skin windows and aspirates of blister fluid failed to reveal any significant accumulation of granulocytes. In vitro studies reveal a striking defect in chemotaxis as well as an inability to ingest C3 or IgG coated particles. The patient's PMNs spread poorly on glass and formed narrow ineffective pseudopods. Actin extracted from the patient's PMNs would not polymerize normally upon stimulation with KCl, suggesting that this critical contractile protein was abnormal. To my knowledge this is the only reported PMN defect related to such an abnormality in contractile proteins. The patient died of infection.

H. Chediak–Higashi Syndrome

Patients with the Chediak–Higashi syndrome (CHS) have striking oculocutaneous albinism, large lysosomal granules, and recurrent infections (Blume and

Wolfe, 1972). Clark and Kimball (1971) first observed a defect in PMN chemotaxis in this disorder, using a micropore filter assay and a skin window technique. A significant reduction was noted in the number of cells accumulating at the skin window in the CHS patients. Furthermore, in the micropore filter assay employing a $5\text{-}\mu M$ pore size, the chemotactic activity of the patients cells equaled 41.2% of that of the controls. When the filter size was decreased to 1.2 μM, chemotaxis of the patients cells was only 9.5% of that of the controls. This finding suggested to these investigators that the large size of the granules could be impairing migration. Subsequently Oliver et al. (1975) found that the PMNs of beige mice, which have a similar disease, formed spontaneous caps when incubated with fluorescinated Con A, suggesting that microtubular polymerization was impaired. Additional studies indicated that cyclic adenosine monophosphate (cAMP) levels within the cells of a human patient with the disorders were increased compared with concentrations of cGMP (Boxer et al., 1976). Conflicting results on the presence of such a microtubule defect in CH leukocytes have appeared (White and Clawson, 1979), and there is considerable controversy over whether the defect can be corrected with agents such as ascorbate (Boxer et al., 1976; Weening et al., 1981; Gallin et al., 1979). Recently Nath et al. (1980) have demonstrated abnormal tyrosylation of the α-chain of tubulin in two brothers with the disorder, who have decreased numbers of centriole-associated microtubules. This finding constitutes more direct evidence that, at least in some patients, the functional disorders are related to abnormal microtubule function.

I. Wiskott–Aldrich Syndrome

Patients with Wiskott–Aldrich syndrome have marked eczema, thrombocytopenia, and recurrent infection. They also often have hyperimmunoglobulinemia E. Altman et al. (1974) found defective monocyte chemotaxis in these patients. In addition, they documented increased circulating levels of a lymphocyte derived chemotactic factor in their serum. These workers postulated that activated lymphocytes in the patients were releasing soluble factors that were deactivating the patients' PMNs and MNs. Although others have confirmed the defect in PMN and MN chemotaxis in these patients, no additional insights into the mechanism involved have appeared.

J. Chronic Mucocutaneous Candidiasis

Defective PMN and MN chemotactic responses have been described in a variety of patients with chronic mucocutaneous candidiasis (CMC) (Snyderman et al., 1973; Van Scoy et al., 1975; Clark et al., 1973; Fischer et al., 1980). The phagocyte abnormality may accompany or occur in the absence of associated lymphocyte dysfunction. In one case we observed normal cell-mediated immunity to *Candida* antigen in an infant with CMC whose only defect was in PMN chemotactic responsiveness (Van Scoy *et al.,* 1975). Later abnormal lymphocyte responses to *Candida* antigen developed in this child, suggesting that chronic *Candida* colonization and infection may eventually suppress lymphocyte reactivity to this organism.

K. Miscellaneous Disorders of Cellular Motility

Kartagener's syndrome is a relatively common (1 in 40,000) autosomal recessive genetic disorder in which patients suffer recurrent sinopulmonary infections and have situs inversus (Gallin, 1981). Males with the syndrome are sterile, and defects in sperm motility have been documented. The abnormality is most likely due to a deficiency of dynein arms, which are proteins with ATPase activity that are bound to microtubules and may be critical in their function. Caleb *et al.* (1977), employing both a Boyden chamber assay and a radiolabeled technique, first reported that the PMNs of these patients have defective directed and random movement. Others have subsequently confirmed these results (Gallin *et al.,* 1980; Afzelius *et al.,* 1980).

One additional patient has been described by Gallin *et al.* (1978) whose defect may be related to abnormal microtubule function. This patient had defective PMN and Mn chemotaxis, increased numbers of microtubules, and elevated levels of cellular cGMP.

Komiyama *et al.* (1979) reported a 7-year-old girl who had recurrent episodes of abscesses, otitis and mastoiditis. The nuclei of circulating PMNs were kidney shaped or bilobed like Pelger–Huet cells, and no or few secondary granules were detected. Chemotaxis and bactericidal activity of the patient's PMNs were decreased. The mechanisms behind this abnormality are unknown.

Pahwa *et al.* (1978) reported defective PMN and Mn chemotaxis in two of four patients with severe combined immunodeficiency disease. Bone marrow transplantation abolished the abnormality. Again, the mechanisms of the defect are entirely unknown.

Steerman *et al.* (1971) reported defective PMN chemotaxis in a patient with sex-linked agammaglobulinemia. The patient, a 3-year-old boy, had suffered from recurrent abscesses and pneumonia. In addition to a depression in chemotactic function, the patient's cells demonstrated less NBT dye reduction upon phagocytic challenge than did control PMNs. Bactericidal activity was also decreased for *Staphylococcus aureus* but not *E. coli.* The reduced activity against staphylococci was due primarily to decreased phagocytosis of the organisms, however.

Two extremely unusual cases have been described by Shurin *et al.* (1979). These patients suffered marked gingivitis, oral ulcerations, and erosive lesions of bone. Neutrophils from the patients failed to orient properly, and locomotion was less than 50% of normal cells. *Capnocytophaga,* a gram-negative anaerobe, was cultured from these patients. After eradication of the organism, neutrophil morphology and function returned to normal. A dialyzable substance was recovered from sonicates and culture filtrates of the organisms which affected PMNs in a similar matter after *in vitro* exposure. Obviously, this is an extremely interesting factor that may be valuable in dissecting the chemotactic response.

Defective neutrophil chemotactic responses have also been described in individuals with the juvenile form of periodontitis (Cianciola *et al.*, 1977; Clark *et al.*, 1977; Lavine *et al.*, 1979; Van Dyke *et al.*, 1979; Genco *et al.*, 1980). Cianciola *et al.* (1977) first demonstrated depressed PMN chemotaxis in nine patients with the localized form of juvenile periodontitis (LJP). Subsequently, a number of associated diseases, such as generalized juvenile periodontitis and postlocalized juvenile periodontitis, have also been found to have chemotactic defects (Van Dyke *et al.*, 1979). In contrast, patients with adult periodontitis seldom have depressed PMN chemotactic responsiveness (2 of 23) and may even have enhanced activity (10 of 23). The chemotactic defect observed in the juvenile periodonititis patients is usually an intrinsic cellular one and is present when a variety of chemoattractants are employed (Genco *et al.*, 1980). Cell directed inhibitors of chemotaxis have also been detected in the serum of periodontitis patients, but usually in a minority of the patients studied (Lavine *et al.*, 1979). Similarly, depressed monocyte chemotaxis has been observed, but it does not appear to affect many subjects with LJP.

The precise mechanism of defective PMN chemotaxis in juvenile periodontitis patients is unknown. Decreased adherence or deformability do not appear to play a role in the defect (Genco *et al.*, 1980). Of interest is the fact that unaffected family members of some of the patients also have depressed chemotactic responses, suggesting a genetic predisposition to the disorder (Genco *et al.*, 1980).

Congenital deficiency of neutrophil specific granules has been described and is associated with defective adhesion and chemotaxis, probably due to a lack of lactoferrin, a critical factor in cell attachment (Breton-Gorius *et al.*, 1980; Komiyama *et al.*, 1979; Strauss *et al.*, 1974).

Depressed chemotaxis has also been described in children with recurrent otitis media (Giebink *et al.*, 1979). No indications of the mechanisms behind these abnormalities have been presented.

L. Systemic Diseases Associated with Abnormalities of Phagocyte Movement

An ever-increasing number of systemic diseases are being reported to be associated with defects in phagocyte chemotactic activity. In evaluating the significance of these reports one should ask (1) whether patients with the disorder suffer from infections like those associated with phagocyte dysfunction; and (2) whether the degree of depression of phagocyte function is sufficient to account for the infections observed. In the absence of positive findings for these two factors, it is very unlikely that the abnormality has any clinical significance.

1. Diabetes Mellitus

It is unclear whether diabetics suffer more frequent infections, but there is no question that when infection does occur in such patients it is more severe and complicates control significantly. Diabetics do tend to suffer from cutaneous abscesses, mucocutaneous candidiasis and respiratory infection (Hill, 1979b).

Diabetes mellitus has been associated with deficiencies of PMN and monocyte chemotaxis in adults and children (Mowat and Baum, 1971b; Miller and Baker, 1972; Hill et al., 1974c, 1983; Hill, 1979b). The presence of the abnormality does not appear to correlate with the duration of disease, degree of control or with the presence of complications. Insulin has been reported to correct the PMN defect in vitro (Mowat and Baum, 1971b; Hill et al., 1974c), but has little effect in vivo (Miller and Baker, 1972). Recently, Hill et al. (1983) reported that Mn chemotaxis is also decreased in diabetics. In contrast to the results with PMNs, insulin had no effect on the diabetic Mn. Additional studies indicated that the diabetic Mn produces enhanced quantities of chemiluminescence and superoxide when challenged (Kitahara et al., 1980). This may be the result of sustained hyperglycemia commonly observed in diabetics. It is conceivable, therefore, that the defect in chemotaxis observed in the diabetic is related to auto-oxidative membrane damage resulting from enhanced respiratory burst activity of diabetic phagocytes. Treatment of diabetic individuals with the antioxidant vitamin E has recently been reported to improve chemotactic function in a limited number of patients (Hill et al., 1983).

2. Rheumatoid Arthritis and Other Collagen Vascular Diseases

To my knowledge, patients with rheumatoid arthritis do not generally suffer from cutaneous abscesses, mucocutaneous candidiasis, recurrent gastrointestinal infections, or pulmonary infections. They do, however, have an increased incidence of death from systemic infection as compared with controls. Mowat and Baum (1971a) as well as Beeuwkes and Bulsma (1974) have indicated that chemotaxis as measured by micropore filter techniques is depressed in rheumatoid arthritis, systemic lupus erythematous (SLE), and polymyositis. In general, depression averaged around 40% of that of control PMNs. Incubation of normal PMNs in rheumatoid sera or with purified rheumatoid complexes decreased chemotactic function suggesting that phagocytosis of rheumatoid factor may account for the defect observed (Mowat and Baum, 1971a). Given the degree of depression observed as well as the lack of infections typical of PMN disorders, the significance of this defect is open to some question.

3. Mannosidosis

Deficiency of α-mannosidase activity results in a marked accumulation of mannose in cells. Patients who lack this enzyme may suffer from repeated infections and can have defective PMN chemotaxis (Desnick et al., 1976). Although the precise mechanism of this defect has not been fully elucidated, it has been suggested that excessive mannose alters cell surface receptors for chemotactic factors.

4. Shwachmann's Syndrome

Shwachmann's syndrome includes pancreatic insufficiency, marrow hypoplasia and neutropenia, chondrodysplasia, growth retardation, and frequent infections. Aggett et al. (1979), studied 14 patients with the syndrome and found significantly depressed chemotaxis and random migration in 12. No other immune abnormality was detected except for occasional hypogammaglobulinemia and neutropenia in 10 of the patients. Parents of the patients had an intermediate level of chemotactic responsiveness suggesting a familial pattern of transmission of the defect.

5. Thermal Injury

Patients with severe burns have severe depression of PMN and MN chemotaxis proportional to the size and severity of the burn (Warden et al., 1974; Altman et al., 1977a,b). After sustaining burns, patients may lose the specific granules from their PMNs, resulting in a decrease in PMN levels of lysozyme and elevated levels of this enzyme in their plasma (Gallin et al., 1980; J. M. Davis et al., 1980). A correlation has been observed between PMN lysozyme levels and chemotactic responsiveness. Alternatively, products released by the injured skin or even topical medications used in burn therapy may affect cell movement.

6. Hemodialysis Patients

Patients undergoing hemodialysis and renal transplantation have been reported to have decreased chemotactic responses (Warden and Maxwell, 1976). In general the degree of depression paralleled the elevation in BUN and creatinine observed in the patients or could be correlated with steroid doses in transplant patients. Hemodialysis leukopenia and decreased random motility of PMNs has been attributed by Henderson et al. (1975) to the use of cellulose membranes. Klempner and associates (1980) have suggested that hemodialysis induced neutropenia activates complement, which then interacts with circulating PMNs and depletes a population of cells that possess receptors for the Fc fragment of IgG. This leaves nonreceptor bearing, less active PMNs in the circulation and results in the observed depression of chemotaxis.

7. Viral Infections

Viral infections including those due to measles, herpesvirus, and influenzae have been reported to depress PMN and Mn chemotaxis (R. Anderson *et al.,* 1976*b;* Abramson *et al.,* 1982; Snyderman and Pike, 1978). The mechanism of the depression of chemotaxis by viruses is not known. Abramson *et al.* (1982), have suggested, however, that exposure of PMNs to influenza A inhibits lysosome–phagosome fusion.

8. Malnutrition

Malnutrition has been reported to depress PMN chemotactic responses; however, other studies have suggested that concurrent infection was more responsible for the defect in cell movement than the malnutrition *per se* (Rosen *et al.,* 1975). Rich *et al.* (1977) studied 13 age-matched nourished and malnourished children in Ghana and report normal to enhanced chemotactic activity in these children. It is conceivable that mild malnutrition may actually enhance immune function in some cases. Alternatively, low-grade or chronic infection may actually enhance rather than depress phagocyte function.

9. Bacterial Infection

Although several investigators have reported defective chemotactic respones in patients with infection (Mowat and Baum, 1971*c;* McCall *et al.,* 1971), these patients have either been studied later in their course, after antimicrobial therapy, or when severely ill with toxic granulations in their PMNs (Hill and Quie, 1974*a*). When otherwise healthy persons with cutaneous (Hill *et al.,* 1974*b*), respiratory (Hill *et al.,* 1974*e*), and systemic bacterial infection (Hill *et al.,* 1974*a*) are studied, PMN chemotactic function is generally found to be enhanced.

M. Humoral Defects Resulting in Defective Phagocytic Migration

Defective production of the complement associated chemotactic factor, C5a, is associated with total absence of C3 and C5 and results in defective inflammatory responses and severe and recurrent infections (Alper *et al.,* 1972, 1976; Ballow *et al.,* 1975; Rosenfeld *et al.,* 1976). Crohn's disease has also been associated with defective chemotaxis, which may result from faulty *in vivo* generation of inflammatory mediators (Segal and Loewi, 1976).

Ward and associates have described and characterized a serum inactivator of chemotactic factors in several diseases including Hodgkin's disease, sarcoidosis, leprosy, and cirrhosis (Ward and Berenberg, 1974; Ward *et al.,* 1976; Ward and Ozols, 1976; Maderazo *et al.,* 1975, 1976). The activity is present in normal human serum in low levels but increases in the diseases mentioned above. The factor irreversibly inhibits chemotactic factors, probably through an aminopeptidase activity. Patients with high levels of the factor generally have depressed *in vivo* skin test responses. Van Epps *et al.* (1974) also have described a serum inhibitor of chemotactic factors that is apparent in the serum of patients with anergy.

A cell-directed inhibitor of chemotactic function was described in a patient who was later found to also have a marked defect in microbicidal activity (Ward and Schlegel, 1969). Clark and Klebanoff (1978) reported two patients, a male and female, with the autosomal recessive form of CGD who also had defective PMN chemotactic responses. Each had a high-molecular-weight cell-directed inhibitor of chemotaxis in the serum. Smith *et al.* (1972) and Soriano *et al.* (1973) described two patients with a serum inhibitor of chemotaxis that was reversed by the addition of normal plasma. The authors attributed this unusual phenomena to the presence in plasma of a normal antagonist to a serum inhibitor of chemotaxis; a very difficult mechanism to understand, to say the least. Neither of these "inhibitors" has been further defined, and the mechanism of their action is unknown.

The monoclonal immunoglobulin observed in IgA myeloma has also been reported to inhibit phagocyte chemotaxis (Van Epps and Williams, 1978). In addition, Snyderman and Pike (1978) have shown that tumors may produce factors that inhibit chemotaxis of monocytes and allow progression of the malignancy.

Patients with nephritis and nephrotic syndrome have been reported to have circulating chemotactic factors in their serum and depressed PMN motility (Norman and Miller, 1973, 1974). Defective chemotaxis probably results from the presence of these circulating factors, which serve to deactivate PMNs.

Kramer *et al.* (1980) described a fascinating 46-year-old man who had a 20-year history of recurrent cutaneous staphylococcal infections. An IgG was isolated from the patient's serum that irreversibly inhibited chemotaxis and random migration of normal PMNs without affecting adherence, phagocytosis, degranulation, or superoxide formation.

IV. CLINICAL ABNORMALITIES OF PHAGOCYTIC INGESTION

PMNs and Mns are voracious eaters that ingest most properly opsonized particles without delay. Moreover, the phagocytic response is a strong one that persists intact after considerable manipulation or damage to the cell. Abnormalities of ingestion have been described, but in only a few cases have these been well documented. Clearly, the patient with the actin dysfunction syndrome mentioned earlier (Boxer et al., 1974) had markedly decreased to absent phagocytic uptake. Less striking decreases in uptake have been reported in severely iron-deficient children (MacDougall et al., 1975) and in malnourished persons with infection (Schopfer and Douglas, 1976). Hyperalimentation with attendant hypophosphatemia has also been reported to decrease uptake of particles as well as cell movement (Craddock et al., 1974). Except in the instance of actin dysfunction, it is highly unlikely that the degree of phagocytic dysfunction in these syndromes is sufficient to cause clinical abnormalities. Phagocytic or ingestion disorders are therefore of relatively minor importance.

V. CLINICAL ABNORMALITIES OF MICROBICIDAL ACTIVITY

In general, the infections suffered by patients with profound intracellular microbicidal defects are more severe than those associated with defects in phagocyte movement. It does not matter how slow a phagocyte arrives at an area of bacterial invasion; once it ingests an offending microbe, it still has the power to kill it, if microbicidal mechansims are intact. In contrast, in the severe microbicidal defects the PMN, Mn and Mac cannot kill ingested microorganism and this leads to severe persistent infections, poor wound healing, and granuloma formation. Chronic granulomatous disease was once termed fatal granulomatous disease (Berendes et al., 1957) because of the marked granulomatous lesions that appeared and the almost universal fatal outcome. Fortunately, as we have come to understand the basic pathophysiology of these syndromes, it has been possible to devise more rapid and more efficacious therapeutic regimens so that many patients with the disorder survive well into adulthood.

Deep-seated cutaneous, visceral, and bone abscesses are not uncommon in these disorders, as are chronic sinopulmonary infections. In many cases the deep location of the abscesses may preclude appropriate diagnostic procedures, and infection readily becomes indolent and persistent. Both the respiratory and gastrointestinal tracts, in which phagocytes are particularly important, are heavily involved in most patients. In general, viral infections are not a major problem, although at least one of our patients with a profound bactericidal defect has suffered from severe progressive varicella and what was probably herpesvirus encephalitis. It should be noted that cell-mediated immune function including natural killer cell activity in this patient was normal. Thus, at least in my opinion, these patients should be watched closely during viral infections, and one should be very cautious in using live virus vaccines in such patients. Several unreported reactions to such immunizations have occurred.

A. Chronic Granulomatous Disease

1. Clinical Presentation

The major clinical manifestations of CGD include recurrent pulmonary infections, cutaneous and visceral abscesses, lymphadenitis, osteomyelitis, liver abscesses, and obstructive phemomena from granuloma formation (Mills and Quie, 1980; Johnston and Newman, 1977). Pulmonary infection tends to be presistent and pneumonias often become encapsulated. Liver abscesses are extremely common, as are episodes of osteomyelitis of the small bones of the hands and feet. Diarrhea and perianal abscess occur in the up to 20% of patients (Mills and Quie, 1980). Malabsorption is not uncommon, and irregular-shaped brownish yellow histiocytes are characteristically observed in the lamina propria of the small bowel (Ament and Ochs, 1973). In general the major pathogens are catalase-producing organisms or ones that fail to produce H_2O_2, such as *Staphylococcus, Klebsiella, Escherichia coli, Serratia, Pseudomonas, Aspergillus, Candida,* and *Salmonella* (Johnston and Newman, 1977). Several patients have also been infected with *Nocardia* and *Mycobacterium*, both of which are extremely difficult to eradicate. Fungal infections with agents such as *Aspergillus, Torulopsis,* and *Cadida* are also common (Cohen *et al.*, 1981). In general these patients are resistant to streptococci, *Hemophilus influenzae*, and other organisms that produce H_2O_2 and no catalase.

Dermatitis and lymphademitis is extremely common in CGD, and cystitis with bladder granulomas has been reported in the literature. Dysuria associated with such bladder lesions was the only presenting finding in a 5-year old-patient of ours with CGD. Granuloma formation can result in gastric outlet obstruction (Griscom *et al.*, 1974), a finding that has occurred in two of our patients. Obstruction within the genitourinary tract by granuloma is also not uncommon. Esophagitis, otitis, arthritis, and even sepsis occasionally occur, and chorioretinal lesions have been described (Johnston and Newman, 1977). The patients are usually detected within the first 2 years of life, although patients have attained young adulthood (23 years) before actual diagnosis (Balfour *et al.*, 1971). A number of patients have not lived into middle age. In those who have not survived, pulmonary disease has been the major cause of death.

2. Functional Abnormalities

In spite of the fact that this disease was intitally described as early as 1954, we still do not precisely understand the underlying defect in the disorder. Quie *et al.* (1967) first described the abnormality in intracellular killing by the PMN of these patients. Holmes *et al.* (1967) then documented a defect in oxidative metabolism and the lack of hexose monophosphate shunt stimulation and H_2O_2 production by the PMNs. In addition, these patients fail to reduce NBT dye to a blue-black deposit within their PMNs. Production of $^{14}CO_2$ from $[1\text{-}^{14}C]$ glucose is also absent due to the failure of $NADP^+$ to stimulate the hexose monophosphate shunt. Chemiluminescence production is essentially absent (Fig. 3) because of the failure to produce O_2^-, H_2O_2 and other high-energy oxygen radicals.

In most cases, other PMN functions such as chemotaxis, adhesion, degranulation, and lysosomal enzyme release are normal in CGD PMNs (Mills and Quie, 1980). However, Ward and Schlegel (1969) and Clark and Klebanoff (1978) have reported a total of three CGD patients with decreased chemotactic responses due to cell-directed serum inhibitor(s) of chemotaxis. In their original report, Quie et al. (1967) suggested that degranulation might also be abnormal in the CGD PMN. Gold et al. (1974) later reported delayed degranulation responses during the first 15 min after ingestion of particulate matter; no abnormality was detected after 30 min of incubation, however. Recently, Ingraham et al. (1981) have shown by electron spin resonance that CGD PMNs fail to show an increase in membrane fluidity following particle uptake.

3. Mechanisms

The underlying mechanism behind the microbicidal defect in CGD is related to a failure to generate sufficient superoxide anion (O_2^-) hydrogen peroxide, and other oxygen intermediates essential in bacterial killing (Curnutte et al., 1975; Briggs et al., 1977). All forms of CGD have this defect in oxidative metabolism and carriers of the X-linked type have intermediate levels of superoxide generation (Borregaard et al., 1979). The abnormality is expressed by a variety of cells throughout the body, including PMNs, Mns, lymphocytes, and perhaps fibroblasts, which has led some workers to suggest that the disease might be diagnosed prenatally (Newburger et al., 1979; Peerless and Stiehm, 1983).

The disease occurs most commonly in males (6:1) and is sex linked (Johnston and Newman, 1977). Female carriers may be detected by their intermediate level of NBT dye reduction, chemiluminescence generation, superoxide production, and intracellular microbicidal activity. In spite of the partial defect, carriers are most often said to be asymptomatic. A recent report on 15 carrier females did, however, indicate that five suffered from what appeared to be discoid lupus erythematosus, and five others had recurrent apthouslike stomatitis (Borregard et al., 1981). A survey of 10 discoid lupus patients revealed that two were actually carriers of CGD; a fact that should be kept in mind. One additional carrier of CGD was also a chronic carrier of Salmonella (Moellering and Weinberg, 1970).

At least in the sex-linked form of the disease, the major defect appears to be in a deficiency of NADPH oxidase activity which catalyzes the one electron reduction of molecular oxygen to superoxide anion (Hohn and Lehrer, 1975; McPhail et al., 1977). While actual deficiency of the enzyme has been reported, other papers have implicated a defective enzyme with altered affinity or kinetic characteristics (Lew et al., 1981). The enzyme appears to be closely associated with the cell membrane, although it may be present in a granule fraction. Of interest is the fact that there appears to be a close linkage between the sex-linked form of CGD and the lack of an X-linked, Kell-related surface antigen, Kx (Densen *et al.*, 1981). This antigen is normally present on the surface of PMNs, suggesting that there may be some relationship between the absence of this surface antigen and oxidase activity.

Segal *et al.* (1978) initially reported that four patients with CGD and that two carrier mothers had absence or gross abnormalities in a cytochrome *b* that is a component of the oxidase system that transports electrons to molecular oxygen. Subsequent studies (Segal *et al.*, 1983) have found that the cytochrome *b* was absent in all 19 of 19 male patients with CGD and markedly reduced in all the heterozygous carriers. Thus, absence of this cytochrome may be the molecular defect in the sex-linked form of CGD.

Chronic granulomatous disease also occurs in female patients (Holmes *et al.*, 1970), initially thought to be the result of glutathione peroxidase deficiency. Because of the absence of this enzyme, H_2O_2 would be expected to build up in the cell, less $NADP^+$ would be generated (Fig. 2), and auto-oxidative damage to the cell would occur. Bass *et al.* (1977) have subsequently shown, however, that PMNs of animals completely lacking glutathione peroxidase maintain the postphagocytic respiratory burst and have bactericidal activity. Moreover, other CGD patients, including some males, with a similar inheritance pattern have been shown to have normal levels of this enzyme (Johnston and Newman, 1977). Mills, *et al.* (1980*a,b*) more recently indicated that mothers of female cases of CGD may also have intermediate metabolic responses when a luminol-enhanced chemiluminescence assay is employed. The phenotypic variation in the disease, evidence of two leukocyte populations in patients and their mothers with this form of the disease, low but detectable CL in the patients, and an intermediate level in the mothers suggest an X-linked inheritance with X-chromosome inactivation, according to the Lyon hypothesis. Of great interest is the report of Segal *et al.* (1983) mentioned above, which indicated that patients with the autosomal recessive form of the disease have cytochrome *b* but it is nonfunctional. Thus, absence or malfunction of this heme-containing protein responsible for electron transfer may be the critical defect in these two forms of CGD.

A third form of the disease was first reported by Gray *et al.* (1973) in patients with a complete abscence of erythrocyte and leukocyte glucose 6-phosphate dehydrogenase (G6PD). Three male siblings in a Canadian family suffered from chronic nonsperocytic hemolytic anemia, recurrent lymphadenitis and were found to have a defect in PMN bactericidal and metabolic activity. The mother had intermediate abnormalities. The infections suffered by these patients were generally less severe than in the other forms of CGD, and one sibling was even free from infection. The absence of G6PD, the first enzyme in the hexose monophosphate shunt, would be expected to result in failure to regenerate NADPH, which is critical in the initial reduction of O_2 to O_2^-. Thus, the initial step in the generation of microbicidal activity would be arrested in these patients. In general the metabolic and killing defect in G6PD deficiency is not as severe as it is in the classical forms of CGD. The patients' cells failed to reduce significant amounts of NBT (< 1%) while the mothers had intermediate values (42%, 55%, and 72% versus 90% in the unaffected father.)

A subsequent patient described by Corberand *et al.* (1978) had recurrent infections associated with decreased leukocyte G6PD (< 3%) but normal erythrocyte G6PD. The patient's PMNs failed to reduce NBT and to kill *Staphylococcus aureus*. The mother's leukocytes had intermediate levels of G6PD and functional activity. Rutenberg *et al.* (1977) have reported multiple enzyme defects involving G6PD in a family with CGD.

B. Lipochrome Histiocytosis

Ford *et al.* (1962) described a syndrome of lipochrome pigmentation of histiocytes, hypergammaglobulinemia, pulmonary infiltrates, splenomegaly, rheumatoid arthritis, and susceptibility to infection, which shared several characteristics with CGD. The patients did not, however, show the development of granulomatous lesions. Rodey *et al.* (1970) subsequently demonstrated that two sisters with the disorder had a defect in PMN oxidative metabolism like that in CGD. Furthermore, their PMNs failed to kill staphylococci. The mother and an unaffected female siblings had normal PMN function and oxidative metabolism.

C. Myeloperoxidase Deficiency

Deficiency of myeloperoxidase has been described as a hereditary disorder with autosomal recessive inheritance (Lehrer and Cline, 1969). Myeloperoxidase (MPD), a lysosomal enzyme, catalyzes the reaction between H_2O_2 and a halide ion to form a hypohalite compound such as ^-OCl. This reaction is probably important in bactericidal, fungicidal, and tumoricidal activity. The patient described by Lehrer and Cline (1969) had infections with *Candida albicans* and was shown to have a defect in bactericidal and fungicidal mechanisms. Subsequently, A. T. Davis, *et al.* (1971) reported a 58-year-old male patient with acute myelomonocytic leukemia who had infection, with *C. albicans* and markedly decreased levels of MPO in his PMNs, as determined by histochemical staining techniques. The pateint's cells also demonstrated an early 30 and 60 min) defect in bactericidal activity that disappeared after 4 hr of incubation. Approximately 15 patients with markedly decreased to absent levels of MPO have been described in the literature according to Mills and Quie (1980), four of whom have had serious or prolonged *Candida* infections. Other patients with marked deficiency of myeloperoxidase have not, however, demonstrated any unusual susceptibility to infection, so the precise role of this enzyme in the host defense mechanism has not been determined.

Rosen and Klebanoff (1976) reported that the chemiluminescence response and superoxide production by myeloperoxidase deficient PMNs are different from normals in that (1) the peak is lower and occurs slightly later, and (2) the fall-off in chemiluminescence or O_2^- production is less rapid, so that overall O_2^- generation is actually higher in the MPO-deficient cells. This could account for the early defect in microbicidal activity followed by the return to normal killing over a 4-hr period.

Patients with Chediak–Higaski (CH) syndrome (Section III. H) have a defect in lysosomal granule release into phagocyte vacoules, which results in a relative deficiency of MPO. This is probably due to abnormal microtubule function in these patients and may contribute to their increased susceptibility to infection. Shortly after phagocytic ingestion, there is little peroxidase activity present in phagocytic vacoules of the CH patients. Later some activity may be present but, in general, bactericidal and candicidal activity is depressed. Alterations in cAMP: cGMP ratios have been described in the PMNs of patients with the syndrome, which could potentially explain the microtubule defect (Boxer *et al.*, 1976) and offer at least some hope for successful therapeutic intervention.

D. Bilobed Nucleus Syndrome

Two patients with intermittent neutropenia and recurrent infection have been reported by Komiyama *et al.* (1979) and Strauss *et al.* (1974). These patients had peculiar bilobed or kidney bean-shaped nuclei in their PMNs, decreased specific granules, defective chemotaxis, and impaired bactericidal activity. Nitroblue tetrazolium dye reduction and phagocytic uptake were normal. The reasons for the observed abnormalities are unclear at this time.

E. Glutathione Synthetase Deficiency

Glutathione participates in the detoxification of H_2O_2 within phagocytes. Deficiency of this substance could conceivably result in a buildup of H_2O_2 and result in auto-oxidative cell damage. Gluthathione synthetase deficiency has been reported in association with increased susceptibility to infection (Spielberg *et al.*, 1979). The PMNs from the patients had normal phagocytosis, chemotaxis, and glucose oxidation, but with increased levels of H_2O_2. Depressed bactericidal activity was observed as well as abnormal microtubule formation, which probably resulted from exposure to high levels of H_2O_2.

Partial gluthathione reductase deficiency has also been described in two female patients and one male patient (Roos *et al.* 1979). The patients had no particular problem with recurrent infections but suffered episodes of hemolysis associated with oxidant stress and had early development of cataracts. Bactericidal activity of the patients' PMNs were normal. Oxygen uptake, H_2O_2 production, and hexose monophosphate shunt activity (HMP) shut off after 5 to 15 min. This was presumably due to the buildup of H_2O_2 within the cell, leading to damage and the lack of $NADP^+$ formation.

F. Miscellaneous Deficiencies of Microbicidal Activity

A number of miscellaneous defects in microbicidal activity have been described that do not fit into any known category. In general, these have been isolated case reports, and little is known about the mechanisms involved.

Van der Meer *et al.* (1975) described what appeared to be a familial defect in microbicidal activity that was the result of the absence of a cell surface receptor on phagocytes. Three members of the family had early onset of recurrent, cutaneous, and respiratory infections, and the father suffered from perianal fistulas. The patients' cells responded with increased respiratory burst activity when exposed to IgG-coated particles, but did not respond in a similar fashion to unopsonized latex particles. Thus, such persons may lack a cell surface component necessary for respiratory burst activation, but have one that is responsive to IgG-coated particles. In contrast, Harvath and Anderson (1979) described a 2-year-old boy with recurrent bacterial infection whose PMNs failed to respond to opsonized particles. Respiratory burst activity after exposure to soluble stimulants such as PMA and sodium fluoride was normal, however. Such cases suggest that there may be individual mechanisms for initiating the respiratory burst that may become defective.

Patients with Down's syndrome have been reported to have a variety of PMN abnormalities, including defects in attachment, chemotactic, and bactericidal activity (Rosner *et al.*, 1973; Gregory *et al.*, 1972). In general the bactericidal capacity of the Down's syndrome patient's PMNs may be decreased, especially for *Staphylococcus aureus*. The depression is variable, however, and no specific metabolic defect has been defined to explain the abnormality.

Defective bactericidal activity has also been reported in patients with severe infections and toxic granulations (McCall *et al.*, 1971) and in patients with isolated defects in staphylococcal killing (Mandell, 1972; W. C. Davis *et al.*, 1968). Stressed human neonates (Shigeoka *et al.*, 1979; 1981; Mills *et al.*, 1979; Wright *et al.*, 1975) and patients with diabetes mellitus (Hill, 1979b) may also have decreased bactericidal activity and decreased metabolic responses. The reasons for these abnormalities are unclear; however, autooxidative damage to the PMN is one distinct possibility in both cases (Shigeoka, *et al.*, 1981; Hill *et al.*, 1983).

VI. THERAPY OF PHAGOCYTE DISORDERS

A. General Measures

Management of patients with granulocyte disorders is often quite difficult, since no specific curative therapeutic regimens are known. It is essential, however, that the functional and biochemical defect be defined as specifically as possible. Such information is critical to appropriate genetic counseling but, in addition, defining the exact defect has usually led to a better prognosis and improvement in the quality of life for most patients. If the underlying defect is known, the most likely type of infection can be induced and early more appropriate therapy instituted. Furthermore, invasive procedures such as surgery to drain an abscess or remove an infected lymph node can be limited in diseases such as CGD, in which healing is notoriously poor.

B. Antimicrobial Therapy

An aggressive approach to the diagnosis of the specific infectious agent is essential in these patients. Needle aspiration, biopsy, and other means of obtaining infected tissue are indicated so that one can select the most appropriate antimicrobial agent. In addition to determining routine antibiotic sensitivities in order to select appropriate antimicrobial agents, one must also consider penetration of the drug into phagocytes, especially in microbicidal defects. Recent studies have suggested that a number of antibiotics, including clindamycin, sulfa, sulfamethoxazole/trimethoprim, and rifampin, actively concentrate (4–40 X) in PMNs and reach levels cidal to organisms that are not commonly sensitive to these agents (Seger et al., 1981; Gmünder and Seger, 1981; Klempner and Styrt, 1981; Ezer and Soothill, 1974). In general, the duration of antimicrobial therapy needs to be longer than in normal persons, since persistence and relapse is a common problem.

C. Leukocyte, Blood, or Plasma Therapy

Granulocyte transfusions have been employed in patients with CGD and deep-seated infection with some success (Raubitschek et al., 1973). Blood, plasma, and granulocyte transfusions have also been successful in the treatment of overwhelming sepsis in stressed neonates (Hill, 1981b; Shigeoka et al., 1978; Christensen et al., 1982). Such therapy has not gained widespread use in adult patients, however, probably because it is quite difficult to supply sufficient numbers of PMNs by this technique (Strauss et al., 1981).

D. Prophylaxis

Indiscriminate use of antibiotic prophylaxis is usually of no benefit. Specific prophylaxis when one particular agent such as staphylococci is usually involved, however, is often quite helpful (Philippart *et al.*, 1972). More recently, Johnston *et al.* (1975) suggested that sulfisoxazole may decrease infectious complications in CGD patients and augment the bactericidal activity of their PMNs. The change in killing was not great, however, so that the beneficial effect most likely results from the marked tendency of sulfisoxazole concentrate within phagocytes.

Soderberg-Warner *et al.* (1983) have also suggested that trimethoprim sulfa prophylaxis is effective in patients with the hyperimmunoglobulinemia E syndrome, but their study was limited to two patients with the disorder.

E. Immunomodulation

Ideal therapy of a granulocyte disorders would involve biochemical correction of the basic underlying mechanism. A number of attempts have been made to do this, with some success. Chediak–Higashi syndrome patients have altered cyclic nucleotide metabolism within their phagocytes, which results in poor microtubule function, defective chemotaxis, decreased degranulation, and defective bactericidal activity. Oliver and Zurier (1976) first showed that cholinergic agonist and cGMP could correct the microtubule defect in beige mice and in two patients with CHS. Subsequently, Boxer *et al.* (1976) indicated that ascorbic acid partially reversed abnormal cyclic nucleotide levels in the PMNs of a CHS patient and corrected the functional chemotactic and degranulation defects. Gallin *et al.* (1979), however, found that such therapy had no effect on the clinical course in two patients with the syndrome, despite improved *in vitro* function of their PMNs. Weening *et al.* (1981) reported that ascorbate therapy did improve both the clinical course and functional phagocyte activity of a single patient with the syndrome. Thus, it seems at least worthwhile to attempt a trial of therapy with this agent in CHS. The one report of the development of an accelerated lymphomatous phase in a patient treated with ascorbate probably had nothing to do with the therapy (Saitoh *et al.*, 1981).

Ascorbate has also been employed in patients with the hyperimmunoglobulinemia E syndrome (Hill, 1979*a*), asthma (R. Anderson *et al.*, 1980), and CGD (R. Anderson, 1981; R. Anderson and Dittrich, 1979) with some success. Unfortunately, the natural course of the disease is so variable that it is quite difficult to tell whether therapy is beneficial.

Boxer *et al.* (1979) have reported that vitamin E therapy improves PMN function in glutathione synthetase deficiency by protecting membrane components from toxin oxygen species. Hill *et al.* (1983) reported that such therapy also improved MN chemotactic responsiveness in diabetics. The use of scavengers of toxic oxygen species or enzymes such as catalase or superoxide dismutase may have great potential in the therapy of auto-oxidative disorders.

Levamisole has been reported to improve chemotactic function of PMN and Mns and to alter cellular cyclic nucleotide levels (Hogan and Hill, 1978; R. Anderson et al., 1976a; Wright et al., 1977; Pike and Snyderman, 1976). Several investigators have reported a beneficial effect of this agent in patients with chemotactic defects with and without hyperimmunoglobulinemia E (Rebora et al., 1980; Businco et al., 1981). Recently, however, Donabedian et al., (1982) indicated that levamisole is inferior to placebo in the treatment of the hyper-immunoglobulinemia E syndrome (Job's syndrome). The precise role for this agent in the therapy of granulocyte disorders remains in doubt, especially since it has been reported to cause granulocytopenia (Rosenthal et al., 1976).

If defective chemotactic function in the hyperimmunoglobulinemia E syndrome is related to histamine stimulation of cAMP within PMNs, then a H_2 histamine blocking agent might have an effect in this disorder. In 1976 Hill et al. (1976a) reported that in vitro incubation of such patients cells with the H_2 histamine blocking agent, burimamide, had an effect to increase chemotactic responsiveness. Mawhinney et al. (1980) reported that in vivo therapy with cimetidine in a patient with the hyperimmunoglobulinemia E syndrome abolished the chemotactic defect and decreased the number of infectious complications. Obviously, many more such persons will have to be studied in a controlled fashion before any conclusions can be drawn about the potential efficacy of such agents.

There are, of course, a number of additional immunomodulatory agents under investigation. These include muramyl dipeptide, poly A:U, and other agents that may someday find usefulness in the therapy of these disorders. Meantime, those of us who are interested in phagocytes will continue to probe for the underlying metabolic, biochemical, and genetic abnormalities that result in these devastating diseases. It is hoped that such studies will provide further insights into normal and abnormal host-defense mechanisms and cell biology, in general.

ACKNOWLEDGMENTS

I wish to acknowledge the generous secretarial assistance of Joleen Langston and Jana Lawton.

VII. REFERENCES

Abramson, J. S., Giebink, G. S., and Quie, P. G., 1982, Influenzae A virus-induced polymor-phonuclear leukocyte dysfunction in the pathogenesis of experimental pneumococcal otitis media, Infect. Immun. 36:289.

Afzelius, B. A., Ewetz, I., Palmblad, J., Uden, A. M., and Venizelos, N., 1980, Structure and function of neutrophil leukocytes from patients with the immotile-cilia syndrome, *Acta Med. Scand.* **208**:145.

Aggett, P. G., Harries, J. T., Harvey, B. A. M., and Soothill, J. F., 1979, An inherited defect of neutrophil mobility in Shwachmann syndrome, *J. Pediatr.* **94**:391.

Allen, R. C., and Loose, L. D., 1976, Phagocytic activation of a luminol-dependent chemiluminescence in rabbit alveolar and peritoneal macrophages, *Biochem. Biophys. Res. Commun.* **69**:245.

Allen, R. C., Yevich, S. J., Orth, R. W., and Steel, R. H., 1974, The superoxide anion and singlet molecular oxygen: Their role in the microbicidal activity of the polymorphonuclear leukocyte, *Biochem. Biophys. Res. Commun.* **60**:909.

Allred, C. D., Shigeoka, A. O., and Hill, H. R., 1979, Evaluation of Group B streptococcal opsonins by radiolabeled bacterial uptake, *J. Immun. Methods* **25**:355.

Allred, C. D., Margetts, J., and Hill, H. R., 1980, Luminol induced neutrophil chemiluminescence, *Biochem. Biophys. Acta* **631**:380.

Alper, C. A., Cotton, H. R., Rosen, F. S., Rabson, A. R., MacNab, G. M., and Gear, J. S. S., 1972, Homozygous deficiency of C3 in a patient with repeated infections, *Lancet* **2**:1179.

Alper, C. A., Colten, H. R., Gear, J. S. S., Rabson, A. R., and Rosen, F. S., 1976, Homozygous human C3 deficiency, *J. Clin. Invest.* **57**:222.

Altman, L. C., Snyderman, R., and Blaese, R. M., 1974, Abnormalities of chemotactic lymphokine synthesis and mononuclear leukocyte chemotaxis in Wiskott-Aldrich syndrome, *J. Clin. Invest.* **54**:486.

Altman, L. C., Furukawa, C. T., and Klebanoff, S. J., 1977*a*, Depressed mononuclear leukocyte chemotaxis in thermally injured patients, *J. Immunol.* **119**:199.

Altman, L. C., Furukawa, C. T., and Klebanoff, S. J., 1977*b*, Defective polymorphonuclear leukocyte (PMN) function in thermally injured patients, *Clin. Res.* **25**:117A. (Abstr.)

Ament, M. E., and Ochs, H. D., 1973, Gastrointestinal manifestations of chronic granulomatous disease, *N. Engl. J. Med.* **288**:382.

Anderson, D. C., Hughes, B. J., and Smith, C. W., 1981, Abnormal mobility of neonatal polymorphonuclear leukocytes. Relationship of impaired redistribution of surface adhesion sites by chemotactic factor or colchicine, *J. Clin. Invest.* **68**:863.

Anderson, R., 1981, Assessment of oral ascorbate in three children with chronic granulomatous disease and defective neutrophil motility over a 2 year period, *Clin. Exp. Immunol.* **43**:180.

Anderson, R., and Dittrich, O. C., 1979, Effects of ascorbate on leucocytes. Part IV. Increased neutrophil function and clinical improvement after oral ascorbate in two patients with chronic granulomatous disease, *South Afr. Med. J.* **56**:476.

Anderson, R., Glover, A., Koornhof, H. J., and Rabson, A. R., 1976*a*, In vitro stimulation of neutrophil motility by levamisole: Maintenance of cGMP levels in chemotactically stimulated levamisole-treated neutrophils, *J. Immunol.* **117**:428.

Anderson, R., Rabson, A. R., Sher, R., and Koornhof, H. J., 1976*b*, Defective neutrophil motility in children with measles, *J. Pediatr.* **89**:27.

Anderson, R., Glover, A., and Rabson, A. R., 1977, The in vitro effects of histamine and metiamide on neutrophil motility and their relationship to intracellular cyclic nucleotide levels, *J. Immunol.* **118**:1690.

Anderson, R., Hay, I., Van Wyk, H., Oosthuizen, R., and Theron, A., 1980, The effect of ascorbate on cellular humoral immunity in asthmatic children, *South Afr. Med. J.* **58**:974.

Arnaout, M. A., Pitt, J., Cohen, H. J., Melamed, J., Rosen, F. S., and Colten, H. R., 1982, Deficiency of a granulocyte-membrane glycoprotein in a boy with recurrent bacterial infections, *N. Engl. J. Med.* **306**:693.

Baehner, R. L., 1974, Molecular basis for functional disorders of phagocytes, *J. Pediatr.* **84:** 317.

Baehner, R. L., and Nathan, D. G., 1968, Quantitative nitroblue tetrazolium test in chronic granulomatous disease, *N. Engl. J. Med.* **278:**971.

Bale, J. F., Jr., Wilson, J. F., and Hill, H. R., 1977, Fatal histiocytic lymphoma of the brain associated with hyperimmunoglobulinemia E and recurrent infections, *Cancer* **39:**2386.

Balfour, H. H., Shehan, J. J., Speicher, C. C., and Kauder, E., 1971, Chronic granulomatous disease of childhood in a 23 year old man, *JAMA* **7:**960.

Ballow, M., Shira, J. E., Harden, L., Yang, S. Y., and Day, N. K., 1975, Complete absence of the third component of complement in man, *J. Clin. Invest.* **56:**703.

Bannatyne, R. M., Skawrom, P. N., and Weber, J. L., 1969, Job's syndrome: A variant of chronic granulomatous disease, *J. Pediatr.* **75:**236.

Bass, D. A., DeChatelet, L. R., Burk, R. F., Shirley, P., and Szejda, P., 1977, Polymorphonuclear leukocyte bactericidal activity and oxidative metabolism during glutathione peroxidase deficiency, *Infect. Immun.* **18:**78.

Bassaris, H. P., Lianou, P. E., Shoutelis, A. T., Papavassiliou, J. T., and Phair, J. P., 1982, Defective adherence of polymorphonuclear leukocytes to nylon induced by thalassemic serum, *J. Infect. Dis.* **146:**52.

Baum, J., Mowat, A. G., and Kirk, J. A., 1971, A simplified method for the measurement of chemotaxis of polymorphonuclear leukocytes from human blood, *J. Lab. Clin. Med.* **77:** 501.

Beeuwkes, H., and Bulsma, A., 1974, Reduced chemotaxis of polymorphonuclear leukocytes in sera from patients with rheumatoid arthritis, *Antonïe van Leeuwenhock* **40:**233.

Berendes, H., Bridges, R. H., and Good, R. A., 1957, A fatal granulomatous disease of childhood: The clinical study of a new syndrome, *Minn. Med.* **40:**309.

Berger, M., Kirkpatrick, C. H., Goldsmith, P. K., and Gallin, J. I., 1980, IgE antibodies to *Staphylococcus aureus* and *Candida albicans* in patients with the syndrome of hyperimmunoglobulinemia E and recurrent infections, *J. Immunol.* **115:**2437.

Björksten, B., and Lundmark, K. M., 1976, Recurrent bacterial infections in four siblings with neutropenia, eosinophilia, hyperimmunoglobulinemia A, and defective neutrophil chemotaxis, *J. Infect. Dis.* **133:**63.

Blum, R., Geller, G., and Fish, L. A., 1977, Recurrent severe staphylococcal infections, eczematoid rash, extreme elevations of IgE, eosinophilia, and divergent chemotactic responses in two generations, *J. Pediatr.* **90:**607.

Blume, R. S., and Wolff, S. M., 1972, The Chediak-Higashi syndrome: Studies in four patients and a review of the literature, *Medicine (Baltimore)* **51:**247.

Borregaard, N., Johansen, K. S., and Esmann, V., 1979, Quantitation of superoxide production in human polymorphonuclear leukocytes from normals and 3 types of chronic granulomatous disease, *Biochem. Biophys. Res. Commun.* **90:**214.

Borregaard, N., Kragballe, K., Brandrup, F., Koch, C., and Johansen, E. S., 1981, Relation of monocyte and neutrophil oxidative metabolism to skin and oral lesions in carriers of chronic granulomatous disease, *Clin. Exp. Immunol.* **43:**390.

Bowen, T. J., Ochs, H. D., Altman, L. C., Klebanoff, S. J., Page, R. C., Perkins, W. D., Carter, W. B., Wedgwood, R. J., and Price, T. H., 1980, A cellular chemotactic and adherence defect associated with recurrent bacterial infections, abnormal umbilical cord separation, and severe periodontitis, *Pediatr. Res.* **14:**544.

Boxer, L. A., Hedley-Whyte, E. J., and Stossel, J. P., 1974, Neutrophil actin dysfunction and abnormal neutrophil behavior, *N. Engl. J. Med.* **291:**1093.

Boxer, L. A., Wantanbe, A. M., Rister, M., Besch, H. R., Jr., Allen, J., and Baehmer, R. L., 1976, Correction of leukocyte function in Chediak-Higashi syndrome by ascorbate, *N. Engl. J. Med.* **295:**1041.

Boxer, L. A., Oliver, J. M., Spielberg, S. P., Allen, J. M., and Schulman, J. D., 1979, Protection of granulocytes by vitamin E in gluthathione synthetase deficiency, *N. Engl. J. Med.* **301**:901.

Boyden, S., 1962, The chemotactic effect of mixtures of antibody and antigen on polymorphonuclear leukocytes, *J. Exp. Med.* **115**:453.

Brayton, R. G., Stokes, P. E., Schwartz, M. S., and Louria, O. B., 1970, Effect of alcohol and various diseases on leukocyte mobilization, phagocytosis and intracellular bacterial killing, *N. Engl. J. Med.* **282**:123.

Breton-Gorius, J., Mason, D. Y., Buriot, D., Vilde, J. L., and Griscelli, C., 1980, Lactoferrin deficiency as a consequence of a lack of specific granules in neutrophils from a patient with recurrent infections, *Am. J. Pathol.* **99**:413.

Bridges, R. A., Berendes, H., and Good, R. A., 1959, A fatal granulomatous disease of childhood. The clinical, pathological, and laboratory features of a new syndrome, *Am. J. Dis. Child.* **97**:387.

Briggs, R. T., Karnovsky, M. L., and Karnovsky, M. J., 1977, Hydrogen peroxide production in chronic granulomatous disease, *J. Clin. Invest.* **59**:1088.

Bryant, S. M., Lynch, R. E., and Hill, H. R., 1982, Kinetic analysis of superoxide anion production by activated and resident murine peritoneal macrophages, *Cell Immunol.* **69**:46.

Buckley, R. H., Wray, B. B., and Belmaker, E. Z., 1972, Extreme hyperimmunoglobulinemia E and undue susceptibility to infection, *Pediatrics* **49**:59.

Businco, L., Laurenti, R., Rossi, P., Galli, E., and Aiuti, F., 1981, A child with atopic features, raised serum IgE and recurrent infection treated with levamisole, *Arch. Dis. Child.* **56**:60.

Caleb, M., Lecks, H., South, M. A., and Norman, M. E., 1977, Kartageners syndrome and abnormal cilia. (Letter.), *N. Engl. J. Med.* **297**:1012.

Charette, R. P., and Hill, H. R., 1982, Defects in phagocytic cells, in: *Infections in Children* (R. J. Wedgewood, S. D. Davis, C. G. Ray, and V. C. Kelly, eds.), pp. 109–125, Harper and Row, Philadelphia.

Cheson, B. D., Christensen, R. L., Sperling, R., Kohler, B. E., and Babior, B. M., 1976, The origin of the chemiluminescence of phagocytosing granulocytes, *J. Clin. Invest.* **58**:789.

Christensen, R. D., Rothstein, G., Bradley, P., Priebat, D., Bybee, B., and Anstall, H. B., 1982, Granulocyte transfusions in neonates with bacterial sepsis, neutropenia and depletion of marrow neutrophils, *Pediatrics* **70**:1.

Chusid, M. J., Gallin, J. I., Dale, D. C., Fauci, A. S., and Wolff, S. M., 1976, Defective polymorphonuclear leukocyte chemotaxis and bactericidal capacity in a boy with recurrent pyogenic infections, *Pediatrics* **58**:513.

Cianciola, L. J., Genco, R. J., Patters, M. T., McKenna, J., and Van Oss, C. J., 1977, Defective polymorphonuclear leukocyte function in human periodontal disease, *Nature* **265**:445.

Clark, R. A., and Kimball, H. R., 1971, Defective granulocyte chemotaxis in the Chediak-Higashi syndrome, *J. Clin. Invest.* **50**:2645.

Clark, R. A., and Klebanoff, S. J., 1978, Chronic granulomatous disease: Studies of a family with impaired neutrophil chemotactic, metabolic and bactericidal function, *Am. J. Med.* **65**:941.

Clark, R. A., Root, R. K., Kimball, H. R., and Kirkpatrick, C. H., 1973, Defective neutrophil chemotaxis and cellular immunity in a child with recurrent infection, *Ann. Intern. Med.* **78**:515.

Clark, R. A., Page, R. C., and Wilde, G., 1977, Defective neutrophil chemotaxis in juvenile periodontitis, *Infect. Immun.* **18**:694.

Cohen, M. S., Isturiz, R. E., Malech, H. L., Root, R. K., Wilfert, C. M., Gutman L., and

Buckley, R. H., 1981, Fungal infection in chronic granulomatous disease, *Am. J. Med.* 71:59.

Corberand, J., DeLarrard, B., Vergnes, H., and Carriere, J.-P., 1978, Chronic granulomatous disease with leukocytic glucose-6-phosphate dehydrogenase deficiency in a 28-month-old girl, *Amer. J. Clin. Path.* 70:296.

Craddock, P. R., Yawata, Y., VanSanten, L., Gilberstadt, S., Silvis, S., and Jacobs, H. S., 1974, Acquired phagocyte dysfunction: A complication of the hypophosphatemia of parenteral hyperalimentation, *N. Engl. J. Med.* 290:1403.

Craddock, P. R., Fehr, J., Brigham, K. L., Kronenberg, R. S., and Jacob, H. S., 1977*a*, Complement and leukocyte-mediated pulmonary dysfunction in hemodialysis, *N. Engl. J. Med.* 196:770.

Craddock, P. R., Fehr, J., Dalmasso, A. P., Brigham, K. L., and Jacob, H. S., 1977*b*, Hemodialysis leukopenia—Pulmonary vascular leukostasis resulting from complement activation by dialyzer cellophane membranes, *J. Clin. Invest.* 59:879.

Craddock, P. R., White, J. G., and Jacob, H. S., 1978, Potentiation of complement (C5a)-induced granulocyte aggregation by cytochalasin B, *J. Lab. Clin. Med.* 91:490.

Craddock, P. R., Hammerschmidt, D. E., Moldow, C. F., Yamada, O., and Jacob, H. S., 1979, Granulocyte aggregation as a manifestation of membrane interactions with complement: Possible role in leukocyte margination, microvascular occlusion and endothelial damage, *Semin. Hematol.* 16:140.

Crowley, C. A., Curnutte, J. T., Rosin, R. E., Andre-Schwartz, J., Gallin, J. I., Klempner, M., Snyderman, R., Southwick, F. S., Stossel, T. P., and Babior, B. M., 1980, An inherited abnormality of neutrophil adhesion, *N. Engl. J. Med.* 302:1163.

Curnutte, J. T., Kipnes, R. S., and Babior, B. M., 1975, Defect in pyridine nucleotide dependent superoxide production by a particulate fraction from the granulocytes of patients with chronic granulomatous disease, *N. Engl. J. Med.* 293:628.

Cutler, J. E., 1974, A simple in vitro method for studies on chemotaxis, *Proc. Soc. Exp. Biol. Med.* 147:471.

Dahl, M. V., Greene, W. H., and Quie, P. G., 1976, Infection, dermatitis, increased IgE and impaired neutrophil chemotaxis, *Arch. Dermatol.* 112:1387.

Dale, D. C., Fauci, A. S., and Wolff, S. M., 1974, Alternate day prednisone—Leukocyte kinetics and susceptibility to infections, *N. Engl. J. Med.* 291:1154.

Davis, A. T., Brunning, R. D., and Quie, P. G., 1971, Polymorphonuclear leukocyte myeloperoxidase deficiency in a patient with myelomonocytic leukemia, *N. Eng. J. Med.* 285:789.

Davis, J. M., Dineen, P., and Gallin, J. I., 1980, Neutrophil degranulation and abnormal chemotaxis after thermal injury, *J. Immunol.* 124:1467.

Davis, S. D., Schaller, J., and Wedgwood, R. J., 1966, Job's syndrome: Recurrent "cold" staphylococcal abscesses, *Lancet* 1:1013.

Davis, W. C., Douglas, S. D., and Fudenberg, H. H., 1968, A selective neutrophil dysfunction syndrome: Impaired killing of staphyloccocci, *Ann. Intern. Med.* 69:1237.

Densen, P., Wilkinson-Kroovand, S., Mandell, G. L., Oyen, R., and Marsh, W. L., 1981, Kx: Its relationship to chronic granulomatous disease and genetic linkage with Xg, *Blood* 58:34.

Desnick, R. J., Sharp, H. L., Grabowski, G. A., Brunning, R. D., Quie, P. G., Sung, J. H., Gorlin, R. J., and Ikonne, J. V., 1976, Mannosidosis: Clinical, morphologic, immunologic and biochemical studies, *Pediatr. Res.* 10:985.

Donabedian, H., Alling, D. W., and Gallin, J. I., 1982, Levamisole is inferior to placebo in the hyperimmunoglobulin E recurrent infection (Job's) syndrome, *N. Engl. J. Med.* 307:290.

English, D., and McPherson, T. A., 1977, Chemotaxis radioassays: A simplified, quantitative method using technetium 99m radiocolloid labeled granulocytes, *Am. J. Hematol.* 3:245.

Ezer, G., and Soothill, J. F., 1974, Intracellular bactericidal effects of rifampicin in both normal and chronic granulomatous disease polymorphs, *Arch. Dis. Child.* **49**:463.

Fischer, T. J., Gard, S. E., Rachelefsky, G. S., Klein, R. B., Borut, T. C., and Stiehm, R. E., 1980, Monocyte chemotaxis under agarose: Defects in atopic disease, aspirin therapy, and mucocutaneous candidiasis, *Pediatr. Res.* **14**:242.

Ford, D. K., Price, G. E., Culling, C. F. A., and Vassar, P. S., 1962, Familial lipochrome pigmentation of histiocytes with hyperglobulinemia, pulmonary infiltration, splenomegaly, arthritis and susceptibility to infection, *Am. J. Med.* **33**:478.

Friedlander, A. M., 1978, DNA release as a direct measure of microbial killing by phagocytes, *Infect. Immun.* **22**:148.

Gallin, J. I., 1981, Abnormal phagocyte chemotaxis: Pathophysiology, clinical manifestations, and management of patients, *Rev. Infect. Dis.* **3**:1196.

Gallin, J. I., Clark, R. A., and Kimball, H. R., 1973, Granulocyte chemotaxis: An improved in vitro assay employing ^{51}Cr-labeled granulocytes, *J. Immunol.* **110**:233.

Gallin, J. I., Gallin, E. K., Malech, H. L., and Cramer, E. B., 1978, Structural and ionic events during leukocyte chemotaxis, in: *Leukocyte Chemotaxis* (J. I. Gallin and P. G. Quie eds.), pp. 123–140, Raven Press, New York.

Gallin, J. I., Elin, R. J., Hubert, R. T., Fauci, A. S., Kaliner, M. A., and Wolff, S. M., 1979, Efficacy of ascorbic acid in Chediak-Higashi syndrome (CHS): Studies in humans and mice, *Blood* **53**:226.

Gallin, J. I., Wright, D. G., Malech, H. L., Davis, J. M., Klepner, M. S., and Kirkpatrick, C. H., 1980, Disorders of phagocyte chemotaxis, *Ann. Intern. Med.* **92**:520.

Genco, R. J., Van Dyke, T. E., Park, B., Ciminelli, M., and Horoszewicz, H., 1980, Neutrophil chemotaxis impairment in juvenile periodontitis: Evaluation of specificity, adherence, deformability, and serum factors, *J. Reticuloendothelial Soc.* **28**:81s.

Giebink, G. S., Mills, E. L., Huff, J. S., Cates, K. L., Juhn, S. K., and Quie, P. G., 1979, Polymorphonuclear leukocyte dysfunction in children with recurrent otitis media, *Pediatrics* **94**:13.

Gmünder, F. K., and Seger, R. A., 1981, Chronic granulomatous disease: Mode of action of sulfamethoxazole/trimethoprim, *Pediatr. Res.* **15**:1533.

Gold, S. B., Hanes, D. M., Stites, D. P., and Fudenberg, H. H., 1974, Abnormal kinetics of degranulation in chronic granulomatous disease, *N. Engl. J. Med.* **291**:332.

Gray, G. R., and Klebanoff, S. J., Stamatoyannopoulos, G., Naiman, S. C., Kliman, M. R., Klebanoff, S. J., Austin, T., Yoshida, A., and Robinson, G. C. F., 1973, Neutrophil dysfunction, chronic granulomatous disease and non-spherocytic haemolytic anemia caused by complete deficiency of glucose-6-phosphate dehydrogenase, *Lancet* **2**:530.

Gregory, L., Williams, R., and Thompson, E., 1972, Leukocyte function in Down's syndrome and acute leukemia, *Lancet* **1**:1359.

Griscom, N. T., Kirkpatrick, J. A., Girdany, B. R., Berdon, W. E., Grand, R. J., and Mackie, G. G., 1974, Gastric antral narrowing in chronic granulomatous disease of childhood, *Pediatrics* **54**:456.

Hammerschmidt, D. E., Bowers, T. K., Lammi-Keffe, C. J., Jacob, H. S., and Craddock, P. R., 1980, Granulocyte aggregometry: A sensitive technique for the detection of C5a and complement activation, *Blood* **55**:898.

Hammerschmidt, D. E., Weaver, L. J., Hudson, L. D., Craddock, P. R., and Jacob, H. S., 1980, Association of complement activation and elevated plasma-C5a with adult respiratory distress syndrome, *Lancet* **1**:947.

Harvath, L., and Andersen, B. R., 1979, Defective initiation of oxidative metabolism in polymorphonuclear leukocytes, *N. Engl. J. Med.* **300**:1130.

Hayward, A. R., Leonard, J., Wood, C. B. S., Harvey, B. A. M., Greenwood, M. D., and Soothill, J. F., 1979, Delayed separation of the umbilical cord, widespread infections and defective neutrophil mobility, *Lancet* **1**:1099.

Hellum, K. B., and Solberg, C. O., 1977, Human leukocyte migration: Studies with an improved skin chamber technique, *Acta Pathol. Microbiol. Scand. [C]* **85**:413.

Hemming, V. G., Hall, R. T., Rhoades, P. G., Shigeoka, A. O., and Hill, H. R., 1976, Assessment of group B streptococcal opsonins in human and rabbit serum by neutrophil chemiluminescence, *J. Clin. Invest.* **48**:1379.

Henderson, L. W., Miller, M. E., Hamilton, R. W., and Norman, M. E., 1975, Hemodialysis leukopenia and polymorph random mobility—a possible correlation, *J. Lab. Clin. Med.* **85**:191.

Hill, H. R., 1979a, Biochemical control of phagocyte function, in *Pediatric Immunology* (H. Hodes and B. M. Kogan, eds.), pp. 15–28, Science and Medicine, New York.

Hill, H. R., 1979b, Immunity in the diabetic: Impaired or enhanced? (Editorial.) *West. J. Med.* **130**:547.

Hill, H. R., 1980, Laboratory aspects of immune deficiency in children, *Pediatr. Clin. North Am.* **27**:805.

Hill, H. R., 1981a, Granulocyte disorders predisposing to infection, in: *Pediatric Update* (E. R. Stiehm and A. J. Moss, eds.), 3rd ed., pp. 321–337, Elsevier, New York.

Hill, H. R., 1981b, Phagocyte transfusion: Ultimate therapy of neonatal infection, *J. Pediatr.* **98**:59.

Hill, H. R., 1982, The syndrome of hyperimmunoglobulinemia E and recurrent infections, *Am. J. Dis. Child.* **136**:767.

Hill, H. R., and Patriarca, P. 1982, Clinical application of leukocyte function tests, in *Biochemistry and Function of Phagocytes* (F. Rossi and P. Patriarca, eds.), pp. 659–682, *Advances in Experimental Biology.*, Vol. 141, Plenum Press, New York.

Hill, H. R., and Quie, P. G., 1974a, Contradiction in neutrophil chemotaxis in bacterial infection, *J. Pediatr.* **85**:444.

Hill, H. R., and Quie, P. G., 1974b, Raised serum IgE levels and defective neutrophil chemotaxis in three children with eczema and recurrent bacterial infections, *Lancet* **1**:183.

Hill, H. R., Gerrard, J. M., Hogan, N. A. and Quie, P. G., 1974a, Hyperactivity of neutrophil leukotactic responses during active bacterial infection, *J. Clin. Invest.* **53**:996.

Hill, H. R., Kaplan, E. L., Dajani, A., Wannamaker, L. W. and Quie, P. G., 1974b, Leukotactic activity and reduction of nitroblue tetrazolium by neutrophil granulocytes from patients with streptococcal skin infections, *J. Infect. Dis.* **129**:322.

Hill, H. R., Sauls, H. S., Dettloff, J. L., and Quie, P. G., 1974c, Impaired leukotactic responsiveness in patients with juvenile diabetes mellitus, *Clin. Immunol. Immunopathol.* **2**:395.

Hill, H. R., Quie, P. G., Pabst, H. F., Ochs, H. D., Clark, R. A., Klebanoff, S. J., and Wedgwood, R. J., 1974d, Defect in neutrophil granulocyte chemotaxis in Job's syndrome of recurrent "cold" staphylococcal abscesses, *Lancet* **2**:617.

Hill, H. R., Warwick, W. J., Dettloff, J., and Quie, P. G., 1974e, Neutrophil granulocyte function in patients with pulmonary infections, *J. Pediatr.* **84**:55.

Hill, H. R., Hogan, N. A., Mitchell, T. G., and Quie, P. G., 1975, Evaluation of a cytocentrifuge method for measuring neutrophil granulocyte chemotaxis, *J. Lab. Clin. Med.* **86**:703.

Hill, H. R., Estensen, R. D., Hogan, N. A., and Quie, P. G., 1976a, Severe staphylococcal disease associated with allergic manifestations, hyperimmunoglobulinemia E, and defective neutrophil chemotaxis, *J. Lab. Clin. Med.* **88**:796.

Hill, H. R., Williams, P. B., Krueger, G. G., and Janis, B., 1976b, Recurrent staphylococcal abscesses associated with defective neutrophil chemotaxis and allergic rhinitis, *Ann. Intern. Med.* **85**:39.

Hill, H. R., Book, L. S., Hemming, V. G., and Herbst, J. J., 1977, Defective neutrophil chemotactic responses in patients with recurrent episodes of otitis media and chronic diarrhea, *Am. J. Dis. Child.* **131**:433.

Hill, H. R., Augustine, N. H., Rallison, M. L., and Santos, J. I., 1983, Defective monocyte chemotactic responses in diabetes mellitus, *J. Clin. Immunol.* **3**:70.

Hogan, N. A., and Hill, H. R., 1978, Levamisole enhances PMN chemotaxis and elevates cellular cyclic GMP, *J. Infect. Dis.* **138**:437.

Hohn, D. C., and Lehrer, R. I., 1975, NADPH oxidase deficiency in X-linked chronic granulomatous disease, *J. Clin. Invest.* **55**:707.

Holmes, B., Page, A. R., and Good. R. A., 1967, Studies of the metabolic activity of leukocytes from patients with a genetic abnormality of phagocyte function, *J. Clin. Invest.* **46**:1422.

Holmes, B., Park, B. H., Malawista, S. E., Quie, P. G., Nelson, D. L., and Good, R. A., 1970, Chronic granulomatous disease in females: A deficiency of leukocyte glutathione peroxidase, *N. Engl. J. Med.* **283**:217.

Hosea, S., Brown, E., Hammer, C., and Frank, M., 1980, Role of complement activation in a model of adult respiratory distress syndrome, *J. Clin. Invest.* **66**:375.

Ingraham, L. M., Boxer, L. A., Haak, R. A., and Baehner, R. L., 1981, Membrane fluidity changes accompanying phagocytosis in normal and in chronic granulomatous disease polymorphonuclear leukocytes, *Blood* **58**:830.

Issekutz, A. C., Lee, K. Y., and Bigger, W. D., 1978, Neutrophil chemotaxis in two patients with recurrent staphylococcal skin infections and hyperimmunoglobulinemia E, *J. Lab. Clin. Med.* **92**:640.

Jacob, H. S., Craddock, P. R., Hammerschmidt, D. E., and Moldow, C. F., 1980, Complement-induced granulocyte aggregation, *N. Engl. J. Med.* **302**:789.

Jacobs, J. C., and Norman, M. E., 1977, A familial defect of neutrophil chemotaxis with asthma, eczema, and recurrent skin infections, *Pediatr. Res.* **11**:732.

Janeway, C. A., Craig, J., Davidson, M., Downey, W., Gitlin, D., and Sullivan, J. C., 1954, Hypergammaglobulinemia associated with severe recurrent and chronic nonspecific infection, *Am. J. Dis. Child.* **88**:388.

Johansen, K. S., Borregaard, N., Koch, C., Taudort, E., Wandall, J. H., and Repine, J. E., 1982, Chronic granulomatous disease presenting as xanthogranulomatous pyelonephritis in late childhood, *J. Pediatr.* **100**:98.

Johnston, R. B., and Newman, S. L., 1977, Chronic granulomatous disease, *Pediatr. Clin. North Am.* **24**:365.

Johnston, R. B., Jr., Klemperer, M. R., Alper, C. A., and Rosen, F. S., 1969, The enhancement of bacterial phagocytosis by serum: The role of complement components and two cofactors, *J. Exp. Med.* **129**:1275.

Johnston, R. B., Wilfert, C. M., Buckley, R. H., Webb, L. S., De Chatelet, L. R. and McCall, C. E., 1975, Enhanced bactericidal activity of phagocytes from patients with chronic granulomatous disease in the presence of sulphisoxazole, *Lancet* **1**:824.

Keller, H. U., Wilkinson, P. C. Abercrombie, M., Becker, E. L., Hirsch, J. G., Miller, M. E., Ramsey, W. S., and Zigmond, S. H., 1977, A proposal for the definition of terms related to locomotion of leukocytes and other cells, *Clin. Exp. Immunol.* **27**:377.

Kimura, G. M., Miller, M. E., Leake, R. D., Raghunathan, R., and Cheung, A. T. W., 1981, Reduced concanavalin A capping of neonatal polymorphonuclear leukocytes (PMNs), *Pediatr. Res.* **15**:1271.

Kitahara, M., Eyre, H. J., and Hill, H. R., 1980, Monocyte functional and metabolic activity in malignant and inflammatory diseases, *J. Lab. Clin. Med.* **93**:472.

Klein, R. B., Fischer, T. J., Gard, S. E., Biberstein, M., Rich, K. C., and Stiehm, E. R., 1977, Decreased mononuclear and polymorphonuclear chemotaxis in human newborns, infants, and young children, *Pediatrics* **60**:467.

Klempner, M. S., and Styrt, B., 1981, Clindamycin uptake by human neutrophils, *J. Infect. Dis.* **144**:472.

Klempner, M. S., Gallin, J. I., Balow, J. E., and VanKammen, D. P., 1980, The effect of hemodialysis and C5a des arg on neutrophil subpopulations. *Blood* 55:777.

Komiyana, A., Morosawa, H., Nakahata, T., Miyagawa, Y., and Akabane, T., 1979, Abnormal neutrophil maturation in a neutrophic defect with morphologic abnormality and impaired function, *J. Pediatr.* 94:19.

Kramer, N., Perez, H. D., and Goldstein, I. M., 1980, An immunoglobulin (IgG) inhibitor of polymorphonuclear leukocyte motility in a patient with recurrent infection, *N. Engl. J. Med.* 303:1253.

Lavine, W. S., Maderazo, E. G., Stolman, J., Ward, P. A., Cogen, R. B., Greenblatt, I., and Robertson, P. B., 1979, Impaired neutrophil chemotaxis in patients with juvenile and rapidly progressing periodontitis, *J. Periodont. Res.* 14:10.

Leber, T., 1888, Ueber die entstehung der entzündung und die wirkung der entzundungserregenden Schädlichkeiten, *Fortschr. Med.* 6:460.

Lehrer, R. I., and Cline, M. J., 1969, Leukocyte myeloperoxidase deficiency and disseminated candidiasis: The role of myeloperoxidase in resistance to *Candida* infection, *J. Clin. Invest.* 48:1478.

Lentnek, A. L., Schreiber, A. D., and MacGregor, R. R., 1976, Induction of augmented granulocyte adherence in inflammation; mediation by a plasma factor, *J. Clin. Invest.* 57:1098.

Lew, P. D., Southwick, F. S., Stossel, T. P., Whitin, J. C., Simons, E., and Cohen, H. J., 1981, A variant of chronic granulomatous disease: Deficient oxidative metabolism due to a low-affinity NADPH oxidase, *N. Engl. J. Med.* 305:1329.

Lohr, K. M., and Snyderman, R., 1981, Disorders of human leukocyte chemotaxis, *Clin. Immunol. Rev.* 1:67.

MacDougall, L. G., Anderson, R., McNab, G. M., and Katz, J., 1975, The immune response in iron deficient children: Impaired cellular defense mechanisms with altered humoral components, *J. Pediatr.* 86:833.

MacGregor, R. R., 1977, Granulocyte adherence changes induced by hemodialysis, endotoxin, epinephrine and glucocorticoids, *Ann. Intern. Med.* 86:35.

MacGregor, R. R., Spagnuolo, P. J., and Lentnek, A. L., 1974, Inhibition of granulocyte adherence by ethanol, prednisone, and aspirin, measured with an assay system, *N. Engl. J. Med.* 291:642.

MacGregor, R. R., Macarak, E. J., and Kefalides, N. A., 1978, Comparative adherence of granulocytes to endothelial monolayers and nylon fiber, *J. Clin. Invest.* 61:697.

Maderazo, E. G., Ward, P. A., and Quintiliani, R., 1975, Defective regulation of chemotaxis in cirrhosis, *J. Lab. Clin. Med.* 85:621.

Maderazo, E. G., Ward, P. A., Woronick, C. L., Kubik, J., and DeGraff, A. C., 1976, Leukotactic dysfunction in sarcoidosis, *Ann. Intern. Med.* 84:414.

Mandell, G. L., 1972, Staphylococcal infection and leukocyte bactericidal defect in a 22 year old woman, *Ann. Intern. Med.* 130:754.

Mass, M. F., Dean, P. B., Weston, W. L., and Humbert, J. R., 1975, Leukocyte migration *in vivo*: A new method of study, *J. Lab. Clin. Med.* 86:1040.

Matoth, Y., 1952, Phagocytic and ameboid activities of the leukocytes in the newborn infant, *Pediatrics* 9:748.

Mawhinney, H., Killen, M., Fleming, W. A., and Roy, A. D., 1980, The hyperimmunoglobulin E syndrome—a neutrophil chemotactic defect reversible by histamine H2 receptor blockage? *Clin. Immunol. Immunopathol.* 17:483.

McCall, C. E., Caves, J., Cooper, R., and DeChatelet, L., 1971, Functional characteristics of human toxic neutrophils. *J. Infect. Dis.* 135:376.

McCall, C. E., DeChatelet, L. R., Brown, D., and Lachmann, P., 1974, New biologic activity following intravascular activation of the complement cascade, *Nature* 249:841.

McGeady, S. J., and Buckley, R. N., 1975, Depression of cell-mediated immunity in atopic eczema, *J. Allergy Clin. Immunol.* 56:393.

McPhail, L., DeChatelet, L. R., Shirley, P. S., Wilfert, C., Johnston, R. B., and McCall, C. E., 1977, Deficiency of NADPH oxidase in activity in chronic granulomatous disease, *Pediatrics* 90:213.

Metchnikoff, E., 1905, *Immunity in Infective Diseases* (F. G. Binnie, transl.), Cambridge University Press, London.

Miles, A. A., 1964, The acute reactions of injury as an antimicrobial defense, in: *International Symposium on Injury, Inflammation and Immunity* (L. Thomas and J. W. Uhr, eds.), 1st ed., pp. 162–182, Williams & Wilkins, Baltimore.

Miles, A. A., Miles, E. M., and Burke, J., 1957, The value and duration of defense reactions of the skin to primary lodgement of bacteria, *Br. J. Exp. Pathol.* 38:79.

Miller, M. E., 1971, Chemotactic function in the human neonate: Humoral and cellular aspects, *Pediatr. Res.* 5:487.

Miller, M. E., 1973, Leukocyte movement—*in vitro* and *in vivo* correlates, *J. Pediatr.* 83: 1104.

Miller, M. E., 1975, Developmental maturation of human neutrophil motility and its relationship to membrane deformity, in: *The Phagocytic Cell in Host Resistance* (J. A. Bellanti and D. H. Dayton, eds.), pp. 295–302, Raven Press, New York.

Miller, M. E., and Baker, L., 1972, Leukocyte functions in juvenile diabetes mellitus: Humoral and cellular aspects, *J. Pediatr.* 81:979.

Miller, M. E., Oski, F. A., and Harris, M. B., 1971, Lazy-leukocyte syndrome, *Lancet* 1: 1665.

Miller, M. E., Norman, M. E., Koblenger, P. J., and Schonauer, T., 1973, A new familial defect of neutrophil movement, *J. Lab. Clin. Med.* 82:1.

Mills, E. L., and Quie, P. G., 1980, Congenital disorders of the functions of polymorphonuclear neutrophils, *Rev. Infect. Dis.* 2:505.

Mills, E. L., Thompson, T., Björkstein, B., Filipovich, D., and Quie, P. G., 1979, The chemiluminescence response and bactericidal activity of polymorphonuclear neutrophils from newborns and their mothers, *Pediatrics* 63:429.

Mills, E. L., Rholl, K. S., and Quie, P. G., 1980a, Luminol-amplified chemiluminescence: A sensitive method for detecting the carrier state in chronic granulomatous disease, *J. Clin. Microbiol.* 12:52.

Mills, E. L., Rholl, K. S., and Quie, P. G., 1980b, X-linked inheritance in females with chronic granulomatous disease, *J. Clin. Invest.* 66:332.

Moellering, R. C., Jr., and Weinberg, A. N., 1970, Persistent *Salmonella* infection in a female carrier of chronic granulomatous disease, *Ann. Intern. Med.* 73:595.

Mowat, A. G., and Baum, J., 1971a, Chemotaxis of polymorphonuclear leukocytes from patients with rheumatoid arthritis, *J. Clin. Invest.* 50:2541.

Mowat, A. G., and Baum, J., 1971b, Chemotaxis of polymorphonuclear leukocytes from patients with diabetes mellitus, *N. Engl. J. Med.* 284:621.

Mowat, A. G., and Baum, J., 1971c, Polymorphonuclear leukocyte chemotaxis in patients with bacterial infection, *Br. Med. J.* 3:617.

Nath, J., Flain, M., and Gallin, J. I., 1980, Tubulin tyrosylation in normal and Chediak-Higashi syndrome neutrophils, *J. Cell Biol.* 87:1952.

Nelson, R. D., Quie, P. G., and Simmons, R. L., 1975, Chemotaxis under agarose: A new and simple method for measuring chemotaxis and spontaneous migration of human polymorphonuclear leukocytes and monocytes, *J. Immunol.* 115:1650.

Newburger, P. E., Cohen, H. J., Rothchild, S. B., Hobbins, J. C., Malawista, S. E., and Mahoney, M. J., 1979, Prenatal diagnosis of chronic granulomatous disease, *N. Engl. J. Med.* 300:178.

Norman, M. E., and Miller, M. E., 1973, Spontaneous chemotaxis in patients with glomerulonephritis and the nephrotic syndrome, *J. Pediatr.* 83:390.

Norman, M. E., and Miller, M. E., 1974, Spontaneous chemotaxis in acute glomerulonephritis: Demonstration of a positive correlation with disease activity, *J. Pediatr.* 85:20.

O'Flaherty, J. T., Kreutzer, D. L., and Ward, P. A., 1977, Neutrophil aggregation and swelling induced by chemotactic agents, *J. Immunol.* 119:232.

Ogden, B. E., Krueger, G. G., and Hill, H. R., 1979, Lymphocyte suppressor activity in atopic eczema, *Clin. Exp. Immunol.* 35:269.

Oliver, J. M., and Zurier, R. B., 1976, Correction of characteristic abnormalities of microtube function and granule morphology in Chediak-Higashi syndrome with cholinergic agonists—studies *in vitro* in man and *in vivo* in the beige mouse, *J. Clin. Invest.* 57:1239.

Oliver, J. M., Zurier, R. B., and Berlin, R. D., 1975, Concanavalin A cap formation on polymorphonuclear leukocytes of normal and beige (Chediak-Higashi) mice, *Nature* 253:471.

Orr, W., and Ward, P. A., 1978, Quantitation of leukotaxis in agarose by three different methods, *J. Immunol. Methods* 20:95.

Pahwa, S. G., Pahwa, R., Grimes, E., and Smithwick, E., 1977, Cellular and humoral components of monocyte and neutrophil chemotaxis in cord blood, *Pediatr. Res.* 11:677.

Pahwa, S., Smithwick, E. M., Grimes, E. R., O'Reilly, R., Pahwa, R. N., and Good, R. A., 1978, Chemotactic defects in severe combined immunodeficiency, *Pediatrics* 92:43.

Peerless, A. G., and Stiehm, E. R., 1983, Defective red blood cells and T-lymphocyte chemiluminescence in chronic granulomatous disease: Possible global membrane defect, *Clin. Res.* 31:A119.

Philippart, A. I., Colodny, A. H., and Baehner, R. L., 1972, Continuous antibiotic therapy in chronic granulomatous disease: Preliminary communication, *Pediatrics* 50:923.

Pike, M. C., and Snyderman, R., 1976, Augmentation of human monocyte chemotactic response by levamisole, *Nature* 201:136.

Pross, S. H., Hallock, J. A., Armstrong, R., and Fishel, C. W., 1977, Complement and Fc receptors on cord blood and adult neutrophils, *Pediatr. Res.* 11:135.

Quie, P. G., White, J. G., Holmes, B., and Good, R. A., 1967, *In vitro* bactericidal capacity of human polymorphonuclear leukocytes: Diminished activity in chronic granulomatous disease of childhood, *J. Clin. Invest.* 46:668.

Raubitschek, A. A., Levin, A. S., Stites, D. P., Shaw, E. B., and Freidenberg, H. H., 1973, Normal granulocyte infusion therapy for aspergillosis in chronic granulomatous disease, *Pediatrics* 51:230.

Rebora, A., Dallegri, F., and Patrone, F., 1980, Neutrophil dysfunction and repeated infections: Influence of levamisole and ascorbic acid, *Br. J. Dermatol.* 102:49.

Rebuck, J. W., and Crowley, J. H., 1955, A method of studying leukocytic functions *in vivo*, *Ann. NY Acad. Sci.* 59:757.

Repine, J. E., Rasmussen, B. R., and White, J. G., 1979, An improved nitroblue tetrazolium (NBT) test using phorbol myristate acetate (PMA) coated coverslips, *Am. J. Clin. Pathol.* 71:582.

Rich, K. C., Neuman, C. G., and Stiehm, E. R., 1977, Neutrophil chemotaxis in malnourished Ghandian children, in: *Malnutrition and the Immune Response* (Suskind, R. M., ed.), pp. 271–275, Raven Press, New York.

Rivkin, I., and Becker, E. L., 1972, Possible implication of cyclic 3'5'-adenosine monophosphate in the chemotaxis of rabbit peritoneal polymorphonuclear leukocytes, *Fed. Proc.* 31:657.

Rodey, G. E., Park, B. H., Ford, D. K., Gray, B. H., and Good, R. H., 1970, Defective bactericidal activity of peripheral blood leukocytes in lipochrome histiocytosis, *Am. J. Med.* 49:322.

Roos, D., Weening, R. S., Voetman, A. A., van Schaik, M. L. J., Bot, A. A. M., Meerhof, L. J., and Loos, J. A., 1979, Protection of phagocytic leukocytes by endogenous glutathione: Studies in a family with glutathione reductase deficiency, *Blood* 53:851.

Rosen, E. U., Geefhuysen, J., Anderson, R., Joffe, M., and Rabson, A. R., 1975, Leucocyte function in children with kwashiorkor, *Arch. Dis. Child.* 50:220.

Rosen, H., and Klebanoff, S. J., 1976, Chemiluminescence and superoxide production by myeloperoxidase-deficient leukocytes, *J. Clin. Invest.* 58:50.

Rosenfeld, S. I., Baum, J., Steigbigel, R. T., and Leddy, J. P., 1976, Hereditary deficiency of the fifth component of complement in man, *J. Clin. Invest.* 57:1635.

Rosenthal, M., Trabert, U., and Müeller, W., 1976, Leucocytotoxic effect of levamisole, *Lancet* 1:369.

Rosner, R., Kozinn, P. J., and Jervis, G. A., 1973, Leukocyte function and serum immunoglobulins in Down's syndrome, *NY State J. Med.* 73:672.

Rubin, J. L., Griffiths, R. W., and Hill, H. R., 1978, Allergen induced depression of neutrophil chemotaxis in allergic individuals, *J. Allergy Clin. Immunol.* 62:301.

Rutenberg, W. D., Yang, M. C., Doberstyn, B., and Bellanti, J. A., 1977, Multiple leukocyte abnormalities in chronic granulomatous disease: A familial study, *Pediatr. Res.* 11:158.

Saitoh, H., Komiyama, A., Norose, N., Morosawa, H., and Akabane T., 1981, Development of the accelerated phase during ascorbic acid therapy in Chediak-Hagashi syndrome and efficacy of colchicine on its management, *Br. J. Haematol.* 48:79.

Schopfer, K., and Douglas, S. D., 1976, Neutrophil function in children with kwashiorkor, *J. Lab. Clin. Med.* 88:450.

Schopfer, K., Baerlocher, K., Price, P., Krech, V., Quie, P. G., and Douglas, S. D., 1979, Staphylococcal IgE antibodies, hyperimmunoglobulinemia E and *Staphylococcal aureus* infections, *N. Engl. J. Med.* 300:835.

Segal, A. W., and Loewi, G., 1976, Neutrophil dysfunction in Crohn's disease, *Lancet* 2:219.

Segal, A. W., Webster, D., Jones, Q. T. G., and Allison, A. D., 1978, Absence of a newly described cytochrome b from neutrophils of patients with chronic granulomatous disease, *Lancet* 2:446.

Segal, A. W., Cross, A. R., Garcia, R. C., Borregaard, N., Valerius, N. H., Soothill, J. F., and Jones, D. T. G., 1983, Absence of cytochrome b-245 in chronic granulomatous disease: A multicenter European evaluation of its incidence and relevance, *N. Engl. J. Med.* 308:245.

Seger, R. A., Baumgartner, S., Tiefenauer, L. X., and Gmünder, F. K., 1981, Chronic granulomatous disease: Effect of sulfamethoxazole/trimethoprim on neutrophil microbicidal function, *Helv. Paediatr. Acta* 36:579.

Shigeoka, A. O., and Hill, H. R., 1978, Recurrent pseudomonas infection associated with neutrophil dysfunction, *Scand. J. Infect. Dis.* 10:307.

Shigeoka, A. O., Hall, R. T., and Hill, H. R., 1978, Blood-transfusion in group B streptococcal sepsis, *Lancet* 1:636.

Shigeoka, A. O., Santos, J. I., and Hill, H. R., 1979, Functional analysis of neutrophil granulocytes from healthy, infected and stressed neonates, *J. Pediatr.* 95:454.

Shigeoka, A. O., Charette, R. P., Wyman, M. L., and Hill, H. R., 1981, Defective oxidative metabolic responses of neutrophils from stressed neonates, *J. Pediatr.* 98:392.

Shurin, S. B., Socransky, S. S., Sweeney, E., and Stossel, T. P., 1979, A neutrophil disorder induced by *Capnocytophaga*, a dental micro-organism, *N. Engl. J. Med.* 301:849.

Smith, C. W., Hollers, J. C., Dupree, E., Goldman, A. S., and Lord, R. A., 1972, A serum inhibitor of leukotaxis in a child with recurrent infections, *J. Lab. Clin. Med.* 79:878.

Snyderman, R., and Pike, M. C., 1978, Pathophysiologic aspects of leukocyte chemotaxis: Identification of a specific chemotactic factor binding site on human granulocytes and defects of macrophage function associated with neoplasia, in: *Leukocyte Chemotaxis: Methods, Physiology, and Clinical Implications* (J. I. Gallin and P. G. Quie, eds.), pp. 357–378, Raven Press, New York.

Snyderman, R., Altman, L. C., Frankel, A., and Blaese, R. M., 1973, Defective mononuclear leukocyte chemotaxis: A previously unrecognized immune dysfunction. Studies in a patient with chronic mucocutaneous candidiasis, *Ann. Intern. Med.* 78:509.

Soderberg-Warner, M., Rice-Mendoza, C. A., Mendoza, G. R., and Stiehm, E. R., 1983, Neutrophil and T lymphocyte characteristics of two patients with hyper-IgE syndrome, *Pediatr. Res.* 17:820.

Soriano, R. B., South, M. A., Goldman, A. S., and Smith, C. W., 1973, Defect of neutrophil motility in a child with recurrent bacterial infections and disseminated cytomegalovirus infection, *J. Pediatr.* 83:951.

Spielberg, S. P., Boxer, L. A., Oliver, J. M., Allen, J. M., and Schulman, J. D., 1979, Oxidative damage to neutrophils in glutathione synthetase deficiency, *Br. J. Haematol.* 42:215.

Steerman, R. L., Snyderman, R., Leikin, S. L., and Colten, H. R., 1971, Intrinsic defect of the polymophonuclear leukocyte resulting in impaired chemotaxis and phagocytosis, *Clin. Exp. Immunol.* 9:939.

Stevens, P. Winston, D. J., and Van Dyke, K., 1978, In vitro evaluation of opsonic and cellular granulocyte function by luminol-dependent chemiluminescence: Utility in patients with severe neutrogenia and cellular deficiency states, *Infect. Immun.* 22:41.

Stossel, T. P., 1973, Evaluation of opsonic and leukocyte function with a spectrophotometric test in patients with infection and with phagocytic disorders, *Blood* 42:121.

Stossel, T. P., 1974, Phagocytosis, *N. Engl. J. Med.* 290:717, 774, 833.

Strauss, R. G., Bove, K. E., Jones, J. F., Mauer, A. M., and Fulginiti, V. A., 1974, An anomaly of neutrophil morphology with impaired function, *N. Engl. J. Med.* 290:478.

Strauss, R. G., Connett, J. E., Gale, R. P., Bloomfield, C. D., Herzig, G. P., McCullough, J., Maguire, L. C., Winston, D. J., Ho, W., Stump, D. C., Miller, W. V., and Koepke, J. A., 1981, A controlled trial of prophylactic granulocyte transfusions during initial induction chemotherapy for acute myelogenous leukemia, *N. Engl. J. Med.* 305:598.

Van der Meer, J. W. M., Van Zwet, T. L., and Van Forth, R., 1975, New familial defect in microbicidal function of polymorphonuclear leukocytes, *Lancet* 2:630.

Van Dyke, T. E., Reilly, A. A., Horoszewicz, H., Gargliardi, N., and Genco, R. J., 1979, A rapid semiautomated procedure for the evaluation of leukocyte locomotion in the micropore filter assay, *J. Immunol. Methods* 31:271.

Van Epps, D. E., and Williams, R. C., Jr., 1978, Serum inhibitors of leukocyte chemotaxis and their relationship to skin test anergy, in: *Leukocyte Chemotaxis: Methods, Physiology and Clinical Implications* (J. I. Gallin and P. G. Quie, eds.), pp. 237–253, Raven Press, New York.

Van Epps, D, Palmer, D. L., and Williams, R. C., 1974, Characterization of serum inhibitors of neutrophil chemotaxis associated with anergy, *J. Immunol.* 113:189.

Van Scoy, R. E., Hill, H. R., Ritts, R. E., Jr., and Quie, P. G., 1975, Familial neutrophil chemotaxis defect, recurrent bacterial infections, mucocutaneous candidiasis and hyperimmunoglobulinemia E, *Ann. Intern. Med.* 82:766.

Ward, P. A., and Berenberg, J. L., 1974, Defective regulation of inflammatory mediators in Hodgkin's disease, *N. Engl. J. Med.* 290:76.

Ward, P. A., and Ozols, J., 1976, Characterization of the protease activity of the chemotactic factor inactivator, *J. Clin. Invest.* 58:123.

Ward, P. A., and Schlegel, R. J., 1969, Impaired leukotactic responsiveness in a child with recurrent infection, *Lancet* 2:344.

Ward, P. A., Cochrane, C. G., and Müller-Eberhard, H. J., 1965, The role of serum complement in chemotaxis of leukocytes *in vitro*, *J. Exp. Med.* 122:327.

Ward, P. A., Goralnick, S., and Bullock, W. E., 1976, Defective leukotaxis in patients with lepromatous leprosy, *J. Lab. Clin. Med.* 87:1025.

Warden, G. D., and Maxwell, J. G., 1976, Leukocyte chemotaxis in vitro in chronic dialysis patients and after renal transplantation, *Surg. Forum* 27:323.

Warden, G. D., Mason, A. D., Jr., and Pruitt, B. A., Jr., 1974, Evaluation of leukocyte chemotaxis *in vitro* in thermally injured patients, *J. Clin. Invest.* 54:1001.

Weening, R. S., Schoorel, E. P., Roos, D., van Schaik, M. L. J., Voetman, A. A., Bot, A. A. M., Batenburg-Plenter, A. M., Willems, Ch., Zeijlemaker, W. P., and Astaldi, A., 1981, Effect of ascorbate on abnormal neutrophil, platelet and lymphocyte function in a patient with the Chediak-Higashi syndrome, *Blood* 57:856.

Weiblen, B. J., Forstrom, L., and McCullough, J., 1979, Studies of the kinetics of indium-111-labeled granulocytes, *J. Lab. Clin. Med.* 94:246.

Weston, W. L., Humbert, J. R., August, C. S., Harnett, Mass, M. F., Dean, P. B., and Hagen, I. M., 1977, A hyperimmunoglobulin E syndrome with normal chemotaxis in vitro and defective leukotaxis *in vivo*, *J. Allergy Clin. Immunol.* 59:115.

White, J. G., and Clawson, C. C., 1979, The Chediak-Higaski syndrome: Microtubules in monocytes and lymphocytes, *Am. J. Hematol.* 7:349.

Witemeyer, S., and Van Epps, D. E., 1976, A familial defect in cellular chemotaxis associated with redheadedness and recurrent infection, *J. Pediatr.* 89:33.

Wright, D. G., Kirkpatrick, C. H., and Gallin, J. I., 1977, Effect of levamisole on normal and abnormal leukocyte locomotion, *J. Clin. Invest.* 59:941.

Wright, W. C., Jr., Ank, B. J., Herbert, J., and Stiehm, E. R., 1975, Decreased bactericidal activity of leukocytes of stressed newborn infants, *Pediatrics* 56:579.

Zimmerman, G. A., Renzetti, A. D., and Hill, H. R., 1983, Functional and metabolic activity of circulating polymorphonuclear leukocytes from patients with the adult respiratory distress syndrome, *Am. Rev. Respir. Dis.* 127:290.

Addendum to Chapter 2

New information about neutrophil stimulation has accumulated since this review was written. The Ca^{2+} probe Quin 2 has come into general use. There is a rapid rise in intracellular Ca^{2+} to at least μM within 5 sec. The elevation comes largely from intracellular sources, requires occupancy of only $\sim$1 percent of the formyl peptide receptors, but is transient unless new receptors are occupied. The time course of the Ca^{2+} elevation and its dependence on occupancy parallels the generation of O_2^- (Sklar and Hyslop, 1984). However, the elevation of intracellular Ca^{2+} appears to be an insufficient signal for cell activation (Pozzan et al., 1983). The pathway of activation of adenylate cyclase in the neutrophil, analogous to the beta-adrenergic receptor, is further supported by the observation of a formyl-peptide stimulated GTPase (Hyslop et al., 1984). There are now several reports of the rapid turnover of phosphatidylinositol in the neutrophil (Cockroft et al., 1980; Volpi et al., 1983). The recognition that protein kinase C is a receptor for phorbol esters suggests a pathway, potentially independent of Ca^{2+}, for neutrophil activation (Sha'afi et al., 1983).

Two technical developments are noteworthy. A rapid ruffling of the cell surface characterized by a transient alteration in light scattering (Yuli and Synderman, 1983) has been described. A functional enucleated neutrophil "cytoplast" described by Roos and co-workers (1983) promises to be a valuable adjunct to studies of the biochemistry of cell activation.

REFERENCES

Cockroft, S., Bennet, J. P., and Gomperts, B. D., 1980, Stimulus–secretion coupling in rabbit neutrophils is not mediated by phosphatidylinositol breakdown, *Nature* **288**:275.

Hyslop, P. A., Oades, Z. G., Jesaitis, A. J., Painter, R. G., Cochrane, C. G., and Sklar, L. A., 1984, Evidence for *N*-formyl chemotactic peptide-stimulated GTPase activity in human neutrophil homogenates, *FEBS Lett.* **166**:165.

Pozzan, T., Lew, D. P., Wollheim, C. B., and Tsien, R. Y., 1983, Is cytosolic ionized calcium regulating neutrophil activation? *Science* **221**:1413.

Roos, D., Voetman, A. A., and Meerhof, L. J., 1983, Functional activity of enucleated human polymorphonuclear leukocytes, *J. Cell. Biol.* **97**:368.

Sha'afi, R. I., White, J. R., Molski, T. F., Shefcyk, J., Volpi, M., Naccache, P. H., and Feinstein, M. B., 1983, Phorphol 12-myristate 13-acetate activates rabbit neutrophils without an apparent rise in the level of intracellular free calcium, *Biochem. Biophys. Res. Commun.* **114**:538.

Sklar, L. A., and Hyslop, P. A., 1984, Signal transduction and ligand–receptor dynamics in the human neutrophil, *Biophys. J.* **45**:270a.

Volpi, M., Yassin, R., Naccache, P. H., and Sha'afi, R. I., 1983, Chemotactic factor causes rapid decrease in phosphatidylinositol 4.5-biphosphate and phosphatidylinositol 4-monophosphate in rabbit neutrophils, *Biochem. Biophys. Res. Commun.* **112**:957.

Yuli, I., and Snyderman, R., 1983. Rapid perpendicular light scattering: A previously unrecognized response of human neutrophils to chemoattractants, *Clin. Res.* **31**:97a.

Index